If students sit on the sidelines, how can we expect them to change their behavior?

FitWell empowers students to become active participants in their own fitness and wellness through a first-of-its-kind student-centered approach.

To find out what college students really want to know about fitness and wellness, the authors collected more than one thousand questions from students around the country. They use these questions to engage students, make the concepts relevant to them, and motivate them to become active in their own lives.

Through "Myth or Fact?" videos, real-life "Behavior Change Challenge" video case studies, animations, interactive assignments, online labs, and a contemporary magazine-like design, *FitWell* engages students as no other fitness and wellness program has done.

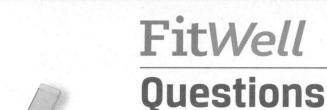

FitWell

Questions and Answers

Active learning.
Active students.

Through active learning, *FitWell* empowers students to become active in their own lives—physically, emotionally, socially, and environmentally—for life

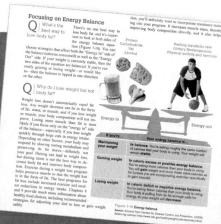

The Right Questions, the Right Answers...

The authors integrated student questions into a proven fitness and wellness framework, along with research-based answers to the questions. The result is a learning system that is relevant, accessible, and appropriate for today's students. The dynamic magazine-style format and online multimedia activities encourage students to be active learners.

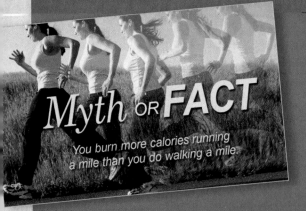

Myth OR FACT
You burn more calories running a mile than you do walking a mile.

The Right Instruction...

Basing their work on tested learning theory and instructional design, the authors use case studies and other real-life examples, videos, animations, and online interactive activities and assessments to engage students and ensure positive learning outcomes.

The Right Time...

With a single sign-on and integrated grade book, *FitWell* can be seamlessly woven within Blackboard courses. The time is right for a flexible hybrid print-digital learning system that meets students online, where they work, play, and live.

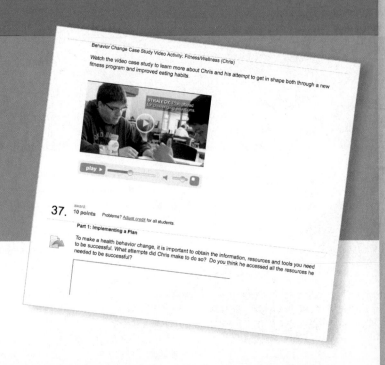

FitWell
Questions and Answers
Active learning. Active students.

Brief Contents

FitWell

AUTHORS
Gary Liguori   Sandra Carroll-Cobb

Vice President, Editorial   **Michael J. Ryan**
Director, Editorial   **Beth Mejia**
Executive Editor   **Christopher Johnson**
Director of Development   **Kathleen Engelberg**
Developmental Editor   **Kirstan Price**
Editorial Coordinator   **Lydia Kim**
Market Development Manager   **Michael McKinney**
Marketing Manager   **Caroline McGillen**
Production Editor   **Melissa Williams**
Manuscript Editor   **Barbara Armentrout**
Art Manager   **Robin Mouat**
Illustrators   **Robin Mouat, John and Judy Waller**
Designers   **Andrei Pasternak and Lisa Buckley**
Cover Designer   **Andrei Pasternak**
Photo Research Coordinator   **Nora Agbayani**
Photo Researcher   **Jennifer Blankenship**
Digital Product Manager   **Sora Kim**
Media Project Managers   **Thomas Brierly and Jami Woy**
Buyer   **Tandra Jorgensen**

Published by McGraw-Hill, a business unit of The McGraw-Hill Companies, Inc., 1221 Avenue of the Americas, New York, NY 10020. Copyright © 2012 by The McGraw-Hill Companies, Inc. All rights reserved. No part of this publication may be reproduced or distributed in any form or by any means, or stored in a database or retrieval system, without the prior written consent of The McGraw-Hill Companies, Inc., including, but not limited to, in any network or other electronic storage or transmission, or broadcast for distance learning. Some ancillaries, including electronic and print components, may not be available to customers outside the United States.

1 2 3 4 5 6 7 8 9 0 QDB/QDB 9 8 7 6 5 4 3 2 1

ISBN: 978-0-07-352370-5
MHID: 0-07-352370-4

The text was set in 10/12 Times New Roman by Thompson Type, Inc., and printed on acid-free 45# Orion Gloss by Quad/Graphics.

Cover images: front cover: (woman) © Dave & Les Jacobs/Getty Images; back cover: Harrison Eastwood/Getty Images

Because this page cannot legibly accommodate all acknowledgments for copyrighted material, credits appear at the end of the book and constitute an extension of this copyright page.

Library of Congress Control Number: 2010938426

Contents

Q | What are the chances of living to 100?

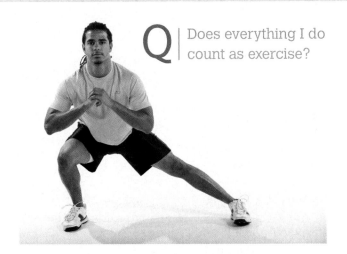

Q | Does everything I do count as exercise?

3 Fundamentals of Physical Fitness   63

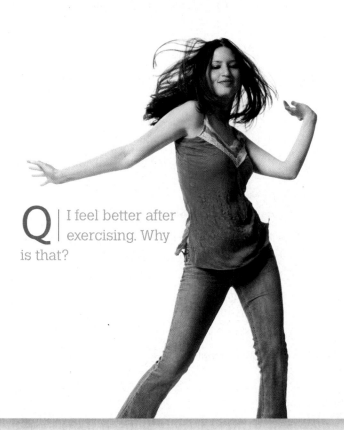

Q | I feel better after exercising. Why is that?

Q | Why should I bother with stretching?

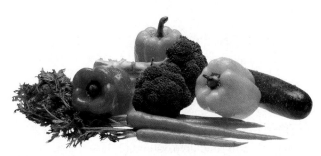

Q | What are the most filling foods with the fewest calories?

10 Stress   343

Q | What is rated as the most stressful thing?

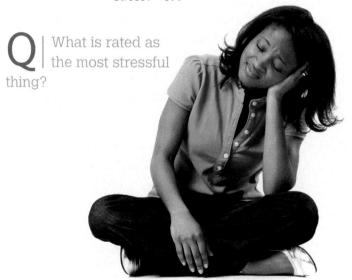

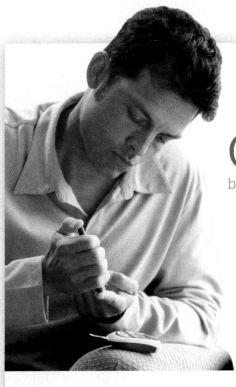

Q | What's bad about high blood sugar?

12 Infectious Diseases   415

11 Chronic Diseases   379

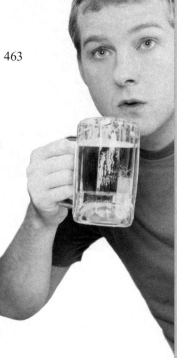

Q | Is recreational drinking safe?

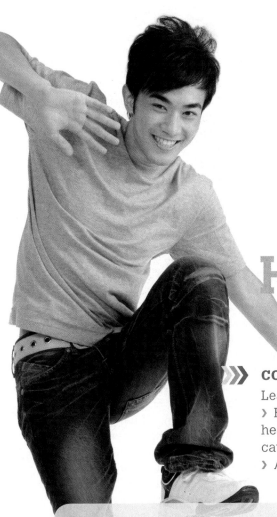

1

Introduction to Health, Wellness, and Fitness

Wellness Connections

What do you think about your health today? If you aren't currently sick, would you describe yourself as "well"? Here are a few things that college students said about their health over the past year:[1]

- 28% reported that stress hurt their academic performance.
- 31% did something they later regretted as a result of drinking.
- 54% saw a doctor for an illness or injury.

Does this sound a little like you? Do you want more for yourself than just making it through the day? The good news is that you—through your choices and actions—can make a huge difference in your health and well-being. But with this opportunity comes the responsibility of choosing healthy lifestyle behaviors.

What are your health habits like? How do they compare to what is recommended? Here's how college students rate on some key health behaviors:[2]

- 6% ate enough fruits and vegetables.
- 44% engaged in regular exercise.

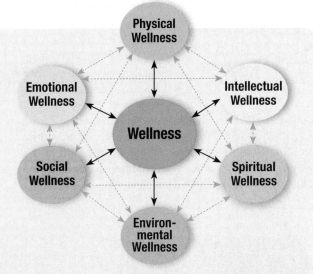

- 71% had never smoked cigarettes.

This text introduces the concepts of health and wellness along with a review of recommended health habits. You'll learn that wellness is more than just physical health or the absence of illness—it encompasses all the dimensions illustrated in the Wellness Integrator including physical, emotional, intellectual, social, spiritual, and environmental wellness. To be truly well, you must develop and balance all the dimensions of wellness. Let's get started!

What is health? Ask ten people this question, and you'll probably get ten different answers. The truth is *health* means different things to different people. If you throw in the terms *wellness* and *physical fitness,* the definition may get even more complex. In order to gain a better understanding of your own health and wellness, it's important to clarify these concepts and to learn more about the various factors that influence them.

This chapter provides a framework for thinking about health and wellness—their dimensions and their connections to your behavior, your environment, and your goals and aspirations. We'll also take a look at key health challenges, both overall and those particularly affecting college students. You'll also have the opportunity to assess your own wellness status and identify potential areas of improvement.

Personal Health and Wellness

Although people talk a great deal about health and wellness, there are no universally accepted definitions. However, the different definitions of these closely related concepts share many characteristics.

Evolving Definitions of Health

Q | I haven't been sick in over a year. Can I rate myself as healthy?

That would depend on your definition of *healthy.* For many people, health is something they think about only if there is a sudden, noticeable change for the worse—for example, an illness or injury. From this perspective, health is an either-or state: You are either healthy or unhealthy, with no middle ground. If you think about health in this way, you'll miss important opportunities to improve your health and well-being throughout your life.

Health comes from the Old English word *hoelth,* meaning "a state of being sound and whole," generally in reference to the body. The ancient Greek physician Hippocrates was one of the first credited with using observation and inquiry to assess health status—rather than considering health to be a divine gift. He and other physicians of his time believed health was a condition of balance or equilibrium; therefore ill health or disease was caused by imbalance among elements in the body. Much of Hippocrates' teachings were based on prevention. He promoted "balance" through means such as good hygiene, exercise, eating well, and moderation in all things—ideas that are still important today.

Many other visions and definitions of health have surfaced over the years. A widely used modern definition comes from the constitution of the World Health Organization (WHO): "Health is a state of complete physical, mental, and social well-being, and not merely the absence of disease or infirmity."[3] This definition emphasizes the important idea that health is more than just the absence of disease. However, some critics point out that *complete* well-being is unrealistic for most people and that health is not a single state but rather a dynamic condition.

Some professionals have modified and expanded the WHO definition to include the idea of health status as a continuum.[4] That is the framework we'll use in this text: **Health** is a condition with multiple dimensions that falls on a continuum from negative health, characterized by illness and premature death, to positive health, characterized by the capacity to enjoy life and to withstand life's challenges.

At different times, your health status may be on different points on the continuum—and it may be moving in either a positive or negative direction (Figure 1-1). Many young adults fall into the positive half of the continuum, experiencing minor, short-term illnesses interspersed with periods of no symptoms. However, in terms of other factors—habits that influence future health risks and current subjective feelings of mood, energy level,

health A condition with multiple dimensions that falls on a continuum from negative health, characterized by illness and premature death, to positive health, characterized by the capacity to enjoy life and to withstand life's challenges.

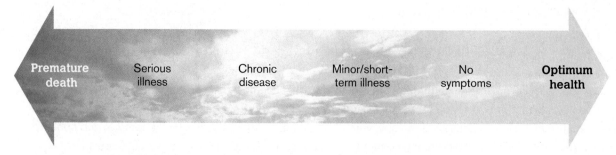

| Premature death | Serious illness | Chronic disease | Minor/short-term illness | No symptoms | Optimum health |

Figure 1-1 The health continuum. At the negative end of the continuum is serious illness and premature death. At the positive end of the continuum is the capacity to enjoy life and to withstand challenges.

Sources: Adapted from Bouchard, C., Shephard, R. J., & Stephens, T. (1994). *Physical activity, fitness, and health: International proceedings and consensus statement.* Champaign, IL: Human Kinetics; *Mental health: A report of the Surgeon General.* (1999). Rockville, MD: U.S. Public Health Service.

Fast Facts

No April Fools

April 7 is World Health Day, the anniversary of the day in 1948 when the World Health Organization's constitution was adopted. On this day around the globe, thousands of events take place demonstrating the importance of health for happy and productive lives. Each year, World Health Day highlights a different area of WHO concern. Recent themes have included maternal and child survival, the impacts of climate change, and the effects of urbanization on health. Visit http://www.who.int for more information.

Behavior Change Challenge

Video Case Study

▶ **WATCH ONLINE** Meet Erika

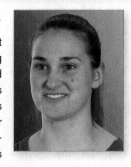

Erika is a 23-year-old student and mother of two young children. She experienced an abusive marriage and is interested in making changes in her life for herself and her children. She also likes participating in research studies and projects, so she is excited to have her progress tracked over the semester for this Behavior Change Challenge case study.

Erika's goal is to train to complete a 5K run; while doing this, she also hopes to return to her pre-marriage weight. Watch the video to learn more about Erika's story and her behavior change plan and strategies. As you watch the video, think about the following questions:

- How did Erika go about developing her plan? What resources did she use? Are similar types of resources available to help you?
- What strategies does Erika use to stay motivated? What role does self-esteem play? What can you learn from Erika's experiences that will help you in your efforts to make positive behavior changes and improve your wellness?

(Connect users can register and access the ebook and other online resources at http://connect.mcgraw-hill.com.)

and sense of well-being—they may not feel "healthy" at all. It is in these areas that the concept of wellness can provide a useful framework for action.

Actively Working Toward Wellness

Q | Are health and wellness the same to some degree?

Yes, health and wellness are closely related, and some people use the terms interchangeably. But in this text, we define **wellness** differently from health. It is a more personalized concept than health and has several additional key characteristics:

- Wellness has multiple, clearly defined dimensions; balance is very important, but you can be at a different level of wellness for each dimension (see the next section).
- Wellness is an active process, meaning you can always be working to improve your wellness status.
- Individual responsibility and choice are critical wellness components; by becoming aware of the factors that affect you and making appropriate choices, you can significantly affect your level of wellness.
- Wellness status is a reflection of your own perceptions about your health and well-being.

Two people at similar places on the health continuum may perceive their wellness status very differently. An individual with a severe illness or impairment may still have a strong sense of well-being and may be living up to her or his full wellness potential. Wellness is determined by the decisions people make about how to live their lives with vitality and meaning.

wellness An active process of adopting patterns of behavior that can improve an individual's health and perceptions of well-being and quality of life in terms of multiple, intertwined dimensions.

Discovering Dimensions of Wellness

Q | Can you be physically unfit but still be happy and social at the same time?

Yes, you can. This question gets at one of the key aspects of wellness—that there are different dimensions and although the dimensions interact, you can be at a different

Mind Stretcher

Critical Thinking Exercise

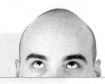

What makes you feel exuberant, vital, joyful, and living to your full potential—characteristics that exemplify a state of wellness? How often do you feel this way and under what circumstances?

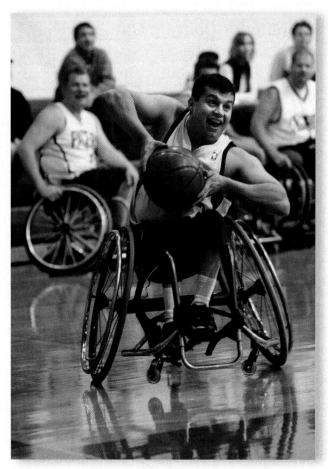

Wellness is determined by the choices people make about how to live their lives with energy and meaning. Someone with a physical impairment can achieve a high level of wellness.

- Do I get enough sleep?
- Do I use alcohol and drugs responsibly?
- Do I make intentional and responsible sexual choices?
- Do I use sunscreen?
- Do I practice safe driving?
- Do I manage injuries and illnesses appropriately, practice self-care, and seek medical assistance when necessary?

Maintaining physical wellness means making informed health decisions on many fronts and offers many opportunities for improving your quality of life.

How does **physical fitness** relate to physical wellness? *Fitness* is the ability to carry out daily tasks with vigor and alertness, without undue fatigue, and with ample energy to enjoy leisure-time pursuits and respond to emergencies.[5] This definition ties closely with wellness and quality of life. But fitness also has components that can be measured, including the strength of your muscles and the flexibility of your joints. Your level of fitness depends on specific physical attributes, including the functioning of your heart, lungs, blood vessels, and muscles. It's also important to note that good fitness doesn't equal good physical wellness; fitness is just one piece of physical wellness, and a person with a high fitness level can have other serious risks to their physical health. For example, being physically fit doesn't prevent the damage that smoking does to lungs, arteries, and other body systems.

For physical wellness, you should strive for a level of fitness that meets your goals for daily functioning and recreational pursuits. A certain level of fitness is needed to obtain its many associated health benefits, such as reduced risk of chronic diseases like heart disease and cancer (see Chapter 3), but you don't need an extremely high level of fitness for health and wellness. People who are sedentary can reap many of the benefits of fitness when they add a modest amount of activity to their daily routine (Figure 1-2). Some individuals strive for high fitness because they have specific goals related to physical performance. For example, the typical person needs a level of flexibility that allows the joints to move freely during activities of daily life; ballet dancers and gymnasts, on the other hand, need a much greater degree of flexibility in order to excel in their chosen sport. Don't be discouraged from physical activity because you think you must exercise very intensely or become extremely fit in order to obtain wellness benefits. Also remember that physical activity has many immediate benefits, including improved mood, reduced stress, and increased energy level.

Although all physical activity can affect wellness, not all activity builds physical fitness—for example, for most people, just walking down the hall doesn't increase measures of fitness.

physical wellness
Dimension of wellness referring to the complete physical condition and functioning of the body; focuses on behaviors that support physical aspects of health, including diet, exercise, sleep, stress management, and self-care.

physical fitness The ability to carry out daily tasks with vigor and alertness, without undue fatigue, and with ample energy to enjoy leisure-time pursuits and respond to emergencies.

level of wellness for each. A person who is unfit might not rate highly on the physical dimension of wellness but may fare much better in other dimensions, such as social or intellectual wellness. On the flip side, someone who is very fit and the picture of what we'd call physical health may in fact rate poorly in terms of the other dimensions of wellness. For true wellness, you need to address all the dimensions. Let's take a closer look at key characteristics and behaviors associated with each of the six dimensions included in our wellness model.

PHYSICAL WELLNESS. Mention **physical wellness** and many will picture someone who is active and looks fit. However, physical wellness isn't only about physical fitness or appearance. Physical wellness is the complete physical condition and functioning of your body—both the visible aspects, such as how fit you look, and those that are not, such as your blood pressure and the density of your bones. Throughout life, physical wellness is reflected in your ability to get through your daily activities and to take care of yourself.

Regular physical activity and healthy eating are the foundation behaviors of physical wellness, but they are just a beginning. Ask yourself these questions:

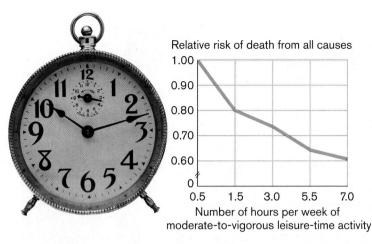

Figure 1-2 **Level of physical activity and risk of death.** The biggest reduction in the risk of death is at the low end of the physical activity spectrum, between people who are sedentary and people whose activity level is low or moderate; additional risk reductions accompany higher levels of physical activity.

Source: Physical Activity Guidelines Advisory Committee. (2008). *Physical Activity Guidelines Advisory Committee report, 2008.* Washington, DC: U.S. Department of Health and Human Services.

That usually requires **exercise**—planned, structured, repetitive body movements specifically designed to develop fitness. You'll learn much more about physical activity, exercise, and physical fitness in later chapters, along with details on how to put together an exercise program that is right for you.

EMOTIONAL WELLNESS. **Emotional wellness** is based in your ability to carry on your day-to-day activities while understanding your feelings and expressing them in constructive and appropriate ways. It involves accepting your feelings, monitoring your emotional reactions, and recognizing your strengths and limitations. It is also exemplified by your ability to cope, manage, and adapt to normal stressors. The following qualities are associated with emotional wellness:

- optimism
- enthusiasm
- trust
- self-confidence
- self-acceptance
- resiliency
- self-esteem

People with a high level of emotional wellness have a generally positive outlook and can meet challenges while maintaining emotional stability. They can deal effectively with strong feelings—they are both flexible and balanced. They can live and work autonomously while also reaching out to others. They also are willing to seek help for emotional problems, if needed.

INTELLECTUAL WELLNESS. **Intellectual wellness** is characterized by the ability to think logically and solve problems in order to successfully meet life's challenges.

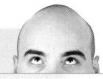

Mind Stretcher
Critical Thinking Exercise

Evaluate a Web site that you use for health and wellness information. Use the criteria described in the chapter—including authorship, sources, potential for bias, and currency—in your evaluation (see p. 6). How does the site rate? Do you think the site is credible? Why or why not?

An active and engaged mind is vital for making sound choices related to all the dimensions of wellness. Do you enjoy learning new skills, solving problems, and exploring ideas? People who enjoy a high level of intellectual wellness are creative, open to new ideas, and motivated to learn new information and new skills. They actively seek ways to challenge their minds and pursue intellectual growth. They can apply critical thinking skills as they gather and evaluate information and use it to make sound decisions.

Every health consumer should know how to use critical thinking to evaluate the quality of online health and wellness information; see the box "Safe Wellness Web-Surfing" for tips.

SOCIAL WELLNESS. Human beings are social by nature—some more than others, but all of us are social creatures. **Social wellness** is defined by the ability to develop and maintain positive,

exercise Planned, structured, repetitive body movements conducted specifically to develop components of physical fitness.

emotional wellness Dimension of wellness that focuses on one's ability to manage and express emotions in constructive and appropriate ways.

intellectual wellness Dimension of wellness that focuses on developing and enhancing one's knowledge base and critical thinking, decision-making, and problem-solving skills.

social wellness Dimension of wellness that focuses on one's ability to develop and maintain positive, healthy, satisfying interpersonal relationships and appropriate support networks.

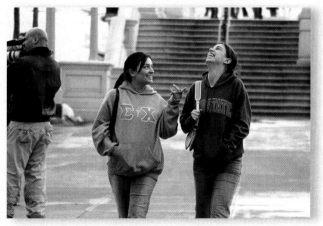

Social wellness is exemplified by positive, satisfying interpersonal relationships.

Practical Prevention

Safe Wellness Web-Surfing

The following are some things to look for when evaluating the quality of health information on Web sites.

Consider the source: Know who is responsible for the content, and look for recognized authorities.

- Look for an "about us" page. Is the site run by a branch of the federal government, a nonprofit institution, a college or university, a professional organization, a health system, a commercial organization, or an individual?
- Use caution if the site doesn't provide a way to contact the organization or webmaster.

Focus on quality and look for the evidence: Look for information that is authored by experts or reviewed and approved by an editorial board before it is posted.

- Use caution on sites that don't identify the author, that rely on testimonials and opinions rather than qualified individuals, research, or organizations.
- Look for sites with HONCode certification, meaning they follow the code of conduct developed by the Health on the Net (HON) Foundation (http://www.hon.ch).

Be a cyberskeptic: Avoid quackery.

- Beware of claims that are too good to be true, such as a remedy that will cure a variety of illnesses, that is a "breakthrough," that will have quick and dramatic results, or that relies on a "secret ingredient."
- Avoid sites that have a sensational writing style (lots of exclamation points, for example) or that use technical jargon or deliberately obscure, "scientific"-sounding language.
- Get a second opinion! Check more than one site.

Check for currency: Look for dates on Web pages. An article on coping with the loss of a loved one doesn't need to be current, but an article on the latest treatment of diabetes does.

Beware of bias: What is the purpose of the site? Who is providing the funding?

- Use caution if the sponsor of the site is selling something, even if the product is only indirectly referred to on the site. Any advertisements that do appear should be labeled; they should say "Advertisement" or "From our Sponsor."
- See if it is clear whether content comes from a noncommercial source or an advertiser is providing it. For example, if a page about treatment of depression recommends one drug by name, the manufacturer of the drug may have provided that information. You should consult other sources to see what they say about the drug and whether others can also be used.

Protect your privacy: Health information should be confidential. Look for a privacy policy that tells you what information the site collects and what they do with it. For example, if the site says "We share information with companies that can provide you with useful products," then your information isn't private.

Consult with your health professional before making any major lifestyle changes or health care decisions.

Source: Adapted from National Library of Medicine. (2006). *MedlinePlus guide to healthy Web surfing* (http://www.nlm.nih.gov/medlineplus/healthy-websurfing.html).

---

healthy, satisfying interpersonal relationships and appropriate support networks. This includes building relationships with individuals and groups both inside and outside your family, as well as contributing to the broader community in which you live. The ability to communicate effectively and develop a capacity for intimacy are key elements of social wellness. Do you have friends or family members who you can confide in and lean on for support? Are people comfortable confiding in you and coming to you for help? Do you get along with others and communicate with respect, despite differences of opinion or values? Are you a good listener?

SPIRITUAL WELLNESS. Wellness involves more than striving for physical health; it is also a search for meaning, purpose, and fulfillment. **Spiritual wellness** means having a set of values, beliefs, or principles that give meaning and purpose to your life and help guide your choices and actions. Compassion, forgiveness, altruism, tolerance, and the capacity for love are all qualities associated with spiritual wellness. Do the choices you make every day reflect your values and priorities? Or do you sometimes act in ways that conflict with your values?

People develop and express spirituality in different ways. For some people, purpose and direction come from organized religion or the belief in a higher power in the universe; they may engage

spiritual wellness Dimension of wellness that focuses on developing a set of values, beliefs, or principles that give meaning and purpose to life and guide one's actions and choices.

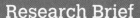

Research Brief

It's Good to Be Good

Many researchers have investigated whether helping others—by participating in organized volunteer work or by providing instrumental support to friends or family members—affects the health of the helper. Most studies have found clear benefits for both physical and mental health. One recent study followed more than 7,000 older adults for eight years. It found that those who were frequent volunteers had significantly reduced mortality. Similar benefits to health and well-being have been found for people of all ages.

How does helping others improve health? The underlying cause isn't clear, but it may relate to reduced levels of stress and the physiological effects of stress, including changes in the levels of hormones and certain chemicals in the brain. Volunteering provides opportunities for so-

cial interaction and support as well as a distraction from your own worries. One caution from researchers is that the helping needs to be voluntary and not overwhelming, or it won't reduce stress.

What does this mean for you? Take time out to help others, even if you can't commit to being a regular volunteer. Try practicing small, random acts of kindness during the day—hold the door open, help someone with their shopping cart, let someone go ahead of you in line, or just smile and say hello.

Source: Harris, A. H., & Thoresen, C. E. (2005). Volunteering is associated with delayed mortality in older people. *Journal of Health Psychology*, *10*(6): 739–752.

---

in spiritual practices such as prayer or meditation. Religion is not the only path to spiritual wellness, however. People may express spirituality through the arts, through volunteer work in their communities, or through personal relationships.

Spirituality may be considered a controversial part of wellness models because it touches on issues or beliefs that some people prefer to keep private and other people feel compelled to share or even to try to bring others around to their ways of thinking. Talking about spirituality or specific religious issues can sometimes make people uncomfortable, but that doesn't make it a topic to be avoided or a less important part of one's wellness. Actually, the fact that many people become so impassioned on the topic speaks to its relevance in their lives. Regardless of your specific beliefs or the propensity for some to create controversy in this area, spirituality—however you express it in your own life—is an essential part of your overall well-being. The values, beliefs, and principles you live by are an indispensable part of the whole you.

ENVIRONMENTAL WELLNESS. Your own wellness depends on your surroundings: Does your physical environment support your wellness or detract from it? Are there hazards in your environment—toxins such as secondhand smoke, a high degree of violence in the local community—that you should be aware of in order to protect yourself? Are there actions you could be taking to make your world a cleaner, safer place? **Environmental wellness** recognizes the inter-

dependence of your wellness and the condition and livability of your surroundings. You can take steps to make sure your lifestyle is respectful of the environment and helps create sustainable human and ecological communities. Do your choices reflect your awareness of the health of the planet and your place on it?

environmental wellness Dimension of wellness that focuses on the condition and livability of the local environment and the planet as a whole.

Assess your wellness status in each of the dimensions by completing Lab Activity 1-2.

OTHER WELLNESS DIMENSIONS. The model of wellness we've adopted in this text incorporates the six dimensions described above—physical, emotional, intellectual, social, spiritual, and environmental wellness. Other models may highlight different dimensions, including two we'll describe briefly here in terms of their relevance to college students: financial wellness and occupational wellness. Both can be important to wellness, and they encompass many

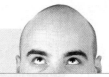

Mind Stretcher
Critical Thinking Exercise

How do you personally define health and wellness? Do you include all the dimensions of wellness described here? Do you include other dimensions? Do you rate all the dimensions equally? Has your personal definition of wellness—or lack of a definition—affected your attitudes, behaviors, and priorities? How?

aspects of the six dimensions we've already discussed.

Financial wellness refers to appropriate management of financial resources, a task that typically requires self-discipline and critical thinking skills. Take advantage of budgeting resources and financial planning help available on your campus and in your community (see the box "Financial Strategies for College Students"). Watch out for common financial pitfalls, including poor choices about which credit cards to get, overuse of credit cards, not setting up a budget, and letting friends or your own unrealistic expectations pressure you into spending more than you should. Working toward wellness doesn't have to be an expensive endeavor; check the Dollar Stretcher tips throughout the text for strategies to save money while you boost your wellness.

Occupational wellness refers to the satisfaction, fulfillment, and enrichment you obtain through work. If you consider the hours, days, and years you're likely to spend at work, you can clearly see why your job choices are important to health and wellness. You want to work in environments that help you increase personal satisfaction, find enrichment and meaning, build useful skills, and contribute to your community. When you think about your potential career choices, consider your values, skills, personal qualities, and goals. Although a high-paying job may sound like the best choice, if you don't value and enjoy what you'll be doing every day, you'll have little satisfaction from your work. Look for opportunities to learn and grow, to engage your personal interests, and to end each day feeling that your time has been well spent.

DOLLAR STRETCHER
Financial Wellness Tip

To get a handle on your finances and plan a budget, start by tracking all your income and expenses for several weeks. Many people find that just by tracking their expenditures, they cut back on nonessentials.

MYTH or FACT?

People spend less money when they use cash instead of a credit card.

▶ WATCH ONLINE

Integrating the Dimensions: Recognizing Connections and Striving for Balance

Q If you change your behavior for fitness, will that help other areas of your life too?

Absolutely. Any activity or choice that affects one dimension of wellness will directly or indirectly affect the other

dimensions, and each dimension is vital in the quest for optimal wellness. For example, engaging in physical activity reduces stress and improves mood (emotional wellness) and is linked to the maintenance of cognitive functioning (intellectual wellness); it also provides opportunities for enjoyable interaction with others (social wellness). The influence also runs in the opposite direction: strong intellectual wellness helps you plan a successful program for building fitness, and your social support system can be a huge plus as you work to change your exercise behavior.

To improve wellness, you must integrate all the dimensions of wellness with the personal choices and actions that affect your health and well-being. Balance among the dimensions is also critical for wellness. Don't focus on a few dimensions and neglect others. Doing that is like removing a few spokes from a wheel: In most ways it still looks like a wheel, but it no longer functions optimally. Figure 1-3 shows the close relationship among the dimensions—and with your own choices and actions. You'll see this Wellness Integrator in the Wellness Connections box at the start of every chapter in your text, along with a description of how that chapter's topic influences, and is influenced by, each dimension of wellness.

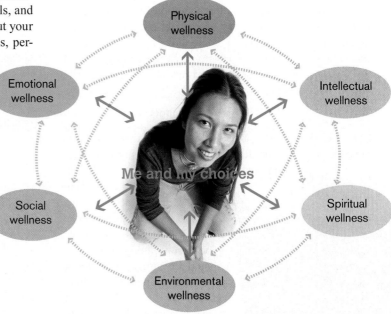

Figure 1-3 **Wellness Integrator.** The dimensions of wellness are linked to each other and to you and your choices.

Wellness Strategies

Financial Strategies for College Students

Financial wellness doesn't refer to being rich but rather to appropriately managing your financial resources—whatever they are. Money doesn't guarantee good health and happiness, but financial difficulties can strain physical, emotional, and social dimensions of wellness and thus reduce your overall well-being. A study conducted at Ohio State University's office of student affairs also correlated increased financial stress with decreased GPA. Financial security provides peace of mind and reduces stress. Live within your financial means and, when possible, save for the future.

For many traditional-age college students, money management is a relatively new experience and, unfortunately, many learn from their mistakes rather than by educating themselves up front. They continue to build up debt while in college, not realizing the long-term implications. Although some accumulation of debt may be necessary (student loans) for long-term benefit, it's important to distinguish between necessary and unnecessary expenses and to manage resources accordingly.

Credit cards are one of the biggest financial pitfalls for college students. The ease of obtaining and using credit cards can lead to unintentional and overwhelming debt. Research indicates 84 percent of full-time undergraduate students have at least one credit card; the average number of cards is 4.6, and the average unpaid balance is nearly $3,200.

Learning to develop and manage a budget is another common challenge for students. The majority of college students do not have a budget, and many who do don't stick to it. As a rule, women are more likely than men to have a budget, married students are more likely than unmarried students to follow a budget, and students over age 35 are most likely to stick to their budgets more often.

There's hope for everyone, though, and it's never too late—or too early—to make choices to improve your financial wellness. Many campuses have resources to help you develop a financial-wellness plan. If assistance is not available on your campus, there are many reputable financial-planning tools available. Check with your bank, credit union, or other financial institution, as many offer free access to Web-based financial management applications; also review the resources from the Financial Literacy & Education Commission (http://www.mymoney.gov). When you do seek financial advice, choose your sources wisely and follow up with knowledgeable individuals you trust.

Here are some specific tips to help college students stay on track financially:

- Track your income and spending carefully; you're less likely to buy on impulse when you become more aware of where your money is going.
- Be frugal: Take advantage of student discounts on everything from pizza to school supplies.
- Keep only one credit card, and use it sparingly.
- Build up an emergency fund; if you run into trouble, many colleges provide grants or emergency loans (just make sure you are using additional loan money for something related to school, like computer repair, and not an expensive spring break trip that you can't really afford).
- Develop a personal budget, and review it often.
- Use caution: Don't give out your personal account or other numbers; don't leave payments in unsecure mail boxes; and review bills and statements carefully.

For additional tips, visit http://www.moneymanagementtips.com/students.htm

Sources: SallieMae. (2009, April). *How undergraduate students use credit cards: National study of usage rates and trends 2009* (http://www.salliemae.com/about/news_info/research/credit_card_study/). Henry, R. A., Weber, J. G., & Yarbrough, D. (2001). Money management practices of college students. *College Student Journal, 35*(2), 244–249.

Health in United States: The Bigger Picture

Most of us think about health and well-being as personal concerns, and we focus on our own health and that of our friends and family members. But health is also an issue for communities and for the nation as a whole. A healthy population is creative and productive, the engine for economic growth. An unhealthy population raises national health care costs and lowers productivity. Tracking the health status of Americans and developing strategies for extending healthy life and reducing the burdens of illness and disability are key goals of federal health agencies.

Measures of Health and Wellness

Q | By what standards is health measured?

There is no single best measure of health. Consider the possible criteria: Is it how long people live? How well they live? What they die from? The rates of specific diseases and injuries? How much money people spend on health care? Different measures of health and wellness show us different things about individuals and the societies they live in.

Q | What are the chances of living to 100?

LIFE EXPECTANCY. It would depend on your age, location, and, of course, your current health status. **Life expectancy** is the average number of years people are expected to live. It depends on your age: A hypothetical average American born in 2006 is expected to live to age 77.7; a person who is 75 in 2005 can expect to live nearly twelve more years, to age 86.6.[6] The longer life expectancy for the 75-year-old reflects the fact that someone who has already lived to age 75 has escaped some of the causes of death common among younger individuals—and has already shown a fairly good degree of health by living to age 75.

The average life expectancy number hides some disparities. Women live longer than men (80 years versus 75 years for those born in 2006), and whites live longer than African Americans (78 years versus 73 years). And if you were wondering how life expectancy in the United States stacks up against other countries, it ranks forty-ninth overall and twenty-ninth among countries with a population of 1 million or more.[7] Obviously, there's room for improvement.

life expectancy The average number of years people born in a given year are expected to live.

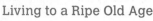

Fast Facts

Living to a Ripe Old Age

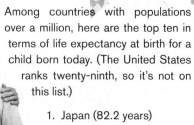

Among countries with populations over a million, here are the top ten in terms of life expectancy at birth for a child born today. (The United States ranks twenty-ninth, so it's not on this list.)

1. Japan (82.2 years)
2. Singapore
3. Hong Kong
4. Australia
5. Canada
6. France
7. Sweden
8. Switzerland
9. Israel
10. New Zealand (80.5 years)

Source: Central Intelligence Agency. (2010). *The world factbook online* (https://www.cia.gov/library/publications/the-world-factbook/index.html).

Q | Why do people live longer now than they used to?

Life expectancy increased dramatically in the past century. A child born in 1900 had an average life expectancy of only 47 years, compared to close to 80 years today. Much of this difference is due to decreased rates of death among infants and children: In 1900, more than 30 percent of all deaths occurred among children under age 5; today that figure is less than 2 percent. Improvements in public health helped fuel this dramatic change in life expectancy:[8]

- Vaccinations for childhood diseases, improved sanitation, safer foods, and the development of antibiotics dramatically decreased deaths from infectious diseases like cholera, typhoid, measles, and tuberculosis.
- Better hygiene, nutrition, and health care reduced maternal and infant mortality by over 90 percent; mothers and babies are much more likely to survive and thrive today.
- Millions of smoking-related deaths were prevented by the recognition that tobacco use is a health hazard and the subsequent anti-smoking campaigns and laws protecting nonsmokers from environmental tobacco smoke.
- Improvements in motor vehicle safety (better designed roads and cars; use of safety belts, child safety seats, and motorcycle helmets) and in workplace safety reduced motor vehicle–related deaths and occupational injuries and deaths.

Later in the chapter, we'll take a closer look at the leading causes of death in the United States today—and the factors that contribute to them. Further improvements in life expectancy are possible, but they will require action by both individuals and health systems.

Q | Why do women usually live longer than men?

The gender gap in life expectancy is due to both behavioral and biological factors. In the developing

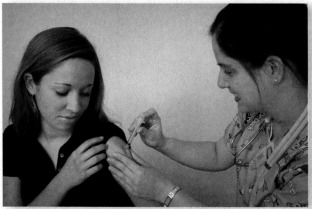

The development and use of vaccines helped increase U.S. life expectancy by dramatically reducing illness and death from infectious diseases such as smallpox, measles, mumps, diphtheria, pertussis (whooping cough), and polio.

world, women do not fare as well as men due to high rates of maternal mortality (deaths related to pregnancy and childbirth). In the developed world, women live on average 5–10 years longer than men; among people over age 100 in the United States, 80 percent are women.[9]

One of the reasons for different death rates for men and women is the number of younger men who die as a result of risky and violent behavior—men are much more likely than women to die from unintentional injuries (accidents), assault (murder), and suicide.[10] Is risky behavior due to some biological factor, such as higher levels of the hormone testosterone, or does it relate to cultural norms for male behavior? Both biology and social factors may play a role. The higher rate of deaths by suicide among men is a function of the choice of method: Women are more likely than men to attempt suicide, but men are much more likely to succeed because they tend to choose more lethal methods (such as a firearm). Higher rates of smoking and excess alcohol consumption among men are likely linked to social norms for behavior.

Another reason women have a longer average life expectancy is that they tend to develop cardiovascular disease, the leading cause of death among Americans, at a later age than men. The reason may be biological differences between the sexes—levels of hormones or iron status, for example. Women also have healthier behaviors on average: They are less likely to smoke, they have healthier diets, and they are more likely to deal with stress in positive ways, such as seeking social support.

Both men and women can take steps to improve their lifestyles and the likelihood that they'll live long and healthy lives.

Q | Do you have to be super healthy to live longer?

QUALITY OF LIFE. Yes and no—it would help, but there is no guarantee either way. A high level of health means that you are free from serious or chronic illness, at least for the moment, so you're on the positive side of the health continuum. However, many people with chronic illness live for many years with symptoms of varying severity. It's important to note that longevity isn't the only goal of health and wellness. You want not only more years but more *healthy* years, more years in which you enjoy a high quality of life.

Your overall perception of your wellness is one way to assess your quality of life. But researchers use more specific measures for research and comparative purposes. One measure is *unhealthy days,* or the estimate of the number of days of poor or impaired physical or mental health in the past 30 days. As you can see from Fig-

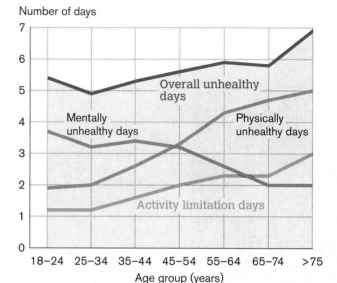

Number of days

Figure 1-4 **Quality of life among Americans: Unhealthy days and activity limitations during a 30-day period.** Overall unhealthy days, physically unhealthy days, and days with activity limitations all increase with age, but mentally unhealthy days are highest for young adults and lowest for older adults.
Source: Centers for Disease Control and Prevention. (2005). Health-related quality of life surveillance—United States. *MMWR, 54*(SS-4).

ure 1-4, young adults report more mentally unhealthy days and older adults report more physically unhealthy days. It is important to recognize that young adults might be on the positive end of the health continuum because they have no symptoms yet rate their stress level so high that they feel unwell several days each month—definite room for improvement in several dimensions of wellness!

A related measure is *years of healthy life.* The difference between life expectancy and years of healthy life is the number of years of less-than-optimal health due to chronic or acute diseases or limitations. Currently, Americans can expect an average of 65 years of healthy life and a life expectancy of 78 years, leaving about 13 years in less-than-optimal health.[11] Good lifestyle choices now can help you not only to live longer but also to have more years of healthy life and more healthy days.

The National Healthy People Initiative

Q | Has there been any substantial improvement in physical health in the past few years in the United States, or are we all just getting less and less healthy?

Some measures of health have improved; others have worsened. If you want all the details, check the data for Healthy People objectives. The national Healthy People initiative,

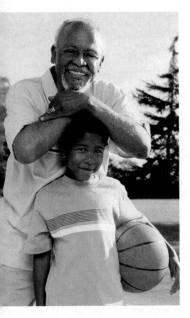

sponsored by the U.S. Department of Health and Human Services, is a broad collaborative effort with the goal of improving health—the health of each individual, the health of communities, and the health of the nation. Healthy People plans, published each decade since 1990, set specific health goals framed on ten-year agendas. Progress is tracked throughout the decade, followed by the updated plan for the next ten years. The most recent plan, *Healthy People 2020,* was released in 2010.

The Healthy People initiative has two broad goals:

■ Increase quality and years of healthy life: Help individuals of all ages increase life expectancy and improve their quality of life.
■ Eliminate health disparities among segments of the U.S. population, including differences that occur by gender, race or ethnicity, education or income, disability, geographic location, or sexual orientation.

Supporting these goals are hundreds of specific objectives, along with a national data collection effort to track our progress. Here are two examples of specific objectives from *Healthy People 2010* and the progress we've made— or not made:[12]

■ Reduce the percentage of children age 6 years and under who are exposed to tobacco smoke at home from a baseline of 27 percent to a target of 10 percent by 2010; the most recent figure of 8 percent means this objective has been achieved.
■ Reduce the prevalence of diabetes from a baseline rate of 40 per 1,000 people to a target rate of 25 per 1,000 people by 2010; the most recent figure of 59 per 1,000 people means that we've moved significantly farther away from achieving this objective.

You can look up the Healthy People 2020 plan or the data on all the Healthy People 2010 objectives by visiting the Healthy People Web site: http://www.healthypeople.gov.

Leading Causes of Death

Q | How does the United States compare to other countries in terms of diseases?

We are very fortunate in this country. Although people in many parts of the world live in poverty and less than desirable, sometimes even deplorable, conditions, people in the United States enjoy a relative abundance of resources. Sometimes, however, abundance can lead to excess. In the developing world, people suffer and die primarily from diseases and conditions related to the lack of necessities and basic public health measures. In developed countries, people are more likely to die from diseases associated with abundance. Even in lower-income areas of the United States, the primary causes of death are considered lifestyle diseases. Diseases such as diabetes and cardiovascular disease are highly correlated with lifestyle choices including overindulgence in such things as fat, sugar, and alcohol.

Figure 1-5 compares the general categories of leading causes of death in developing countries and developed countries. The high percentage of deaths in developing countries from **communicable (infectious) diseases** is similar to what was seen in the United States in 1900.

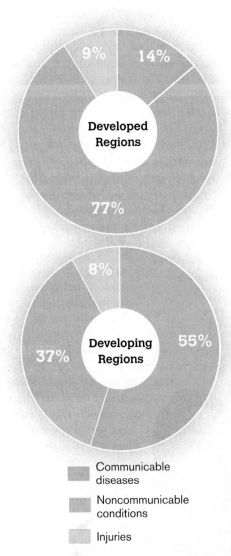

Figure 1-5 Causes of death in developed and developing regions of the world

Source: University of California, Santa Cruz. *The UC atlas of global inequality* (http://ucatlas.ucsc.edu/cause.php).

communicable (infectious) disease A disease that can be passed from one person to another; also known as an infectious disease; typically caused by a pathogen such as a bacterium or virus.

noncommunicable (chronic) disease A disease that is not infectious or contagious; many are chronic diseases that develop over time and are the result of the interplay of genetic, behavioral, and environmental factors. Examples are heart disease and diabetes.

risk factor A behavior or a characteristic that increases susceptibility for the development, onset, or progression of a disease or an injury.

In developed countries, most deaths are now due to **noncommunicable (chronic) diseases.**

Communicable or infectious diseases are those caused by a pathogen such as a bacterium or virus. They typically develop very quickly and are contagious. People who contract an infectious disease, except for serious ones like HIV infection and hepatitis, often recover completely if the appropriate treatment is available.

By contrast, noncommunicable diseases are not caused by pathogens and are not contagious. They are mostly chronic diseases that develop over time from a combination of genetics, environmental factors, and lifestyle choices. They include heart disease, some forms of cancer, and diabetes. People with chronic diseases must often adapt their lives to accommodate the symptoms and effects of the disease. Approximately 70 percent of the people in the United States develop and die from some form of chronic disease. (Chronic and infectious diseases are discussed in greater detail in Chapters 11 and 12.)

Q | It seems like everyone has cancer. Is cancer now the leading cause of death for Americans?

For many age groups, yes—but not overall (Table 1-1). Although deaths from heart disease have fallen significantly in recent decades, heart disease is still the number-one killer of Americans. Cancer tops heart disease as a cause of death in for younger people, but among people age 75 and older, heart disease kills many more than cancer. As you can see from Table 1-1, these two chronic diseases—heart disease and cancer—are responsible for nearly half of all deaths in the United States each year.

Q | What is the leading cause of death for young adults?

Few traditional-age college students die from heart disease and cancer, which are fairly uncommon in young adults. Death rates overall are low among young adults, and the top causes of death—accidents, assault (homicide), and suicide—stem from risky behaviors, violence, and depression (Figure 1-6). The chronic diseases that are the major causes of death for the population as a whole develop over many years, and their symptoms may not appear until middle or later adulthood. That doesn't mean young adults should ignore them! Your habits now have a big influence on whether and when you develop a serious chronic disease.

Q | What can be done to decrease the leading causes of death?

A great deal. You'll have an opportunity to assess your risk for specific chronic diseases in later chapters. For now, it's important to understand the basics about **risk factors,** which are factors that increase your susceptibility for the development, onset, or progression of a disease or an injury. Smoking is an example of a risk factor; people who smoke are far more likely to develop heart disease and cancer than those who don't smoke.

TABLE 1-1 LEADING CAUSES OF DEATH IN THE UNITED STATES, ALL AGES

RANK	CAUSE	NUMBER OF DEATHS	PERCENTAGE OF ALL DEATHS
1	Heart disease	631,636	26.0%
2	Cancer	559,888	23.1%
3	Stroke	137,119	5.7%
4	Chronic lower respiratory diseases	124,583	5.1%
5	Accidents (unintentional injuries)	121,599	5.0%
6	Diabetes	72,449	3.0%
7	Alzheimer's disease	72,432	3.0%
8	Influenza and pneumonia	56,326	2.3%
9	Kidney disease	45,344	1.9%
10	Septicemia (systemic blood infection)	34,234	1.4%

Source: National Center for Health Statistics. (2010). Deaths: Leading causes for 2006. *National Vital Statistics Reports, 58*(14).

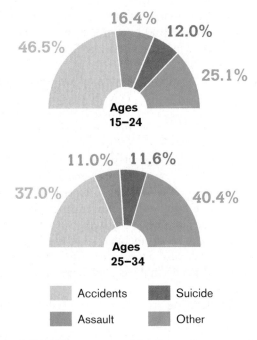

Figure 1-6 Leading causes of death among young adults. Young adults are most likely to die from causes related to risky behavior and violence.

Source: National Center for Health Statistics. (2010). Deaths: Leading causes for 2006. *National Vital Statistics Reports 58*(14).

Not wearing a safety belt is another risk factor; if you don't buckle up, you are far more likely to be seriously injured in a crash than someone who does use a seat belt.

Risk factors can typically be divided into two groups—those that can be changed and those that cannot be changed. Age is a common risk factor for chronic disease that you can't change; for example, years of wear and tear on your joints increase the risk of developing arthritis. However, you can change other risk factors for arthritis, such as excess body weight. Most chronic diseases develop from a combination of risk factors, some of which are under your control. This means that through your own actions, you can reduce your risk for most major chronic diseases and types of injuries. Later in this chapter, we'll review the components of a wellness lifestyle that can help you both increase wellness and reduce the risk of health problems throughout your life.

Q | How many people die from obesity?

Obesity isn't on the list of leading causes of death among Americans. However, it is an important underlying cause of many chronic diseases. Researchers have examined the lifestyle and environmental factors that contribute to the leading causes of death, and they have identified and ranked what they call the *actual* causes of death (Table 1-2). Obesity appears near the top of this list—it contributes to heart disease, cancer, and diabetes, among other serious health conditions. Large

decreases in life expectancy have been seen in people who are obese: Among nonsmokers who were obese at age 40, women lost 7.1 years of life and men lost 5.8 years.[13] Being overweight even though not obese is also associated with reduced life expectancy.

Tobacco use remains the leading preventable cause of death in the United States. The 440,000 deaths attributed to tobacco use every year include 35,000 deaths among nonsmokers exposed to secondhand smoke and 1,000 infant deaths due to maternal smoking. All the factors in Table 1-2 are included in the discussion of a wellness lifestyle on pp. 16–20.

Health and Wellness on Campus

Q | What are the main health and wellness concerns of college students?

Many college students do their best to ignore their health—and to push their limits in terms of stress, lack of sleep, relationship strain, and poor time management.

TABLE 1-2 ACTUAL CAUSES OF DEATH AMONG AMERICANS

CAUSE	NUMBER OF DEATHS PER YEAR	PERCENTAGE OF TOTAL DEATHS PER YEAR
Tobacco	440,000	18.1%
Obesity (poor diet and inactivity)	112,000	4.6%
Alcohol consumption	85,000	3.5%
Microbial agents	75,000	3.1%
Toxic agents	55,000	2.3%
Motor vehicles	43,000	1.8%
Firearms	29,000	1.2%
Sexual behavior	20,000	0.8%
Illicit drug use	17,000	0.7%

Sources: Flegal, K., Graubard, B., Williamson, D., & Gail, M. (2005). Excess deaths associated with underweight, overweight, and obesity. *JAMA, 293*, 1861–1867. Mokdad, A., Marks, J., Stroup, D., & Gerberding, J. (2004). Actual causes of death in the United States, 2000. *JAMA, 291*, 1238–1245 [original study]. Mokdad, A., Marks, J., Stroup, D., & Gerberding, J. (2005). Correction: Actual causes of death in the United States, 2000 (letter). *JAMA, 293*(3), 293–294.

Even if the hectic life of a college student doesn't lead to illness, it can certainly leave him or her feeling exhausted, overwhelmed, and generally unwell. In a recent survey in which over 80,000 college students identified health problems that affected them during the previous school year, back pain and allergies topped the list.

As you can see from Figure 1-7, most of the health problems reported by students aren't of the chronic variety. Many are short-lived and curable. Why then should they be such a concern? Because, although the physical effect on your body may be short-lived, these health problems also affect other areas of your life.

Are the academic, financial, time-management, and relationship effects all short term, or do some have long-term implications? Table 1-3 shows a range of common health issues that affect

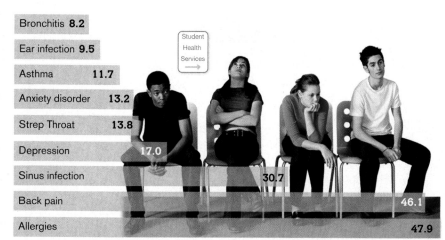

Bronchitis	8.2
Ear infection	9.5
Asthma	11.7
Anxiety disorder	13.2
Strep Throat	13.8
Depression	17.0
Sinus infection	30.7
Back pain	46.1
Allergies	47.9

Percentage of students experiencing the problem within the last school year

Figure 1-7 **Most common health problems reported by college students**
Source: American College Health Association. (2008). *American College Health Association national college health assessment: Reference group executive summary spring 2008.* Baltimore, MD: ACHA.

TABLE 1-3 ACADEMIC IMPACTS OF SELECTED HEALTH PROBLEMS*

	PERCENTAGE OF STUDENTS REPORTING AN ACADEMIC IMPACT
Stress	27.8%
Sleep difficulties	20.0%
Cold/flu/sore throat	19.0%
Anxiety	18.6%
Depression	11.1%
Concern for a troubled friend or family member	10.5%
Relationship difficulties	9.8%
Alcohol use	3.8%
Chronic health problem or serious illness	3.6%

*Academic impacts include a lower grade on an exam or important project; a lower grade in a course; an incomplete or dropping a course; or a significant disruption in thesis, dissertation, research, or practicum work.

Source: American College Health Association. (2009). American College Health Association national college health assessment II: Reference group executive summary fall 2009. Baltimore, MD: ACHA.

the academic life of college students. The high percentages of students reporting these health problems also indicate that students' health behaviors are not optimal and that there is plenty of room for improvement in multiple wellness dimensions. Students whose academic performance is being hurt by stress, sleep difficulties, depression, anxiety, relationships difficulties, or alcohol use are certainly not living up to their full wellness potential.

The truth is that when it comes to your health, any problem may produce longer-term consequences than just a missed class or two. Your finances, your relationships, and your risk for chronic conditions are among the many factors that can be affected. So how do you break the cycle? Or at least interrupt it? It comes back to that issue of risk and responsibility. It's up to you to make good choices and to avoid risk when you can. That's where a wellness lifestyle comes into play: Make choices every day that will help boost your health and well-being now and in the future.

Factors Influencing Individual Health and Wellness

Although this chapter—and the entire text—stresses the role of individual choice and behavior in health and wellness, it's obvious those aren't the only factors. You have the most control over your individual lifestyle choices, but it's important to be aware of all the other influences on your well-being. Even for those you can't control or change, you can make choices to help improve wellness. For example, even though a condition like high blood pressure may be common in your family, increasing your personal risk of developing it, genetics isn't the only risk factor. You can

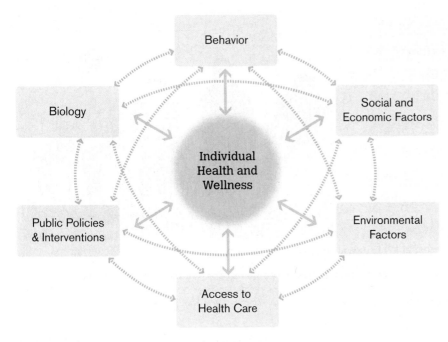

Figure 1-8 **Factors determining health and wellness status**

make choices such as limiting the salt in your diet and getting regular blood pressure checks that can help both to reduce the risk of developing high blood pressure and to limit its adverse effects if you do develop the condition. In this section, we'll review various influences on individual health and wellness, with special attention to health-related behavior choices (Figure 1-8). Just as the dimensions of wellness interact, so do the factors that determine your health and wellness status.

Wellness Behavior Choices

Q | What are the basic things you should do every day or every week for a healthy lifestyle?

The decisions you make and the actions you take every day affect all dimensions of wellness—physical, emotional, intellectual, social, spiritual, environmental—as well as your overall health status and risk for chronic diseases and premature death.

BE PHYSICALLY ACTIVE. Your body is designed to function best when it is active—and busy isn't the same thing as active. Because so much of modern life is tied to technologies that keep us sedentary, most people need to purposely plan time for physical activity. It's well worth the time and effort! People who are physically active live longer and healthier lives (see Figure 1-2). And many of the benefits of physical activity are immediate: It reduces stress and anxiety, helps you sleep better, and boosts your mood and self-esteem. Chapter 3 goes into much more detail about the benefits of physical activity and physical

fitness, and later chapters will guide you in putting together an exercise program that is right for you.

CHOOSE A HEALTHY DIET. Think about *diet* as your daily eating habits and not as a temporary restriction of the foods you eat. Eating well means choosing more healthful foods and fewer harmful foods, most of the time. Nutrition and dietary planning will be discussed in detail in Chapters 8 and 9. General guidelines for healthy eating include the following:

- Eat more fruits, vegetables, legumes, whole grains, fish, and low-fat or nonfat dairy products.
- Consume less sugary foods and drinks, unhealthy fats, refined carbohydrates, salty foods, red meat, and full-fat dairy products.
- Balance your overall energy (calorie) intake with your level of physical activity to prevent weight gain.

A healthy diet will give you the energy and nutrients you need today and limit the substances that increase your risk for chronic diseases in the future.

MAINTAIN A HEALTHY WEIGHT. Achieving and maintaining a healthy weight depends on your diet and activity habits—and on your ability to manage stress and make sound choices. It is perhaps the most challenging lifestyle

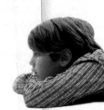

Fast Facts

Too Much TV Is Harmful to Your Health!

Too much time spent sitting—even for people who exercise—has been found to increase the risk of dying, particularly for cardiovascular disease. One study found that every hour spent watching TV each day (three hours versus two hours per day, for example) increased the risk of an early death from heart disease by up to 18 percent. The technologies of modern life may work against efforts to increase physical activity, but you do have control over how you spend your leisure time. Turn off the TV! Move more and sit less!

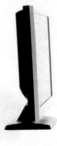

Source: Dunstan, D. W., and others. (2010). Television viewing time and mortality. *Circulation, 121*(3), 384–391.

Research Brief

Healthy Living Counts . . . and Every Choice Matters

A great deal of research has gone into tying specific behaviors to health outcomes—smoking to lung cancer, for example. But it's also important to consider the effects of combinations of lifestyle factors. For example, if you smoke, does it matter if you lose weight? If you exercise regularly, is there really any extra benefit to a healthy diet?

Researchers recently examined data on more than 20,000 adults who were tracked for an average of eight years. They looked at healthy lifestyle factors in relation to the study participants' risk of developing a major chronic disease (diabetes, heart attack, stroke, cancer). In the analysis, participants were awarded one point for each of four healthy lifestyle factors:

- Never having smoked
- Engaging in physical activity for 3.5 or more hours per week
- Having a healthy dietary pattern (high intake of fruits, vegetables, and whole grains and low meat consumption)
- Having a body mass index (BMI) below 30 (BMI is a single number representing weight-to-height ratio;

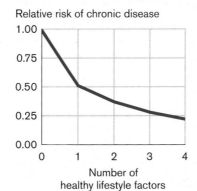

Relative risk of chronic disease

Number of healthy lifestyle factors

a BMI below 30 means the person is not obese)

Researchers found that the risk of developing a chronic disease decreased progressively as the number of healthy factors increased. People with all four healthy factors had nearly an 80 percent lower risk of developing a chronic disease than participants without a healthy factor. But risk was also reduced for people with one, two, or three healthy factors. The risk reduction was most striking for diabetes, for which having one healthy factor reduced risk by more than 60 percent and having all four healthy factors reduced risk by 93 percent compared to having no healthy factors.

This research shows the strong effect that a healthy lifestyle has on the risk for chronic disease. The findings also emphasize that every behavior counts. Even if you feel like you can't change all your unhealthy habits, changing even one is very beneficial to your health.

Source: Ford, E. S., and others. (2009). Healthy living is the best revenge. *Archives of Internal Medicine, 169*(15), 1355–1362.

---

goal to achieve in our society, where environmental influences often work against our efforts. But even modest success at weight management improves health, reduces chronic disease risk, and makes people feel better about themselves. Chapter 7 provides information on assessing body weight and body composition, and Chapter 9 presents healthy eating strategies for weight management.

AVOID TOBACCO IN ALL FORMS. As shown in Table 1-2, tobacco use is the leading preventable cause of death, accounting for about one in five deaths every year.[14] In the short term, smoking impairs your lung function and your immune system; in the long term, it is a major risk factor for eight of the top ten causes of death. Smoking also kills thousands of nonsmokers every year. No form of tobacco use is safe. Although smoking rates have dropped significantly over the past fifty years, about 20 percent of Americans are still smokers. Strategies for quitting smoking are described in Chapter 13.

MANAGE STRESS AND GET ADEQUATE SLEEP. Many college students feel stressed out and short on sleep. Excess negative stress is uncomfortable in the short-term and can have serious health consequences over time.

Fast Facts

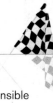

Smoking by the Numbers

- Cigarette smoking is estimated to be responsible for $193 billion in annual health-related economic losses in the United States (for direct medical costs and lost productivity); this translates into $10.47 per pack of cigarettes.
- An estimated 46 million people or 20.6 percent of all adults in the United States currently smoke cigarettes, and smoking kills about 440,000 Americans a year.
- Worldwide, more than 1.3 billion people smoke cigarettes, and smoking kills about 5 million people a year.

Sources Centers for Disease Control and Prevention. (2010). *Smoking and tobacco use* (http://www.cdc.gov/tobacco). World Wellness Organization. (n.d.). *Tobacco free initiative* (http://www.who.int/tobacco).

Learn to recognize the key causes of stress in your life and develop coping strategies—time management, social support, exercise, a relaxation technique. Don't turn to alcohol, tobacco, or overeating in an effort to reduce stress; they are ineffective and harmful to your health in other ways. Adequate sleep is one of the best things you can do to reduce stress and improve your ability to cope. For more on stress management, see Chapter 10.

LIMIT ALCOHOL CONSUMPTION. If you choose to drink alcohol, do so moderately and in situations that don't put yourself or others at risk. Excess alcohol consumption damages the body, and intoxication is linked to a high risk of injuries and violence. See Chapter 13 for more on the health effects of alcohol.

AVOID RISKY BEHAVIORS. Risky behaviors, such as the following, greatly increase the likelihood of an injury or illness:

- Dangerous driving, including driving at high speeds, driving while distracted, and not wearing a safety belt
- Unsafe handling of firearms
- Unprotected sexual activity, which carries the risk of sexually transmitted infections
- Not using appropriate safety equipment during sports and recreational activities (for example, helmets and personal flotation devices) or during work activities (for example, goggles, gloves, helmets)
- Drug or alcohol intoxication, which can be dangerous in itself (for example, alcohol poisoning) and also lead to other risky behaviors, including unintentional injuries and violence

Make safety a priority for yourself and those around you. Most safety-related behaviors aren't complicated, but they can be challenging in some circumstances. Use common sense, plan ahead, and don't let peer pressure or lack of commitment get in the way of safe choices.

Behaviors related to safe driving deserve special mention. Motor vehicle crashes are the leading cause of death for Americans ages 1–35: Someone—driver, passenger, pedestrian—dies from a motor vehicle crash every twelve minutes in the United States.[15] People don't think of driving as a risky behavior, but it is probably the most dangerous thing most of us do on any given day. Treat driving with the attentiveness it deserves, and always drive (or ride) safely. Pay attention, don't speed, wear your seatbelt, don't tailgate, and use signals before turning or changing lanes. Just because you've previously gotten away with driving too

fast—or while distracted by texting, talking, or changing the station—doesn't mean you will next time.

LIMIT EXPOSURE TO RADIATION AND TOXINS. Exposure to pollutants and other environmental toxins is a risk factor for a number of health problems. The most common source of radiation exposure is sunlight. Always use sunscreen, and don't use tanning lamps (see Chapter 11). Have X-rays only when they are medically necessary. If you live or work in an area with high pollution levels—for example, in a building that may have high levels of radon or asbestos—take appropriate steps to protect yourself. You can boost the environmental wellness of your community through such strategies as recycling, reducing driving time, saving energy and water, and disposing of hazardous wastes properly. For more on limiting your exposure to toxins and on

DOLLAR STRETCHER
Financial Wellness Tips

Reduce your spending on beverages! College students spend billions each year on beer and soft drinks. Different choices could benefit your health and your wallet.

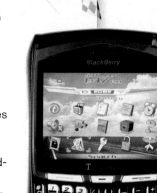

Fast Facts

Hanging Up

- On average, drivers spend about 10 percent of their driving time on the phone.
- Drivers phone and text even at the riskiest times (in bad weather and heavy traffic, for example).
- More than 40 percent of drivers ages 18–29 text while driving, even in states with texting bans.
- People are less likely to talk on hand-held phones in states that ban the practice, but the bans are frequently ignored.
- Using a hands-free phone does not reduce the risk of crashes; the mental distraction of talking on the phone is the same for every type of phone.

For safety, limit all types of distractions while you're driving! Keep your eyes on the road, your hands on the wheel, and your mind on what you're doing. For more information, visit http://www.distraction.gov.

Source: Insurance Institute for Highway Safety. (2010). Phoning while driving. *Status Report, 45*(2), 1–8. Ishigami, Y., & Klein, R. M. (2009). Is a hands-free phone safer than a handheld phone? *Journal of Safety Research, 40*(2), 157–164.

Living with . . .

Migraine Headaches

For those who get migraine headaches, the experience can be debilitating. These recurring, severe headaches cause pulsing or pounding pain, usually on one side of the head, often accompanied by nausea, vomiting, and sensitivity to light and sound. They can last from 6 to 48 hours. For some people, migraines are preceded by warning symptoms known as an aura—visual disturbances consisting of zigzag patterns of flashing lights, blind spots, and tunnel vision. Many people experience a "zombie phase" or "migraine hangover" of fatigue and lethargy after an attack. Migraines can be brought on by a variety of triggers, including bright lights, certain foods and food additives, stress, changes in weather, and hormonal changes (in women).

Although migraines used to be called "vascular headaches" and were thought to be caused by dilation and contraction of blood vessels in the brain, research has revealed that they are related to a wave of nerve cell activity that sweeps across the brain, affecting nerve pathways and brain chemicals. Researchers are beginning to investigate gene mutations that may cause this abnormal activity in brain cells. Migraines may run in families, and they occur more frequently in women than in men.

There is no cure for migraines, but they can be managed. The goal is to identify and avoid triggers. If you get migraines, keep a headache diary for a while and record the following information:

- When you got the migraine and its severity
- What you've eaten
- How much sleep you've had
- For women, where you are in your menstrual cycle
- Other factors that may have an effect, including stress

If you start to get migraine symptoms, act quickly to treat them. You may be able to reduce or prevent further symptoms by taking these steps:

- Drink water to avoid dehydration.
- Rest in a quiet, dark room with your eyes closed.
- Place a cool cloth on your head.

Over-the-counter pain relievers and nausea medicines may help manage symptoms during a migraine. There are also prescription medications that can reduce the number of attacks, stop the headache once it starts, and treat pain and other symptoms.

The best way to prevent migraines is to modify your habits and environment to avoid triggers:

- Avoid the personal triggers you have identified through your headache diary.
- Avoid smoking, alcohol, artificial sweeteners, and other known food-related triggers.
- Get regular exercise.
- Get enough sleep.
- Learn to manage stress.

Don't let migraines stop you from working toward wellness. More information about treatment and support is available from the American Council for Headache Education (http://www.achenet.org), the American Migraine Foundation (http://www.americanmigrainefoundation.org), and the National Headache Foundation (http://www.headaches.org).

Sources: MedlinePlus. (2009). Migraine (http://www.nlm.nih.gov/medlineplus/ency/article/000709.htm). Dodick, D. W., & J. J. Gargus. (2008, August). Why migraines strike. *Scientific American*, 56–73.

improving the environment, visit the Web site for the U.S. Environmental Protection Agency (http://www.epa.gov).

PRACTICE GOOD SELF-CARE. Take care of yourself! To reduce your risk of infections, wash your hands frequently and limit your exposure to people who are ill with colds or the flu. Practice good dental care by brushing and flossing regularly. Use over-the-counter remedies carefully, following the label instructions. For more on avoiding and treating infectious diseases, see Chapter 12.

If you have a chronic or recurring medical condition—asthma, diabetes, or migraine headaches, for example—follow your health care provider's instructions for managing it. Take preventive medications if you need them. Having a chronic condition is challenging but it doesn't mean you can't achieve optimal wellness. Take whatever actions you can to manage your condition and limit its impact on your

life; see the box "Living with . . . Migraine Headaches" in this chapter and look for other Living with . . . boxes throughout the text for tips and strategies about managing common chronic conditions.

SEEK APPROPRIATE MEDICAL CARE. Don't wait to visit a health care provider until you're sick. Get recommended check-ups, screening tests, and immunizations. Don't ignore symptoms that should be evaluated by a doctor; if you aren't sure, you can usually call or e-mail a doctor's office or clinic for advice. And don't neglect your mental health; if symptoms of emotional or psychological problems are interfering with your daily life, seek help. For additional advice on evaluating symptoms, treating minor medical problems, and getting appropriate tests and vaccines, visit the Web site of the American Academy of Family Physicians (http://familydoctor.org).

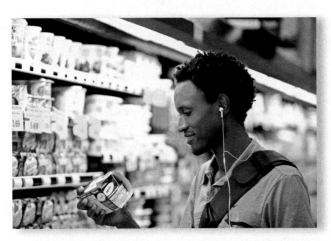

Use your critical thinking skills to read and understand the information on food, supplement, and drug labels—and what that information means for you.

APPLY CRITICAL THINKING SKILLS AS A HEALTH CONSUMER. Evaluating health Web sites (see p. 6) is only one of the ways to use critical thinking skills for health and wellness. A high level of intellectual wellness can also help you navigate the complex U.S. health care system, with its many products, services, and professionals. Other wellness-related tasks that require critical thinking skills include reading food and drug labels, considering the risks and benefits of various tests and treatments, evaluating health insurance plans, and communicating with health care providers. Keep asking questions and searching for answers! See the box "Understanding Health Headlines" to learn more about how to understand the results of medical research studies—and what they mean for you.

CULTIVATE RELATIONSHIPS AND SOCIAL SUPPORT. Strong relationships provide emotional and material support. Spend time with the people who are important to you. Don't neglect family and friends when you are busy— make the time. Be supportive and kind, and expect that friendships will have ups and downs. Communicate acceptance and respect.

TAKE TIME TO NOURISH YOUR SPIRITUAL SIDE. Don't neglect spiritual wellness. Consider the values and principles that are important to you, and ask yourself if you need to make changes in your life to be true to them. When making decisions, stop and consider your options: Which choice is most consistent with your values? Don't allow expediency or peer pressure to have undue influence over your actions. Your choices and actions tell those around you what you stand for.

Are you currently engaging in any spiritual practices or expressing your spirituality in other ways? If you aren't currently doing volunteer work, think about ways you might get more involved in some type of community service. Tutor or coach low-income students, visit home-

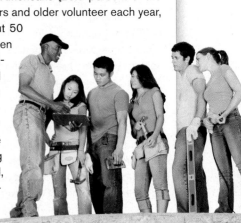

Fast Facts

Be a Volunteer!

More than one in four Americans (26.8 percent of the population) age 16 years and older volunteer each year, for an average of about 50 hours per year. Women are more likely to volunteer than men, and rates of volunteerism also go up with education level. Popular volunteer activities are fundraising, preparing and distributing food, general labor, supervising youth sports teams, and tutoring or teaching. Find an organization and activity you want to support and get involved! You'll boost your wellness as well as serving your community.

Data source: U.S. Department of Labor, Bureau of Labor Statistics. *Current population survey* (http://www.bls.gov).

bound seniors, clean up local roads or beaches, or help at an animal shelter. Find an activity or organization that fits your values and your schedule.

HAVE FUN! Don't make a chore of your efforts to achieve good health and wellness. Wellness is about living with joy and vitality. Cultivate your sense of humor: Laughter improves health and makes you and everyone around you feel better.

How do your health habits compare with the description of a healthy lifestyle in this section? If you're like most people, you are doing well in some areas but could improve in others. You can use Lab Activity 1-1 to help identify areas of concern for you. In Chapter 2, you'll learn more about strategies and techniques for making changes in your health behaviors to improve wellness in both the short and long term.

Other Factors That Influence Wellness

Q | Is health mostly dependent on genes and family history?

Genetic inheritance can affect your risk for certain diseases, but in most cases, your genes are just one factor in your disease risk and

Wellness Strategies

Understanding Health Headlines

Every day, you can find hundreds of news stories related to health. Use your critical thinking skills to evaluate news reports about medical research findings and to determine whether the results might be important for you.

Types of Research Studies and Findings: The Basics

Studies using animals or cells in test tubes can provide important information but don't often lead directly to treatments or lifestyle advice for people. Initial studies about people are often *observational* or *correlation studies,* in which researchers track a group of people over time but don't try to change their behavior or provide special treatments. Observational studies can find associations, but they do not establish cause-and-effect relationships.

Clinical or *experimental studies* look for cause-and-effect relationships by comparing a treatment group with a control group. For example, in tests of a new drug, one group of people is given the drug and the control group is given a *placebo* (an inactive pill); then a specific health outcome between the two groups is compared. The most meaningful clinical studies have a large number of participants, are randomized (meaning participants are randomly assigned to either the treatment or the placebo group), and are double-blind (meaning neither the participants nor the researchers know who is receiving the placebo and who is receiving the treatment).

Research results are often reported in terms of risk:

- *Relative risk* is a ratio or percentage expressing the comparative risk between two groups, such as a 50 percent reduced risk of heart attack in people who took a particular medication or engaged in a particular behavior.
- *Absolute risk* is a number expressing the incidence of a disease or event in a group, such as 25 heart attacks in every 1,000 people.

It's often important to know both numbers. Say your absolute risk of developing a disease is 8 in 1,000. If a treatment reduces the relative risk by 50 percent, then it would reduce your absolute risk to 4 in 1,000. Not a big change, but if the disease in question is very serious or fatal, then any risk reduction might be beneficial.

Questions to Ask About a New Medical Finding

- Was it a study in the laboratory, in animals, or in people? The results of research in people are more likely to be meaningful for you.
- Does the study include people like you? Were the people in the study the same age, sex, educational level, income group, and ethnic background as yourself? Did they have the same health concerns?
- Was it a randomized, double-blind, controlled clinical trial involving thousands of people? This type of study is the most expensive, but it also gives scientists the most reliable results.
- Are the results presented in an easy-to-understand way? They should use absolute risk, relative risk, or some other uncomplicated number.
- If a new treatment was being tested, were there side effects? Sometimes side effects are almost as serious as the disease.
- Who paid for the research? Take special care in evaluating research that was partly or fully funded by a company that stands to gain financially from the results.
- Who is reporting the results? Is the newspaper, television station, or Web site a reliable source of medical news? Was the report written by a reporter who is trained to interpret medical findings?

Talk with your health care provider before changing your lifestyle or medications on the basis of health headlines. Progress in medical research takes years, and findings must be duplicated by other scientists at different locations before they become part of accepted medical practice.

Source: Adapted from National Institute on Aging. (2006, November). *Understanding risk: What do those headlines really mean?* (http://www.nia.nih.gov/HealthInformation/Publications/risk.htm).

---

overall health status. Some relatively rare diseases and disorders are caused by a single gene, but most diseases are caused by a complex combination of biological, behavioral, and environmental factors.

Nevertheless, it is important to know your family health history. If you know you are at higher risk for a particular condition—for example, alcoholism or high cholesterol—you can make informed lifestyle choices to reduce your risk. Someone with a family history of high cholesterol can reduce her personal risk by choosing a diet low in saturated fat and high in fiber and by getting regular exercise.

Sometimes it can be difficult to separate the effects of genetic inheritance from those of health habits; many of us have copied the eating patterns and exercise habits of our parents or caregivers. So, you might have "inherited" both a genetic predisposition for high cholesterol and an eating pattern that increases your risk. Although you can't do anything about your genes, you can change your eating habits for the better.

In the previous section of the chapter, we looked at lifestyle behaviors that affect health and wellness. Let's look next at other factors that influence wellness.

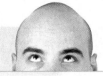

Mind Stretcher
Critical Thinking Exercise

What sorts of health habits did your parents and other family members have when you were growing up? Were they active or sedentary? Did they smoke? What kinds of foods did they eat? How have your own health habits been influenced by those of your family members?

BIOLOGY. Your biology includes your genetic makeup, family health history, and any mental or physical problems you've developed. Certain health habits, such as smoking and drinking, can "change" your biology by altering the functioning of your cells and organs. Your age and gender can also be considered part of your biology—and both have a big effect on your health and wellness. But again, lifestyle choices can help reduce the impact of biology. For example, although bone density inevitably decreases with age, a healthy diet and regular weight-bearing exercise throughout your life help maintain bone density and reduce your risk of falling.

As described on p. 10, the health differences between the sexes may be due to a mix of biological, behavioral, and cultural factors. Gender differences that have a biological basis include the following:

- Men are taller, have more muscle mass, and are more likely to store excess body fat in the abdomen; women are shorter, have relatively less muscle mass (especially in the upper body), and are more likely to store excess body fat around the hips.
- Men have denser bones than women and have lower rates of osteoporosis (loss of bone mass that can lead to fractures).
- Women have a higher risk of lung cancer than men at a given level of exposure to cigarette smoke, and they become more intoxicated at a given level of alcohol intake.
- Women have stronger immune systems than men and are less susceptible to infectious diseases, but they have higher rates of autoimmune disorders.
- Women are more likely than men to be infected with a sexually transmitted disease during intercourse and are more likely to suffer severe effects, including infertility.
- Men are more likely than women to have cardiovascular disease and classic heart attack symptoms like chest pain; women are more likely to have atypical symptoms such as difficulty breathing and extreme fatigue.

What about race or ethnicity? As with gender, health differences among population groups usually stem from a mixture of factors—some biological/genetic and some based on lifestyle, culture, or socioeconomic factors. For example, Latinos have higher rates of diabetes, and African Americans have above-average rates of high blood pressure. Just like knowing your family's health history, it's important to be aware of any health conditions for which you may be at elevated risk due to your ethnicity; in some cases, earlier or more frequent screening may be advisable. For more information, visit the Web site for the CDC Office of Minority Health and Health Disparities (http://www.cdc.gov/omhd).

SOCIAL AND ECONOMIC FACTORS. Your social environment includes all your interactions with people in your community. It also includes social institutions such as schools and law enforcement as well as factors such as the quality of housing, the availability of public transportation, and the level of violence.

The economic level of a community has a big impact on the health of its citizens: Lower-income communities are likely to have a worse physical environment (more pollutants and toxins), higher rates of violence, and lower quality health care than affluent communities. Lower-income people have higher rates of many unhealthy habits, including smoking and poor dietary choices; they are also more likely to be exposed to toxins and to be injured on the job. Income is closely tied to educational attainment. People with low incomes and a low level of education have the worst health status.

ENVIRONMENTAL FACTORS. The physical environment can harm health if it is high in pollutants or physical hazards. Environmental factors can also be positive—for example, if a community has many places to buy fruits and vegetables and an extensive network of walking trails and bicycle lanes. People with lower incomes and educational attainment are more likely to live in communities with harmful environmental factors. Look around your own community for factors or conditions that can enhance or harm health.

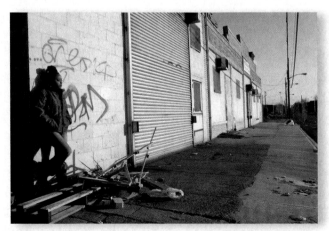

Lower-income communities are usually associated with additional health risks, including more toxins and pollutants in the physical environment, lower quality housing and health care, and higher rates of violence.

Research Brief

The Health Burdens of Poverty and Lack of Education

Poverty and high school dropout rates are often looked at as social or economic problems, but perhaps they are even more important in relation to health. Researchers recently analyzed the impact of selected social and behavioral risk factors on quality of life and life expectancy. They calculated the number of years of healthy life lost from smoking, low income, lack of education, obesity, and other factors. They determined that low income may be even more damaging to health than smoking—and low educational attainment wasn't far behind. Their findings:

- Low income (below 200 percent of the federal poverty line): 8.2 years of healthy life lost
- Smoking: 6.6 years of healthy life lost

- Less than 12 years of education (high school dropout): 5.1 years of healthy life lost
- Obesity: 4.2 years of healthy life lost

It's difficult for individuals by themselves to improve social determinants of health, but you can support efforts in your community to improve nonmedical factors that impact health. Consider supporting poverty reduction programs as well as efforts to reduce class size in elementary schools.

Source: Muennig, P., Fiscella, K., Tancredi, D., & Franks, P. (2010). The relative health burden of selected social and behavioral risk factors in the United States: Implications for policy. *American Journal of Public Health,* e-pub ahead of print.

ACCESS TO HEALTH CARE. Unequal access to quality health care underlies many of the health disparities in the United States. Lack of health insurance and an inability to pay costs out of pocket keeps some people away from health care they need. In lower-income communities, health care services may be very limited or located at an inconvenient distance. Language barriers can also restrict access to health care.

PUBLIC POLICIES AND INTERVENTIONS. Health promotion campaigns and disease prevention services can affect health in positive ways. Laws mandating child safety seats have increased safety for infants and children. Restrictions on smoking have had a positive effect on the health of nonsmokers and also encouraged smokers to quit. You can help promote positive changes to public policy that would improve the health of people living in your community.

Q | What can businesses and the government do to encourage healthy choices? **READ ONLINE**

Wellness: What Do You Want for Yourself—Now and in the Future?

Q | What does it feel like to be well?

It feels great! Wellness is characterized by feelings of energy, vitality, curiosity, empowerment, and enjoyment—a high quality of life. It also means you are consciously engaged in the process of achieving your full potential in all the wellness dimensions.

How do you rate your own levels of health and wellness today? Do you feel optimally healthy? Do you feel you've achieved a high level for each dimension of wellness? How does your lifestyle compare to the healthy lifestyle described in this chapter?

If you're like most young adults, you probably have room for improvement, both in terms of your lifestyle behaviors and how far you've developed all the dimensions of wellness. The good news is that you can decide what kind of future you want. Wellness is something everyone can work on and improve. It comes from the choices you make every day. Any improvements to your wellness behaviors will bring immediate benefits as well as a feeling of empowerment.

Do you want to make changes but aren't sure how to get started? In the next chapter, you'll review principles of behavior change and examine strategies for making positive

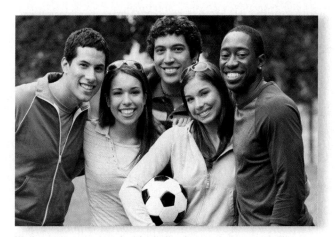

Wellness is associated with vitality, joy, optimism, curiosity, empowerment, and many other characteristics exemplifying a high quality of life.

changes in your own life. You can apply the model of behavior change to any health-related behavior; keep the principles in mind as you work your way through subsequent chapters.

Each chapter that follows will examine a specific area of health or health behavior. You'll see a focus on issues and challenges of particular interest to college students, with answers to questions asked by students like yourself. You'll have an opportunity to assess your status in each area of health and wellness, and you'll find the information you need to make positive changes and improve your overall wellness.

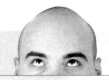

Mind Stretcher
Critical Thinking Exercise

Are you satisfied with your overall level of wellness? If not, in what ways would you like to change it? What do you think are your wellness strengths? In what dimensions of wellness would you most like to improve?

Summary

Health is a condition with multiple dimensions that falls on a continuum from negative health, characterized by illness and premature death, to optimum health, characterized by the capacity to enjoy life and to withstand life's challenges. Wellness is an active process of adopting patterns of behavior that can improve health and perceptions of well-being and quality of life in terms of multiple, intertwined dimensions. The dimensions of wellness—physical, emotional, intellectual, social, spiritual, and environmental—are closely connected and must be developed in a balanced way for overall wellness.

Health status can be assessed through life expectancy, days and years of healthy life, and a review of the leading and underlying causes of death. Healthy lifestyle behaviors include the following:

- Be physically active
- Choose a healthy diet
- Maintain a healthy weight
- Avoid tobacco in all forms
- Manage stress and get adequate sleep
- Limit alcohol consumption
- Avoid risky behaviors
- Limit exposure to radiation and toxins
- Practice good self-care
- Seek appropriate medical care
- Apply critical thinking skills as a health consumer
- Cultivate relationships and social support
- Take time to nourish your spiritual side
- Have fun

Other factors include family history, income and educational attainment, the environment, access to health care, and public policies.

More to Explore

American Academy of Family Physicians (FamilyDoctor.org)
   http://familydoctor.org
Centers for Disease Control and Prevention: Healthy Living
   http://www.cdc.gov/HealthyLiving
Healthy People Initiative
   http://www.healthypeople.gov
MedlinePlus
   http://www.medlineplus.gov
National Wellness Institute
   http://www.nationalwellness.org
Surgeon General's Family Health History Initiative
   http://www.hhs.gov/familyhistory
U.S. Department of Health and Human Services: Prevention
   http://www.hhs.gov/safety/index.html
U.S. Department of Health and Human Services: Quick Guide to Healthy Living
   http://www.healthfinder.gov/prevention

🖳 **SUBMIT ONLINE**

NAME	**DATE**	**SECTION**

This lab activity will help you identify your positive and negative wellness lifestyle behaviors.

Equipment None

Preparation None

Instructions

For each wellness behavior listed below, place a check in the column with the answer that best describes your behavior.

	A Almost always	B Some-times	C Almost never
1. I engage in at least 150 minutes per week of moderate-intensity aerobic exercise.			
2. I perform muscular strength and endurance exercises at least 2 times per week.			
3. I perform stretching exercises at least 2 days per week.			
4. I spend some leisure time each week engaged in physical activity.			
5. I eat at least 7 servings of fruits and vegetables a day.			
6. I avoid skipping meals.			
7. I limit my intake of foods high in saturated and trans fat.			
8. I limit the amount of added sugars I consume from sweetened beverages, desserts, and similar products.			
9. I limit the amount of salt I consume.			
10. For breads, cereals, and other grain-based products, I choose whole-grain foods at least half the time.			
11. I check food labels, ingredient lists, and nutrition information at restaurants in order to make informed choices.			
12. I maintain a healthy weight, avoiding overweight or underweight.			
13. I get 7–8 hours of sleep each night.			
14. I don't smoke cigarettes, cigars, or any other form of tobacco.			
15. I don't use smokeless (spit) tobacco.			
16. I avoid exposure to secondhand smoke.			
17. I use alcohol in moderation (1 drink or less per day for women; 2 drinks or less per day for men) or not at all.			
18. I do not use alcohol or any substance to the point of intoxication.			
19. I use over-the-counter medications as directed.			
20. I use prescription drugs as prescribed.			
21. I avoid unproven, dangerous, and illegal substances, including steroids, as well as unproven health remedies.			
22. I practice good dental care by brushing my teeth two or more times a day, flossing at least once per day, and having a dental checkup at least once a year.			
23. I have medical checkups annually or as suggested by my physician in order to obtain all recommended screening tests.			
24. I get recommended immunizations.			

	A Almost always	B Some-times	C Almost never
25. I obtain only medically necessary X-rays.			
26. I manage any chronic medical conditions (such as asthma, migraines, allergies, diabetes, seizure disorder) according to the advice of my health care practitioner.			
27. I abstain from sex or engage in safe sex practices.			
28. I wash my hands frequently over the course of the day.			
29. I use sunscreen as directed and use protective clothing (e.g., a wide-brimmed hat) as needed when working or playing outside.			
30. I don't try to tan, either from exposure to the sun or through use of tanning lamps or salons.			
31. I keep my computer desk or other workspace set up in a way that allows me to maintain good posture and minimize stress on my body.			
32. I use appropriate protective equipment when participating in recreational activities that require such equipment.			
33. I use appropriate protective equipment for occupational activities that require such equipment.			
34. I am actively responsible for my personal safety by being aware of my surroundings, avoiding being alone in unprotected areas, locking doors and windows when appropriate, and so on.			
35. If I have access to a firearm, I store it securely and use it safely.			
36. I do not talk on the phone, send text messages, or engage in other distracting activities while driving.			
37. I wear a seatbelt when driving or riding in a car.			
38. I avoid driving while under the influence of alcohol or other drugs or riding with others who are under the influence.			
39. I obey the rules of the road by not speeding or tailgating, by always signaling before I turn or change lanes, and by adjusting my speed and driving to road and weather conditions.			
40. I recycle paper, plastic, and other appropriate items, and I reuse items such as shopping bags.			
41. I take steps to conserve energy and water (turning off lights and faucets, carpooling, and so on).			
42. I avoid environmental toxins and areas or times of day with high pollution levels.			
43. I manage stress in positive ways (e.g., physical activity, time management, deep breathing).			
44. I have or would seek help for depression or another mental health concern.			
45. I maintain a group of close friends I can confide in and ask for help or support.			
46. I manage my anger in ways that are not harmful to myself or others.			
47. I resolve conflicts with family, friends, co-workers, and fellow students in positive, respectful ways.			
48. I feel a sense of connectedness with others.			
49. I accept responsibility for my own feelings.			
50. I accept responsibility for my own actions.			
51. I engage in activities that are consistent with my beliefs and values.			

	A Almost always	B Some-times	C Almost never
52. I spend time each day in prayer, meditation, or personal reflection.			
53. I participate in university and/or community events, or I volunteer.			
54. I like my job.			
55. I take at least a little time each day to relax and engage in a hobby or other activity I enjoy.			
56. I make a budget, track my spending, and keep my finances under control.			
57. I manage my time well through strategies such as setting priorities, creating to-do lists, and managing my schedule using a planner.			
58. I am motivated to learn new information and skills, and I actively seek ways to challenge my mind and seek intellectual growth.			
59. I gather and evaluate information in order to make sound decisions about health and wellness.			
60. I am able to set realistic goals for myself and work toward them.			
TOTAL NUMBER OF RESPONSES IN EACH COLUMN			

Results

To calculate your score, add up the total number of responses in each column and copy them onto the appropriate lines below. Multiply the total for column A by 2, the total for column B by 1, and the total for column C by 0. Add the final three numbers together for your total score, and then find your rating on the table.

Total for column A ☐ × 2 points = ☐

Total for column B ☐ × 1 point = ☐

Total for column C ☐ × 0 point = ☐

Total Score ☐

Rating	Total score
Excellent	110–120
Good	90–109
Fair	60–89
Needs attention	Less than 60

Reflecting on Your Results

How did you score? Were you surprised by number of wellness lifestyle behaviors you currently engage in—or don't engage in? Do your results give you encouragement or cause concern?

Select two behaviors of concern for you—something for which you checked "Almost never" or something for which you checked "Sometimes" but which you know is a problem for you (for example, smoking, drinking until intoxicated, never exercising). For each behavior, make a list of how it affects the different dimensions of wellness—positively as well as negatively. For example, smoking is physically and environmentally harmful, but it may make you feel better physically and emotionally in the short term; you may enjoy smoking with certain friends, but you may miss out on other social activities due to your habit.

Behavior 1: _____

How it impacts the dimensions of wellness:

Behavior 2: _____

How it impacts the dimensions of wellness:

Planning Your Next Steps

Any behavior for which you didn't check "Almost always" is a possible candidate for change and improvement. Choose five behaviors from the assessment that you are most interested in changing and list them below. For each, give one reason why you'd like to change the behavior.

Behavior 1: _____

Reason to change:

Behavior 2: _____

Reason to change:

Behavior 3: _____

Reason to change:

Behavior 4: _____

Reason to change:

Behavior 5: _____

Reason to change:

SUBMIT ONLINE

NAME	DATE	SECTION

This activity will help you identify wellness strengths and the behaviors that support or detract from each dimension.

Equipment None

Preparation None

Instructions

For each dimension, fill in the characteristics, attributes, or abilities you currently possess that you think represent your *strengths*. Also fill in your lifestyle behaviors that support and detract from each dimension; if needed, review Lab Activity 1-1 for ideas. Because behaviors affect multiple dimensions, you can enter a particular lifestyle behavior under more than one dimension. After you complete the chart for a dimension, rate yourself for that dimension by assigning a score from 1 to 10 (1 is low, 10 is high).

Physical wellness—The complete physical condition and functioning of the body		My score: _____
Physical wellness strengths (*e.g., muscular strength, healthy blood pressure*)	Behaviors that support physical wellness (*e.g., adequate sleep, regular exercise*)	Behaviors that detract from physical wellness (*e.g., binge drinking, tanning salon use*)

Emotional wellness—The ability to manage and express emotions in constructive and appropriate ways		My score: _____
Emotional wellness strengths (*e.g., optimism, trust, self-confidence*)	Behaviors that support emotional wellness (*e.g., writing in a journal every week*)	Behaviors that detract from emotional wellness (*e.g., using food to manage stress*)

Intellectual wellness—Developing and enhancing critical thinking, decision-making, and problem-solving skills		My score: _____
Intellectual wellness strengths (*e.g., common sense, curiosity, creativity*)	Behaviors that support intellectual wellness (*e.g., keeping up-to-date on health-related recommendations*)	Behaviors that detract from intellectual wellness (*e.g., getting product information from commercial Web site*)

Social wellness—The ability to maintain positive, healthy, satisfying interpersonal relationships		My score: _____
Social wellness strengths (*e.g., supportive, compassionate, trustworthy*)	Behaviors that support social wellness (*e.g., regularly contacting friends*)	Behaviors that detract from social wellness (*e.g., being a poor listener*)

Spiritual wellness—Developing a set of values, beliefs, or principles that give meaning and purpose to life and guide your actions and choices		My score: _____
Spiritual wellness strengths (*e.g., faith, tolerance, altruism*)	Behaviors that support spiritual wellness (*e.g., prayer, volunteer work*)	Behaviors that detract from spiritual wellness (*any behavior that goes against personal values*)

Environmental wellness—The condition and livability of the local environment and the planet as a whole		My score: _____
Environmental wellness strengths (*e.g., awareness of environmental effects of actions*)	Behaviors that support environmental wellness (*e.g., recycling, taking public transit*)	Behaviors that detract from environment wellness (*e.g., buying products with lots of packaging*)

Results

Enter the scores (1–10) you assigned for each level of wellness

	SCORE (1–10)		SCORE (1–10)		SCORE (1-10)
Physical wellness		Intellectual wellness		Spiritual wellness	
Emotional wellness		Social wellness		Environmental wellness	

Reflecting on Your Results

What is your wellness status? What are your strongest and weakest dimensions, and why? When you thought about each dimension individually, were you surprised—positively or negatively—by how many strengths and supportive behaviors you were able to identify? Do you feel balanced in terms of all of the dimensions of wellness?

Planning Your Next Steps

Choose one dimension in which you'd like to improve, and describe at least three specific strategies that would help you build wellness in that area.

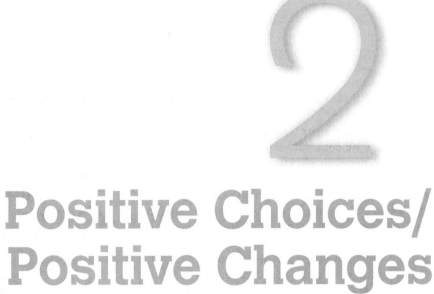

Positive Choices/ Positive Changes

COMING UP IN THIS CHAPTER

Identify the factors that influence your wellness behaviors › Develop strategies for increasing your motivation to change for the better › Learn how to apply techniques that match your stage in the change process › Develop a personalized plan for successful behavior change, including appropriate goals and strategies for overcoming barriers

Wellness Connections

The link between behavior change and the dimensions of wellness is clear—making positive changes in your health habits can improve your level of wellness in every dimension. But the relationship works both ways. The dimensions of wellness also influence how—and how well—your behavior change plans and programs progress. A high level of intellectual wellness will help you develop a sound plan and identify strategies for overcoming barriers to change. Emotional and spiritual wellness help you understand and address values and feelings that affect your behavior and ability to change; changing your behavior to bring it in line with your personal values can be a key motivational factor. Your physical wellness—your overall health and fitness and your ability to care for yourself—affects the choices and strategies available to you for some types of behavior change programs.

Satisfying and supportive relationships, the hallmarks of social wellness, are another critical component for successful behavior change. The people

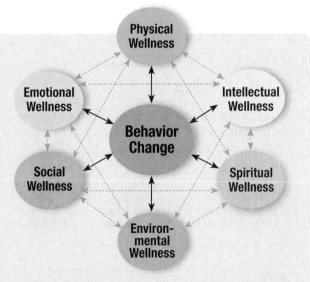

in your life can have a huge influence on your ability to adopt and maintain positive health habits. All aspects of your physical environment also affect behavior change—your local environment may support change (for example, safe places to exercise, many places to shop for healthy foods) or it may include obstacles to change. As an individual, you can develop strategies to deal with environmental challenges and work to improve the environment for yourself as well as everyone in your community.

We each are responsible for the choices we make every day that so greatly influence our personal health and well-being, for good or bad. Yet, although almost everyone wants to look and feel their best—inside and out, now and in the future—actually doing all the things that lead to personal wellness is not so easy. Why is that? Why do we make negative health choices? There is no simple answer.

Sometimes we don't have the information we need to make the best decisions and plans. Sometimes we have the knowledge, but other factors—such as peer pressure, social norms, emotions, motivation, or environment—get in the way of making a good decision. A good decision produces healthy behaviors and has a positive effect on one or more components of our wellness and our collective well-being. Examples from the wellness dimensions are the decision to exercise, to wear a seatbelt, to end a negative relationship, to respond appropriately when angry, to study for a test, and to recycle.

In this chapter you'll learn about the variety of factors that contribute to your health behaviors and your ability to sustain positive behavioral changes. Once you know about the stages and processes of making a behavior change, you can stack the odds in your favor. Additionally, you'll review guidelines for setting appropriate goals for change, overcoming barriers to change, and developing strategies for success.

Factors Influencing Health Behavior and Behavior Change

Psychologists have long studied motivation and behavior. Why, in spite of all of the information about preventable chronic diseases and the importance of good lifestyle choices, do so many people still make poor choices? Why, even when we know we shouldn't, do we still often choose unhealthy behaviors? The fact is knowledge alone isn't enough to make us change our behavior for the better. Even knowledge coupled with good intentions will likely not be enough. In order to improve your chances of succeeding at behavior change, you need to understand some key concepts about behavior in general and the factors that help shape it.

Factors Inside and Outside Your Control

Q | Why is behavior change so hard?

Your behavior is influenced by many factors, some of which can be difficult to recognize or control. Behavior change requires commitment and effort—if it was really easy to always engage in positive health behaviors, everyone would do it!

A *behavior* is an observable action or response. A behavior that recurs, often unconsciously, and develops into a pattern is what we call a *habit*. Health behaviors, or health habits, are all the actions that affect any area of your health or wellness. Your health behaviors, both good and bad, result from a combination of influences. Some of these influences are under your control, and others are not. It's important to identify and be aware of the factors that affect your behavior—even those outside your control (Figure 2-1). You can often make adjustments in other areas to help deal with factors that can't be controlled or planned for. Consider the following behavioral influences:

- **Heredity/genetic make-up:** We don't get to choose our genetic makeup, and genetically based variability makes any given health behavior or goal easier for some and harder work for others.

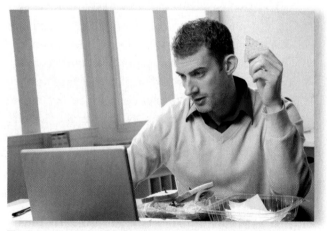

Think first! Habits are just that—so deeply engrained that we often don't consider or even notice what we're doing. A good first step in positive behavior change is simply becoming more aware of your actions . . . before you eat that next chip, smoke that next cigarette, or park yourself in front of the television or computer.

Wellness Strategies

Helping Children Develop Healthy Behaviors

- Practice healthy habits yourself—be a positive role model.
- Be active together—but don't expect all kids to like or want to participate in the same activities. Play together, but also encourage each child to pursue her or his interests.
- Don't reward kids with food. Find other ways to celebrate good behavior.
- Limit screen time, including television, video games, and Web surfing and other computer activities.
- Make dinner time a family time—in addition to ensuring children have a healthy meal, you can make dinner a time to talk about what happened during the day, a time to address issues and reduce stress.

- Involve children in planning and preparing meals and snacks. Help children develop skills like reading food labels, measuring portion sizes, and practicing making food choices.
- Be an advocate for daily physical education classes in school and healthy food choices in the school cafeteria.
- Be supportive and celebrate even small successes!

Sources: Adapted from American Heart Association. (2010). Help children develop healthy habits. *Healthier Kids* (http://www.heart.org/HEARTORG/GettingHealthy/HealthierKids/HowtoMakeaHealthyHome/Help-Children-Develop-Healthy-Habits_UCM_303805_Article.jsp). U.S. Department of Agriculture. (2009). Developing healthy eating habits. *MyPyramid.gov* (http://www.mypyramid.gov/Preschoolers/HealthyHabits/index.html).

- **Gender:** Although there's no known biological cause, research consistently shows women are more likely than men to exhibit health-promoting behaviors and avoid risky behaviors, such as substance abuse.

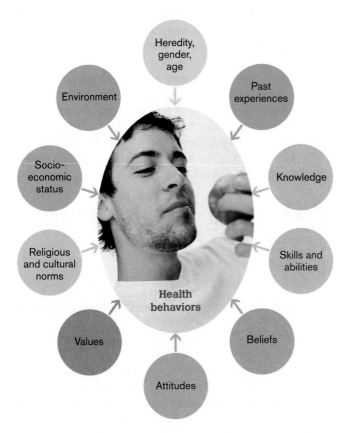

Figure 2-1 Factors that influence health behaviors
Source: Adapted from Hayden, J. (2009). *Introduction to health behavior theory.* Boston, MA: Jones and Bartlett.

- **Childhood and past experiences:** Some children are exposed to better role-modeling of healthy living and get more support for healthy choices (see the box "Helping Children Develop Healthy Behaviors"). Your experiences throughout your life shape your behavior; for example, you might not have worn a bike helmet until you were injured in a crash.
- **Knowledge, skills, abilities:** Information alone may not be sufficient to make us make healthy choices, but it is necessary in shaping our behavior. We must also have the skills and abilities to act on wellness-enhancing choices.
- **Age:** Children haven't had the same opportunities as adults to develop knowledge, skills, and abilities about healthy behaviors. Additionally, they have less control and fewer choices than adults.
- **Beliefs:** Your ideas about what is real or true influence your behavior in many ways. For example, although you may know that lack of exercise is a poor health habit, you may not believe you are susceptible to the potential consequences of a sedentary lifestyle—heart disease, for example—or that the consequences of using tanning booths will be particularly severe for you (see the box "Skin Damage from Tanning").
- **Attitudes:** Your evaluation and judgment (opinion) of objects, people, and actions influence your behavior. For example, what is your attitude toward spit tobacco? Toward people who are very fit or very unfit? Toward use of meditation for stress reduction?
- **Values:** Your values help guide your choices and prioritize your activities. For health-behavior change, it can be useful to identify conflicts between your values and your behavior.
- **Religious and cultural norms and practices:** Your values, attitudes, and beliefs are shaped by religious

Research Brief

Skin Damage from Tanning: Will It Really Happen to Me?

Surveys have consistently found high rates of indoor tanning booth use among college students. Most students say they tan because they want to change their appearance—they associate a tan with attractiveness and health. Do they know about the risks? More than 90 percent of college students using tanning booths report being aware that possible complications include premature skin aging and skin cancer. Why do they continue to tan? Do they believe that, somehow, they won't be affected?

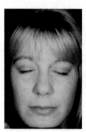 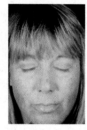

In a recent study of a group of college students who were users of tanning booths, researchers showed them ultraviolet (UV) photographs of their faces. UV photographs reveal damage to facial skin caused by previous UV exposure—damage that often isn't yet visible in ordinary light. In follow-up sessions, researchers found that students who were shown their UV photographs reported less tanning booth use than the control group, who didn't see their photos. One explanation for this difference is an alteration in the students' beliefs about the consequences of tanning. The hypothetical risks became more clear and real for those who saw their UV photos: They now believe that they are personally susceptible to the consequences of tanning—and that those consequences are severe.

A takeaway from this research is that strengthening your belief in the personal consequences of your health behaviors can help you make and maintain positive changes.

Source: Gibbons, F. X., Gerrard, M., Lane, D. J., Mahler, H. I., & Kulik, J. A. (2005). Using UV photography to reduce use of tanning booths: A test of cognitive mediation. *Health Psychology, 24*(4), 358–363.

---

and cultural norms as well as by your family environment. Together, all these factors influence behavior.

- **Socioeconomic status (income, education, occupation):** Socioeconomic status affects your resources and opportunities as well as many of the other factors listed above. For example, negative health behaviors such as smoking are strongly associated with low levels of educational attainment.

- **Environment:** Environmental influences on behavior may be in or out of your control—for example, you can remove unhealthy snacks from your residence but you can't change the fact that your neighborhood has twelve fast food restaurants but no place to buy fruit. It's important to recognize environmental factors that affect your behavior—even if you can't change them, you can develop strategies to minimize their influence.

The ten factors illustrated in Figure 2-1 that shape your behaviors can also enhance or inhibit your ability to change

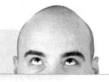

Mind Stretcher
Critical Thinking Exercise

Examine one of your own health behaviors—positive or negative. Look at the categories of influences listed in Figure 2-1, and identify ways each factor influences that behavior.

your behaviors. If you answered the question in "Mind Stretcher," you likely have already begun to realize this. Although some behavioral influences are outside your control, many of them, including the most powerful ones, are under your control. And even some of the uncontrollable influences such as family role-modeling and support become much less significant as people reach adulthood and become independent. Just as some students may have to study harder than other students to get a good grade, some people need to work a bit harder to achieve their wellness goals. That's reality. The good news is that health behavior change is doable for anyone. Our choices and plans—along with our attitudes, beliefs, and values—are factors we can control.

Predisposing, Enabling, and Reinforcing Factors

Q | Is there some way I can bribe myself into making a change in my habits?

Sometimes a "bribe," or an external reward, can be a helpful support for behavior change. Just make sure it is an appropriate reward—not too expensive and not an obstacle to change. For example, allowing yourself to buy and download one song for each day or week you stick with a new healthy behavior is a more realistic and affordable reward than something like an overseas vacation.

Rewards are a form of *reinforcement*. To plan how best to use rewards for behavior change, it helps to examine behavioral influences in another way—looking beyond whether they are controllable. The factors described in the previous section can also be grouped and categorized as predisposing, enabling, or reinforcing factors (Figure 2-2).

- **Predisposing factors** are those that you bring to the table. Your culture, age, gender, past experiences, beliefs, values, and attitudes are all predisposing, or existing, factors.
- **Enabling factors** are ones than help you change your behavior. They include your knowledge, skills, and abilities as well as various resources available to you.
- **Reinforcing factors** are ones that encourage or discourage your new behavior.

Reinforcing factors can be divided into external and internal factors. External reinforcing factors include encouragement and support from family and friends, worksite policies that make it easier for you to continue the desired behavior, and an established reward system such as the downloaded songs described above. In the early stages of changing a health behavior, external reinforcement can be very helpful. However, as you continue with a new behavior, it's important to focus on internal reinforcement, such

DOLLAR STRETCHER
Financial Wellness Tip

Rewards in a behavior-change program don't need to be elaborate or expensive. Think of free things that you enjoy, such as taking a study break to talk to a friend, watching a favorite TV show, or spending some time on a video game. Inexpensive rewards—a song download, a rented movie, a favorite book or magazine—are also effective.

as enjoyment of your new lifestyle or the sense of accomplishment that succeeding in your goals can bring.

External reinforcement, or bribes, can certainly help you succeed, but they are not always feasible—or necessary for success. You're the key. As you institute positive changes in your health habits, focus on your own personal reasons for change.

Motivation for Behavior Change

Q How can you find motivation?

Motivation comes from within yourself. It is one of the most challenging aspects of health behavior change, but there are many concrete strategies and techniques to help you boost motivation.

Motivation can be thought of as an energized state that directs and sustains behavior. People will put out more effort and persist in the face of difficulty when their motivation is high, and they'll give up more readily or not even try at all when their motivation is low. Motivation is not something a lucky few are born with. It's a dynamic quality we all have that rises and falls because of internal and external factors, many of which we can

predisposing factors Preexisting factors such as heredity, gender, beliefs, attitudes, values, and knowledge that influence health behavior.

enabling factors Factors that make it possible or easier for an individual to change a health behavior.

reinforcing factors Factors such as rewards that follow a behavior and either increase or decrease the likelihood of repeating the behavior.

motivation An energized state that directs and sustains behavior.

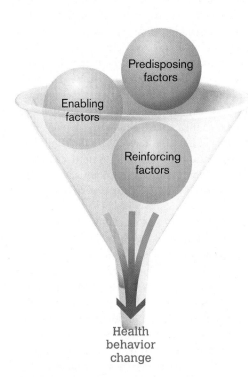

Figure 2-2 **Factors affecting behavior change**

Predisposing factors

Enabling factors

Reinforcing factors

Health behavior change

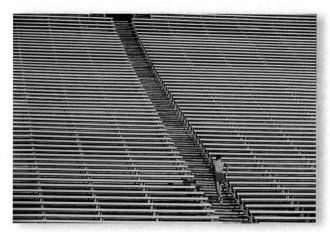

Motivation for behavior change must come from within you, but there are many strategies that will help you boost your level of effort and persistence, and increase your chance of achieving your goals.

control. For example, satisfying your hunger with a healthy snack before you shop for groceries increases your motivation to resist buying the wrong foods. Increasing factors that boost motivation and decreasing factors that interfere with motivation will help you increase your effort, persistence, and success in attaining your goals. Factors affecting motivation are locus of control, self-efficacy, goal setting, and decisional balance.

Locus of Control: Do You Feel in Charge?

Q | What's the point of all the effort? Practically everyone in my family gets diabetes about when they hit age 40.

You can do many things to reduce your risk of diabetes and other chronic diseases, no matter what happens to your family members. How much control you feel you have over your life and behavior affects whether you will be motivated to change. Researchers investigating perceived control distinguish between people who exhibit an internal locus of control and those who exhibit an external locus of control.[1] People with an **internal locus of control** believe that their personal outcomes largely depend on what they do and how hard they try. They are higher in their perception of personal control. Conversely, those with an **external locus of control** believe that factors outside their control largely determine the outcomes of what they do. They are lower in their perception of personal control.

The extent to which people take and perceive personal control affects both their success in their endeavors and their sense of well-being. Researchers have found that people who believe how well they do in life is mostly up to them—not 100 percent, but mostly—have better health, better health habits, greater happiness, less stress, greater resiliency to setbacks, and overall better mental health.[2]

How does locus of control affect health decisions and behaviors? Let's take the example of the student with several older relatives who have diabetes. A person with an external locus of control may believe she is fated by her genes to get diabetes and that nothing she does will make any difference—and therefore she does nothing to reduce her risk. A person with an internal locus of control, on the other hand, may believe that she can control her risk for diabetes and therefore takes many positive steps to reduce her risk—such as regular physical activity, healthy diet, and control of body weight.

As with motivation, your locus of control may vary over time and in different situations. To boost your sense of personal control, take the time to examine your beliefs about the situations you encounter, especially the frustrating ones. Evaluate each situation realistically, and don't think in absolutes ("nothing I do will make any difference"). It may be that no good choices are available, but you can brainstorm actions that you might take and then act according to your own choices. If nothing else, you can change and control your attitude.

Also, act based on facts—or at least on the best available information. For example, in response to surveys asking people to identify major causes of cancer, many more people list air pollution than diet or excess body fat as cancer risk factors.[3] This finding indicates that it's easier to believe things outside our control, like air pollution, pose more risk than factors we have more personal control over. In reality, air pollution contributes to only about 2 percent of cancer deaths, whereas diet and obesity contribute to 30 percent.[4] It's important to recognize and accurately evaluate the risks you can influence—and take personal control of your related health behaviors.

Self-Efficacy: Do You Anticipate Success?

Q | I start a workout program for two weeks, and then I just stop. How do I keep motivated?

Do you start your program expecting to succeed or to fail? Your personal expectations have a big effect on your motivation level. Expecting a positive outcome leads to greater effort and persistence.[5] When it is looked at as a personality trait, expecting success is referred to as *optimism*. Optimism combines a positive focus with positive expectations for how things will turn out.

Although being an optimistic person is associated with trying harder and being more effective in changing behavior, no one is optimistic about everything. People who are optimistic about most things can still lack confidence in their ability to lose weight or quit smoking, for example. For this reason, measuring people's tendency to be optimistic versus pessimistic may not predict their success in losing weight or quitting smoking. A more accurate predictor would be to ask them whether they specifically expect to succeed at losing weight or quitting smoking.

SELF-EFFICACY EXPECTATIONS. Your expectations regarding your ability to perform behavior leading to a specific outcome is called **self-efficacy.** Self-efficacy is a control-related concept formalized by psychologist Albert Bandura that has helped clarify the influence of expectations on behavior.[6] People high in self-efficacy for a particular behavior are confident they can execute it successfully—they believe they can achieve that particular goal. People low in self-efficacy lack confidence in their ability to execute a particular behavior leading to an outcome they want. In general, someone with a high level of self-efficacy views difficult tasks as challenges rather than

internal locus of control Belief that the source of power or control in one's life resides in oneself—in one's own hard work, attributes, actions, and choices.

external locus of control Belief that the source of power or control in one's life resides outside oneself—in chance, fate, and the actions of others.

self-efficacy Belief in one's capability to perform a task that leads to a specific outcome.

Wellness Strategies

Self-Efficacy for Health Goals

Circle a number between 0 and 100 on the scale below to rate your degree of confidence for reaching your specific health goal.

0	10	20	30	40	50	60	70	80	90	100

Highly certain   Moderately certain   Highly certain
  I can't do it   I can do it   I can do it

If you're not highly certain (score of 90 or more) that you can reach your health-behavior-change goal, ask yourself why. See if you can identify the barriers and other controllable factors that could possibly get you off track in terms of your goal pursuit.

    Here are some tips for boosting self-efficacy:

- Set realistic final and interim goals for behavior change.
- Monitor your behavior with a journal, log, or other tracking method.
- Identify potential obstacles to change and plan how to overcome them.

- Find a role model—someone similar to yourself who engages in your target behavior.
- Ask friends and family to support you and encourage your efforts.
- Make a mental picture of success by imagining yourself engaging in your target behavior.
- Recognize and celebrate your successes; attribute them to your own efforts.

Take charge. Develop a behavior-change plan that you have confidence in!

---

as things to be avoided, sets high goals and stays committed to them, perseveres when the going gets tough, and bounces back quickly from setbacks and failures. On the other hand, people with low self-efficacy avoid challenges, set the bar low when choosing goals and show little commitment to reaching them, doubt their abilities, give up quickly in the face of difficulties, and recover slowly from failures.[7]

Self-efficacy is different from belief. You might believe that losing weight will improve your self-confidence and want to lose weight very much. Yet, if your personal expectations for successfully losing weight are low, you may not even try. If you don't have confidence that your efforts to achieve a particular health goal will be successful (low self-efficacy), your motivation—and with it, your effort level—goes down.

This is how self-fulfilling prophecies are formed. People who expect to succeed tend to try harder and persist longer than people who aren't sure they can succeed. So, people with strong expectations of succeeding tend to be more successful partly because they try harder—and make their prediction of success come true. Conversely, by not trying as hard and giving up more easily, people with lower self-efficacy can make their prediction of failure come true.

Take the quiz in the box "Self-Efficacy for Health Goals" to gauge your level of self-efficacy for your targeted health-behavior change—whether it is to increase physical activity, improve your diet, quit smoking, or another behavior you identified. If your score is 90 percent or more, then you rate very highly in self-efficacy. But don't worry if your score is lower; there are many strategies you can try to boost your self-efficacy.

HOW SELF-EFFICACY DEVELOPS—AND CAN BE INCREASED. You can build up your self-efficacy and

with it your motivation and odds of success. Self-efficacy expectations develop from a combination of past performance, observational learning, verbal persuasion, and cognitive processing of cues such as emotional and physiological arousal.[8]

Past Performance: Direct experience is the strongest influence on self-efficacy expectations.[9] If you've succeeded in the past at controlling a similar behavior or outcome, then your self-efficacy will be higher for the current behavior. Conversely, past failures to control relevant specific outcomes will lower your self-efficacy. Success breeds success, and failure breeds failure.

Direct experience is not only the most powerful influence on self-efficacy expectations, but it is also the factor you have the most control over. Set a series of small, realistic goals that build toward your final goal. For example, if you are currently sedentary and your goal is to add 30 minutes of physical activity to each day, start off with a less ambitious goal—10 minutes of walking three times a week. Keep track of your progress through self-monitoring so that you have a record of your activities. By succeeding

Success breeds success! Your past experiences in changing a similar behavior have the most powerful influence on your self-efficacy. Start with a small change and build your confidence for the next step.

Wellness Strategies

Sample SMART Goals: Specific, Measurable, Achievable, Realistic, Time-Bound

- I'm going to increase my consumption of fruits and vegetables from an average of 3 servings per day to an average of 6 servings per day. I'll start on September 1 and reach my final goal by December 1. I will increase from 3 to 4 servings by October 1 and from 4 to 5 servings by November 1. I will use a log to track my progress, noting the number of servings I eat per day.

- I'm going to increase my current activity level from no exercise to walking for 30 minutes per day, 5 days a week. I will start by walking for 10 minutes, twice a week, on January 15. I will increase to 15 minutes, 3 days a week, on February 15; to 20 minutes, 4 days a week, on March 15; and to my final goal by April 15. I will use an online journal to track my progress.

at small initial steps, you build your confidence for the next step—and then the next.

Observational Learning: Watching the actions and outcomes of others—vicarious experiences—also influences self-efficacy, though not as strongly as direct experience.[10] You might see someone walking on the school track during a break between classes and realize that you could do that, too. Or you might see someone packing his or her own lunch and say to yourself, "Hey, that doesn't look so hard." Seeing someone else do something successfully can increase your own expectations for success—your self-efficacy. Try to find people similar to yourself to observe. For example, if you are a beginning exerciser, make your model another beginning exerciser taking a short walk rather than an elite athlete running in a marathon.

Persuasion: Under some circumstances, people can be persuaded that they're going to do well, and this persuasion can increase their self-efficacy expectations. Generally though, persuasion is a less powerful influence on self-efficacy than either direct or vicarious experience. Someone's ability to persuade us that we really can do something rests on the degree to which we see their comments as true. When someone we view as sincere and credible believes in us—that we can do something—it can increase our self-efficacy.

Interpreting Internal Cues: In uncertain situations, people actively look for clues about how something will go. For example, a person who has never worked out in a gym in front of people might feel anxious when thinking about it. The images you create and the thoughts you entertain about how you are going to do influence your emotions and motivation. Imagining yourself failing can increase your anxiety and lower your self-efficacy; on the other hand, imagining yourself succeeding can decrease your anxiety and increase your self-efficacy.[11] Strategies for increasing positive self-talk are discussed in more detail later in the chapter; see also the cognitive stress-management strategies in Chapter 10.

Goal Setting: What Are You Trying to Achieve?

Q | How do you come up with a good goal that fits you as an individual? An appropriate goal is essential to successful behavior change. One strategy for developing goals is to apply what's called the SMART principle—your goal should be specific, measurable, achievable, realistic, and time-bound (see the box "Sample SMART Goals").

SPECIFIC GOALS. What *exactly* are you going to do? Cut back on smoking, exercise more, and eat better are all goals—but they aren't specific enough for the basis of a behavior-change program. Reframe your goal with specific numbers; for example:

- Reduce cigarette smoking from 2 packs per day by 2 cigarettes every other day until I reach zero, and then keep it at zero.
- Increase my current activity level from no exercise to walking for 30 minutes per day, 5 days per week.
- Increase my consumption of fruits and vegetables from an average of 3 servings a day to an average of 6 servings a day.

Notice that these goals have both a starting point and an endpoint. If you haven't already done so, monitor your current behavior to obtain a baseline measure. How many minutes of physical activity do you currently engage in? How much sleep do you average a night? How many fast food meals do you buy each week?

MEASURABLE GOALS. Your goal must be measurable in order for you to monitor your progress and see if you are on track. Develop a measure or standard for your progress, such as the number of cigarettes smoked, minutes of exercise completed, steps taken, or servings of vegetables consumed. Tracking is also a great motivational tool—you can see just how much progress you've made. Many people also find that having to record their behavior improves

Research Brief

New Year, New You: Do New Year's Resolutions Work?

The beginning of a new year often inspires people to want to begin anew. In fact, almost half of Americans make resolutions at the beginning of a new year. But do such resolutions work?

A study followed two groups of people for six months; the two groups were similar in demographics, histories, and goals, and all wanted to make changes in their lives. The first group, called *resolvers*, made New Year's resolutions. The second group, called *nonresolvers,* were people who desired to make changes in their lives but not by way of New Year's resolutions.

After six months, almost half (46 percent) of the resolvers had maintained their resolutions. Research indicated these participants used more positive behavior change strategies than the nonresolvers. And only 4 percent of the nonresolvers were successful at the six-month mark.

Longer studies are needed. However, this research supports the importance of specific goals and start dates for implementing specific behavior-change strategies.

Source: Norcross, J., Mrykalo, M., & Blagys, M. (2002). Auld lang syne: Success predictors, change processes, and self-reported outcomes of New Year's resolvers and nonresolvers. *Journal of Clinical Psychology,* 397–405.

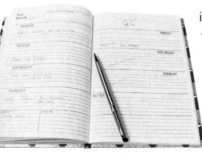

it—for example, you pass up a donut because you don't want to write in your food journal that you ate it—and self-monitoring does increase the likelihood of successfully changing health behavior.[12] Pick a tracking tool that is simple to use and works well for you.

ACHIEVABLE GOALS. Your goal should be meaningful and inspiring, but also something that you can actually do. Consider your limitations—such as your physical condition and available and affordable resources—when setting your goal. For example, improving skiing ability might not be an achievable goal for a man with a knee injury who lives a long distance from ski facilities and who could not easily afford the travel and ski rentals. Likewise, losing weight to wear a size 2 is not an achievable goal for a woman with an average body type.

REALISTIC GOALS. Goals should also be realistic. Your goal should be ambitious and challenging—but not impossible. You want to stretch yourself, but you should also be confident that you can reach your goal. Don't set yourself up to fail: Goals that aim too high or require too much, too quickly are unrealistic and cause frustration. Realistic goals allow steady progress, which is what you want. Build on your success to increase self-efficacy and motivation.

TIME-BOUND GOALS. A time-bound goal has a time frame for action. Your plan for behavior change should have a start date and a goal completion date. You should also break up your goal into several steps, each with its own date. As described above, a series of smaller, achiev-

able goals can give you opportunities for success and help keep you motivated over time. If, for example, your goal is to increase servings of fruits and vegetables from 3 to 6 per day over the course of 12 weeks, set short-term goals, evenly spaced throughout your target time frame.

Once you have a goal that meets the SMART criteria, take a second look at it. Does it accurately reflect what you want to accomplish? Will achieving it give you the outcome you want? When you think about your goal, does it make you feel challenged but motivated to get to work? A good goal should help inspire you to take action (see the box "New Year, New You"). Lab Activity 2-1 will help you create a personal SMART goal.

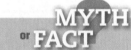

Frequently reevaluating and changing goals is a clear indication that a behavior-change program is failing.

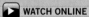 WATCH ONLINE

Decisional Balance: What Are the Pros and Cons of Change?

Q | What if someone doesn't have any motivation to do anything?

No motivation to do anything at all? That's unlikely. If you feel that way about health-behavior change, it may be that you don't perceive the benefits of change as significant or that the obstacles to change seem overwhelming. There is also the problem of behaviors that seem like good choices in the short term but are unhealthy in the long run.

Self-defeating behaviors are those that accomplish one goal (usually a short-term goal) but interfere with the chances of reaching more important goals (usually longer-term goals).[13] Examples abound. Avoiding premature death from smoking is a more important goal than reducing the short-term discomforts of the effort to quit smoking. Yet many people who are struggling to quit give in to the short-term benefit of decreasing the discomfort caused by nicotine cravings, at the expense of the more important benefit of a longer and healthier life. Similarly, wanting to lose weight commonly runs up against the desire to satisfy a craving for a favorite food when we're hungry or tired. And just like giving in to nicotine cravings, sometimes the immediate desire wins out over the more important plans to maintain a healthy weight. Doing what we know is best for us is often difficult.

One strategy that can help focus your energies and boost your motivation is to analyze the pros and cons of the change you want to make. On your list of pros, include all the benefits of change; on your list of cons, include barriers to change that you feel hold you back. Highlight the benefits that are most personally relevant to you—those that you are most excited about. Focusing on these can help shift your view about the benefits of change and increase your motivation. You can use your list of barriers later to brainstorm strategies to address them. See the sample pros-versus-cons analysis in Figure 2-3.

The Behavior-Change Process: The Transtheoretical Model

There are many models and theories about how people change their behaviors. One of the better-known models, one that combines many processes and principles of change from different theories, is the Transtheoretical Model, or TTM. The model was developed in the early 1980s and was originally used to study people who were trying to quit smoking. It has since been applied to a broad range of health and wellness behaviors. TTM is sometimes referred to as the "stages of change" model because one of its main ideas is that people must go through stages as they work to change a habit or adopt a new behavior. In this section, we'll review the stages of change and the processes and techniques that can help you move forward to successfully change your behavior.

Stages of Change

Q | How do I get organized, motivated, and focused to change my behavior?

Find out where you stand—and get started! Once you determine which stage of change you are currently in for your target behavior, you can choose appropriate strategies to move forward (see the box "What's My Stage?"). The stages in the transtheoretical model each have unique attributes and build on one another (Figure 2-4). Because slips and relapses between stages of change are common, the model can be viewed as a spiral rather than a straight line.

PRECONTEMPLATION. The first stage of change in the transtheoretical model is *precontemplation.* People in this stage engage in a problem behavior and aren't yet actively thinking about change. They may be choosing to rationalize their behavior, be afraid of change, be unsure of their ability to change, or be unaware of the full consequences of their behavior and the need for change. Or they may have tried and failed to change and now avoid thinking about their high-risk behavior.

Benefits I want to enjoy:

- *Feel better in body, mind, and spirit*
- *Reduce feelings of stress and tension*
- *Feel less tired*
- *Sleep better*
- *Maintain a healthy weight*
- *Shed abdominal fat*
- *Feel better about my body*
- *Reduce my risk of heart disease, diabetes, and osteoporosis*
- *Become stronger*
- *Try new activities and participate in more activities*
- *Set a good example for my family*

Barriers to change:

- *Difficulty finding time for activity*
- *Not wanting another challenge*
- *Feeling too tired*
- *Having other things I'd rather do during the time*
- *Had a bad experience with exercise in the past*
- *Sometimes find that exercise is difficult and boring*
- *Don't want to spend money on a gym or special equipment*
- *Don't want to work out in front of other people*
- *Don't like getting sweaty*
- *Feel unmotivated*
- *Afraid of failure*

Pros   **Cons**

Increasing physical activity

Figure 2-3 Sample pros-versus-cons analysis for behavior change
Source: Adapted from Centers for Disease Control and Prevention / The Cooper Institute. (n.d.). *Personal Empowerment Plan (PEP) kit: Physical activity precontemplation.* Dallas, TX: The Cooper Institute

Wellness Strategies

What's My Stage?

Which of the following statements best describes you in terms of your target behavior?

☐ I do not intend to take action to change my behavior within the next 6 months.
   Your stage = precontemplation

☐ I do intend to change my behavior within the next 6 months.
   Your stage = contemplation

☐ I intend to take action within the next month and have already taken steps to make changes.

   Your stage = preparation

☐ I have taken action and made changes in my behavior within the past 6 months.
   Your stage = action

☐ I have maintained my targeted behavior change for more than 6 months.
   Your stage = maintenance

Source: Adapted from Prochaska, J. O., Redding, C. A., & Evers, K. E. (2008). The transtheoretical model and stages of change. In K. Glanz, B. K. Rimer, & K. Viswanath, Eds. *Health behavior and health education: Theory, research, and practice* (4th ed.). San Francisco: Jossey-Bass.

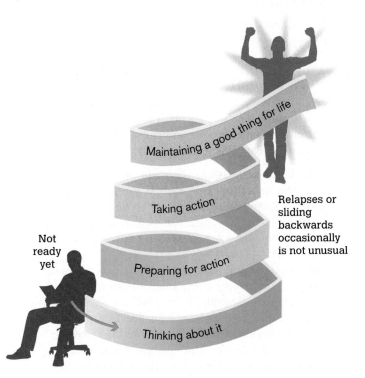

Figure 2-4 Stages of change in the transtheoretical model of behavior change

Source: Adapted from Centers for Disease Control and Prevention / The Cooper Institute. (n.d.). *PEP kit: Physical activity precontemplation.* Dallas, TX: The Cooper Institute.

CONTEMPLATION. *Contemplation* is the "thinking" stage. Here people recognize and acknowledge a problem and have begun to think about change. Many things can lead us to recognizing there's a problem, including new medical information, communication with others, and media messages. In this stage people must weigh the pros and cons of taking action and then decide whether to proceed with trying to change a behavior. It's important to note that some people spend longer in this "thinking" stage than others. In fact, some people never get out of this stage. Others, though, just need more time to process all the information. When people do decide to make a change, they move into the next stage.

PREPARATION. The *preparation* stage is the "planning and getting ready" part of change. In this stage you take a realistic look at where you are in relation to where you want to be and then make a specific plan to reach your destination. Base your plan on accurate information and appropriate tools. The preparation stage is a turning point for many people—when they move from thinking to doing.

ACTION. Once the preparation or planning is complete, it's time to move into the *action* stage. This is when people implement the plan and behavior change actually begins. They start increasing their fruit and vegetable consumption or the number of steps they take daily, or they start cutting back on the number of cigarettes they smoke. If they continue with their goal behavior for about six months, they move into the next stage.

MAINTENANCE. For most behaviors, *maintenance* is the final stage. In this stage, people continue to work to maintain their new behavior and avoid relapse. It is similar to the action stage, but because people have already been successful at maintaining their behavior for a while, they typically don't have to apply as many techniques and strategies to keep going. They are increasingly confident in their ability to maintain their new healthy behavior—no matter what comes along. External rewards are less important than they were earlier, because the new behavior (and all its benefits) is the true reward of behavior change.

Once you successfully change one behavior, your chance of success in making other changes increases significantly. If you make it to the maintenance stage, ask

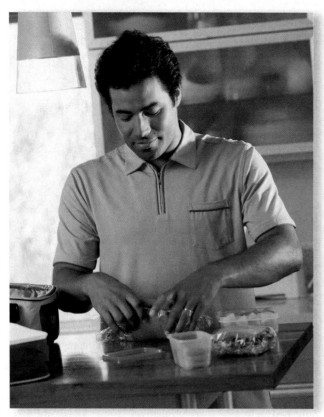

For people in the maintenance stage, their new healthy behavior is well-established and serves as its own reward.

yourself what other positive changes you could make. Keep working to improve wellness!

Q | Is it possible to modify behavior beyond the point of relapse?

Possibly—but only for a small number of people and only for certain types of behaviors. Researchers studying health-behavior change have found that few people ever reach a condition of zero temptation and total self-efficacy.[14] The transtheoretical model includes a final stage called *termination,* but its criteria of zero chance of relapse isn't considered realistic for most people and most health behaviors, including exercise and diet.

It may be best to consider yourself in a lifetime state of maintenance: You are confident in your ability to maintain your behavior, but you are also ready to apply new strategies and work to overcome any lapses that might occur in response to changes in your life. An example is someone

who has been a regular exerciser for eight years but then gets a new job that completely changes his schedule. He can continue to be active, but he'll likely need to cycle back and use strategies from the preparation and action stages to develop his new exercise plan.

This example brings up an important point about the transtheoretical model. Lapses and relapses are common—so don't get discouraged if you experience one. In most cases, people who lapse don't fall all the way back to the initial stage of precontemplation, and they can move more quickly back up through the other stages. Moving through the stages gives you a taste of a success—thereby raising your self-efficacy, motivation, and chances of success when you try again!

Processes and Techniques of Change

Q | According to the quiz, I'm in the contemplation stage. Now what?

Your stage represents how far you've progressed in making a change. Now it's time to take a look at the processes and techniques that can help you move forward to the next stage. The transtheoretical model includes ten general change processes or strategies, each associated with a number of specific techniques.[15]

- **Consciousness raising:** Increase your knowledge about the unhealthy habit and its causes and consequences, including learning more about your status in regard to the behavior and how its consequences relate to you personally. Ask yourself what things you do that are unhealthy—and why you do them.
- **Emotional arousal (dramatic relief):** Experience the worry, fear, and other strong negative emotions that go along with an unhealthy behavioral risk (see the box "'Super Size' Your Behavior-Change Effort"). Techniques for dramatic relief include observing someone's personal testimony or reading a vivid case history of someone who has experienced a problem due to the target behavior—or someone who has made the change you want to make.
- **Self-reevaluation:** Look at yourself with and without the unhealthy habit and evaluate the differences cognitively (thinking) and affectively (feeling). Imagine the consequences that are most meaningful to you. What will your life be like as a more active person, for example? What will it be like if you continue as a couch potato? Also think about whether your current behavior is in line with your

DOLLAR STRETCHER
Financial Wellness Tip

For a behavior change that will save you money, such as quitting smoking or cutting back on eating out, consider setting aside all the money you save and buying yourself something special once you reach the maintenance stage. Have a friend hold the money or keep it in a special bank account.

Research Brief

"Super Size" Your Behavior-Change Effort

Would you watch a movie to help you get information and motivation for behavior change? Researchers tested a group of young adults for their knowledge of fast food and certain psychosocial measures, including their stage of change, self-efficacy, and locus of control for healthy weight. They then showed part of the group the film *Super Size Me,* which provides information about fast food and recounts the filmmaker's experience in eating only fast food for all meals for thirty days. The control group watched an unrelated film.

The two groups had similar scores to start. But follow-up testing showed that the group who watched *Super Size Me* scored higher on knowledge of fast food and on nearly all the psychosocial measures, including stage of change. The experience of watching the film worked as a technique for two stage-of-change processes—consciousness raising and emotional arousal.

Even if fast food isn't related to your target behavior, you can use ideas from this study to identify techniques for change. Watch a relevant movie or TV special. Read a biography. Find interviews on YouTube. Be creative in your efforts to increase your knowledge about your behavior and to engage your emotions.

Source: Cottone, E., & Byrd-Bredbenner, D. (2007). Knowledge and psychosocial effects of the film *Super Size Me* on young adults. *Journal of the American Dietetic Association, 107*(7), 1197–1203.

---

values. Highlight the benefits of change for yourself—emphasize the reasons it will be a step worth taking.

- **Environmental reevaluation:** Look at yourself with and without the unhealthy habit and imagine the effects on your environment, both physical and social. For example, consider how smoking hurts air quality and the health of people you care about—and then consider the effects of quitting. What kind of role model do you want to be for your family, friends, and community?

- **Commitment (self-liberation):** Believe in your ability to change a behavior and make a firm commitment to that change. Refer to the final section of the chapter for more on developing a plan for change that you are confident in.

- **Helping relationships:** Seek out and use social support for your behavior change. Think about how the people you spend time with can support your efforts. The box "Dealing with an Unsupportive Significant Other" offers advice to encourage support from the people closest to you.

- **Countering:** Find or learn healthy behaviors that can substitute for the unhealthy behavior. For example, use a relaxation technique instead of a cigarette to combat stress. Countering also includes substituting more positive thinking patterns. Instead of "I'm too tired to exercise," try "I'm tired, but I'll feel better after my workout."

- **Reinforcement management (rewards):** Enforce the consequences for behavior by increasing the rewards for the desired behavior and decreasing the rewards of the unhealthy behavior. You can set up a formal system of rewards for reaching program milestones as well as punishments for unhealthy behaviors. As a rule,

rewards work better than punishment, and they work best when associated with positive changes—choosing to adopt a healthy behavior as opposed to discontinuing an unhealthy one. Also use positive self-talk for reinforcement; congratulate yourself for every program success, and think about what you enjoy about your new, healthier behavior.

- **Environment control:** Remove cues and triggers that prompt the unhealthy behavior and add new cues and triggers to encourage the healthy behavior. For example, if you are trying to cut back on big, unhealthy snacks after work, remove those foods from your home to avoid the temptation. Keeping small, healthy snacks at work to reduce hunger will also help. By restructuring your environment, you can support your new healthy behavior and reduce the risk of relapse.

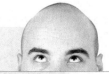

Mind Stretcher
Critical Thinking Exercise

Think about the last time you did something you knew to be unhealthy primarily because those around you were doing it. How could you have restructured the situation or changed the environmental cues so that you could have avoided the behavior? Identify several possible actions that will help you avoid the unhealthy behavior the next time you're in a similar situation.

Wellness Strategies

Dealing with an Unsupportive Significant Other

Everyone wants a supportive significant other. Behavior change is difficult enough without having to face negativity or lack of support at home. If you find yourself lacking support, try these simple steps.

1. Share your plans. People can't help you if they don't know what you're trying to do. (If it's appropriate, invite them to join you. You may be just the motivation they need.)
2. If your significant other still isn't helpful, it may be because he or she simply doesn't know how to help. Say specifically what you would find helpful—whether it is something you need him or her to do or to stop doing.
3. If neither of these suggestions work, remember that the responsibility for your behavior ultimately lies with you. If your significant other can't or won't help, you have to decide how to adjust your plans so that you're still moving toward your goal.

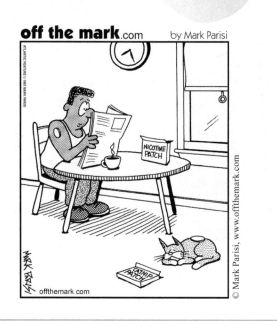

- **Social liberation:** Seek different or additional social alternatives to the unhealthy behavior. Recognize when social norms and public policies provide support for healthy behavior change—such as smoke-free buildings, bike lanes, and workplace health-promotion programs.

Certain processes lend themselves to particular points in the stages of change and can make your efforts at change more effective (Table 2-1). Throughout the stages, work on your pros-versus-cons analysis (see the section on decisional balance earlier in the chapter). As you apply the processes and work your way forward through the cycle of change, you'll notice that the pros on your list start to outweigh the cons. Consider keeping a journal with your pros-versus-cons analysis and descriptions of the techniques for change that you try; take note of what works best for you.

TABLE 2-1 PROCESSES AND TECHNIQUES OF CHANGE

PROCESS OF CHANGE	EXAMPLES OF TECHNIQUES OF CHANGE
	PRECONTEMPLATION
CONSCIOUSNESS RAISING Increasing knowledge about the behavior and its causes and consequences	■ Do research about the behavior in reputable sources; look especially for information on the immediate benefits of change. ■ Examine your attitudes and self-talk about the behavior; ask yourself if you minimize the consequences of your behavior, rationalize reasons for not changing, or avoid thinking about it at all. ■ Ask other people about how they perceive your behavior and its consequences; also ask if they notice defense mechanisms that block change.

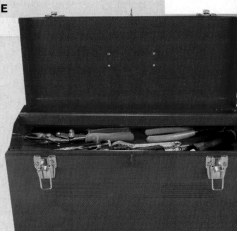

EMOTIONAL AROUSAL Experiencing negative emotions associated with an unhealthy behavior	■ Watch a film or read a story related to the behavior; observe personal testimony or read a case history. ■ Create some personally relevant propaganda; for example, blow smoke from a cigarette into a white cloth, have someone film you while sitting on the couch eating, pile up all the junk food you eat in a week or month (but take care not to overwhelm yourself with negative messages).
ENVIRONMENTAL REEVALUATION Imagining the effects of behavior on the physical and social environment	■ Link the benefits of change to your values and priorities in terms of how your behavior affects other people and your environment. ■ Ask yourself what kind of role model you are and what kind you want to be.
CONTEMPLATION	
SELF-REEVALUATION Imagining the effects of current and goal behavior on your life cognitively and affectively	■ Link the benefits of change to your values and priorities, what you want for yourself. ■ Create a new self-image by imagining your life in detail after you've made the change. ■ Keep a journal of your current behavior. ■ To break the reflexive nature of your behavior, think before you act — ask yourself if you really want to smoke a cigarette, eat a cookie, or sit instead of working out. ■ Work on your pros-and-cons list, incorporating what you've learned about yourself and your behavior.
PREPARATION	
COMMITMENT Making a firm commitment to change	■ Obtain information and tools you need. ■ Develop a detailed plan for change that includes small intermediate steps toward your final goal. ■ Create and sign a contract. ■ Tell friends and family about the change you're making.
ACTION AND MAINTENANCE	
HELPING RELATIONSHIPS Seeking out and using social support	■ Find a buddy to work with on the same behavior change. ■ Arrange for supportive meetings, calls, or e-mails from a friend; ask people for the type of support you want. ■ Join a formal support group or meet with a counselor; if face-to-face support isn't available, consider an online support group.
COUNTERING Identifying healthy behaviors that can substitute for unhealthy behaviors	■ Divert your attention when temptation arises; exercise and relaxation are good countering strategies for many behaviors. ■ Brainstorm ideas for overcoming obstacles to change. ■ Refocus your energy on positive behavior change. ■ Examine your thinking patterns for self-defeating and negative thoughts; substitute rational and positive self-talk.
REINFORCEMENT MANAGEMENT (REWARDS) Enforcing consequences for behavior to increase the reward for the desired behavior	■ Develop a formal system of rewards for reaching milestones; build them into your program plan. ■ Track your behavior. ■ Engage in positive self-talk for sticking with the program.

(continued)

ACTION AND MAINTENANCE *(continued)*	
ENVIRONMENT CONTROL Changing cues and triggers so they prompt the healthy behavior and not the unhealthy behavior	▪ Avoid temptations (objects, places, people) and add cues and reminders to trigger your healthy behavior. ▪ Check your residence and work space for triggers and make appropriate changes (for example, remove junk food and place healthy snacks in plain sight, put exercise shoes by the door). ▪ Examine your daily routine for triggers and make adjustments (for example, go for a walk after dinner instead of smoking a cigarette or having a big dessert).
NOT TIED TO ANY PARTICULAR STAGE	
SOCIAL LIBERATION Seeking social alternatives to the unhealthy behavior	▪ Look for social norms or public policies that can support you (for example, bike lanes, smoke-free zones). ▪ Look for enabling conditions in your environment (such as free access to the campus gym or a stress-management workshop, availability of fruits and vegetables at local stores, self-help groups sponsored by your school or online).

Sources: Adapted from Prochaska, J. O., Redding, C. A., & Evers, K. E. (2008). The transtheoretical model and stages of change. In K. Glanz, B. K. Rimer, & K. Viswanath (Eds.), *Health behavior and health education: Theory, research, and practice* (4th ed.). San Francisco, CA: Jossey-Bass. Prochaska, J., Norcross, J., & Diclemente, C. (1994). *Changing for good.* New York, NY: Morrow.

Q | What are ways to really change a "toxic" environment for wellness?

🔲 **READ ONLINE**

Overcoming Common Barriers to Change

Q | What is the greatest obstacle to overcome in dealing with behavioral change?

The biggest obstacle to change is different for each person and her or his particular target behavior. Is lack of time your problem? Or stress and a negative outlook? Although each of us is unique, we're also alike in many ways. This section describes some of the most common barriers to health-behavior change and offers some strategies for overcoming them. To every barrier there is a solution.

Remember, changing health habits isn't easy—especially because we want our change to last a lifetime, not just a few weeks or months. Many people go through all the work of quitting smoking, losing weight, or getting in shape, only to revert back to where they started. It's an all-too-common and frustrating scenario. You can greatly improve your odds for success both in the short and long terms by having a good plan. Simply starting out with a SMART goal improves your odds, as many failures are due to unrealistic or poorly defined goals. Developing a plan that anticipates common barriers to success likewise improves your odds. Identify barriers ahead of time and plan how you will address them—put yourself in control!

I Don't Have Enough Time

Complaints about lack of time are most relevant for goals that require time—for example, cooking more meals at home or getting more exercise. Everyone has the same

Fast Facts

The Lesson of the Ever-Filling Soup Bowl

For successful behavior change, you need to manage environmental cues and think carefully about your choices. Consider this example: Researchers compared two groups of people who were served soup—one group ate from a normal bowl and one group ate from a bowl that (unknown to the participants) was continually refilled. People who ate from auto-refilling bowls consumed substantially more soup, but they didn't believe they'd eaten more and didn't perceive themselves as more sated than those who ate from the normal bowls. They were eating with their eyes and not their stomachs. Your behavior is influenced by many factors—and you need to recognize them and develop a plan for managing them in order to change your health habits.

Source: Wansink, B., Painter, J. E., & North, J. (2005). Bottomless bowls: Why visual cues of portion size may influence intake. *Obesity Research, 13*(1), 93–100.

24 hours in a day, but some people have more commitments and obligations than others. In today's complex and fast-paced world, time management skills are critical. The more commitments you have, the more essential effective time management becomes. By managing your time well, you'll have more time to relax and have fun.

The purpose of time management is not to fit more into your schedule. It's about planning and prioritizing so that you spend your time wisely. Give priority to activities that are important to your core values and long-term well-being. Scheduling and making time for important activities and goals allows you to better meet your overall needs and achieve a healthy balance in your life.

Start by tracking your current activities and then take a close look at where your time goes. Identify activities and demands you can cut back on to make time for activities that should have a higher priority. Use a calendar—paper or electronic—that has room for writing in plans and reminders. Writing things down and making a schedule are basics of good time management. Just writing something down increases the likelihood you will do it.

Talk to people who engage in the healthy behavior you are trying to incorporate into your lifestyle—ask them how they make time. Also look for ways to combine activities: For example, can you combine physical activity with your commute to school or with time you spend with friends or family? See Chapter 10 for more information on time management.

I Can't Get Motivated

If you're not sure that you really want to make a change, or that the health goal is really worth all the effort, your motivation will suffer. To address this, review the discussion of motivation presented earlier in the chapter. Write out a pros-versus-cons analysis, focusing on your reasons for wanting to make this change. Behavior change is a lot of work and you need to be clear why you're doing it. If the cons still outweigh the pros of change, work through some of the processes and techniques associated with contemplation and planning in the stages-of-change model. If you decide that you really want to change this health habit *now,* then you can make use of all the suggestions in this chapter for planning and for overcoming barriers to keep motivated and moving forward.

Remember that goals need to be personal and realistic. If they're not, your motivation will suffer. Consider the example of a young woman whose doctor told her that she should lose at least fifty pounds. She'd like to do that, but it seemed like such an unreachable target that she felt discouraged before she even started. After all, she'd tried before and failed. She lacked motivation to try to lose that much weight. After reading about goal setting and behavior change strategies, she changed her goal. Instead of focusing on weight loss, which is an outcome and not a behavior, she planned to change several specific behaviors, and she felt more confident about succeeding.

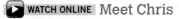

Behavior Change Challenge
Video Case Study

▶ **WATCH ONLINE** Meet Chris

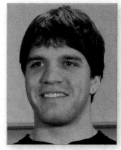

Chris is a 20-year-old student who attends classes four days a week and works long hours during the rest of the week. He recently injured his shoulder and feels that he's now completely out of shape—which he hates. He wants to start a new type of exercise program and improve his eating habits, but he has many potential barriers to change—especially his work schedule and environment. Watch the video to learn more about Chris and his plans for change. As you watch, think about the following:

- What barriers and challenges does Chris encounter, and what strategies does he employ to try to overcome them?
- What can you learn from Chris's experiences, especially in terms of how to maintain motivation and commitment and to overcome challenges?

She decided to keep only healthier foods and snacks in her home, to eat a healthy snack before she shopped for groceries and before she left her work so that she wouldn't be too hungry to be disciplined when she got home. She scheduled times and ways to do more walking, including walking on the campus track before her first class. She also signed up for a free cooking class with a friend to learn how to make food she loves that has fewer calories. She didn't make dramatic changes. Rather, by starting out with small, doable steps that she was confident she could accomplish (high self-efficacy), she found that her motivation was much better. She used SMART goals and built on success.

I'll Get Around to Changing—Later

Is procrastination your problem? Have you decided you'll start to exercise once your life is less busy? That you'll quit smoking when you're 30 (or 50)? That you don't need to improve your diet until your older—and only when you eventually develop health problems?

Procrastinating, rationalizing, and minimizing the effects of your behavior are hallmarks of the precontemplation stage of behavior change. Refer back to Table 2-1 for suggestions and techniques that can help you make progress in behavior change. Don't fool yourself into thinking that your life will get less busy or that your current unhealthy behaviors won't have an effect. Talking yourself into maintaining

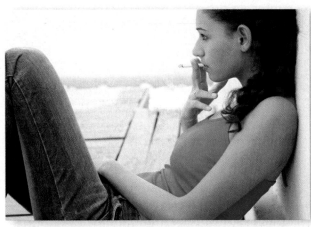

Don't wait to change your behaviors for the better! Although change at any age is beneficial, not all the effects of negative health behaviors are reversible. Many young smokers believe that they'll quit "later" and won't suffer any ill effects from smoking. But quitting is very difficult, and some risks from smoking may be permanent.

unhealthy behaviors doesn't help you. There's no better time to improve your health habits than right now!

I Don't Know How

If you're reading this text and attending college, you're in the perfect position to learn not only what to do but how to do it and how to find support for doing it. Your text provides up-to-date information on a wide variety of wellness goals and behaviors; refer to Chapter 1 for suggestions for quality health information online. Once you've clarified what you want to change, you then can use the information and the step-wise process described in this chapter to create your behavior change plan. Your instructor and student health service may have additional advice and help to offer. If you have specific health concerns, speak with your health care provider.

I Don't Have Enough Money

Joining a health club can be expensive, and a healthy meal in a restaurant can cost significantly more than a burger and fries from the dollar menu at one of the fast food chains. However, getting in shape doesn't require belonging to a health club, and packing a lunch can provide you with a healthy, low-cost meal.

The fact is that healthy lifestyles are generally less expensive, not more expensive than unhealthy

ones. Smoking is a perfect example. Not smoking is much healthier—and dramatically cheaper. In the same vein, walking and biking are free and can even save money on gas and transit fare. Likewise, cooking healthy meals at home is generally far less expensive than eating out or buying prepackaged meals. If your money is tight, look for ways to improve your health habits that don't stretch your budget—or that even save you money. Check the "Dollar Stretcher" tips throughout the text and brainstorm even more money-saving ideas.

I Lack Willpower

Some situations tempt you more than others—a basic fact that you can use to your advantage. For example, it's easier to resist buying unhealthy foods if you don't shop when you're hungry, and it's easier to not eat the wrong foods if they're not right in front of you. The key is to identify and control the situations and stimuli that trigger behaviors you want to decrease or eliminate. If an alcoholic drink triggers the desire for a cigarette at the same time it reduces decision-making capacity, then avoid drinking alcohol when cigarettes are available.

Having healthy—or healthier—alternatives available also helps us resist temptation. If you carry healthy snacks with you, you're less likely to make a bad choice if you get hungry at school, work, or home. This is an example of the strategy of relapse prevention, in which you plan ahead for challenging situations. For example, if you know you will have trouble keeping up with your exercise program when you travel, develop an alternative plan in advance. The same goes for finals week, Thanksgiving with the family, severe weather, campus or office parties, and any other challenging circumstance or situation.

You can also use some temptations—for example, to watch TV instead of exercising—as rewards. It just takes a bit of planning and effort—finish your workout without procrastinating, then watch a favorite show without guilt. Remember though, the behavior you want to increase must be done *before* you get the reward.

DOLLAR STRETCHER
Financial Wellness Tip

Support for behavior change can be free! Use customizable e-cards to send a supportive message to yourself or a friend, to let others know you're trying to make a change, or to let someone know you care and would support them if they tried to make a change:
http://www.smokefree.gov/ecards/index .aspx
http://www2c.cdc.gov/ecards

It's Too Hard— and No Fun

A number of factors act together to influence how difficult a behavior change seems—factors you can alter in your favor. First, remember to personalize your goal. Goals that reflect your values and choices are more motivating and yield greater persistence.[16] Once you've selected a change that is personally important, develop a realistic plan and build in concrete rewards

Research Brief

Self-Control Can Be Contagious

Study after study has confirmed the effects of social networks and peer groups on poor health behaviors—meaning that people copy the behavior of those around them, whether that be smoking, drinking, or overeating. But what about the effects of others on healthy behaviors and self-control?

Researchers recently completed a series of studies with college students that looked at whether thinking about or watching someone with good self-control might actually make someone more likely to exert self-control. Here are brief descriptions of three of those studies:

■ Students were randomly assigned to two groups and observed people they were told were taste testing; the taste-test actors were presented with a plate of cookies and a plate of carrot sticks. One group watched people who ate carrots and not cookies; the other observed people who ate cookies and not carrots. The group that watched the carrot eaters scored higher on a later test of self-control.

■ Participants were asked to make a list of friends that included a person with very good self-control and a person with very bad self-control. The students were then given a computer-based test that measures self-control. Prior to the presentation of each test item on the screen, the participants were subliminally primed with the name of the person they identified as either very good or very bad at self-control (the name flashed on the screen very briefly). The participants who were primed with the name of their friend with good self-control scored better.

■ Students were divided into three groups and asked to write about a friend with good self-control, a friend with bad self-control, or a friend who is moderately extroverted. On a follow-up test of self-control, those who wrote about a friend with good self-control did best, those who wrote about a friend with bad self-control did worst, and those who wrote about an extroverted friend scored in the middle.

These study results suggest that self-control is, indeed, contagious. If you want to make positive health behavior changes, surround yourself with people with good self-control. Interestingly, anyone you observe—not just the friends you hang out with by choice—can have an impact (remember the study with the carrot eaters). And it doesn't matter what the context or behavior: Thinking about or watching someone exhibit self-control related to one behavior can affect your actions related to a different behavior. You should also consider what these study results say about the effects your actions have on others: People you care about may be influenced by any lack of self-control that you display. Your own examples of good and bad self-control may be contagious!

Source: van Dellen, M. R., & Hoyle, R. H. (2010). Regulatory accessibility and social influences on state self-control. *Personality and Social Psychology Bulletin, 36*(2), 251–263.

---

for reaching program milestones. As a rule, small, positive steps are easier to accomplish and maintain than are big, quick changes. The idea that you can *never* eat your favorite foods or skip a workout is unrealistic. What matters is your behavior over the long term—if you generally eat healthy and exercise daily, that's fine. Of course, if your goal is to never restart drinking or smoking, then it's more about planning for situations that might trigger those impulses.

Activities you enjoy are easy to initiate and maintain. Therein lies yet another answer to behavior changes. Make your new health habits enjoyable. Find ways of exercising that you enjoy—perhaps getting involved in team sports will help, or try walking with friends who you wish you could spend more time with. If you hate jogging, don't jog for exercise; instead, find an activity you do enjoy. For goals related to weight control, learn what healthy foods

taste fantastic. It's so much easier to get yourself to do the right thing when it's something you like.

I'm Too Tired

Are you a morning person or night owl? Everyone has energy rhythms, and variations in your mood and energy level will affect your motivation. Do things that require the most energy when you are at your highest energy level. If you aren't sure when that typically is, take a week to keep a log of your energy levels to get an idea of your personal pattern. Also, pay attention to what factors influence your energy level. If you feel tired by the time you're through with school or work, do something fun or social to get revitalized. Many times the fatigue people feel at the end of a day is due to tension. Become one of the countless people who've discovered how exercising at the end of a long day can release tension and boost energy levels. Big meals also have a tendency to make people sleepy. Instead, try some light exercise and a healthy snack to increase energy. Remember that your energy level will likely improve as you get into better physical condition. It gets easier!

I Can't Say "No"

We are responsible for our own choices and values. If the inability to say no or "not now" keeps you from sticking with your goals, work on developing a more assertive communication style. You can improve your communication skills and assertiveness. Most colleges offer classes and other student services that help students develop effective communication skills. See Chapter 10 for more on assertive communication.

I Have a Negative Outlook

Imagine two people with brisk walks as part of their fitness plan. One says to himself, "I don't want to do this . . . I'm so tired . . . I need to just relax." The other person thinks, "OK. Let me get this done and I'll feel better. Five minutes into this walk, I won't feel tired anymore. Once I'm done, I can relax." You don't need to know anything about psychology to know which one would be more likely to do the exercising. If you approach work (and behavior change is work) thinking about how much you dislike it and how much you do not want to do it, you set up inner resistance to the task. It becomes harder and more stressful, and your focus is less productive. Approaching your goals with a positive attitude makes it easier. Starting your actions with thoughts such as "I can do this" and "I'm doing this for me" leads to less inner resistance and improved effort.

If you catch yourself talking yourself out of doing something you should do, try reframing your self-talk. Consciously change what you're saying to yourself to support staying on track with your goals. You might find it helpful to write out negative thoughts so that you can examine them for their flaws. Replace inaccurate, negative self-talk with realistic, positive self-talk that will help you move toward your goal. Situations and patterns of thinking repeat; Table 2-2 gives examples of a few common patterns. If you identify what you can say that would be more positive, you'll likely get plenty of opportunities to practice your more positive inner dialogue in similar situations

TABLE 2-2 EXAMPLES OF NEGATIVE AND POSITIVE PATTERNS OF SELF-TALK

PATTERN OF DISTORTED THINKING	EXAMPLE OF DISTORTED, NEGATIVE SELF-TALK	EXAMPLE OF MORE REALISTIC, POSITIVE SELF-TALK
ALL-OR-NOTHING THINKING	Since I skipped two workouts this week, my exercise program and I are both complete failures. I give up.	I'm disappointed with myself that I skipped two workouts this week. Part of the problem was that I didn't make time for them in my schedule. I've scheduled them in my calendar next week so I can do better.
BLAMING OTHERS	I wouldn't have eaten so much pizza if I hadn't been with those friends. It's all their fault.	I'm responsible for my own food choices. Next time, I'll suggest a different restaurant, or I'll eat just one piece. I'm a strong person and I can be in control.
OVERGENERALIZING	My roommate was so rude to me this morning. He really hates me.	My roommate was really upset this morning. He's usually in a much better mood. I'm going to talk to him about what's upsetting him.
JUMPING TO CONCLUSIONS	Our class TA asked to meet with me tomorrow. I must have done something awful on that last assignment, or maybe I'm failing the class.	Our class TA asked to meet with me tomorrow. It's the first time that's happened, but I'll just wait and see what's up.
DWELLING ON NEGATIVES	I can't believe I ate that piece of chocolate this afternoon. That's one of my old habits I'm supposed to be breaking. I'm such an idiot.	Too bad I ate that chocolate today—that's one of my old habits. But I've done great on my eating plan all week, so I'm not going to stress about it. For next time I'll carry a better snack with me to have instead.

Wellness Strategies

Behavior-Change Support at Your Fingertips

We all know a wealth of information is available on the Internet—good and bad. Research findings have been mixed about the benefits of online support for behavior change, but Web-based tools seem to be improving. In general, Web-based tools have been found less effective than programs involving human interaction—but they are better than no intervention at all. If you don't have an effective face-to-face support system, or if you are a private person, a Web-based program could be a good place for you to get started on behavior change. First, though, ask yourself if a Web-based program is a good fit for you: Will you be just as committed if your support is long distance? Will you be more or less likely to drop out?

A few things to look for in online behavior-change program:

- *A personalized or tailored approach,* based on your current behavior and situation (for example, based on your stage of change and your current fruit and vegetable consumption); look for some type of initial self-assessment.

- *Frequent feedback or engagement*—via e-mails, text messages, e-newsletters, and so on; look for an initial motivational interview or consultation.
- *An approach with a sound theoretical base;* look for a program based on behavior change principles like those discussed in this chapter (such as stages of change, health beliefs, self-efficacy, and motivation).
- *Health information from reputable sources;* look for a program with recommendations from a recognized organization or government program (for example, the American College of Sports Medicine or the American Dietetic Association).

Sources: Alexander, G. L., and others. (2010). A randomized clinical trial evaluating online interventions to improve fruit and vegetable consumption. *American Journal of Public Health, 100*(2), 319–326. Norman, G., Zabinski, M., Adams, M., Rosenberg, D., Yaroch, A., & Atienza, A. (2007). A review of e-health interventions for physical activity and dietary behavior. *American Journal of Preventive Medicine,* 336–345. Spittaels, H., De Bourdeaudhuij, I., & Vandelanotte, C. (2007). Evaluation of a website-delivered computer-tailored intervention for increasing physical activity in the general population. *Preventive Medicine,* 209–217.

in the future. Changing mental habits isn't easy, but it has been shown to be both doable and effective in improving emotions and behavior.

I Don't Feel Supported

College campuses generally have a range of programs that support personal wellness available to interested students—including a variety of health services, fitness programs, activity clubs, and intramural events. Unfortunately, not enough students make use of them. Many of them are funded in part—if not fully—by student fees, so take advantage!

In addition to college programs and services, social support is an important variable. Goals supported by important people in our lives tend to produce more satisfaction and more sustained effort.[17] In contrast, pursuing goals that are not socially supported or that result in relationship conflict decreases goal satisfaction and makes goals harder to achieve. This does not mean that unsupported goals should never be pursued, but simply that attaining goals is harder when it is done without the support and encouragement of significant others.

Let friends and family know what you're trying to accomplish with your health behavior change, and ask for their support. Doing this will also likely heighten your motivation, because your goals are now more public. If, for example, friends know you've quit smoking, they will be less likely to offer you a cigarette and you'll be less tempted to accept if one is offered.

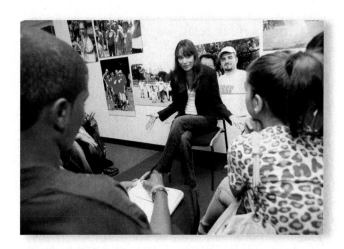

There are also support groups and programs available in many communities, hospitals, and churches. Support programs such as Weight Watchers and Alcoholics Anonymous, for example, have been around for decades and have helped thousands of people with their health goals. If you can't find support locally, look online (see the box "Behavior-Change Support at Your Fingertips").

I Do OK at First and Then Backslide

Remember, there are stages to health habit change, and lapses are a normal part of the process. Maintaining positive

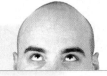

Mind Stretcher
Critical Thinking Exercise

Survey the available services and resources available on campus or in your community. Does the student health services offer groups for students wanting to quit smoking? What physical education classes are offered at your school? Are there walking, jogging, or biking groups you can join? What free exercise facilities are available? What about walking paths? What are all the food options on campus? Colleges are often great places to find support, guidance, and resources for healthy lifestyle changes.

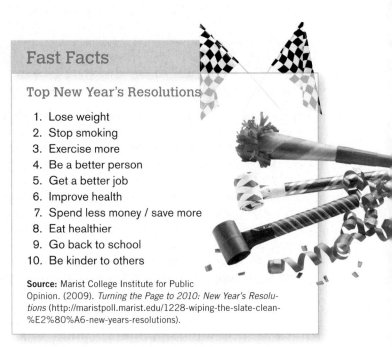

Fast Facts

Top New Year's Resolutions

1. Lose weight
2. Stop smoking
3. Exercise more
4. Be a better person
5. Get a better job
6. Improve health
7. Spend less money / save more
8. Eat healthier
9. Go back to school
10. Be kinder to others

Source: Marist College Institute for Public Opinion. (2009). *Turning the Page to 2010: New Year's Resolutions* (http://maristpoll.marist.edu/1228-wiping-the-slate-clean-%E2%80%A6-new-years-resolutions).

changes is the final stage of the transtheoretical model. Without consciousness and planning for this final stage, it is easy to slide back into old habits. Schedule check-ins with yourself periodically to assess whether your goals and your behavior changes are still on track. Are you exercising as much as you were when you first started your fitness plan? Is your consumption of junk food creeping up? For some people, the maintenance phase is the easy part: They are enjoying their new lifestyle and wouldn't go back to their old ways if you paid them. For others, maintenance takes conscious renewal. Things that are important should not be taken for granted. It's true for romantic relationships, and it is true for long-term health.

Q | How does a person who grew up with bad habits change now? I'm older, and I work and have less time to do things properly. 🔲 **READ ONLINE**

Developing a Personalized Behavior Change Program

Q | What is the best way to start if I am trying to change a behavior? | If you've identified a behavior to change and are already thinking about how to go about it, then you've already started! If you haven't yet picked a behavior to focus on, review the information on wellness lifestyle behaviors in Chapter 1, your results for Lab Activity 1-1, or the ideas in the box "Top New Year's Resolutions." Choose a behavior that will enhance your health and wellness, such as increasing physical activity, reducing fast food consumption, increasing fruit and vegetable intake, quitting smoking, or getting more sleep.

To help keep your behavior-change efforts efficient and on track, this section describes a step-by-step method for developing and implementing a plan that will help focus your attention, time, and energy (see the box "Planning and Implementing a Change"). A good plan is like a good map; it helps you get where you want to go more reliably. Clear, specific plans improve motivation because they give you confidence that you can succeed—your fear of failure goes down, and your expectations for success go up.[18]

The steps outlined here are based on the principles and theories described in the chapter, and they can be used again and again. The general steps are the same whether the goal is developing a good career, improving physical endurance, or maintaining a healthy weight. Indeed, the steps are the same whether we're talking about the goals of individuals or of corporations seeking to solve a company-wide problem. So, although the focus here will be on health-behavior changes, these same steps can be applied to a wide range of goals such as boosting self-esteem, enjoying life more, and improving relationships.

1. Complete a Pros-versus-Cons Analysis

Write up a detailed analysis of the pros and cons of changing your behavior. Your analysis should include the effects of both your current behavior and the new health habit you'd like to adopt. Your pros list should include the benefits you want to enjoy by changing your behavior; this list will help keep you motivated while you work to make a change. Your cons list should incorporate barriers to change—the factors and issues you think most keep you from changing. Think in both the short term and the long

Wellness Strategies

Planning and Implementing a Change

1. Complete a pros-versus-cons analysis.
2. Monitor your current behavior.
3. Set SMART goals and plan rewards.
4. Develop strategies for overcoming obstacles and supporting change.

5. Identify helpers and resources.
6. Put together your program plan.
7. Make a commitment—and act on it.
8. Track your progress and modify your plan as needed.

term when developing your lists. Also consider the effects of changing your behavior (and not changing it) on both yourself and on others. If needed, do additional research on your target behavior to flesh out your analysis. Refer to the sample pros-versus-cons analysis in Figure 2-3.

2. Monitor Your Current Behavior

To help develop a successful program for change, track your current behavior to learn more about it and the factors that influence it. Getting more detailed information about your behavior will also help you to create a more personalized goal and to develop appropriate strategies for change. You want to identify what you're doing that's helpful, as well as anything you're doing that is counterproductive. In addition to your behavior—your food choices, for example, or your activity habits—monitor other relevant factors, such as who you were with when you over-ate or smoked and how hungry you were or how badly you wanted a cigarette.

If you're trying to add a new behavior, such as increased physical activity, you might keep a daily activity record for a week to help you identify times for exercise. For example, how much time do you spend watching TV or surfing the Web? How often do you drive or take an elevator when you could walk or take the stairs? A general activity log is also important for successful time management.

Track your behavior during a usual week (or longer, if appropriate) so that your log or journal truly represents your typical behavior. For example, you likely wouldn't want to

keep track over spring break or during finals week. That said, it's possible as you move through the planning process, some of your strategies may relate to atypical periods—relapse prevention is important. If a relapse is likely, then tracking during these weeks may make sense. In general, however, you'll want to gather information about your typical behavior—particularly if you're just getting started.

People sometimes find this step monotonous and time consuming and are tempted to skip over it. Although it can be a little tedious, it's a very important step in the process. Many people think they already know their habits and behaviors but discover surprising truths when they take the time to track their actions and thoughts. Done well, this step makes the next steps easier and potentially much more effective.

3. Set SMART Goals and Plan Rewards

Next, it's time to set your goal. Use the information you gained by tracking your current behavior as a baseline measure. Refine your goal until it meets all the SMART criteria—specific, measurable, achievable, realistic, and time-bound. Once you've refined your goal, give it another check to ensure that it accurately reflects what you really want to achieve.

When you develop the target time frame for your program, be sure to include several milestones, each with an associated reward. Your rewards should be meaningful to you and relatively inexpensive. Also consider giving yourself small rewards for each day or week you stick with your program, as well as lots of positive self-talk.

4. Develop Strategies for Overcoming Obstacles and Supporting Change

After you've completed your pros-versus-cons analysis and tracked your current behavior, you should have a pretty good idea about the obstacles and challenges to changing your behavior. Next, you want to brainstorm all of

Mind Stretcher
Critical Thinking Exercise

How do you feel about the idea of putting together and carrying out a plan for changing some part of your behavior? Have you ever taken this kind of deliberate action before? Do you feel uneasy about the idea? Or is it exciting and motivating?

the possible things that might help you overcome these obstacles and reach your goal. When you brainstorm, you don't have to decide if the ideas you generate are good or bad. Instead, be open and creative to give yourself lots of options. Your list of strategies might include the following:

- Continue or increase things you are already doing that help your goal pursuit
- Remove cues and triggers that prompt your unhealthy behavior
- Add new cues and triggers that prompt your new, healthy behavior
- Make changes in habits that are linked to your unhealthy behavior

Recheck the list of barriers you identified to ensure you've developed strategies for all the major barriers. Think about potential obstacles in both your physical and social environments. Also think about circumstances most likely to cause lapses, and plan ahead.

Next, look at your list and make some choices. Pare down the possible strategies to a list of actions that reflect what you personally want to do and can do—in essence, what you *will* do. This final list will reflect your knowledge of your personal likes and dislikes, as well as your abilities and resources. For example, someone wanting to be more physically active might make plans to walk more but reject the option of joining a gym (for now) because of costs or logistics; another person with different concerns might decide that joining a gym is the way to go (see the sample in Figure 2-5). The point is that the options you choose should reflect your appraisal of what is most realistic and likely to work for you. We're not all alike, and a plan that is too demanding and unrealistic will fail. Be choosy, and pick the ingredients that are best for you.

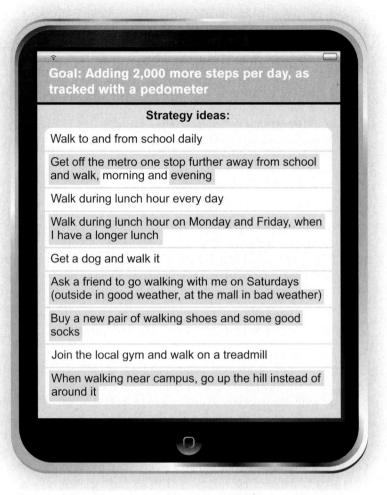

Figure 2-5 **Brainstorming strategies for change.** After identifying as many strategies as possible, select those you think are most realistic and helpful for you.

5. Identify Helpers and Resources

Think about the people in your life: Who can help you with behavior change, and how can they help? Is there someone trying to make the same change who can act as a "buddy" and participate in your program? Is there someone who has already successfully made a change who can serve as a role model and offer advice? Is there a friend or family member who can provide daily or weekly support (phone chats, e-mails)?

Tell people about the change you are trying to make, and ask for their support in specific ways. If someone acts in ways that sabotage your efforts—by pushing you to skip your workout, snack on midnight pizza, or smoke—ask him or her to stop. Remember to use assertive communica-

tion and make clear, constructive requests. If needed, avoid problem people temporarily until you are further along in the cycle of change and better able to resist their influence. As a last resort, consider avoiding the problem people permanently if your health or safety is compromised.

In addition to helpers, also check your resources. Do you have all the information you need? All the equipment? Have you checked your campus and community for resources—a free stop-smoking program, reduced-cost gym time, a stress management workshop, and so on? Gather all the tools you need, and take advantage of the available resources.

6. Put Together Your Program Plan

Using all the information you've gathered, put together a specific program plan. Write out your plan—your goals and rewards, the strategies and techniques you've identified, the helpers and resources that will help you succeed, and so on. See Lab Activity 2-2 for a sample program plan format.

7. Make a Commitment . . . and Act on It

Mentally commit yourself to your behavior change program and goal. Tell people about the change you are trying to make. If you find it helpful, sign a formal contract with yourself. Then get started on change! When the start date of your program arrives, give your plan the time and energy it needs to be successful.

8. Track Your Progress and Modify Your Plan as Needed

As described earlier in the chapter, monitoring your behavior and your progress are key strategies for success. Keep track of your behavior to assess your progress, to keep your motivation high, and to help modify your plans as needed. Use whatever form of log, journal, or graph works for you. Carry a small paper journal, create a spreadsheet, or find an application for your phone or PDA. See the example in Figure 2-6.

Don't be discouraged by small slips and lapses—those are normal. Not every problem or snag can be anticipated, and change may require more time than you initially anticipated. Your overall goal may need to be broken into smaller, more manageable chunks. Your timeline may need to be revised. As long as your goal feels important and attainable, make whatever modifications you need to stay on track. Most plans need to be modified or revitalized along the way. When it comes to personal wellness, the goal is always a permanent lifestyle change, not a temporary change in habits.

Q | How much can I say or do to encourage a family member to quit smoking or lose weight?

Good for you for wanting to help! Keep in mind that helping others change health habits is difficult: You alone can't make someone else change their behavior. A good first strategy is to try to determine what stage of change the friend or family member is in for their unhealthy habit. If he or she is thinking about, planning, or

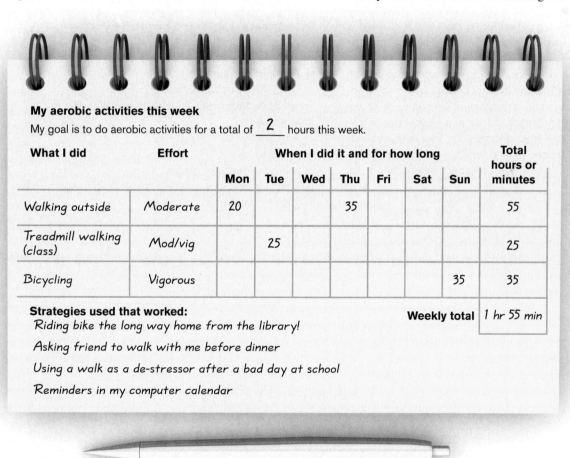

Figure 2-6 Sample behavior change log
Source: Adapted from Department of Health and Human Services. (2008). *2008 physical activity guidelines for Americans: Keeping track of what you do each week.* ODPHP Pub No. U0050. Rockville, MD: Office of Disease Prevention and Health Promotion.

working on making a change, you can offer to help in a concrete way, by providing support or practical help. If he or she is in the precontemplation stage, it's trickier, because you don't want to push a person to act if he or she isn't ready. Some strategies for helping people in the pre-contemplation stage include the following:[19]

- Encourage their inclination to change, but don't push them to act.
- Recommend change frequently, but not too frequently; don't nag, but don't give up—be patient.

- Try discussing specific instances of the problem behavior and its consequences (for example, being unfit meant skipping a fun outing with friends; things said while drunk hurt someone's feelings).
- Acknowledge any positive instances of healthy behavior.

Remember, your own healthy behaviors can be a role model to the people in your life and in your community. Wellness for all!

Summary

Each of us is responsible for our own choices and behaviors. Our behaviors develop over time, based on many contributing factors. When you want to change a behavior, it's important to understand what influences your ability to change—including predisposing, enabling, and reinforcing factors. Motivation directs and sustains your effort for behavior change, and it is influenced by locus of control, self-efficacy expectations, the goals of your program, and how you evaluate the pros and cons of change. For successful change, it's also important to identify your stage in the cycle of change and to apply appropriate processes and techniques of change to overcome key barriers and challenges. Steps in a successful behavior change program include monitoring your behavior, setting SMART goals, and putting together a detailed plan for change that includes strategies, helpers, rewards, and a firm commitment.

More to Explore

American On the Move
http://americaonthemove.org
Centers for Disease Control and Prevention: Healthy Living
http://www.cdc.gov/HealthyLiving
Department of Health and Human Services Physical Activity Guidelines
http://www.health.gov/paguidelines
MyPyramid Tracker
http://www.mypyramidtracker.gov
Small Step: Improving the Health and Well-Being of America
http://www.smallstep.gov
SmokeFree
http://www.smokefree.gov
See also the resources listed in chapters covering the behavior you plan to change.

SUBMIT ONLINE

NAME	DATE	SECTION

Developing a clear goal for your behavior change program is critical for success. You should also identify specific strategies and techniques to support your efforts at change.

Equipment: None

Preparation: None

Part 1: Goals

Instructions: Begin by writing out your general goal for behavior change; if you still need to choose a behavior to focus on, review the results of the assessments in Chapter 1.

Briefly explain why you've chosen this behavior and this goal for your change program. Why is this goal meaningful to you? What benefits do you expect to enjoy when you achieve this goal?

Next, apply the SMART principle to your goal. Below, work on refining your goal, and explain how it meets each of the SMART criterion:

☐ Specific   Explain: _____

☐ Measurable   Explain: _____

☐ Achievable   Explain: _____

☐ Realistic   Explain: _____

☐ Time-bound   Explain: _____

As you refine your goal and develop a time frame for your program, break your final, overall goal into several smaller short-term goals, each with their own target start and completion dates. If your plan includes rewards, choose a reward for each short-term goal and your final goal.

Final goal:

Start date: _____   End date: _____   Reward: _____

Short-term goal 1:

Start date: _____ End date: _____ Reward: _____

Short-term goal 2:

Start date: _____ End date: _____ Reward: _____

Short-term goal 3:

Start date: _____ End date: _____ Reward: _____

Reflecting on Your Goal: On a scale of 0–100, how confident are you that you can achieve your goal as you set it out? [   ]

Explain:

Part 2: Pros versus Cons of Change

Instructions: Based on the goal you've set, complete an analysis of the pros versus cons of making a change. You can use the pros as a source of motivation; the cons will help you identify barriers to change that you'll need to overcome in order to be successful.

PROS: BENEFITS I WANT TO ENJOY	CONS: BARRIERS TO CHANGE

Reflect on Your Analysis: Do you think the pros of change outweigh the cons? If so, what benefits of change are most important to you? If not, what do you think you could do to overcome some of the cons and tip the decisional balance in favor of change?

What is your current stage of change (see p. 41 in the chapter)? [   ]

Part 3: Strategies and Techniques for Change

Instructions: Start by brainstorming—think up as many strategies and techniques as you can that would support your behavior change program. Think about your current actions and environment as well as the suggested techniques for the processes appropriate for your stage of change. What can you do to restructure your (physical and social) environment to help support change? What can you do to overcome key barriers to change? Use your pros versus cons analysis and the following categories to help in your brainstorming activity. Remember, this is brainstorming; just let your ideas flow.

Increase current actions that support the healthy behavior:

Decrease, eliminate, or manage cues and triggers that prompt the unhealthy behavior; include strategies for countering and for preventing lapses in challenging situations:

Add or increase cues and triggers that prompt the new, healthy behavior:

Strategies to overcome key barriers—consider what you learned by tracking your current behavior and by reviewing the list of common barriers in the chapter; check off your key barriers and brainstorm strategies for them:

☐ lack of time   ☐ lack of willpower   ☐ lack of support

☐ lack of motivation   ☐ lack of enjoyment   ☐ problems with maintenance

☐ procrastination   ☐ lack of energy   ☐ other: _____

☐ lack of information   ☐ unable to be assertive   ☐ other: _____

☐ expense   ☐ negative self-talk   ☐ other: _____

Reflecting on Your Strategies Lists: Next, go back and identify (circle) the strategies that you will use—select those that best fit you and your needs and preferences. You'll use these strategies when you complete your program plan in Lab Activity 2-2.

LAB ACTIVITY 2-2 Program Plan for Behavior Change

SUBMIT ONLINE

NAME ______ SECTION ______ DATE ______

Complete this program plan with details on your specific plan for behavior change.

Equipment: None

Preparation: None

Target behavior (the behavior you want to change) ______

Your final goal and your short-term goals (see Lab Activity 2-1)

Final goal: ______

Start date: ______ End date: ______ Reward: ______

Short-term goal 1: ______

Start date: ______ End date: ______ Reward: ______

Short-term goal 2: ______

Start date: ______ End date: ______ Reward: ______

Short-term goal 3: ______

Start date: ______ End date: ______ Reward: ______

Your key strategies and techniques for change (see Lab Activity 2-1)

Your helpers and resources

Who will help with your program and how will they help?

What campus or community resources will support your program?

Make a commitment (sign the statement below to make your plan a formal contract or describe your own plan for making a firm commitment to change)

I _____ commit to achieving the following goal: _____

_____

Signature: _____ Date: _____

OR *describe your plan for making your commitment (telling others, sending e-cards, etc.):*

Plan for monitoring behavior and tracking progress

Describe the journal, log, or other tracking method you plan to use:

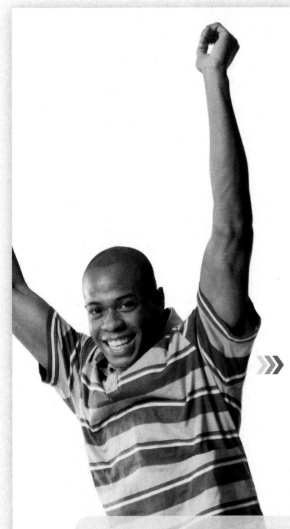

3

Fundamentals of Physical Fitness

>> **COMING UP IN THIS CHAPTER**

Learn the differences among physical activity, physical fitness, and exercise › Identify the benefits of physical activity and fitness › Become familiar with the components of fitness related to health and to skill › Explore methods of assessing fitness › Discover how to apply key training principles › Learn to adapt a fitness program to different environmental conditions

Wellness Connections

How does fitness relate to overall wellness? The relationship to physical wellness is clear—physical activity and physical fitness are critical to a long and healthy life. In terms of emotional wellness, exercise elevates your mood, decreases your stress level, and enhances your sense of well-being. Additionally, increased fitness can lead to greater self-esteem, which in turn can boost interpersonal relationships and social wellness—or perhaps it's camaraderie that gets you motivated to exercise in the first place.

President John F. Kennedy summed up the connection to intellectual wellness when he stated, "Physical fitness is not only one of the most important keys to a healthy body, it is the basis of dynamic and creative intellectual activity." Fitness helps keep your mind sharp; in turn, critical thinking and planning skills help you develop a sound activity plan. Fitness is also linked to the basic tenets of spiritual wellness—your beliefs and values. The connection here is as basic as the value you place on health, on

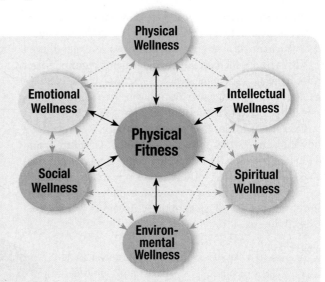

physical activity, and on socializing through activities. Spiritual beliefs may also influence your choice of activities. Finally, consider the environmental dimension: Depending on where you live, your activity options may be many or few because of factors such as weather and available facilities. Environment can also be a wonderful source of motivation—whether you can exercise in a beautiful outdoor setting or in a secure and high-quality indoor fitness facility.

This chapter presents basic information about physical activity and physical fitness. You'll learn more about the benefits of activity, different types and components of fitness, methods of assessing your individual level of fitness, and important training principles. With this foundation, Chapters 4–6 will provide an in-depth look at designing and fine-tuning a fitness program that fits your individual needs and preferences.

Physical Fitness, Physical Activity, and Exercise

Q | Does all activity count as exercise?

Not exactly, no. Physical fitness, physical activity, and exercise are closely related but distinct concepts. **Physical fitness** is a set of attributes that allows a person to carry out daily tasks with vigor and alertness, without undue fatigue, and with ample energy to enjoy leisure-time pursuits and respond to emergencies.[1] People live longer if they are fit, and they can enjoy a higher level of wellness in all dimensions. Some attributes or components of fitness relate to health, and others are tied more to performance in sports or specific activities.

Physical activity is just that—any movement of the body. Physical activity requires work by the body's muscles, which in turn requires energy (calorie expenditure). Physical activity includes all the movements required to get through the day—at home, work, and school. It also includes any activities you engage in during your free time, which is typically referred to as "leisure-time physical activity."

Exercise is a subset of physical activity; it is repetitive body movements that have been planned, structured, and conducted specifically to develop components of physical fitness (Figure 3-1). A difference to remember is that all physical activity involves movement and energy expenditure, but not all physical activity develops or increases physical fitness.

Q | Will I really lose years of my life if I'm unfit?

Yes. Both physical activity and physical fitness are linked to a longer life and a healthier life. People who are active live on average several years longer than their sedentary counterparts, and they have lower rates of many major diseases.[2] Quality of life is also improved, with physical activity linked to better mood, better sleep, and greater self-esteem. Benefits of physical activity are summarized in Table 3-1. Although many people think about activity in terms of reduced risk of chronic disease, the benefits range beyond the physi-

cal; see the box "Exercise Makes You Smarter" for just one such example.

Q | I'm never going to be super-fit—there's just no way. Is there any point in exercising if I can't become really fit?

Yes, absolutely. You may not be able to become as fit as an Olympic athlete, or work out as hard as one, but you can increase physical activity and exercise and improve your health and fitness. The biggest gains in health benefits come when someone who is sedentary becomes moderately active. And some physical activity is better than none. Don't get discouraged by thinking you must do difficult or high-intensity activities. Set realistic goals for improvement and gradually increase the amount of exercise you do.

Q | Don't you think the "couch potato" thing is overblown? It seems like I see more people exercising all the time.

In spite of the many wonderful benefits of physical activity, most American adults don't engage in much activity dur-

physical fitness Ability to carry out daily tasks with vigor and alertness, without undue fatigue, and with ample energy to enjoy leisure-time pursuits and respond to emergencies.

physical activity Bodily movement involving contraction of skeletal muscles and requiring calorie expenditure.

exercise Planned, structured, repetitive body movements conducted specifically to develop components of physical fitness.

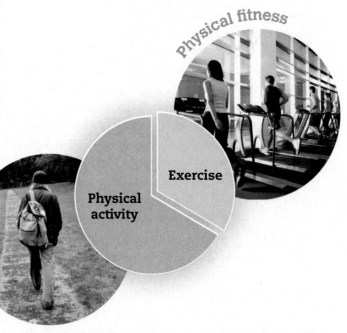

Figure 3-1 Physical activity, exercise, and physical fitness. Exercise is a subset of physical activity specifically designed to develop physical fitness.

Research Brief

Exercise Makes You Smarter

Exercise doesn't just make you feel and look better. New research suggests exercise may also make you smarter by stimulating the production of new brain cells. It was once believed humans were born with a finite number of brain cells that gradually died over the lifespan, but there is now definitive evidence that the human brain can continue to produce new brain cells throughout life.

A recent study focused on the hippocampus, an area of the brain that is critical for memory and learning. Using magnetic resonance imaging (MRI) to create maps of the brain and blood flow, researchers followed a group of adults as they completed a three-month exercise program; participants also took fitness and cognitive tests. The study found that exercise increased markers for the production of new brain cells. In addition, the participants also improved their scores on cognition tests, and the amount of cognitive improvement was tied to the degree of improved fitness. More research is needed, but this study adds to the evidence that physical activity and fitness are important for intellectual wellness.

Source: Pereira, A. C., and others. (2007). An *in vivo* correlate of exercise-induced neurogenesis in the adult dentate gyrus. *Proceedings of the National Academy of Sciences, 104*(13), 5638–5643.

ing their leisure time. And rates of activity have been holding steady or dropping—not what public health officials want to see. Take a look at Figure 3-2 to see how your level of physical activity compares with the nation as a whole and with different population groups.

Types of Fitness

So, how do you add more physical activity, especially exercise to boost physical fitness, to your life? The first step is to learn more about types of fitness and the training

TABLE 3-1 BENEFITS OF PHYSICAL ACTIVITY

- Lower mortality from all causes—that is, active people have lower overall death rates
- Better cardiorespiratory functioning and less risk of heart disease and stroke
  - Lower blood pressure, in some cases enough to reduce or eliminate the need for medication
  - Better blood fat levels—higher levels of high-density lipoprotein ("good cholesterol") and lower levels of triglyceride
  - Lower resting heart rate and blood pressure
  - Stronger heart and lungs, better blood flow
- Less risk of cancer, especially colon cancer and breast cancer
- Less risk of type 2 diabetes
  - Better control of body fat
  - Better blood sugar and insulin levels
  - Less need for insulin by people with type 2 diabetes
- Less risk of osteoporosis and related fractures
  - Better bone density
  - Less risk of falls
- Lower risk of gallbladder disease
- Better body composition
  - Less total body fat, particularly abdominal fat
  - Prevention of weight gain
  - Maintenance of weight after weight loss
- Better mental well-being
  - Better quality of sleep (active people fall asleep more quickly and sleep more deeply)
  - Higher self-esteem and better mood
  - Improvement of mild-to-moderate depression and anxiety
- Better performance in work, leisure, and sport activities
- Better quality of life and increased ability to live independently for older adults

Sources: American College of Sports Medicine. (2009). *ACSM's resources manual for guidelines for exercise testing and prescription* (6th ed.). Baltimore, MD: Lippincott Williams & Wilkins. U.S. Department of Health and Human Services. (2008). *2008 physical activity guidelines for Americans*. ODPHP Pub. No. U0036. Rockville, MD: Office of Disease Prevention and Health Promotion. Haskell, W. L., and others. (2007). Physical activity and public health: Updated recommendations for adults from the American College of Sports Medicine and the American Heart Association. *Circulation, 116,* 1081–1093.

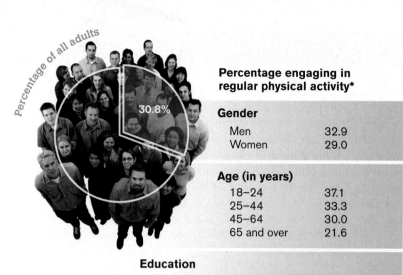

Percentage of all adults

Percentage engaging in regular physical activity*

30.8%

Gender	
Men	32.9
Women	29.0

Age (in years)	
18–24	37.1
25–44	33.3
45–64	30.0
65 and over	21.6

Education	
No high school diploma or GED	46.7
High school diploma or GED	21.8
Some college or more	38.0

Income relative to poverty level	
Below 100%	19.7
100% to less than 200%	23.0
200% or more	34.6

*Regular leisure-time physical activity means three or more sessions per week of vigorous activity lasting at least 20 minutes or five or more sessions per week of light or moderate activity lasting at least 30 minutes.

Figure 3-2 Rates of regular leisure-time physical activity among Americans
Source: National Center for Health Statistics. (2009). *Health, United States, 2008, updated trend tables* (http://www.cdc.gov/nchs/hus/updatedtables.htm).

principles that will help you make the best use of your time and energies.

Fitness components are typically divided into two major categories: health-related fitness and skill-related fitness. **Health-related fitness** components have a direct effect on your health status, disease risk, and day-to-day functioning. **Skill-related fitness** components or attributes influence your performance level in various activi-

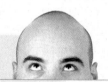

Mind Stretcher
Critical Thinking Exercise

Why are rates of leisure-time physical activity so low, given its many benefits? What do you think are the key reasons for sedentary behavior? If you were a public health official, what would you do to promote physical activity in your community? Think of at least two strategies that might work on your campus or in your community.

ties and are less directly related to health. This section of the chapter provides a brief introduction to the different components of fitness. The health-related components are discussed in much more detail in Chapters 4–7.

Skill-Related Fitness

Q | How is skill related to fitness?

Skill-related fitness, sometimes referred to as motor fitness or performance-related fitness, includes fitness components or attributes that contribute to your ability to function in a more skilled and efficient way. They can result in an increased desire to participate in physical activities. In this indirect way, increased skill-related activity can affect your health.

Skill-related fitness components include agility, balance, coordination, power, reaction time, and speed. Unless you are a skilled athlete wanting to improve a particular skill, you may not even think about these components of fitness. Skill-related fitness is often taken for granted because, through normal development, we typically acquire enough balance, coordination, and so on for daily living. Although not everyone develops to the same level for each component, most people—unless they are ill or have a disability or other limitation—develop adequate levels of skill-related fitness. Typically, the levels of these components are inadequate only at the beginning of life and again in later years. As very young children, we learn these skills through trial and error and continued practice. The natural aging process, often along with decreased use, can take its toll on these skills. Older adults become susceptible to difficulties with balance, reaction time, coordination, and other skill-related abilities.

AGILITY. Agility is the ability to change the direction and position of the body in a quick and precise manner. Agility is important in many sports. Quick, controlled changes in direction are needed for successful performance in individual activities, such as gymnastics and diving, as well as in individual and team sports such as tennis, basketball, and football. Your agility is partly determined by heredity; however, agility can be improved through practice.[3]

BALANCE. Balance is the ability to maintain equilibrium when sitting,

health-related fitness Components or areas of fitness that have a direct effect on overall health and disease risk.

skill-related fitness Components or areas of fitness that contribute to the ability to function in a skilled and efficient way and don't have a direct effect on overall health; also called performance-related fitness.

agility Ability to change the direction and position of the body in a quick and precise manner.

balance Ability to maintain equilibrium when sitting, standing, or moving.

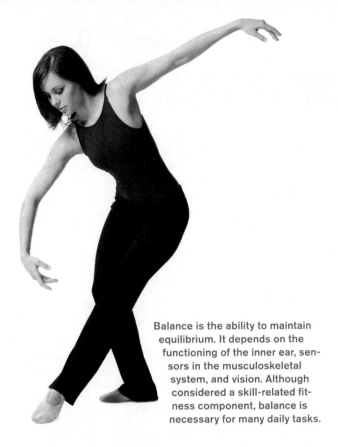

Balance is the ability to maintain equilibrium. It depends on the functioning of the inner ear, sensors in the musculoskeletal system, and vision. Although considered a skill-related fitness component, balance is necessary for many daily tasks.

standing, or moving. Maintenance of equilibrium while in a stationary position such as sitting or standing is known as static balance; maintenance of equilibrium during movement is known as dynamic balance. Each type of balance is important for many specialized activities as well as for routine daily activities.

Balance is controlled by the semicircular canals in the inner ear, musculoskeletal-system sensors known as proprioceptors, and the eyes. The inner ear is very sensitive and has the ability to detect motion and gravity. Proprioceptors in the muscles, tendons, and joints detect a limb's position in space by interpreting muscle contractions and joint angles. Your brain uses signals from each of these sensory organs as well as your ability to see and interpret images to assess any imbalance. The brain sends the data needed for correction back to the appropriate muscles—thus helping you to regain balance. Maintaining equilibrium requires this constant messaging. Balance can be trained by simple movements, such as standing on one leg and reaching forward, or by specialized exercises and equipment such as balance boards.

COORDINATION. Coordination is the ability to synchronize multiple movement patterns into sequenced, efficient, controlled movement. An example is throwing a ball: Multiple movement patterns (arm action, stepping action, hip rotation, and so on) are coordinated to produce a sequenced, efficient movement. Any movement patterns that require hand-eye or foot-eye transactions utilize coordination; the more complex the patterns, the greater the amount of co-

coordination Ability to synchronize multiple movement patterns into sequenced, efficient, controlled movements.

ordination needed. Coordination includes the use of, and is therefore somewhat dependent on, balance, agility, speed, and reaction time.[4]

POWER. Power is the ability to exert a maximum amount of force in a minimum amount of time. It is often described in terms of explosive types of movements, such as the vertical jump. Power requires both strength and speed and therefore typically is greater in those with greater muscle mass. Because strength is one of the contributors, power is sometimes included on the list of health-related fitness components.

REACTION TIME. Reaction time is the amount of time between a stimulus and your response to it. As a rule, young children have very slow reaction times (a longer time between the stimulus and response), but neurological changes during development enable faster processing time. In sports and leisure activities, reaction time shows up in starting a sprint or moving to block a goal in soccer or hockey. In day-to-day activities, you need good reaction time to brake when the car in front of you comes to a sudden stop.

SPEED. Speed is the ability to perform a movement in a short period of time—the shorter the time, the greater the speed. The movement may be of a single body part or your entire body.

power Ability to exert a maximum amount of force in a minimum amount of time.

reaction time Amount of time between a stimulus and your response to that stimulus.

speed Ability to perform movement in a short period of time.

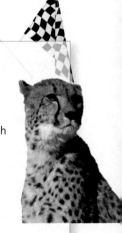

Fast Facts

Faster than a Speeding . . .

The record holders for speed in the animal kingdom:

Flying bird: Peregrine falcon (in a dive)	200 mph
Land mammal: Cheetah	70 mph
Fish: Sailfish	68 mph
Land bird: Ostrich	45 mph
Water mammal: Dall's porpoise	35 mph

Compare these animal records with top human speeds:

Sprint split time (fastest 10 meters)	28 mph
Sprint from standing start (fastest 100 meter run)	23 mph
Mile run	16 mph

Sources: Smithsonian National Zoological Park. (n.d.). *Animal Records* (http://nationalzoo.si.edu/Animals/AnimalRecords). International Association of Athletics Federations. (n.d.). *World Records* (http://www.iaaf.org/statistics/records/inout=O/index.html).

Research Brief

Exercise Keeps You Young

Research suggests that exercise not only helps to delay the onset of age-related diseases but may also actually affect the aging process itself. One recent study examined telomere length at the end of chromosomes in white blood cells of over 2,400 twins. Telomeres of this type typically shorten progressively over time as we age. Even after adjustments for body mass index, smoking, and other potential complicating factors, telomere length in the most active individuals was significantly longer than that in the least active individuals. In fact, the active individuals had telomere lengths equivalent to sedentary individuals ten years younger. Much research needs to be done in this area, but these results suggest that people who are physically active are "biologically younger" than people who are sedentary.

Source: Cherkas, L., Hunkin, J., Kato, B., Richards, J., Gardner, J., Surdulescu, G., Kimura, M., Lu, X., Spector, T., & Aviv, A. (2008). The association between physical activity in leisure time and leukocyte telomere length. *Archives of Internal Medicine,* 154–158.

Like reaction time, speed develops during childhood. Increases in speed level off for most girls between ages 8 and 12, but boys may continue to increase speed throughout adolescence due to their increasing body size and levels of testosterone.

Health-Related Fitness

Q | I'm terrible at sports and have no interest in them. Are there other ways to be just as fit and healthy?

You don't have to be an athlete to be healthy and fit. Instead of focusing on the development of skill-related fitness components you can focus on the health related fitness components—those things that have a direct effect on your overall functional health.[5] These include:

- cardiorespiratory endurance
- muscular strength
- muscular endurance
- flexibility
- body composition

Without a sufficient level of fitness in each of these areas, your health—and your ability to function at capacity in your day-to-day life—may be inhibited. Additionally, you may be at greater risk for some chronic diseases as well as for early onset of diseases. Conversely, adequate levels help to protect against illness and disease and contribute to a better quality of life—more years of healthy life!

The health-related fitness components are defined briefly below. Each is described in greater detail—including contributing factors, benefits, assessment, and appropriate exercises—in Chapters 4–7.

CARDIORESPIRATORY ENDURANCE. Cardiorespiratory endurance is the ability of the circulatory and respiratory systems to sustain physical activity by supplying oxygen to working muscles. The heart, lungs, and entire network of blood vessels work together to provide oxygen to the muscles in order for them to continue working. The lungs take in oxygen, which blood cells pick up and deliver to muscles throughout the body as the blood is pushed through blood vessels via the pumping action of the heart. The same systems carry carbon dioxide, a by-product of the chemical reactions that produce energy for physical activity, in the reverse direction, eliminating it from the body. Cardiorespiratory endurance thus depends on the capacity of the lungs to take in oxygen, the ability of the circulatory system to carry and transport the oxygen, and the force of the heart's pumping action. The terms *cardiorespiratory fitness, cardiovascular endurance, cardiovascular fitness, aerobic endurance,* and *aerobic fitness* are often used interchangeably.

Cardiorespiratory fitness is developed by what are called *aerobic* (with oxygen) activities. This category includes activities like brisk walking, jogging, swimming, and cycling that put stress on the cardiorespiratory system but that can be maintained for a long time. Chapter 4 describes cardiorespiratory fitness training in detail.

cardiorespiratory endurance Ability of the respiratory and circulatory systems to provide oxygen to muscles for sustained physical activity; also called cardiorespiratory fitness.

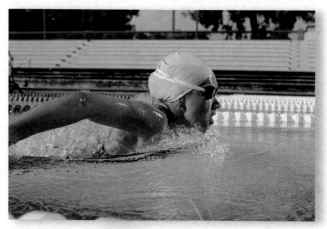

Cardiorespiratory endurance depends on the functioning of the heart, lungs, and blood vessels. It is developed through aerobic activities such as swimming.

MUSCULAR STRENGTH. Muscular strength is the ability of a muscle or group of muscles to generate or apply force. If, when you hear the phrases *muscular strength* or *ability to apply force,* you think only of someone with huge, bulging muscles, you need to reshape your thinking. Muscular strength is something everyone needs. No matter your size or your typical activities, a certain amount of strength is necessary for day-to-day living—thus, the inclusion of this component in the health-related fitness category. For example, it requires a certain amount, maybe even a significant amount, of muscular strength to lift your book bag or backpack safely and without injury.

Activities that increase muscular strength involve the application of force against resistance. Weight training is often the chosen means of developing muscular strength, but calisthenics and other activities that use the body's own weight as resistance can also be effective strengthening exercises.

MUSCULAR ENDURANCE. Muscular endurance is the ability of a muscle or group of muscles to sustain an effort for an extended time; it may take the form of a single continuous exertion or repeated exertions. Muscular endurance is related to strength. For example, lifting your book bag, like many other daily tasks, requires a certain amount of muscular strength. However, simply being able to lift your bag isn't enough. You need to carry it to class, the library, your residence, or wherever you are headed. Lifting the bag or backpack (exerting force) requires strength; carrying it with you (continued exertion) requires muscular endurance. Both are necessary for your daily activities. Together, muscular strength and muscular endurance, as well as some other muscle attributes, are often referred to collectively as *muscle fitness.*

Like strength, endurance improvement requires resistance exercises. However, how you perform these exercises will differ depending on whether you want to emphasize strength or endurance in your training program. Chapter 5 describes muscle-fitness training in detail.

FLEXIBILITY. Flexibility is the ability of a joint to move through its full range of motion. A certain amount of flexibility is needed for day-to-day activities and to help prevent injuries that can be caused by a restricted range of motion. Flexibility of the lower back and hamstrings may be particularly important for some people to help prevent low-back pain and other related problems. For this reason, flexibility is most commonly tested in the lower back. Flexibility is best maintained or improved through stretching exercises. Chapter 6 has more on flexibility training and the lower back.

muscular strength Ability of a muscle or group of muscles to generate or apply force, often by contracting against resistance.

muscular endurance Ability of a muscle or group of muscles to sustain an effort for an extended time.

flexibility Ability of a joint to move through its full range of motion.

body composition Relative amounts of muscle, fat, bone, and other vital tissues of the body.

BODY COMPOSITION. Body composition is just that—the makeup of your body. How much of each of the various types of tissues make up your body? Body composition is usually defined as the relative amounts of muscle, fat, bone, and other vital tissues of the body and is stated in terms of a percentage.[6] Too much or too little fat can negatively affect your health, including an increased risk for various diseases. For this reason, when assessing body composition, fat is typically separated out, and all the other tissues are grouped under the heading of fat-free mass. Body composition testing reports the percentage of body weight that is fat.

Body composition can be affected by diet as well as various types of physical activities. Both aerobic and resistance types of exercise can change overall body composition.

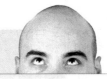

Mind Stretcher
Critical Thinking Exercise

When you think about exercise, do you think about developing all the components of health-related fitness? Do you rate some components as more important than others? Where do you think your ideas come from? Has the media shaped your views? What about your peers? Has your view of the relative importance of different fitness components affected your exercise habits in the past?

Physical Activity Readiness Questionnaire (PAR-Q) A widely used assessment tool developed by the Canadian Society for Exercise Physiology which guides people in determining whether to seek medical clearance prior to beginning or increasing an exercise program.

Assessing Physical Activity and Fitness

Before beginning any type of fitness program, it's important to know your current fitness status. If you are healthy enough for fitness testing, then you should determine your fitness level in each of the health-related fitness components and in all the skill-related components you plan to train. This will help you develop an appropriate training program and assess your progress after you begin to train.

Medical Clearance

Q | Is it safe for anyone to exercise?

Starting or gradually increasing physical activity is safe for most people. If you are between the ages of 15 and 69 with no complicating health factors, you should be fine. Completing the **Physical Activity Readiness Questionnaire (PAR-Q)** in Lab Activity 3-1 will help you to be sure. If you answer yes to any of the questions, if you are not used to being very active, or if you are outside the age range listed, you should check with your

Living with . . .

a Disability

More than 50 million Americans have some type of chronic disability, including those from injury or illness and those present at birth. Here are a few examples among adults age 18 and older:

- Number with vision trouble: 25.2 million
- Number unable (or able with great difficulty) to walk a quarter mile: 16.0 million
- Number with any physical functioning difficulty: 33.1 million

Assistive and adaptive technologies can help people with disabilities with daily tasks and recreational pursuits. If you have a disability and want to be more active, start by checking with your health care provider about the amounts and types of physical activity that are appropriate for you. The Department of Health and Human Services' *2008 Physical Activity Guidelines for Adults* includes a special section for adults with disabilities:

- Adults with disabilities, who are able to, should get at least 150 minutes a week of moderate-intensity, or 75 minutes a week of vigorous-intensity aerobic activity, or an equivalent combination of moderate- and vigorous-intensity aerobic activity. Aerobic activity should be

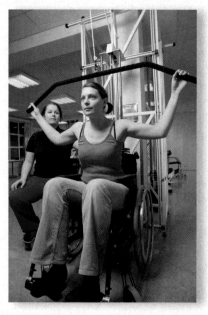

performed in episodes of at least 10 minutes, and preferably, it should be spread throughout the week.

- Adults with disabilities, who are able to, should also do muscle-strengthening activities of moderate or high intensity that involve all major muscle groups on 2 or more days a week, because these activities provide additional health benefits.
- When adults with disabilities are not able to meet the guidelines, they should engage in regular physical activity according to their abilities and should avoid inactivity.

For more information on physical activity and disability, visit the ACSM's Web site *Your Prescription for Health,* which provides informational flyers on many health conditions: http://www.exerciseismedicine.org/YourPrescription.htm. Additional information is available from the National Center on Physical Activity and Disability: http://www.ncpad.org.

Sources: National Center for Health Statistics. (2009). *Disability and functioning (Adults)* (http://www.cdc.gov/nchs/fastats/disable.htm). U.S. Department of Health and Human Services. (2008). *2008 physical activity guidelines for Americans.* ODPHP Publication No. U0036. Rockville, MD: Office of Disease Prevention and Health Promotion.

doctor before starting a new activity program or significantly increasing your current level of physical activity. Depending on your situation, your physician may simply ask you additional questions, or she or he may want to perform additional tests. In any case, your doctor's goal will not be to keep you from participating but rather to help you participate in the safest manner possible. Physical activity is a key strategy for managing or treating many chronic diseases.

Q | My mother-in-law has arthritis in her knees. Is she supposed to do any exercise?

Yes, although she may need to modify a basic exercise program to be appropriate for her. Physical activity can be beneficial for many people with arthritis and other chronic health conditions that affect mobility, cardiorespiratory functioning, and strength. According to the National Center on Physical Activity and Disability, exercise is for everyone. People with disabilities typically lead less active lifestyles,

although appropriate physical activity can help prevent secondary conditions and boost overall wellness. For arthritis, physical activity can reduce joint pain and swelling, improve overall functioning, and help maintain a healthy weight, which reduces pressure on the joints. Anyone with a chronic condition or health concern should check with her or his health care provider about designing an activity program that maximizes the benefits and minimizes the risks; see the box "Living with . . . a Disability."

Assessing General Physical Activity Levels

Q | What do sedentary and active actually mean? I'm busy all the time, so I feel really active.

Unfortunately, busy and active aren't the same. Many people feel as though they are rushing around all day, but all this hurrying doesn't necessarily mean they are *physically* active.

There is no technique that is both simple and precise to judge your overall level of physical activity. One technique that can provide an approximate measure, as well as some motivation, is to wear a pedometer and record the number of steps you take each day. Pedometers provide a rough measure of activity, although they can't differentiate between types of activity (jogging versus walking or walking on a flat surface versus up hills or stairs). There are about 2,000 steps in a mile, and walking at a pace of about 100 steps per minute is considered moderately intense for many adults.[7]

The frequently promoted goal of 10,000 or more steps per day is a reasonable one for most healthy adults (Table 3-2). However, you need to consider your current activity level in setting goals. For example, if you are currently taking 5,000 steps per day, you'll want to set a more modest goal, at least initially. On the other hand, if you are already averaging 10,000 steps a day, then you'll need to set a higher goal in order to increase your level of physical activity. Lab Activity 3-2 takes you through the steps of determining your baseline activity level and setting appropriate goals for improvement. Figure 3-3 summarizes a simple program for increasing physical activity using a pedometer.

Aim	To increase physical activity.
Clip	The pedometer to your waistband midway between your side and the center crease line of your pants.
Reset	The counter to zero at the beginning of each day.
Walk	For a week, counting steps, to establish your baseline.
Set Goal	For stepping that takes your baseline into account; see Table 3-2.
Add	To your daily steps; increase every two weeks by an average of 500–1,000 per day until you reach your final goal.
Track	Your progress toward your goal by keeping a log of your daily steps.

Figure 3-3 **A basic pedometer-based stepping program for increasing physical activity**

Sources: National Institutes of Health. (2004). General guidelines for pedometer use. *Division of Nutrition Research Coordination* (http://dnrc.nih.gov/move/pedometer_use.shtml). Anders, M. (2006). Do you do 10K a day? *American Council on Exercise Fitness Matters, 12*(4). American College of Sports Medicine. (2005). *Selecting and effectively using a pedometer.* Indianapolis, IN: ACSM.

Assessing Fitness

Q | What types of fitness assessments are available?

There are many types of fitness tests to assess and evaluate each component of fitness. Some are simple and require little equipment. Others require more specialized equipment, a lab, and a skilled administrator. Chapters 4–7 include a variety of tests you can perform to assess your fitness for each of the components of health-related fitness. Skill-related fitness

components are not addressed in depth, but your instructor can refer you to appropriate tests.

Principles of Training

Understanding the different types and components of fitness is only the first step to improving your fitness. It's also important to know some of the basic principles of fitness and training. These principles relate to all the fitness components, and understanding and applying them will help you reap the greatest benefits from your training.

Progressive Overload

Q | How do I improve my fitness level?

In order to improve in any area of fitness, the body must do more than it's used to doing. This is known as the principle of **progressive overload.** The body must be exposed to a greater amount of activity than normal. For example, if your current activity limit is walking half a mile in 10 minutes, then to improve fitness, you would need to walk farther or faster, or both. If you can currently do ten push-ups, then you would need to increase that number in order to improve muscular strength and endurance. The amount of overload or stress you place

progressive overload The principle that the body will respond to a gradual application of increasing amounts of stress (load) during exercise training by increasing fitness.

TABLE 3-2 PHYSICAL ACTIVITY LEVEL BASED ON PEDOMETER TRACKING

AVERAGE STEPS PER DAY	ACTIVITY LEVEL
Less than 5,000	Sedentary
5,000 to 7,499	Low active
7,500 to 9,999	Somewhat active
10,000 to 12,500	Active
Over 12,500	Highly active

Source: Tudor-Locke, C., Hatano, Y., Pangrazi, R. P., & Kang, M. (2008). Revisiting "How many steps are enough?" *Medicine and Science in Sports and Exercise, 40*(7 Suppl): S537–S543.

Research Brief

A Step in the Right Direction: Pedometers Improve Health

Pedometers aren't just for gathering data about the number of steps you take each day. They may also motivate you to take more steps and be more active. Researchers recently reviewed data collected from twenty-six studies that included over 2,700 adult participants. They reviewed the number of steps participants took and also evaluated their health in terms of body weight, hypertension, and other factors.

Results revealed that among people who wore pedometers and had a specific step goal, there was a 27 percent increase in activity, corresponding to about 2,000 more steps per day, compared with control groups. Those who wore pedometers also improved in terms of measures of health—their body mass index (a method of assessing body weight) declined, as did their systolic blood pressure. More research is needed, but findings to date support the use of pedometers as an effective activity tool.

Key motivational factors are setting a step goal and using a step diary. So, if you choose to use a pedometer as a tool for increasing physical activity, be sure you set goals and track your progress.

Source: Bravata, D., Smith-Spangler, C., Sundaram, V., and others. (2007). Using pedometers to increase physical activity and improve health: A systematic review. *JAMA, 298*(19), 2296–2304.

on the body is important—too little, and fitness won't improve; too much, and you may be injured.

The "progressive" part of progressive overload means that the amount of overload needs to be increased gradually. As your fitness improves, you will reach a new norm—say, fifteen push-ups—and you'll need to do more to continue to improve fitness. Once you reach a goal fitness level, you can maintain it by continuing to train at that level—say, twenty-five push-ups. To avoid injury, you shouldn't add too much stress or overload at once; gradual increases are best for training. If you are not currently active, start slowly and progress gradually.

The amount of overload needed is specific to the individual. Someone who has high muscle fitness in their arms isn't going to improve strength or endurance by doing ten push-ups. However, this may be a good level of overload for someone who hasn't done any muscle-fitness training. Individual differences also have a genetic component—some people can achieve higher levels of strength and endurance because of physiological characteristics they inherited. When you develop your fitness program, it's important to determine and use an amount of overload appropriate for your own fitness level and goals. Later in this section, we'll look specifically at the components of overload, including intensity and frequency of training.

Q | Is there a limit on how fit a person can be?

Yes. You can improve fitness significantly, but there is a limit. Human physiology has limits, and people's fitness limits are influenced by genetics and training. Most people don't need to train to an extremely high fitness level, because many of the health benefits from physical activity occur at lower levels of training (see Figure 3-4). Also, doing lots of very intense training increases the risk for injury. For safe improvement of fitness, you should slowly increase the amount you train

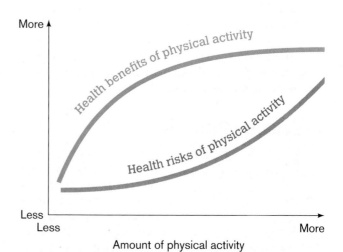

Figure 3-4 **Health benefits and risks of increasing levels of physical activity.** Most of the health benefits of physical activity occur with at least 150 minutes per week of moderate-intensity activity such as brisk walking. More activity brings additional benefits, but high levels of very intense training increase the risk of injury.

until you reach a desired level of fitness—one that helps ensure good health—and then maintain that level. In Chapters 4–6, you'll learn how to set a starting level of training for each component that is right for you and how to adjust your program over time to safely and effectively increase fitness. These program adjustments follow the principle of progressive overload.

Reversibility

Q | If I stop exercising for a while, will I lose fitness?

Unfortunately, yes. "Use it or lose it" is true when it comes to fitness. Just as an increase in activity will improve fitness levels, a decrease in activity or a period of inactivity causes a decline in fitness levels. This is known as the principle of **reversibility.** It is the opposite of the overload principle. Though declines are typically slow at first, it is possible to return to pretraining levels of fitness within a couple of months.[8]

Recovery

Q | Is it harmful to fitness to work out every day?

It can be, depending on the type of training you do. With the increase in activity (overload) comes the need for rest and **recovery.** When the body is overloaded, tissues break down. The body then adapts by repairing and improving the tissues—increasing strength, endurance, and so on (see Chapters 4 and 5 for more information). Without a recovery period, there is no time for rebuilding and improving. This recovery period should not be confused with the inactivity described in answer to the previous question. Fitness declines or reverses as a result of sustained periods of inactivity. Recovery is much shorter—often just a day or two. In terms of training, after a tough workout, your body may need a day to fully recover and be ready to train at a high level again. Most people can do stretching and low-to-moderate intensity exercise daily, but more intense exercise requires a recovery period to maximize the benefits of training and to avoid injury. You'll find more information on program design later in the chapter.

Specificity

Q | What kinds of activities do I need to do to increase fitness?

The effects of training are directly related to the types of activities. This is known as the principle of **specificity.** For example, you will not achieve cardiorespiratory fitness by performing stretching exercises; instead, you need to perform exercises that stress the cardiorespiratory system. Similarly, you will not see any significant changes in flexibility if you are working to build muscular strength.

Specificity also applies *within* particular fitness components. Pull-ups build strength in specific muscles in the upper body only, not general strength. The most effective skill training is to practice what you want to perform—play basketball to improve your basketball skills. A complete exercise program should include exercises to build all the health-related components of fitness and, for muscle fitness and flexibility, all the major muscle groups and joints. Depending on your goals, you may also need to include activities to develop skill-related fitness.

reversibility The principle that a decrease or discontinuance of activity will cause a decline in fitness.

recovery The time needed by the body to rebuild and improve tissues weakened from increased activity (overload).

specificity The principle that the body adapts to the specific types and amounts of stress placed on it.

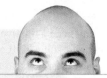
Individuality

Q | Could everyone be as fit as, say, Lance Armstrong, if they worked hard enough?

Unfortunately, no. Everyone can improve, and some could no doubt become highly fit and highly skilled. But, not everyone can be Lance. In fact, no one can be exactly like Lance. Many factors play a role in our ability to achieve and maintain various levels of fitness. Our overall health, past activities, body type, genes, and a number of other factors determine what we can accomplish physically and physiologically. The factors having the greatest effect on each component of health-related fitness are addressed in Chapters 4–7.

The FITT Formula

Q | What types of exercise should I do, and how much?

The easiest way to address these questions is to apply what is commonly referred to as the **FITT formula.** FITT is an acronym for frequency, intensity, time, and type. These training principles can be applied to the different fitness components, and they form the foundation for your exercise program. This section introduces the basics of the FITT formula; more detail on applying FITT to each fitness component can be found in Chapters 4–6.

Q | How many times per week should I work out?

FREQUENCY: HOW OFTEN. How often, or how frequently, you should exercise depends on the component you are training, your goals, and your current fitness level. The optimal frequency of exercise is also affected by the other parts of the FITT formula. For example, if you exercise at a high intensity, a lower frequency is appropriate to allow your body to recover. Also, when starting a new program,

FITT formula Acronym for the foundational components of exercise training and program design: frequency (how often), intensity (how hard), time (how long), and type (what kind of activity).

you may need a relatively low frequency to allow your body to rest and adjust to the new level of activity. As your body becomes more accustomed to the activity or as your goals change, you may choose to increase your frequency.

Guidelines from the American College of Sports Medicine (ACSM) suggest the following frequency of exercise:[9]

- Cardiorespiratory endurance training: 3–5 days/week
- Muscle fitness training: 2–3 days/week
- Flexibility training: At least 2–3 days/week

The guidelines from the ACSM are widely recommended and are consistent with those from other organizations and agencies, including the *2008 Physical Activity Guidelines for Americans* from the Department of Health and Human Services. Additional recommendations will be discussed in later chapters.

Q | How do you know if your workout is hard enough for you?

INTENSITY: HOW HARD. In basic terms, in order to improve, you must do more than you're used to doing. How much more than normal depends on the type of fitness you're working on and what you wish to accomplish. You're trying to reach your threshold and target zone. **Target zone** is the optimal or ideal intensity for achieving maximum benefit from your activity. The **threshold** is the doorway into the target zone—it is the minimum intensity for achieving specific fitness benefits. As Figure 3.5 shows, exercising at an intensity below this threshold will burn calories and contribute to your overall activity level, but it will not cause fitness improvements. There is also an upper limit for intensity, above which fitness improvements continue but injury becomes more likely.

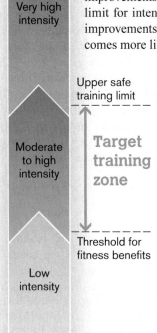

Very high intensity

Upper safe training limit

Target training zone

Threshold for fitness benefits

Moderate to high intensity

Low intensity

Training intensity

Figure 3-5 **Target zone for training intensity**

How is intensity measured? Many people think of target zones only in terms of measuring heart rate for cardiorespiratory training—and that is one way to measure the intensity of a cardiorespiratory workout. However, there is a target zone for exercises that address the other fitness components as well. Intensity target zones also apply to the degree of a stretch during flexibility training and to the amount of resistance during strength training. Specifics for determining the appropriate intensity for each type of fitness training are covered in Chapters 4–6.

Q | How long should I exercise, per day and per week?

TIME: HOW LONG. A training session is typically measured in number of minutes or number of exercises. The amount of time you spend in each session will depend on the fitness components and intensity you choose, the design of your program, and your goals. For example, if you exercise at a high intensity, your training session will be shorter than if you work out at a lower intensity—for example, 45 minutes of brisk walking versus 20 minutes of fast jogging. Also, if your goal includes weight loss and changes in body composition, you'll likely need to spend more time engaging in physical activity than someone who wants to maintain their current weight. For strength and flexibility training, the time is typically determined by the number of exercises and the number of repetitions of each exercise. A stretching program that includes eight different stretches might take 10–15 minutes.

Q | What is the best kind of exercise?

TYPE: CHOICE OF ACTIVITIES. In the FITT formula, *type* refers to the type of activities. You'll select activities based on the fitness component as well as your goals related to that component. Remember the principle of specificity? Different activities are needed to develop each of the health-related components of fitness. That means aerobic activities like brisk walking or cycling for cardiorespiratory endurance, resistance training for muscular strength and endurance, and stretching for flexibility.

You can choose activities for your program based on your fitness level and goals, personal preferences, and environment. You want to choose activities that are convenient and that you enjoy. For example, if you don't like exercising in a group, choose an activity you can do on your own. If you love to play tennis but have access to a court only once per week, then you'll want to choose alternative or additional activities to supplement your tennis workouts. You can stick with one activity for each component or mix things up for variety; see the box "Motivation for Physical Activity" for more suggestions.

target zone Optimal intensity range for achieving maximum fitness benefits from exercise.

threshold The minimum intensity for achieving a specific fitness benefit; the doorway to the target zone.

Wellness Strategies

Motivation for Physical Activity: Move More!

- Set achievable goals for your program.
- Pick activities that you like to do and that are convenient.
- Team up with friends or family members to make activity more fun. If you work out alone, listen to music if you can do so safely.
- Work activity into your daily routine—for example, walk or bike to work and use the stairs instead of the elevator.

- Start slowly, and add activity gradually. Don't push yourself too hard and make your workouts unpleasant.
- Try a variety of activities.
- Track your time and progress to help your program stay on track.

For more information on motivation and goal setting, see Chapter 2.

Q | **What is the best fitness program?**

APPLYING THE FITT FORMULA. A lot depends on you! Knowing the FITT formula is important, but the definitions alone still don't answer the questions "What should I do?" and "How much should I do?" As noted above, the frequency, intensity, time, and type of exercise are related to what you hope to accomplish. Chapters 4–6 go into detail to help you set specific goals and apply the FITT formula for each of the health-related fitness components. A summary of the ACSM FITT guidelines appears in Table 3-3. There are as many ways to combine and vary activities as there are people!

Putting Together a Complete Workout

A safe and effective workout has several phases, but there are many ways to combine them.

Q | **What does a complete workout look like?**

PHASES OF A WORKOUT. An exercise training session includes the following phases:

- warm-up
- conditioning (endurance or resistance exercise, according to the FITT formula) or sport-related activities

- cool-down
- stretching (after the warm-up or cool-down)

The placement of stretching exercises in your program is up to you. Stretching is a separate activity from the warm-up or cool-down. As explained in detail in Chapter 6, some types of stretching just before an activity requiring force and power may reduce performance during the activity. Therefore, if the conditioning portion of your workout includes an activity requiring significant muscular strength and if high performance is a goal, you might be better off stretching after the cool-down phase. However, if the conditioning phase of your workout includes a moderate-intensity activity like brisk walking, stretching before the workout isn't likely to have an impact.

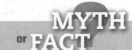

It is best to work out in the morning, because morning workouts elevate your metabolism more than afternoon or evening workouts do.

 WATCH ONLINE

Mind Stretcher
Critical Thinking Exercise

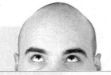

What types of physical activity do you like best? What is it about them that you enjoy? Is it something about the activity or how it makes you feel? Does it relate to the setting or to the people you're with? Are there other activities with the same characteristics that you could try?

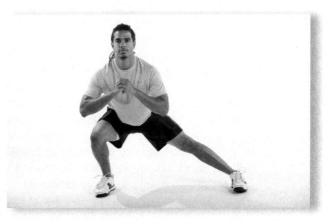

Stretching exercises are best done when muscles are warm, either after the active part of your warm-up or after your cool-down. If your conditioning activity requires significant force or power, it's best for high performance to stretch after your workout.

TABLE 3-3 SUMMARY OF ACSM FITT GUIDELINES

FITNESS COMPONENT	FREQUENCY	INTENSITY	TIME	TYPE
CARDIORESPIRATORY ENDURANCE (see Chapter 4)	3–5 days per week (3 days if vigorous intensity, 5 days if moderate intensity)	Target heart rate zone (lower end for moderate, higher end for vigorous)	20–90 minutes per day 60–300 minutes per week (total depends on intensity and goals)	Rhythmic, aerobic exercise of at least moderate intensity that involves large muscle groups (brisk walking, jogging, cycling, etc.)
MUSCULAR STRENGTH AND ENDURANCE (see Chapter 5)	2–3 nonconsecutive days per week	Enough resistance to cause muscle fatigue after 8–12 repetitions *Note: Resistance and repetitions should be adjusted for strength training vs. endurance training*	8–12 repetitions per exercise per set; 2–4 sets per exercise	Resistance exercises that use multiple joints and target more than one muscle group (shoulder press, curl-up, squat, etc.); the program should include exercises for all major muscle groups
FLEXIBILITY (see Chapter 6)	2–3 days per week, at a minimum	Stretch to the point of mild tightness without significant discomfort	15–60 seconds per stretch 4 or more repetitions of each stretch	Stretching exercises involving the major muscle/tendon groups (neck, shoulders, upper back, etc.)

Source: Adapted from American College of Sports Medicine. (2009). *ACSM's Guidelines for Exercise Testing and Prescription* (8th ed.). Baltimore, MD: Lippincott Williams & Wilkins.

Q | Why do I sometimes feel a bit dizzy after exercise?

WARM-UP AND COOL-DOWN. It's likely that you aren't doing a proper cool-down after your workout. About 5–10 minutes each of warm-up and cool-down are essential for any training session. Both warming up and cooling down are related to exercise intensity. You can't just jump into and out of your target zone. It's important for your body to have time to gradually adapt as you make your way from a resting state to your training intensity, and then again as you transition back to a resting state. **Warm-up** and **cool-down** activities prepare your body for what's coming next (see Table 3-4).

The dizziness you sometimes feel relates to the shift in blood flow distribution and changes in blood vessels that occur during exercise. To help working muscles get the oxygen they need, the heart pumps fast and the blood vessels widen in active muscles, including those in your legs. If you suddenly stop exercising, your heart slows quickly, but the blood vessels take more time to return to their normal size. For this reason, some blood may pool in your legs, creating a feeling of light-headedness. A cool-down will prevent this. If you get really dizzy, check with your physician.

Putting Together a Complete Program

Q | What is the best weekly exercise routine for health?

There are many ways to plan a routine. You can find more information and sample training routines for each health-related fitness component in Chapters 4–6. However, if you're just getting started, you may still be trying to wrap your head around how this all fits together. The examples in Figure 3-6 provide good models for incorporating recommended activities into a weekly schedule of workouts. Examples

warm-up 5–10 minutes of low-intensity activity that prepares the body for exercise.

cool-down 5–10 minutes of slower paced activity that helps the body transition to a normal or resting state after a session of exercise.

TABLE 3-4 WARM-UPS AND COOL-DOWNS SUMMED UP

WARM-UP	COOL-DOWN
5–10 minutes of low- to moderate-intensity aerobic and muscular endurance activities	5–10 minutes of low- to moderate-intensity aerobic and muscular endurance activities
Perform before a training session	Perform after a training session
Purposes: ■ Increase core body and muscle temperature ■ Redirect blood flow to working muscles ■ Gradually increase heart and breathing rate ■ Reduce the chance of after-exercise muscle soreness or stiffness	Purposes: ■ Gradual recovery of heart rate ■ Gradual reduction of blood pressure ■ Redistribution of blood flow ■ Removal of metabolic end products such as carbon dioxide from muscles used during the conditioning phase

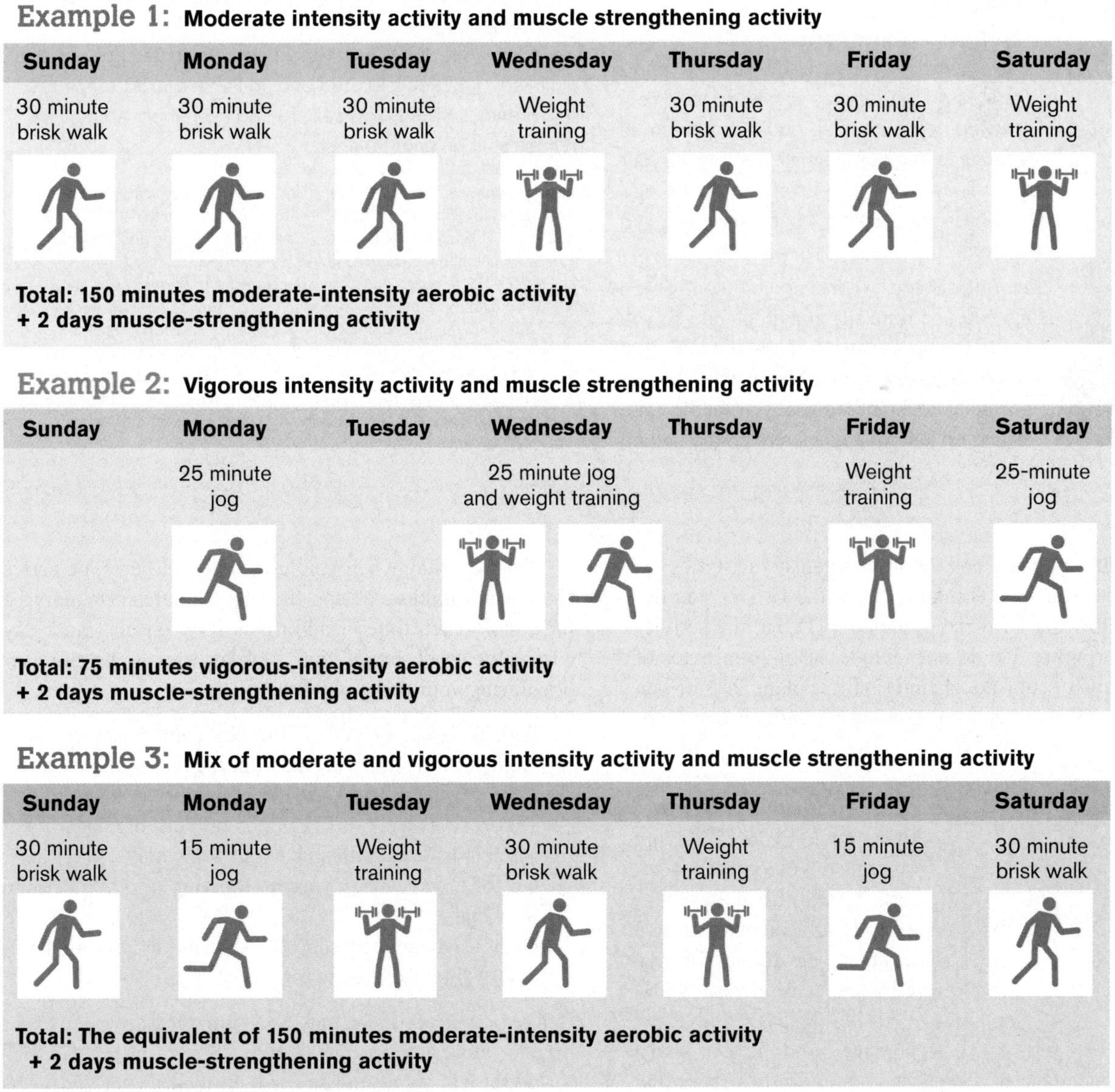

Example 1: Moderate intensity activity and muscle strengthening activity

Sunday	Monday	Tuesday	Wednesday	Thursday	Friday	Saturday
30 minute brisk walk	30 minute brisk walk	30 minute brisk walk	Weight training	30 minute brisk walk	30 minute brisk walk	Weight training

Total: 150 minutes moderate-intensity aerobic activity + 2 days muscle-strengthening activity

Example 2: Vigorous intensity activity and muscle strengthening activity

Sunday	Monday	Tuesday	Wednesday	Thursday	Friday	Saturday
	25 minute jog		25 minute jog and weight training		Weight training	25-minute jog

Total: 75 minutes vigorous-intensity aerobic activity + 2 days muscle-strengthening activity

Example 3: Mix of moderate and vigorous intensity activity and muscle strengthening activity

Sunday	Monday	Tuesday	Wednesday	Thursday	Friday	Saturday
30 minute brisk walk	15 minute jog	Weight training	30 minute brisk walk	Weight training	15 minute jog	30 minute brisk walk

Total: The equivalent of 150 minutes moderate-intensity aerobic activity + 2 days muscle-strengthening activity

Figure 3-6 **Sample fitness program design**

Source: Centers for Disease Control and Prevention. (2009). *Physical activity for everyone: Adding physical activity to your life* (http://www.cdc.gov/physicalactivity/everyone/getactive/index.html).

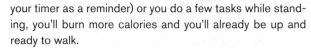

Wellness Strategies

Surviving a Desk Job

A desk job has some advantages such as temperature-controlled air and pleasant surroundings, but it also has its disadvantages. Being tied to a desk not only makes you feel tired and stressed, but it increases your risk for obesity and disease. According to *BizTimes.com,* 70 percent of America's workforce sits on the job, and many of us sit most of the workday. Whether you already have a desk job or you've chosen a major that will likely put you at a desk most of the day, plan for some "office activity" in your day. This added activity doesn't replace the need for regular exercise, but any activity improves circulation, decreases stress, and burns a few calories. Try these strategies.

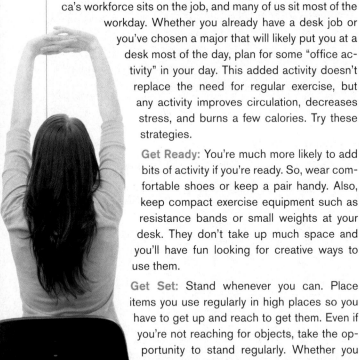

Get Ready: You're much more likely to add bits of activity if you're ready. So, wear comfortable shoes or keep a pair handy. Also, keep compact exercise equipment such as resistance bands or small weights at your desk. They don't take up much space and you'll have fun looking for creative ways to use them.

Get Set: Stand whenever you can. Place items you use regularly in high places so you have to get up and reach to get them. Even if you're not reaching for objects, take the opportunity to stand regularly. Whether you stand up just for a quick stretch (try setting your timer as a reminder) or you do a few tasks while standing, you'll burn more calories and you'll already be up and ready to walk.

Get Going: It's not just your computer that goes into standby mode when idle; so do the fat-burning enzymes in your body. So, take a walk:

- Hand-deliver a report or message.
- Make frequent trips to the fax or copier.
- Get a phone headset so you can stand and walk while talking.
- Take a walking break rather than a coffee break.
- Take a walk and eat your lunch outside the office.
- If practical, schedule a walking meeting instead of a sit-down meeting.

And of course, don't forget to keep your water bottle full. You'll keep yourself hydrated and you'll take extra steps refilling it and "unfilling" yourself. To add even more steps, use the restroom on another floor.

Sources: Brophy, A. (2007). Sitting good: Proper ergonomics reduce workplace injuries. *BizTimes.com* (http://www.biztimes.com/news/2007/10/12/sitting-good). Exercise at work. (n.d.). *Campbell's Nutrition and Wellness* (http://www.campbellwellness.com/article.aspx?id=37). Mayo Clinic staff. (2009, September 24). Office exercise: How to burn calories at work. *MayoClinic.com* (http://www.mayoclinic.com/health/office-exercise/SM00115). Hamilton, M., Hamilton D., & Zderic, T. (2007). Role of low energy expenditure and sitting in obesity, metabolic syndrome, type 2 diabetes, and cardiovascular disease. *Diabetes, 56,* 2355–2360. Mummery, W., Schofield, G., Steele, R., Eakin, E., & Brown, W. (2005). Occupational sitting time and overweight and obesity in Australian workers. *American Journal of Preventive Medicine, 29*(2), 91–97.

for moderate-intensity and vigorous-intensity activities are included as well as a combination of the two. If you decide to follow one of these, remember (1) that the activity minutes in Figure 3-6 do not include the 5–10 minutes of warm-up and of cool-down, and (2) these plans assume you are incorporating stretching exercises into the warm-up or cool-down.

Q I don't exercise at all, and I'm crazy busy. Does any amount of activity help, even five minutes?

Yes. Any activity is better than none. Even if it's not enough to increase your fitness level, it still has benefits. If all you have is five minutes, be active for five minutes. Go for a walk. Walking is easy and inexpensive, and it can burn calories, tone muscles, strengthen bones, improve stamina, reduce stress, and lower your risk for disease. What better way to spend five minutes?

Then one day when you have seven minutes, be active for seven minutes . . . and then ten minutes. Try doing a little more each time or adding activity on one more day during the week. In addition, look for ways to be more active during your daily activities:

- Park your car or get off the bus some distance away from your destination and walk the rest of the way.
- Take the stairs instead of the escalator or elevator.
- Take a short walk during lunch or work breaks.
- Stretch or do calisthenics while you watch TV.
- Go for a walk when you are meeting up with a friend for a chat.
- Do at least one active chore—such as vacuuming, laundry, or mowing the lawn—every day.

Before you know it, you may find yourself wanting to make time for more activity. See the box "Surviving a Desk Job" for additional suggestions. For help identifying and overcoming barriers to activity in your life, complete Lab Activity 3-3.

Other Considerations When You're Starting a Fitness Program

You're almost ready to start your fitness program. You're familiar with the components of health-related fitness and how to determine your current status in each one. You're also acquainted with some essential fitness principles that will help you design a safe and successful exercise program. Before you begin, however, there are a few more things to consider. Some of the concerns addressed here may not be applicable to you at this time. Review the topics and focus on those most relevant to your personal preferences, resources, and geographic location.

Clothing and Safety Gear

Q Why is some clothing considered especially appropriate for exercise?

In most cases, special clothing is not required for exercise—especially if you're just starting out. Loose-fitting, comfortable clothing will usually suffice. However, special exercise clothes can make you more comfortable during your workout, which might help you stick with your program. Some people also find that a new set of exercise clothes helps motivate them to start an exercise program. One of the benefits of new types of synthetic exercise clothing is its ability to "wick" moisture away from the skin. This means that while you sweat, the fabric will move the moisture from your skin to the outer surface of your fancy new shirt, where it can evaporate more quickly. This eliminates the icky, heavy feeling of a cotton T-shirt soaked with sweat.

If you exercise before or after school or work, you are often heading out in the dark. Use caution if you exercise alone, and avoid areas that are unlighted, suspicious, or make you feel uncomfortable. Whatever your route, make it as easy as possible for others to see you. Wear light-colored clothing with as much reflective fabric as possible. Some clothing manufacturers put reflective materials directly into their products. You can also purchase reflective straps to go around your lower arm or leg; small, flashing LED safety lights to loosely wrap around your upper arm or a piece of equipment; reflective

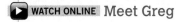 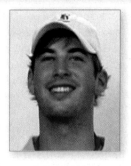

Behavior Change Challenge
Video Case Study

▶ WATCH ONLINE Meet Greg

Greg is a 21-year-old college sophomore who lives in a fraternity. Greg considers himself inactive compared to his high school days. He wants to start an exercise program to try to get back into shape and to avoid the weight gain he's seen in other members of his family. Watch the video to learn more about Greg, his behavior-change goals and plan, and his success over the initial weeks of his program. As you watch the video, think about the following questions:

- How realistic are Greg's goals and his starting program plan?
- Do you think Greg has enough motivation and environmental support for his program? What do you think his biggest barriers and challenges will be?
- What worked for Greg, and what parts of the program caused difficulties for him? What can you learn from Greg's experience that will help you in your behavior-change efforts?

stickers to place almost anywhere; and reflective vests to go over any clothing.[10]

Q Do I need different shoes for different activities? That's way too expensive.

Probably not, even though fitness footwear comes in a dizzying array of choices. There are shoes specific to almost any activity you can think of, cross-training shoes meant to do it all, and shoes for every different foot type, male or female. Where do you start? That might depend on your budget.

Shoes are important because they cushion some of the impact force that occurs when your feet hit the ground. If you don't have good shoes, you increase your risk of injury. Also, poorly fitting shoes can lead to a number of other orthopedic problems, from bunions to knee, back, and hip pain.

Practical Prevention

Put Your Best Foot Forward: Choosing the Right Exercise Shoe

Athletic shoes are essential for exercise but, with so many choices available, how do you know which shoe is right for you? If you're just getting started and plan to try a variety of activities, a cross-training shoe is a good choice. A knowledgeable salesperson can help you narrow down the possibilities, and then it will be up to you to choose the best shoe for you.

When looking for and trying on new shoes, apply the **S-T-R-E-T-C-H** test.

S – Wear the same type of ***socks*** you will wear for your activities.
T – ***Try them out.*** Run or walk a few steps or simulate some of your activity movements to make sure the shoes are comfortable.
R – ***Re-lace*** the shoes, beginning at the toe-end and applying even pressure as you lace in a crisscross fashion.
E – Try on shoes at the ***end of the day,*** when your feet are at their largest.
T – Do the ***toe test.*** There should be three-eighths to one-half inch of space between your longest toe and the end of your shoe. You should have enough room to wiggle your toes comfortably.
C – Your shoes should be ***comfortable*** right away; they shouldn't require stretching out or breaking in. Choose a shoe by how it fits the shape of your foot and not by the shoe size number.
H – Make sure your ***heels*** are hugged snugly by the shoes. Your heels shouldn't slip as you move.

Always take the time to evaluate shoes carefully because (1) shoes and brands vary greatly, and (2) your feet change over time. Also keep in mind that there are many types of shoes for a reason—aside from sales. Shoes that are specially designed for a particular activity maximize proper functioning. If you decide you like one activity more than others and you participate in it three or more times a week, it's worth investing in a specialized shoe.

You should also evaluate your shoes regularly. If they feel or look worn, they are—and it's time for a replacement pair. Although this can be a bit costly, it can save you time, pain, and money in the long run. Rough guidelines for shoe replacement are every 300–500 miles of running or walking, or every 3–6 months depending on your level of activity.

For more information about specific types of athletic shoes and their recommended characteristics, visit the Web sites of the American Academy of Podiatric Sports Medicine and the American Academy of Orthopaedic Surgeons.

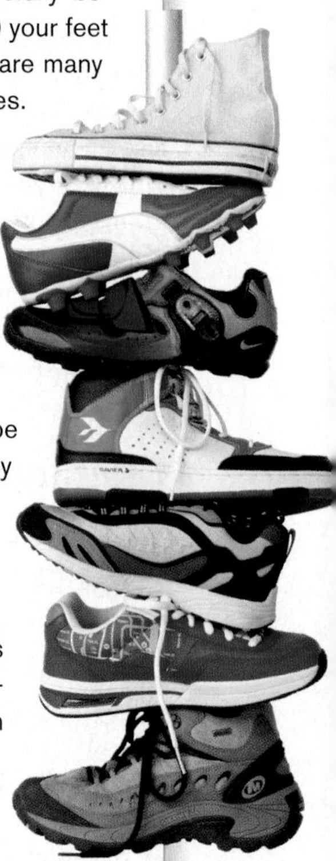

Sources: American Academy of Orthopaedic Surgeons. (2001). Athletic shoes. *Your Orthopaedic Connection* (http://orthoinfo.aaos.org/topic.cfm?topic=A00318). American Academy of Podiatric Sports Medicine. (n.d.) Selecting an athletic shoe (http://www.aapsm.org/fit_shoes.htm).

So, what is the best shoe? There really isn't one. Before buying, consider the activities you'll be doing, what you can afford, your foot type, and the surface you exercise on. Shoes specific to running aren't very good for other activities, especially those requiring side-to-side movements. Cross-training shoes aren't ideal for running, but if you don't run much and have normal foot biomechanics, they should be fine. A large sporting goods store will have the best selection, but a specialty shoe store might provide you with the most care in determining your foot type. See the box "Put Your Best Foot Forward: Choosing the Right Exercise Shoe" for guidelines.

Q Do knee pads really help that much? I think they look goofy.

Yes. You'll look a lot better in the pads than you'll look if you crash without them. For some activities, you need special gear to increase your comfort and performance as well as provide safety. Common types of safety equipment include the following:[11]

- *Elbow and wrist guards and knee pads* are often worn for in-line skating, scooter riding, and skateboarding as well as indoor activities in which there is risk for bumps and falls. Guards and pads protect you not only from cuts and scrapes but also from fractures and breaks.
- *Helmets* should always be worn when biking, skating, or engaging in similar activities. Wear a helmet made specifically for your activity. It should fit snugly on your head, with no forward or backward slipping. Look for the sticker indicating that the helmet meets Consumer Product Safety Commission (CPSC) standards. If your helmet is quite old (perhaps bought at a garage sale or handed down from Mom or Dad), it might be time to upgrade; a good helmet doesn't have to cost much more than $35 or $40.
- *Eye protection* should be worn for contact sports and other activities with heavy or fast flying objects. Face masks are required for some activities, but goggles will suffice for many others. Most goggles are made of polycarbonate plastic. They should fit securely with cush-

ions above the eyebrows and over the nose. If you wear glasses, prescription goggles may be necessary. You should not rely on your regular glasses for protection.

- *Mouth guards* may be required for contact sports and other sports in which there is risk for head injury. Mouth guards protect the mouth, teeth, and tongue. They can be purchased at sporting goods stores or specially fitted by a dentist.
- *Athletic supporters* provide protection from the stresses of vigorous movement, and *athletic cups* also provide protection against direct contact. Men should wear athletic cups for contact sports, and they should wear supporters for noncontact sports. An experienced coach or a doctor can advise you if you are unsure about the appropriate type of support.
- *Sports bras* provide additional support and protection against the stresses of vigorous movement. They come in a variety of styles and can be purchased at most department and sporting goods stores.

Other activities may require even more specialized gear. Check with local organizations and experienced coaches and trainers for more information on the latest and best gear.

Exercise Equipment and Facilities

Q | How should I pick a pedometer?
[READ ONLINE]

Q | What's the best type of home exercise equipment?

The best piece of equipment is one that you will use. Home exercise equipment can be very beneficial and is an excellent choice for some exercisers. To decide if it's for you, consider both the personal and financial factors related to such a purchase. Equipment can range from very simple and inex-

pensive (pedometers, jump ropes, free weights) to high-tech and expensive (treadmills, complete home gyms). If you plan to make a significant financial investment in a piece of equipment, do some research. Local sporting equipment dealers and consumer-ratings magazines and Web sites can help you sort through the specific features. The American College of Sports Medicine (http://www.acsm.org) also provides guidelines for selecting equipment.

In addition to the data gathering, you'll also want to consider personal preferences. Exercising at home is private and convenient, and you're protected from bad weather. But be sure this is what you want. Do you like working out at home, alone? Have you tried exercising at home to be sure that investing in home exercise equipment is the right choice for you? Do you have an appropriate space for the equipment—not just enough room but a place that is appealing and well ventilated? Do you know how to use the equipment properly? Improper form can hinder your results (and possibly cause injury) regardless of how much you exercise. Always try out equipment before making a purchase decision to be sure you like it and to be sure you know how to use it.[12] Some popular home exercise equipment choices are described in Table 3-5.

Q | Should I join a gym?

Deciding whether to join a health club or gym depends on your personal preferences, your environment, and your budget. If you like to exercise in public in a fitness facility, then a local health club or gym may be a good choice

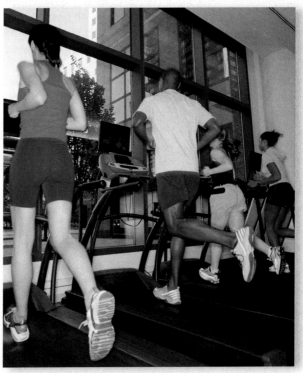

If you decide to join a fitness or health club, shop around first and find one that best fits your schedule and needs. Ask for a free pass or trial membership.

TABLE 3-5 HOME EXERCISE EQUIPMENT OPTIONS

MOTORIZED TREADMILL	Good for improving cardiovascular fitness and lower-body muscle tone. Most allow changes in speed and incline to change exercise intensity. Lower impact than walking or running outdoors. Cost ranges from $500 to $1,500.
STATIONARY CYCLE	Provides non-impact aerobic training. Many have devices for increasing intensity as well as measuring distance, speed, and calories burned. Some can simulate road, mountain, or racing conditions. Recumbent bikes may be more comfortable for people with back problems or those who are large. Cost ranges from $100 to $1,200.
ELLIPTICAL TRAINER	Good for improving cardiovascular fitness and upper- and lower-body muscles. Lower impact than a treadmill; may be a good choice for people with knee problems. Cost ranges from $500 to $3,000.
STAIR-CLIMBING MACHINE	Good for improving cardiovascular fitness and leg strength with less stress to knees. Many have monitors that display steps per minute, time, and calories burned. Some allow for increasing resistance. Cost ranges from $200 to $700.
CROSS-COUNTRY SKI MACHINE	Helps to develop cardiovascular fitness and muscle tone in legs and arms. Most include heart monitors. Some allow increase in incline ability to increase intensity. Cost is about $300 and up.
HOME GYM (ALL-IN-ONE WEIGHT MACHINE)	Provides a variety of strength-training options. Designed to make setup and changing of weights easier. Cost ranges from $200 to $3,000 depending on features.

Sources: American Academy of Orthopaedic Surgeons. (2007). Selecting home exercise equipment. *Your Orthopaedic Connection* (http://orthoinfo.aaos .org/topic.cfm?topic=A00415). Cardiovascular exercise machines: What's right for you. (2009, March). *UC Berkeley Wellness Letter.*

for you. According to the International Health, Racquet and Sportsclub Association (IHRSA), there are more than 30,000 health clubs in the United States, with more than 45 million members.[13] Not all clubs are created equal, however. Facilities range from small and quaint to large and state of the art.

Shop around to find the facility that best meets your needs. A large, flashy facility isn't necessarily the best choice or bargain if you use only a small number of its amenities. Do you want to participate in Pilates classes? Take swimming lessons? Select from a wide variety of weights and weight machines? Become a better racquetball player? Think about your goals, find facilities that meet your needs, and then do some comparison shopping. Ask around. Does each facility have a good reputation? Of those that do, how does each rate on the following characteristics?[14]

- **Location and hours:** Is the location convenient? Do the operating hours meet your needs? Are the classes and equipment you want available at the times you can visit the facility, or is it very crowded at the times you're free?
- **Environment:** Is the environment friendly and welcoming? Is it clean? Is this a place you'll want to go—even when you're tired?
- **Equipment and classes:** Do the offerings meet your needs? Is the equipment in good shape? Are classes offered at convenient hours?

- **Staff:** Is the staff friendly and knowledgeable? Do they display credentials?
- **Amenities:** Does it provide other services that you need (such as parking, towels, and child care)?
- **Cost and policies:** Is the price within your budget? Are convenient payment or billing methods offered? Are the membership contracts and cancellation policies reasonable?
- **Trial:** As with home exercise equipment, you should try out the facility to see if it really meets your needs. Most reputable facilities offer visitor passes or trial memberships.

Many types of equipment and facilities are available, but remember, exercise doesn't have to be expensive. Don't forget to check out your campus facility. Most campuses have adequate facilities, and many are available at low or no cost to students.

Weather

If you choose to exercise outdoors, weather is likely to complicate your fitness program at some point. Of course, common sense tells us not to go out in a hurricane or a blizzard, but what about the average days? It's important to understand how factors such as temperature, humidity, and wind speed change your environment and affect your body.

Q | Is exercising in hot and humid conditions unsafe?

HEAT. It can be, and you may need to adjust your workouts when it's hot and humid. If you're outside regularly, your body naturally acclimates as spring turns into summer. But if you haven't been outside regularly and the weather has already turned hot, you should very gradually increase exercise intensity and time. Withstanding heat is not a test of strength or toughness, and you can always choose to exercise inside on very hot days.

Exercising in the heat places extra stress on the body. The increase in external temperature increases your body temperature, potentially to dangerous levels. Elevated body temperature triggers changes, including more blood circulating to the skin in an effort to cool the body, leaving less blood to flow to your working muscles. In turn, this leads to an increase in heart rate. Your body's natural cooling system, sweat and its evaporation, helps to alleviate some of these stresses, enabling you to acclimate to the heat. However, high humidity can make high temperatures even more difficult to adapt to. Humidity is the amount of water vapor in the air; high humidity doesn't allow sweat to evaporate as easily, so your body temperature increases and you feel hotter than the outside temperature indicates. The National Weather Service has developed the **heat index** (Figure 3-7) to help people assess the risks of the combination of temperature and humidity. When high temperatures and high humidity are combined, the risk of a serious heat-related disorder increases.

Warm temperatures don't necessarily mean you can't exercise outdoors, but it is important to take the appropriate precautions. Assuming your doctor has not advised against it, guidelines for safely exercising in hot weather include the following:

heat index Guide that combines outside air temperature and humidity into a single measure of perceived temperature (how hot it feels).

- Check the heat index on local or national weather channels and Web sites. If the heat index is in the danger zone or higher, you should consider exercising inside in a location with air conditioning. If the heat index is below the danger zone but still very high, you should still take appropriate precautions.
- Work out in the cooler morning or evening hours, if possible. Consider lowering your intensity or duration of exercise.
- Wear appropriate clothing. Lightweight, loose-fitting clothes allow sweat to evaporate more easily and air to pass through more freely for extra cooling. Choose light-colored clothing rather than dark colors, which absorb the sun's heat. A shirt made of moisture-wicking material will likely keep you cooler than a cotton shirt (or no shirt).
- Wear a light-colored hat to shade your face and help to keep your head cool; also wear sunglasses.
- Don't skimp on safety gear; if it's very hot, you may want to limit activities that require heavy or tight-fitting gear.
- Use plenty of sunscreen and use it often. Even waterproof and sweatproof formulas dissipate quickly, so reapply often. Sunburn not only causes damage to your skin, but it also decreases your body's ability to cool itself.[15]
- Keep yourself well hydrated to replace the moisture you lose through sweating.
- Take frequent breaks, preferably in the shade.

Q | How much water should I drink during a workout?

Proper hydration is always important but particularly so during exercise—not only for performance but also for health. The loss of body fluids causes a drop in blood volume, which makes the heart work harder to circulate the blood. Inadequate fluid intake,

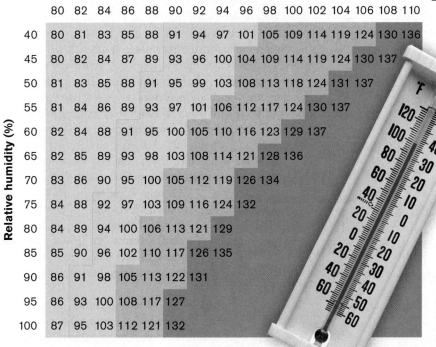

Figure 3-7 Heat index
Source: NOAA, National Weather Service. (2010, May 27). *Heat: A major killer* (http://www.nws.noaa.gov/om/heat/index.shtml).

TABLE 3-6 HYDRATION RECOMMENDATIONS FOR EXERCISE

HYDRATION BEFORE EXERCISE	HYDRATION DURING EXERCISE	HYDRATION AFTER EXERCISE
■ Drink about 17–20 fl. oz. 2–3 hours before exercise ■ Drink about 7–10 fl. oz. 10–20 minutes before exercise	■ Drink enough fluids to prevent dehydration ■ Customize fluid replacement rate by monitoring body weight changes during workouts	■ Weigh yourself before and after exercise and replace fluid losses ■ Drink 20–25 fl. oz. for every 1 pound lost

Sources: American College of Sports Medicine. (2007). Exercise and fluid replacement. *Medicine and Science in Sports and Exercise, 39*(2), 377–390. Casa, D. J., and others. (2000). National Athletic Trainers' Association position statement: Fluid replacement for athletes. *Journal of Athletic Training, 35*(2), 212–224.

excessive sweating, length of exercise session, weather, and altitude can all affect your hydration. General guidelines for hydration appear in Table 3-6. It's best to develop a hydration plan that fits your personal sweat rate and intensity of exercise as well as the environmental conditions. The risk of dehydration increases with length and intensity of exercise.

Q | Are sports drinks a good option?

Sports drinks can help replace losses of sodium, potassium, and other electrolytes. However, electrolytes are usually not significantly depleted during a typical workout. Additionally, many sports drinks are high in sugar. For workouts lasting less than an hour, water is an adequate fluid replacement. For longer or particularly intense workouts, you can consider using a sports beverage for hydration. Choose one with about 4–8 percent carbohydrates, because higher concentrations can slow the absorption of fluid.

Q | Is it bad for you to run in cold air?

COLD. For most people, exercising in cold weather is safe. However, it can be a problem for people with health concerns such as high blood pressure or other heart-related problems. Because the cold puts extra strain on the heart, it's important to follow your doctor's advice if you have these conditions. If you are otherwise healthy, you should be fine exercising in cold temperatures, provided you dress appropriately and follow basic safety guidelines.

When exercising in cold weather, dress in layers. A bottom layer made from synthetic material such as polypropylene helps draw sweat away from the body; synthetic layers are safer than cotton, which can quickly chill you if it becomes wet. Top the synthetic layer with one or more warming layers, such as fleece or wool. These mid-layers should be snug but not too tight and should have the ability to wick moisture. If needed, top your warming layers with a final breathable, waterproof layer. Wearing a hat and gloves is also essential for maintaining warmth; the best kinds are windproof and water resistant and have wicking capabilities. Covering your mouth with a scarf will help warm the air you breathe. Choose footwear that will aid in traction. And, as always, wear sunscreen on sunny days and other safety gear appropriate to the activity.[16] Avoid going straight into the wind, if you can. In contrast to hot weather, in cold weather, it is often best to wait until midday to exercise, when the temperature is at its peak.

As on hot days, the thermometer doesn't tell the full story. On cold days, high winds carry heat away from the body very quickly, causing skin temperature to drop. The temperature your body perceives, known as the **wind chill index** or wind chill factor, is lower than the actual temperature. Figure 3-8 shows how air temperature and wind speed combine to give you that chill. You can find information about the wind chill in your area on local or national weather channels and Web sites.

Lastly, keep in mind that sometimes it's just too cold. If the temperature is far below zero or the wind chill is below –20, it's best to stay inside. Select indoor activities until the outside weather warms up.[17]

When it comes to weather, safety is paramount. Prolonged exposure to extreme temperatures of any kind can cause short- and long-term problems; see Table 3-7 for more information.

wind chill index (factor) Guide that combines outside air temperature and wind speed into a single measure of perceived temperature (how cold it feels).

DOLLAR STRETCHER
Financial Wellness Tip
Don't buy bottled water. Water from the tap is safe . . . and free! Carry a reusable bottle, and you'll always have water when you are exercising or on the go. It's a good choice for the environment, too; bottled water produces over a million tons of plastic waste each year.

Temperature (°F)

Calm	40	35	30	25	20	15	10	5	0	−5	−10	−15	−20	−25	−30	−35	−40	−45
5	36	31	25	19	13	7	1	−5	−11	−16	−22	−28	−34	−40	−46	−52	−57	−63
10	34	27	21	15	9	3	−4	−10	−16	−22	−28	−35	−41	−47	−53	−59	−66	−72
15	32	25	19	13	6	0	−7	−13	−19	−26	−32	−39	−45	−51	−58	−64	−71	−77
20	30	24	17	11	4	−2	−9	−15	−22	−29	−35	−42	−48	−55	−61	−68	−74	−81
25	29	23	16	9	3	−4	−11	−17	−24	−31	−37	−44	−51	−58	−64	−71	−78	−84
30	28	22	15	8	1	−5	−12	−19	−26	−33	−39	−46	−53	−60	−67	−73	−80	−87
35	28	21	14	7	0	−7	−14	−21	−27	−34	−41	−48	−55	−62	−69	−76	−82	−89
40	27	20	13	6	−1	−8	−15	−22	−29	−36	−43	−50	−57	−64	−71	−78	−84	−91
45	26	19	12	5	−2	−9	−16	−23	−30	−37	−44	−51	−58	−65	−72	−79	−86	−93
50	26	19	12	4	−3	−10	−17	−24	−31	−38	−45	−52	−60	−67	−74	−81	−88	−95
55	25	18	11	4	−3	−11	−18	−25	−32	−39	−46	−54	−61	−68	−75	−82	−89	−97
60	25	17	10	3	−4	−11	−19	−26	−33	−40	−48	−55	−62	−69	−76	−84	−91	−98

Wind (mph)

Frostbite times   30 minutes   10 minutes   5 minutes

Figure 3-8 **Wind chill index**
Source: NOAA, National Weather Service (2009, December 17). *NWS wind chill index* (http://www.weather
.gov/os/windchill/index.shtml).

TABLE 3-7 TEMPERATURE-RELATED PROBLEMS, SIGNS, AND TREATMENTS

HEAT PROBLEMS		
WHAT IT IS	**WHAT IT LOOKS LIKE**	**WHAT TO DO**
Heat Cramps		
Muscle pains and spasms due to loss of moisture and salt caused by heavy sweating; an early signal that the body is having difficulty with the heat.	Moderate to severe muscle pains and spasms, typically in the abdomen, arms, or legs.	**Help the heated person:** Have the person rest in a cool place in a comfortable position. The person should lightly stretch cramped areas and rehydrate by slowly drinking water—½ glass every 15 minutes. Avoid alcoholic and caffeinated beverages.
Heat Exhaustion		
A mild form of shock, which usually occurs upon heavy exertion in hot, humid places where body fluids are lost through heavy sweating. Blood flow to the skin increases, causing a decrease in blood flow to vital organs. If left untreated, may lead to heat stroke.	Cool, moist, pale, or flushed skin; heavy sweating; headache; nausea or vomiting; dizziness; and exhaustion. Body temperature near normal.	**Help the heated person:** Get the person out of the heat and to a cooler place to rest. Remove or loosen tight clothing and apply cool, wet cloths. The person should rehydrate by slowly drinking water—½ glass every 15 minutes. Avoid alcoholic or caffeinated beverages. Rest in a comfortable position and watch for changes in condition.

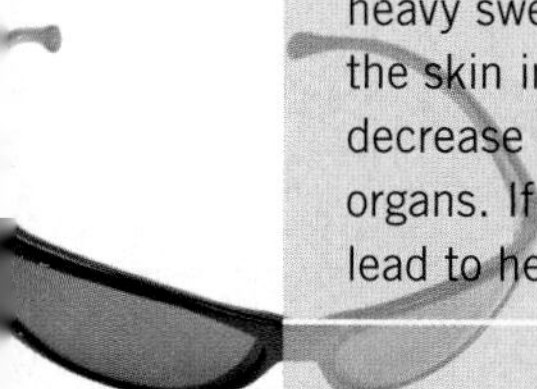

(continued)

TABLE 3-7 *(continued)*

HEAT PROBLEMS *(continued)*		
WHAT IT IS	**WHAT IT LOOKS LIKE**	**WHAT TO DO**
Heat Stroke		
A life-threatening condition that occurs when the body's temperature-control system stops working and sweat (which cools the body) is no longer produced. High temperatures can lead to brain damage and death.	Hot, red skin; changes in consciousness; rapid, weak pulse; rapid, shallow breathing. Body temperature can be as high as 105°F. Skin may feel dry, unless there is sweating from heavy work or exercise.	**Call 9-1-1 and help the heated person:** Move the person to a cooler place to lie down; quickly cool the body by immersing in a cool bath, by wrapping in cool wet sheets and fanning the body, or in any other way possible. **Also:** Watch for signs of breathing difficulties. Do not give anything to drink if there is vomiting or changes in consciousness.

COLD PROBLEMS		
WHAT IT IS	**WHAT IT LOOKS LIKE**	**WHAT TO DO**
Hypothermia		
Abnormally low body temperature due to prolonged exposure to cold, causing the body to lose heat faster and eventually use up the body's stored energy; likely in very cold temperatures but can occur at cool temperatures above 40°F if the person is chilled from rain or sweat or submerged in cold water. 	Shivering, exhaustion, confusion and memory loss, fumbling hands, slurred speech, and drowsiness. In severe cases, unconsciousness, weak pulse, and faint breathing. A body temperature below 95°F indicates an emergency requiring immediate medical attention.	**Seek medical help. If medical care is not available, help the chilled person:** Get the person to a warm room or shelter; remove any wet clothing; warm the center of the body first—including the chest, neck, head, and groin—using an electric blanket, skin-to-skin contact, layers of clothing and blankets, or any means possible. The person should drink warm beverages except those containing alcohol or caffeine. **Also:** Keep the person wrapped warmly including the head and neck even after temperature begins to rise, and get medical attention as soon as possible. If the person is unconscious, check for breathing and pulse. Perform CPR if warranted while warming.
Frostbite		
Injury caused by freezing, most often affecting the nose, ears, cheeks, chin, fingers, or toes; causes a loss of feeling and color in the affected area and can lead to permanent damage; severe cases may require amputation. **Note:** Hypothermia is a more serious medical condition and should be treated prior to any suspected frostbite.	First signs are redness or pain; additional signs include white or grayish-yellow skin, firm or waxy-feeling skin, and numbness.	**Seek medical help. If medical care is not available, help the chilled person:** Get the person to a warm room or shelter. The person should avoid walking on frostbitten feet and toes if possible; do not rub them with snow or massage; warm the affected area by immersing in warm—not hot—water or by using body heat; avoid warming with heating pads, lamps, or the heat from stoves, fireplaces, or radiators as this may unintentionally burn numbed skin.

Source: Adapted from Centers for Disease Control and Prevention. (2005). *Extreme cold: A prevention guide to promote personal health and safety* (http://www.bt.cdc.gov/disasters/winter/pdf/cold_guide.pdf). American Red Cross. (2009). *Be Red Cross ready: Heat wave safety checklist.* Washington, DC: American Red Cross.

Air Quality

Q | Can I exercise on smoggy days?

Often you can, but special precautions may be necessary depending on the level of smog and on whether you have any health conditions that are adversely affected by smog or other types of pollution. Similar to the wind-chill and heat indexes, there is an **air quality index (AQI)** that rates daily air quality and indicates if there is a risk to health. The AQI measures five major air pollutants, including ground-level ozone (the key component of smog), particle pollution, and carbon monoxide. These pollutants can irritate or inflame airways, as well as increase the production of mucus. Breathing may be more difficult, and the body's oxygen-carrying capacity may decrease. Exposure to unhealthy air can aggravate asthma and other respiratory conditions, and it can be dangerous to people with cardiovascular and other diseases.

air quality index (AQI) Guide that rates the quality of the air at a given location; calculated with the ratings of five major air pollutants.

There are six levels in the AQI, each with an associated health risk (Figure 3-9). If pollution is a concern where you live, check the AQI (visit http://www.airnow.gov), and adjust your exercise program as needed. Some tips for exercise in areas with poor air quality include the following:

- Avoid congested streets and heavy traffic, especially heavy bus and truck traffic.
- Work out in the early morning or later in the evening, when it is cooler and smog levels are lowest.
- Avoid combinations of high temperature, high humidity, and a high AQI level.
- Exercise indoors if possible; keep outdoor workouts short.
- Exercise at a lower intensity if needed. Mouth breathing during intense exercise bypasses the nasal passages, which filter air for the body, thereby increasing contact with pollutants.
- Stop exercising immediately and seek medical attention you have difficulty breathing or experience other symptoms.

Injury Prevention and Management

Q | If a person is not physically active at all but would like to be, what is the best way to start?

It's always better to start slowly in order to reduce the risk of injury. More is not better if it is too much! Follow these general safety guidelines for participating in physical activity:[18]

- If you haven't been active in a while, start slowly and build up.
- Learn about the types and amounts of activity that are right for you.
- Choose activities that are appropriate for your fitness level.
- Increase your overall activity time (duration) before switching to activities that take more effort.
- Use the right safety gear and sports equipment, and make sure safety gear and shoes fit well.
- Choose a safe place to do your activity.
- See a health care provider if you have a health problem.

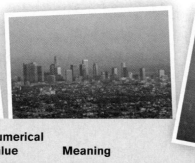

Air Quality Index Levels of Health Concern	Numerical Value	Meaning
Good	0–50	Air quality is considered satisfactory, and air pollution poses little or no risk.
Moderate	51–100	Air quality is acceptable; however, for some pollutants there may be a moderate health concern for a very small number of people who are unusually sensitive to air pollution.
Unhealthy for sensitive groups	101–150	Members of sensitive groups may experience health effects. The general public is not likely to be affected.
Unhealthy	151–200	Everyone may begin to experience health effects; members of sensitive groups may experience more serious health effects.
Very unhealthy	201–300	Health alert: everyone may begin to experience more serious health effects.
Hazardous	>300	Health warnings of emergency conditions. The entire population is more likely to be affected.

Figure 3-9 Air quality index

Source: AIRNow. (2009). *Air Quality Index (AQI)* (http://www.airnow.gov).

TABLE 3-8 COMMON ACTIVITY-RELATED INJURIES

ANKLE SPRAIN	A sprain is a stretching or tearing of ligaments. Ankle sprain most often occurs when the foot turns inward, damaging the tissues on the outside of the ankle.	For immediate care of sprains and strains, use the PRICE method: ■ **Protection:** Protect the joint from further injury. ■ **Rest/restrict activity:** Choose alternate activities that do not place additional stress on the injured area. ■ **Ice:** Cold reduces inflammation; use ice 15–20 minutes every couple of hours for the first 24–48 hours or until the swelling subsides. ■ **Compression:** Use an elastic bandage to apply compression in order to reduce swelling, being careful not to wrap too tightly and hinder circulation. ■ **Elevation:** Elevate the injured area above the heart (especially at night) to help reduce swelling. Over-the-counter medications may be helpful for minor pain relief. See a doctor if there is excessive swelling or pain.
GROIN PULL (STRAIN); HAMSTRING STRAIN	A strain is a stretching or tearing of a muscle or tendon. Groin strains most often occur when pushing off in a side-to-side motion causes damage to the inner thigh. Strains of the hamstrings (the collection of muscles that form the back of the thigh) are typically caused by movements that lead to overstretching of the muscles.	
SHIN SPLINTS	Pain in the shins is most often caused by the trauma of continued running on hard pavement.	■ Rest ■ Ice ■ Over-the-counter pain medication, if needed
KNEE INJURIES	A number of knee injuries can result from overuse, improper exercise, or mishaps. The most common injury is the anterior cruciate ligament (ACL) tear, which typically occurs as a result of sudden stops, sudden changes in direction, or the knee being hit from the side.	■ If an ACL tear is suspected, see a doctor. ACL tears can be serious. Complete tears require surgery.

Source: Adapted from Hoffman, M. (2007). The seven most common sports injuries. *WebMD* (http://men.webmd.com/guide/seven-most-common-sports-injuries).

Q | Are you supposed to pop blisters? READ ONLINE

Q | Is ice or heat better for a sprain?

Ice is often the best initial treatment—but prevention is always best! Most exercise injuries among both new and experienced exercisers are caused by overuse. Knowing the causes and treatments of the most common injuries can reduce lost activity time or prevent injury altogether (Table 3-8). Be sure to obtain medical attention for any serious symptoms, such as significant pain (indicating a possible broken bone or torn ligament), chest pain, fainting, or heat illness.

Q | What can I do about sore muscles?

Sore or stiff muscles are often the result of too much activity, so reducing frequency or intensity of activity might help in the future. To help reduce pain and tenderness, try the following strategies:[19]

■ Massage the affected muscles gently.
■ Engage in some low-intensity movement; for example, if your legs are sore, try slow walking.
■ Take an over-the-counter pain medication.

Allow your body to fully recover after a tough workout—it will help you build more fitness and make your exercise program more enjoyable.

Summary

Physical activity includes all bodily movement. *Exercise* is physical activities conducted specifically to develop components of physical fitness. These components may be performance/skill-related or health-related. Developing a sufficient level of health-related fitness can decrease risk of disease and mortality and increase physical functioning and quality of life.

Physical fitness is developed through planned exercise. Prior to beginning a program, you should be sure you are physically and medically ready for moderate to vigorous activity. Next, you should assess your fitness level to determine an appropriate starting point. Finally, you can establish a program by applying the FITT formula and other training principles. When implementing the program, you should also consider environmental factors, such as weather and air quality, that may affect training.

More to Explore

American College of Sports Medicine
http://www.acsm.org

American Council on Exercise: *Fit Facts*
http://www.acefitness.org/fitfacts

Department of Health and Human Services: *2008 Physical Activity Guidelines for Americans*
http://www.health.gov/paguidelines

President's Council on Physical Fitness and Sports
http://www.fitness.gov

Department of Health and Human Services: *Small Step Adult and Teen*
http://www.smallstep.gov

🖳 **SUBMIT ONLINE**

NAME	DATE	SECTION

Physical Activity Readiness
Questionnaire - PAR-Q
(revised 2002)

PAR-Q & YOU

(A Questionnaire for People Aged 15 to 69)

Regular physical activity is fun and healthy, and increasingly more people are starting to become more active every day. Being more active is very safe for most people. However, some people should check with their doctor before they start becoming much more physically active.

If you are planning to become much more physically active than you are now, start by answering the seven questions in the box below. If you are between the ages of 15 and 69, the PAR-Q will tell you if you should check with your doctor before you start. If you are over 69 years of age, and you are not used to being very active, check with your doctor.

Common sense is your best guide when you answer these questions. Please read the questions carefully and answer each one honestly: check YES or NO.

YES	NO	
☐	☐	1. Has your doctor ever said that you have a heart condition <u>and</u> that you should only do physical activity recommended by a doctor?
☐	☐	2. Do you feel pain in your chest when you do physical activity?
☐	☐	3. In the past month, have you had chest pain when you were not doing physical activity?
☐	☐	4. Do you lose your balance because of dizziness or do you ever lose consciousness?
☐	☐	5. Do you have a bone or joint problem (for example, back, knee or hip) that could be made worse by a change in your physical activity?
☐	☐	6. Is your doctor currently prescribing drugs (for example, water pills) for your blood pressure or heart condition?
☐	☐	7. Do you know of <u>any other reason</u> why you should not do physical activity?

If

you

answered

YES to one or more questions

Talk with your doctor by phone or in person BEFORE you start becoming much more physically active or BEFORE you have a fitness appraisal. Tell your doctor about the PAR-Q and which questions you answered YES.

• You may be able to do any activity you want — as long as you start slowly and build up gradually. Or, you may need to restrict your activities to those which are safe for you. Talk with your doctor about the kinds of activities you wish to participate in and follow his/her advice.

• Find out which community programs are safe and helpful for you.

NO to all questions

If you answered NO honestly to <u>all</u> PAR-Q questions, you can be reasonably sure that you can:

• start becoming much more physically active — begin slowly and build up gradually. This is the safest and easiest way to go.

• take part in a fitness appraisal — this is an excellent way to determine your basic fitness so that you can plan the best way for you to live actively. It is also highly recommended that you have your blood pressure evaluated. If your reading is over 144/94, talk with your doctor before you start becoming much more physically active.

→ **DELAY BECOMING MUCH MORE ACTIVE:**
• if you are not feeling well because of a temporary illness such as a cold or a fever — wait until you feel better; or
• if you are or may be pregnant — talk to your doctor before you start becoming more active.

PLEASE NOTE: If your health changes so that you then answer YES to any of the above questions, tell your fitness or health professional. Ask whether you should change your physical activity plan.

<u>Informed Use of the PAR-Q</u>: The Canadian Society for Exercise Physiology, Health Canada, and their agents assume no liability for persons who undertake physical activity, and if in doubt after completing this questionnaire, consult your doctor prior to physical activity.

No changes permitted. You are encouraged to photocopy the PAR-Q but only if you use the entire form.

NOTE: If the PAR-Q is being given to a person before he or she participates in a physical activity program or a fitness appraisal, this section may be used for legal or administrative purposes.

"I have read, understood and completed this questionnaire. Any questions I had were answered to my full satisfaction."

NAME _____

SIGNATURE _____ DATE_____

SIGNATURE OF PARENT _____ WITNESS _____
or GUARDIAN (for participants under the age of majority)

Note: This physical activity clearance is valid for a maximum of 12 months from the date it is completed and becomes invalid if your condition changes so that you would answer YES to any of the seven questions.

CSEP
SCPE © Canadian Society for Exercise Physiology   Supported by: Health   Santé
                                                                    Canada   Canada

General Personal Health Profile: To help further determine if you have any special exercise concerns, complete as much of the following as possible.

Results from Recent Medical Exams and Tests

Fill in any of the following that you can. Date of last physical/medical exam: ☐

Height: ☐   Weight: ☐   Any recent weight changes? If so, describe: ☐

Blood pressure: ☐   Cholesterol: ☐   Glucose: ☐

Other tests (describe):

Are your immunizations up to date (*circle*)? Yes   No   Not sure

Medical Conditions or Treatments

Any current acute illnesses (cold, flu, etc.):

Any current injuries (sprains, broken limbs, etc.):

Any past illnesses, injuries, surgeries that affect your health today:

Any current chronic conditions (hypertension, diabetes, allergies, depression, etc.):

Prescription medications (name, dosage, how long used):

Over-the-counter medications and supplements (name, dosage, how long used):

Current Health Habits

Activity habits (approximate level of physical activity, any regular exercise):

General eating habits or dietary pattern (e.g., vegetarian, all fast food, no breakfast):

Sleep habits (hours per night on weekdays and weekends):

Tobacco use (type and amount):

Alcohol use (frequency and amount):

Caffeine use (frequency and amount):

Use of other drugs (describe):

Reflecting on Your Results: Did the PAR-Q indicate that exercise is safe for you? Do you think there is anything in your general personal health profile that would be a special concern for starting or continuing a fitness program? If you are not currently active, do you have any additional concerns about becoming more active? (If you're unsure about whether exercise is safe for you, be sure to consult your health care provider.)

SUBMIT ONLINE

NAME	DATE	SECTION

As described in the chapter, a pedometer can be helpful in tracking overall physical activity and your progress toward a goal. Pedometers can also be great motivational tools.

Equipment:

Pedometer

Preparation

- Medical clearance for physical activity (if needed)
- Pedometer accuracy check: Position the pedometer according to the directions that came with it, set the counter to 0, and then take 20 steps at your usual walking pace. If the pedometer reads between 18 and 22, then it is reasonably accurate. If it is outside this range, try it in a different position. If it continues to fail this "test," consider replacing it.

Instructions

1. Determine Your Baseline

Wear the pedometer all day, every day for a week, keeping your usual routine. Record the number of steps you take each day. At the end of the week, calculate your average daily step total. This average will be your baseline.

DAY 1	DAY 2	DAY 3	DAY 4	DAY 5	DAY 6	DAY 7	AVERAGE
Date:	Date:	Date:	Date:	Date:	Date:	Date:	
Steps:	Steps:	Steps:	Steps:	Steps:	Steps:	Steps:	Steps:

2. Set Step Goals

Next, you'll need to set a final goal and then some interim goals. The frequently promoted goal of 10,000 or more steps per day is a reasonable one for most healthy adults (see the table). However, you need to consider your current activity level in setting your goal. For example, if you are currently taking 4,000 steps per day, you'll want to set a more modest goal, at least initially. On the other hand, if you are already averaging 10,000 or more steps a day, then you'll need to set a higher goal in order to increase your level of physical activity. Plan to increase your steps by an average of 500–1,000 per day, every two weeks, until you reach your final goal.

First step goal: _____   Target date: _____

Second step goal: _____   Target date: _____

Third step goal: _____   Target date: _____

Include additional interim step goals as needed for your program.

Final daily step goal: _____   Target date: _____

PHYSICAL ACTIVITY LEVEL BASED ON PEDOMETER TRACKING

AVERAGE STEPS PER DAY	ACTIVITY LEVEL
Less than 5,000	Sedentary
5,000 to 7,499	Low active
7,500 to 9,999	Somewhat active
10,000 to 12,500	Active
Over 12,500	Highly active

Source: Tudor-Locke, C., Hatano, Y., Pangrazi, R. P., & Kang, M. (2008). Revisiting "How many steps are enough?" *Medicine and Science in Sports and Exercise, 40*(7 Suppl): S537–S543.

3. Make a Plan for Increasing Steps

OK, you've set your goal. What strategies will you use to increase your steps by 500–1,000 per day during each segment of your program? Can you add three 10-minute walks to your daily schedule? Can you walk instead of drive when you run certain errands? Develop at least five strategies for increasing daily steps:

1. _____

2. _____

3. _____

4. _____

5. _____

Results: Keep track of your daily steps using the chart at the end of this lab or a different tracking method.

Reflecting on Your Results: After the second week of your program, review your results to date. On average, have you achieved your stepping goal?

Goal for week 1: _____   Average steps week 1: _____

Goal for week 2: _____   Average steps week 2: _____

What strategies are working for you? What barriers have you encountered to meeting your goals?

Do you find that using the pedometer, setting a goal, and tracking your steps motivates you? Why or why not?

Planning Your Next Steps: Keep moving! If you have met your goals so far, briefly describe what you'll do in the coming weeks to keep your program on track. If you haven't met your goals, make any needed adjustments to your program plan, goals, or strategies; briefly describe what you plan to do differently over the next few weeks to improve your chances of success.

```



```

Pedometer Program Variations to Consider

1. **Tracking distance milestones**

   Some people find it motivational to translate their steps into approximate distance measures. Some pedometers allow you to enter an approximate step length and then automatically estimate the distance you travel each day. You can do a similar estimate yourself by walking for a measured distance—say a quarter mile around a track—and counting the number of steps required. You can also use an online mapping site to calculate the distance you traveled during a fitness walk. Calculate the distance you travel each day and plot your path across your state—or the country.

2. **Walk for cardiorespiratory fitness**

   You can use a pedometer-based walking program to improve cardiorespiratory fitness. However, just accumulating more steps over the course of the day won't necessarily increase cardiorespiratory fitness—you must incorporate FITT considerations. The following advice from the U.S. Department of Health and Human Services *2008 Physical Activity Guidelines for Americans* can help you create a walking program to build cardiorespiratory fitness:

   - Episodes of brisk walking that last at least 10 minutes count toward meeting the Guidelines.
   - People generally need to plan episodes of walking if they are to use a pedometer and step goals appropriately.
   - As a basis for setting step goals, it's preferable that you know how many steps you take per minute of a brisk walk. A person with a low fitness level, who takes fewer steps per minute than a fit adult, will need fewer steps to achieve the same amount of walking time. One way to set a step goal is the following:
     1. Determine baseline activity level (see above). Suppose the average is about 5,000 steps a day.
     2. While wearing the pedometer, the person measures the number of steps taken during 10 minutes of an exercise walk. Suppose this is 1,000 steps. Then, for a goal of 40 minutes of walking for exercise, the total number of steps would be 4,000 (1,000 × 4).
     3. To calculate a daily step goal, add the usual daily steps (5,000) to the steps required for a 40-minute walk (4,000), to get the total steps per day (5,000 + 4,000 = 9,000). Each week the person gradually increases the time walking for exercise until the step goal is reached.

   (continued)

TRACKING LOG

WEEK	Steps								
	GOAL	SUN	MON	TUES	WED	THURS	FRI	SAT	WEEKLY AVERAGE
1									
2									
3									
4									
5									
6									
7									
8									
9									
10									
11									
12									

Sources: U.S. Department of Health & Human Services. (2008). *2008 Physical Activity Guidelines for Americans*. ODPHP Publication No. U0036. Rockville, MD: Office of Disease Prevention and Health Promotion. Division of Nutrition Research Coordination of the NIH. (2004). *General Guidance for Pedometer Use* (http://dnrc.nih.gov/move/pedometer_use.shtml). Anders, M. (2006). Do you do 10K a day? *American Council on Exercise Fitness Matters, 12*(4). American College of Sports Medicine. (2005). *Selecting and effectively using a pedometer*. Indianapolis, IN: ACSM.

SUBMIT ONLINE

NAME	DATE	SECTION

"Not enough time." "Bad weather." "I don't want to embarrass myself." What's your reason for not being active—or more active? Complete this quiz and critical thinking activity to help identify and overcome your personal barriers to physical activity.

Equipment: None

Preparation: None

Instructions: Listed below are reasons people give for not getting as much physical activity as they think they should. Please read the following statements and indicate how likely you are to say each of them:

How likely are you to say?	Very likely	Somewhat likely	Somewhat unlikely	Very unlikely
1. My day is so busy now, I just don't think I can make the time to include physical activity in my regular schedule.	3	2	1	0
2. None of my family members or friends like to do anything active, so I don't have a chance to exercise.	3	2	1	0
3. I'm just too tired after work to get any exercise.	3	2	1	0
4. I've been thinking about getting more exercise, but I just can't seem to get started.	3	2	1	0
5. I'm getting older so exercise can be risky.	3	2	1	0
6. I don't get enough exercise because I have never learned the skills for any sport.	3	2	1	0
7. I don't have access to jogging trails, swimming pools, bike paths, etc.	3	2	1	0
8. Physical activity takes too much time away from other commitments—time, work, family, etc.	3	2	1	0
9. I'm embarrassed about how I will look when I exercise with others.	3	2	1	0
10. I don't get enough sleep as it is. I just couldn't get up early or stay up late to get some exercise.	3	2	1	0
11. It's easier for me to find excuses not to exercise than to go out to do something.	3	2	1	0
12. I know of too many people who have hurt themselves by overdoing it with exercise.	3	2	1	0
13. I really can't see learning a new sport at my age.	3	2	1	0
14. It's just too expensive. You have to take a class or join a club or buy the right equipment.	3	2	1	0
15. My free times during the day are too short to include exercise.	3	2	1	0
16. My usual social activities with family or friends do not include physical activity.	3	2	1	0
17. I'm too tired during the week and I need the weekend to catch up on my rest.	3	2	1	0
18. I want to get more exercise, but I just can't seem to make myself stick to anything.	3	2	1	0
19. I'm afraid I might injure myself or have a heart attack.	3	2	1	0
20. I'm not good enough at any physical activity to make it fun.	3	2	1	0
21. If we had exercise facilities and showers at work, then I would be more likely to exercise.	3	2	1	0

Results: To score yourself, enter the circled number in the spaces provided, writing your number for statement 1 on line 1, statement 2 on line 2, and so on. Add the three scores on each line. The barriers to physical activity fall into one or more of seven categories; a score of 5 or above in a category shows that it is an important barrier for you to overcome.

_____ + _____ + _____ = _____   _____ + _____ + _____ = _____
1   8   15   Lack of time   5   12   19   Fear of injury

_____ + _____ + _____ = _____   _____ + _____ + _____ = _____
2   9   16   Social Influence   6   13   20   Lack of skill

_____ + _____ + _____ = _____   _____ + _____ + _____ = _____
3   10   17   Lack of energy   7   14   21   Lack of resources

_____ + _____ + _____ = _____
4   11   18   Lack of motivation or willpower

Reflecting on Your Results: What are your biggest barriers to physical activity? Are they what you expected?

Planning Your Next Steps: Now that you've identified your key barriers, your next step is to develop strategies to overcome them. Refer to the chart of suggestions and brainstorm strategies that might work for you. Choose one of your barriers, and list three strategies for addressing it.

Barrier:

Strategies:

1.

2.

3.

Suggestions for Overcoming Physical Activity Barriers	
Lack of time	Identify available time slots. Monitor your daily activities for one week. Identify at least three 30-minute time slots you could use for physical activity.
	Add physical activity to your daily routine. For example, walk or ride your bike to work or shopping, walk the dog, exercise while you watch TV, park farther away from your destination, etc.
	Select activities requiring minimal time, such as walking, jogging, or stairclimbing.
Social influence	Explain your interest in physical activity to friends and family. Ask them to support your efforts.
	Invite friends and family members to exercise with you. Plan social activities involving exercise.
	Develop new friendships with physically active people. Join a group, such as the YMCA or a hiking club.
Lack of energy	Schedule physical activity for times in the day or week when you feel energetic.
	Convince yourself that if you give it a chance, physical activity will increase your energy level; then, try it.
Lack of motivation	Plan ahead. Make physical activity a regular part of your daily or weekly schedule and write it on your calendar.
	Invite a friend to exercise with you on a regular basis and write it on both your calendars.
	Join an exercise group or class.
Fear of injury	Learn how to warm up and cool down to prevent injury.
	Learn how to exercise appropriately considering your age, fitness level, skill level, and health status.
	Choose activities involving minimum risk.
Lack of skill	Select activities requiring no new skills, such as walking, climbing stairs, or jogging.
	Take a class to develop new skills.
Lack of resources	Select activities that require minimal facilities or equipment, such as walking, jumping rope, or calisthenics.
	Identify inexpensive, convenient resources available in your community (community education programs, park and recreation programs, worksite programs, etc.).

Source: CDC Division of Nutrition and Physical Activity. (1999). *Promoting physical activity: A guide for community action.* Champaign, IL: Human Kinetics.

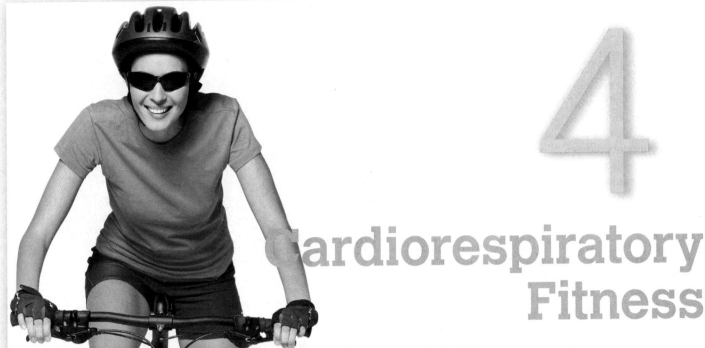

4

Cardiorespiratory Fitness

>> **COMING UP IN THIS CHAPTER**
Learn how your cardiorespiratory system works and what affects its functioning ❯ Discover the benefits of cardiorespiratory fitness ❯ Assess your level of cardiorespiratory fitness ❯ Develop a personalized cardiorespiratory fitness program

Wellness Connections

How does cardiorespiratory fitness relate to overall wellness? A fit heart, lungs, and circulatory system—the physical hallmarks of cardiorespiratory fitness—are keys to health, boosting longevity and reducing the risk of chronic disease. Cardiorespiratory fitness and the activities that build it are linked to emotional and social wellness: Endurance exercise raises mood and self-esteem, reduces stress and anxiety, and provides opportunities for positive interaction with others. It can also be connected to spiritual wellness and personal values. Do you value cardiorespiratory health and fitness—what it allows you to do and how it makes you feel? Is the time you spend developing it, alone or with others, important to you?

Cardiorespiratory fitness also benefits intellectual wellness: It is linked to academic success in the young and improved memory in the old. To boost your brain power throughout life, be active! On the flip side, good use of your intellect, especially your critical thinking skills, can help you maintain a suc-

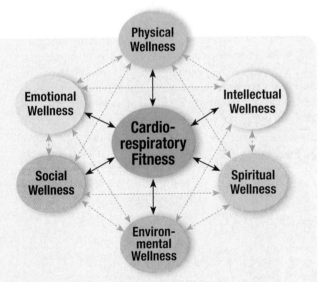

cessful cardiorespiratory-fitness program throughout your life. Environmental wellness also influences, and is influenced by, fitness. A safe and healthy environment can provide many opportunities for endurance activities—as well as a greater variety of activity options. In addition, the more you interact with your environment, the more likely you are to work to provide more positive opportunities for exercise—for you and everyone else in your community.

Cardiorespiratory fitness is key to overall fitness, health, quality of life, and longevity. Numerous studies and reports over the past few decades, including the landmark 1996 Surgeon General's report on physical activity and health,[1] have confirmed the importance of achieving and maintaining a sufficient level of cardiorespiratory fitness. High levels of cardiorespiratory fitness protect against most chronic diseases affecting adults today and also aid in the performance of many daily activities: from yard work and shoveling snow to playing with children, walking to class, and participating in sport and recreation. Even during ancient times, great thinkers saw the value of regular daily exercise. Hippocrates (460–370 BC), the ancient Greek known as the father of medicine, said, "If we could give every individual the right amount of nourishment and exercise, not too little and not too much, we would have found the safest way to health."

Times have changed since 400 BC—and even since the middle of the twentieth century. Today, an abundance of technological conveniences makes our lives somehow better. But this newly engineered world also has the unfortunate side effect of less utilitarian physical activity; we have less need to walk, run, or perform physical labor on a daily basis. In fact, in the United States today, we can accomplish almost everything without ever having to leave our car, office, or home! Because of this decrease in day-to-day utilitarian physical activity, we all have an increased need for regularly planned physical activity, including exercise.

Regular exercise is not always easy to fit into a day. However, we need its benefits. Therefore, this chapter, and this entire text, provides encouragement, tips, motivation, and critical information to help you to understand the benefits of activity, start an exercise program, make exercise more enjoyable, and ultimately improve your health and well-being through exercise. We can't change the society we live in, but with a little knowledge and persistence, we can change how we live in our society.

cardiorespiratory fitness (CRF) Ability of the respiratory and circulatory systems to provide the necessary oxygen to skeletal muscles to sustain regular physical activity; also known as cardiorespiratory endurance, aerobic endurance, and aerobic fitness.

cardiorespiratory (CR) system The heart, lungs, and network of blood vessels.

vascular system The body's network of blood vessels (arteries, veins, capillaries); blood travels in the vascular system throughout the body, delivering oxygen and nutrients and picking up carbon dioxide and other waste products.

Factors Affecting Cardiorespiratory Fitness

By definition, **cardiorespiratory fitness (CRF)** is one of the five health-related components of physical fitness (see Chapter 3). More specifically, CRF is the ability of the circulatory and respiratory systems to sustain physical activity. Cardiorespiratory fitness is also called *cardiorespiratory endurance, aerobic fitness,* or *aerobic endurance.* CRF is a complex physiological state influenced

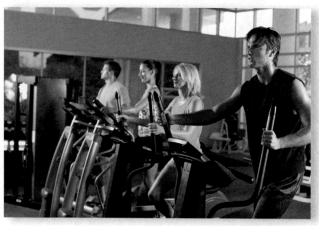

Your cardiorespiratory fitness is influenced by your age, gender, heredity, health status, and, especially, whether you regularly engage in aerobic activities.

by many factors, but everyone has the potential to improve their fitness.

Q I have a friend on the track team. I tried running with her once and felt like I was going to die. Why is it so easy for her?

It probably wasn't always so easy. Your friend has likely been training for many years and has a well-developed cardiorespiratory system. If you have never trained before, regardless of your genetic endowment, the first time you run will be difficult—and your results may be disappointing. The condition of your cardiorespiratory system, including each of the primary players (heart, lungs, blood vessels), is the foundation of CRF. If any of these components are not working optimally, then your CRF cannot be optimal.

The production of sustainable energy, which largely depends on training status and nutrition, is also critical: Without enough energy, there won't be much performance. Disease, genetics, gender, and age are also factors that affect the performance of the cardiorespiratory (CR) system. This section reviews these CRF factors in more detail.

So how does your friend make it look so easy? She has likely been blessed with good genes, no diseases, a strong CR system, and good food—and she's done lots and lots of training.

The Condition of the Cardiorespiratory System

Q So what are the parts of the system that make my muscles go?

The major components of the **cardiorespiratory (CR) system** are the heart, the lungs, and a vast network of blood vessels, collectively called the **vascular system** (Figure 4-1). They each play a role in cardiorespiratory fitness:

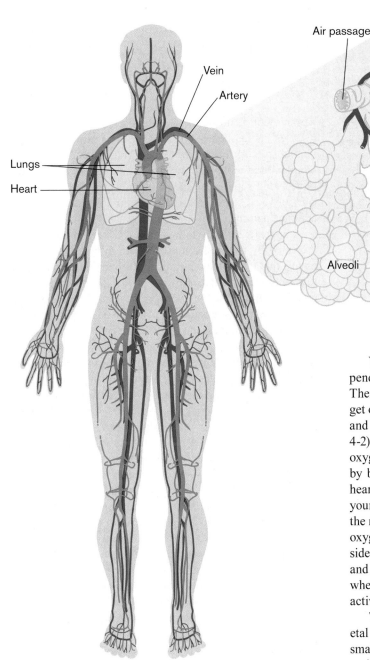

Air passage

Vein

Lungs

Heart

Vein

Capillary

Artery

Alveoli

Figure 4-1 **The cardio-respiratory system.** The cardiorespiratory system consists of the heart, air passages, lungs, and the body's vast network of blood vessels. The exchange of oxygen and carbon dioxide takes place in the alveoli in the lungs. Capillaries are tiny blood vessels that can deliver oxygen from arteries to surrounding tissues and pick up waste products that are carried away by veins.

- The heart acts as a muscle pump to keep blood circulating.
- The lungs take in oxygen from the atmosphere and expel carbon dioxide (a waste product of metabolism); this exchange of gasses takes place in the **alveoli,** tiny sacs deep in the lungs that are covered by blood vessels. Together, your air passages, lungs, and breathing muscles are called the **respiratory system.**
- The vascular system circulates blood to the lungs as well as around the body; it consists of **arteries,** which carry blood away from the heart; **veins,** which carry blood toward the heart; and **capillaries,** tiny blood vessels with walls so thin that substances can pass between the blood they carry and the surrounding cells and tissues.

Your ability to sustain physical activity, or CRF, depends on the availability of oxygen to the working muscles. Therefore, your cardiorespiratory system does its best to get oxygen from the atmosphere, move it through the body and into the skeletal muscles, and then back out (Figure 4-2). First, your lungs must bring oxygen into your body, which you do by breathing. At the same time, your heart pumps oxygen-deficient blood to your lungs, where the blood picks up the newly delivered oxygen. Next, this oxygenated blood returns to the left side of your heart and is pumped out and circulated throughout your body, where it can deliver the oxygen to the active skeletal muscles.

To get from the heart to the skeletal muscles, the blood travels through smaller and smaller arteries and eventually the capillaries. The capillaries are tiny and lie extremely close to muscles, enabling the transfer of oxygen (from blood to muscle) and carbon dioxide (from muscle to blood). Muscle cells use the oxygen to generate energy, a process that produces carbon dioxide as a waste product. The carbon dioxide is picked up by the blood and carried back to the heart via the veins. The carbon dioxide–rich blood then passes quickly through the heart on its way to the lungs, where the carbon dioxide is exhaled and more muscle-enriching oxygen is in inhaled, starting the cycle over again.

alveoli Tiny sacs in the lungs covered by blood vessels, where oxygen is exchanged for carbon dioxide.

respiratory system The lungs, air passages, and breathing muscles; enables gas exchange, with the body taking in oxygen and eliminating carbon dioxide.

arteries Elastic vessels throughout the body that carry oxygen-rich blood away from the heart to the muscles.

veins Elastic vessels throughout the body that store most of the blood at rest and return blood to the heart.

capillaries The smallest blood vessels, with walls so thin that substances can pass between the blood they carry and the surrounding cells and tissues; they are where oxygen and carbon dioxide are transferred between skeletal muscle cells and the bloodstream.

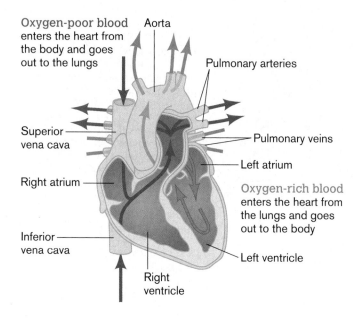

Oxygen-poor blood enters the heart from the body and goes out to the lungs

Aorta

Pulmonary arteries

Superior vena cava

Pulmonary veins

Left atrium

Oxygen-rich blood enters the heart from the lungs and goes out to the body

Right atrium

Inferior vena cava

Left ventricle

Right ventricle

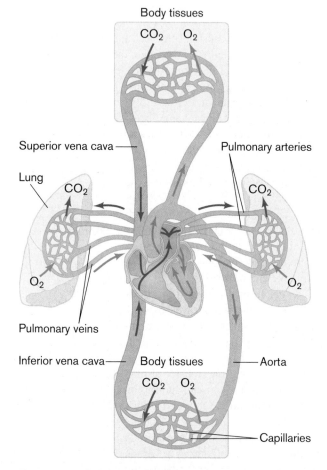

Body tissues

CO_2 O_2

Superior vena cava

Pulmonary arteries

Lung

CO_2

CO_2

O_2

O_2

Pulmonary veins

Inferior vena cava

Body tissues

Aorta

CO_2 O_2

Capillaries

Figure 4-2 **Circulation of oxygen and carbon dioxide.** The heart is a four-chambered pump that circulates blood to the lungs and throughout the body. The right side of the heart pumps oxygen-deficient blood to the lungs, where the blood picks up oxygen. Blood returns to the left side of the heart, where it is pumped out and circulated throughout the body. Oxygen is delivered to active muscles and carbon dioxide and other waste products are picked up and returned to the heart. Carbon dioxide is eliminated when the oxygen-deficient blood is again pumped to the lungs.

Q My heart gets going pretty fast sometimes when I run. Is this normal?

Yes. The body's demand for oxygen constantly changes, and the cardiorespiratory (CR) system must adjust accordingly. When you exercise, your muscles must work harder—and to do so, they need more oxygen. To meet the muscles' increased need for oxygen, your entire CR system must also work harder. Your heart beats faster to get the blood around more quickly. The higher your heart rate, the more blood supplied to the active muscles. But your heart can only beat so fast; therefore, maximum heart rate limits aerobic endurance.

The heart's ability to beat quickly, however, is not determined by training status; it's determined by age. This means that trained and untrained 20-year-olds can achieve the same maximum heart rate, about 200 beats per minute.[2] So training has no effect on maximum heart rate. But training enables you to maintain a high heart rate for a longer time, which in essence is cardiorespiratory fitness!

Q When I try to run fast, why does it feel like I can't breathe?

Your breathing rate, or ventilation, must also adjust to the increased demands of exercise. As described above, your heart rate increases during physical activity, and this increase tends to occur in a linear fashion from rest to maximum exercise. At the same time, ventilation also increases. The increase in ventilation, however, tends to be more curvilinear than the increase in heart rate, especially once you exceed about 50 percent of maximum intensity.[3] Part of the reason for the accelerated breathing rate is the buildup of excess CO_2 in the blood as a by-product of processing more carbohydrate for energy at higher relative intensities. The body's normal response is to increase ventilation to lower the blood CO_2 level. Therefore, the greater the exercise intensity, the faster the ventilation rate. More fit individuals avoid this due to their higher level of conditioning, which allows them to perform at submaximum levels of exercise for a longer period of time.

In a highly conditioned person, the cardiorespiratory system operates very efficiently, matching oxygen supply and demand for a long time. People who are sedentary have a harder time maintaining an adequate oxygen supply, and their CR system can't sustain its effort for very long. The muscles aren't receiving enough oxygen, the heart can't keep up its pace, **lactic acid** and CO_2 accumulate quickly, and ventilation is extremely fast. (Lactic acid is a by-product of energy production in the body, and at high levels, it is associated with muscle fatigue.) To avoid this unpleasant experience, it is wise to exercise at a much lower intensity and use periodic bursts of higher intensity (this is called interval training) to help increase your conditioning level—but more about

lactic acid A chemical by-product of adenosine triphosphate (ATP) production; at low levels, it can be reconverted into ATP, but at high levels it is detrimental to performance.

training programs later. Just know that the increased efficiency of your CR system is a direct function of your increased training: the more you train, the better your system gets, and everyone is capable of improving their CRF.

Q | Is it really true that I shouldn't eat before I exercise?

If you were about to engage in an ultra-marathon then yes, you probably would want to eat something. If you were about to jog two miles, probably not. Is eating before exercise bad for you? It's not necessarily good or bad. However, many people feel uncomfortable if they eat shortly before they go for a jog or some similar type of exercise.

What leads many to advise "Don't eat before exercise" is that the blood vessels open and close during exercise to redirect blood to the active muscles. When you begin to run, your leg muscles crave more oxygen-rich blood, so the body responds by beginning to redirect blood flow away from less critical areas. (Don't worry, your brain is always well protected!) As the intensity of exercise increases, so does the amount of blood being redirected, and the gut is a primary area for redirection. So, as you exercise harder, less is blood available to help you digest food still in your stomach, and this may lead to the dreaded "side stitch,"[4] which can have a detrimental effect on your performance.

So, should you eat before exercising? Well, maybe if you are really, really hungry. But stick to something that is easy to digest (a banana or other fruit, for example) and won't hold you back.

Energy Production

Q | I feel tired all the time. What can I do to get more energy?

There is a difference between how energetic you feel and your body's ability to produce energy. Your energy level mostly depends on the amount of sleep you get, the quality of your diet, how you manage stress, and whether you are regularly physically active. Your body's ability to produce energy, on the other hand, depends on your fitness level, cellular efficiency, and food intake; this energy production is critical for the overall performance of the CR system. For strategies to boost your energy level, see Chapters 3, 8, and 10. To understand how your body produces energy, read on.

Q | What is ATP, and why is it so important for exercise?

Adenosine triphosphate, or ATP, is the fuel for your muscles. All muscles, including the heart muscle, receive their energy from the breakdown of ATP. ATP is formed when the foods we eat are **catabolized** and the energy released is used to manufacture ATP. Catabolism is a metabolic process in which complex substances (proteins, carbohydrates, and fats) are broken down into to simple molecules. These molecules then take part in chemical reactions that release energy in the form of ATP, the fuel for almost every energy-requiring activity of the body.

For ATP production to occur, carbohydrate, protein, or fat must be present. Each of the three substances has unique properties, with carbohydrate being the most readily converted to ATP. Carbohydrates that are circulating in the blood (**glucose**) and carbohydrates that are stored in the liver and skeletal muscle (**glycogen**) can be converted to ATP. There is, however, a limit on how much carbohydrate can be stored. The body's capacity for storing fat is unlimited, but fat is more difficult for the body to catabolize into ATP. The same inefficiency exists for protein, which also has limited storage. Thus, carbohydrates are the body's preferred energy source for ATP creation. However, the limit on carbohydrate storage means that at some point, a person can run out. If you run out during exercise, energy demand is usually too urgent for protein or fat to supply much, so you "hit the wall," signaling a physiological end to your effort. This is not a common experience for the recreational

adenosine triphosphate (ATP) A complex chemical compound formed with the energy released from food; produced in the mitochondria of cells, it is the main energy source of most cellular functions.

catabolize To break down large, complex molecules into simpler compounds through a chemical process; the simpler compounds can be oxidized, releasing energy.

glucose A form of carbohydrate (simple sugar) circulating in the blood; used by the body for energy (ATP) production; derived from food sources.

glycogen A form of stored blood sugar (glucose) typically derived from food; stored in limited amounts in skeletal muscle, liver, and brain.

athlete or even the weekend competitor, but it may occur in marathons, long triathlons, and other ultra-endurance events.

The Three Energy Systems

Energy is the ability to do "work"—lift a heavy weight, take a shower, fly a kite, or ride your bike. It's the cells in your body that do the work, and the cells need energy to accomplish their tasks. In the body, energy is stored in, and released from, chemical bonds: As atoms bond together to form molecules, energy is absorbed; when bonds break apart, energy is released. So when you eat food and break down the molecules in it, energy is released. Similarly, as ATP is created, energy is absorbed, and when ATP bonds are broken, as is done during physical activity, energy is once again released. The body has three systems that can produce ATP and thus create and release energy:

- ATP-CP energy system
- anaerobic energy system
- aerobic energy system

As you'll see in the following sections, each of these three systems involves a different means of producing ATP, and all can assist with energy needs under certain circum-

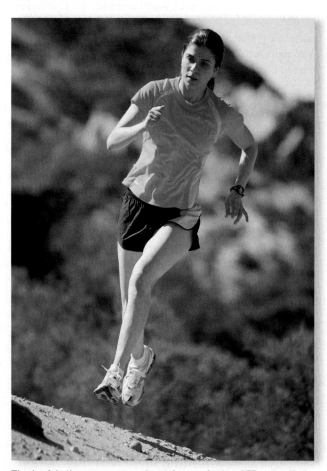

The body's three energy systems for producing ATP are called into action under different circumstances. The aerobic energy system is most important for cardiorespiratory fitness.

stances. The aerobic energy system is most important for developing cardiorespiratory fitness.

Q | Does what I've eaten recently matter for energy during long or short exercise?

ATP-CP ENERGY SYSTEM. The duration of the activity does matter when it comes to what you have eaten lately. When you need a quick burst of energy, your last twenty-four hours of food intake will have little if any effect. But if you want to run a 10K, then your food intake will be important.

The **ATP-CP energy system** is ideally suited for extremely short bouts of activity, such as jumping, throwing, lifting, or sprinting for the bus—anything lasting less than about 10 seconds. This system relies on stored ATP and creatine phosphate to deliver energy. Once these stores run out, which happens quickly, the effort is done. However, this system can replenish itself almost as quickly, and in a matter of a few minutes, you are ready to go again. What you've just eaten plays a minimal role in the ATP-CP system. Having an adequate store of creatine is important, but this is something most people acquire in a typical American diet.

Q | Doesn't anaerobic mean "no oxygen"? Can I hold my breath while working out?

ANAEROBIC ENERGY SYSTEM. Yes, it means "no oxygen"; but no, you probably don't want to hold your breath while you exercise. Anaerobic exercise is possible because the body can produce energy (ATP) for 90–120 seconds without any oxygen being used in the chemical reactions. This is a long time to hold your breath while doing nothing, much less while exercising! And holding your breath has other effects on the body—an increase in blood pressure and a drop in heart rate—that have a bad effect on exercise performance.

Important differences between anaerobic and aerobic energy production include the speed and efficiency of fuel production. In the **anaerobic energy system,** the creation of ATP using the energy within a glucose molecule occurs during a process known as **glycolysis.** This system doesn't require oxygen, but it also doesn't produce much ATP. In fact, glycolysis requires two ATP molecules to get started and in the end produces four ATP molecules— a net gain of only two ATP molecules! Although this doesn't seem particularly efficient, the other end

ATP-CP energy system The immediate energy system that powers activities requiring an immediate burst of energy (no more than 10 seconds); powered by stored adenosine triphosphate (ATP) and creatine phosphate.

anaerobic energy system The system responsible for initial production of energy; it requires glucose but no oxygen and produces a net of only two ATP molecules; it can provide energy for only short periods of physical effort; also known as glycolysis.

anaerobic Occurring in the absence of oxygen.

glycolysis An anaerobic chemical reaction that converts glucose into pyruvate, yielding a small number of adenosine triphosphate (ATP) molecules.

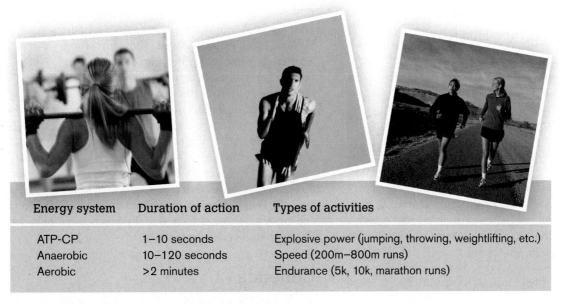

Energy system	Duration of action	Types of activities
ATP-CP	1–10 seconds	Explosive power (jumping, throwing, weightlifting, etc.)
Anaerobic	10–120 seconds	Speed (200m–800m runs)
Aerobic	>2 minutes	Endurance (5k, 10k, marathon runs)

Figure 4-3 **Time span of action of the three energy systems**

pyruvic acid An end product of glycolysis; in aerobic metabolism, pyruvic acid can aid in the production of ATP; in anaerobic metabolism, pyruvate can be converted to lactic acid.

aerobic Occurring in the presence of oxygen.

aerobic energy system The system responsible for most energy production in the body through the Krebs cycle and the electron transport system; takes place in the mitochondria and requires glucose and oxygen; also known as aerobic respiration.

product of glycolysis, **pyruvic acid,** is quite important for further energy production (see the next section).

Under some conditions, pyruvic acid is converted into lactic acid. Although lactic acid can be converted by the liver to a source of fuel for exercise, if it accumulates in the muscles, the result can be fatigue and a noticeable decrease in exercise performance. Well-trained athletes can offset this, because they are better able to convert pyruvic acid to ATP, to use lactic acid as fuel, and to tolerate the uncomfortable effects of lactic acid accumulation. Because the aerobic energy system has the potential to produce lots of lactic acid and is relatively inefficient at generating ATP, glycolysis is best suited for activities that last less than about 90 seconds (Figure 4-3).

Q | What's the difference between aerobic and anaerobic activities?

AEROBIC ENERGY SYSTEM. Both ATP-CP and glycolysis are anaerobic because they occur without oxygen and are best suited for short-term efforts. To build cardiorespiratory fitness (CRF) though, you'll need to perform activities that primarily use the **aerobic** energy system—the one that allows for longer, sustained effort.

The **aerobic energy system** requires oxygen and doesn't produce ATP fast enough for an all-out intense effort. However, when oxygen is present, the potential for ATP production increases dramatically. The pyruvic acid that was

generated at the end of glycolysis is now used to start a complex series of chemical reactions for large-scale ATP production. This process takes place primarily in structures within cells called **mitochondria.** Like the anaerobic energy system, the aerobic energy system also uses up ATP. However, the net production of ATP from the aerobic system is much greater—32 ATP molecules—compared to just two ATP molecules from the anaerobic system.

Production of energy through the aerobic system depends largely on the number of mitochondria in muscle cells and the availability of oxygen. Regular physical training involving aerobic activities like brisk walking, running, and cycling helps in both areas by increasing the number of mitochondria and making the cardiorespiratory system better at delivering oxygen. You also need to have enough carbohydrate present for fuel; a well-rounded diet with plenty of complex carbohydrates will ensure this criterion is met (see Chapter 8).

mitochondria Structures within cells in which most of the chemical reactions in cellular (oxidative) respiration occur; these cellular "power plants" are the location for most adenosine triphosphate (ATP) production.

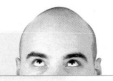

Mind Stretcher
Critical Thinking Exercise

Consider your daily routine. Do you engage in activities that use all three energy systems? Make a list of your typical activities that use the different energy systems. How often do you think you engage in activities using the aerobic energy system?

Diseases Affecting the Cardiorespiratory System

Diseases of the heart, lungs, and blood vessels can all have a negative impact on the cardiorespiratory system. Lung diseases may limit the ability to move air in and out of the body, thereby decreasing the capacity for physical activity. Heart disease takes may forms, including some that decrease the pumping ability of the heart or inhibit blood flow. Although each of these conditions may be an obstacle to an active lifestyle, they need not rule it out. In fact, physical activity is an important part of the management of many chronic diseases. With a physician's clearance, some careful planning and program adjustments, and possibly some supervision, most people with heart or lung disease can remain quite active.

Q | Can you still achieve cardio fitness if you have something like asthma?

ASTHMA AND OTHER CHRONIC RESPIRATORY CONDITIONS. The most common lung diseases are asthma, chronic bronchitis, and emphysema. **Asthma** is characterized by varying and recurring symptoms affecting the air passages (bronchi). During an attack, symptoms of airway inflammation and bronchoconstriction increase, causing difficulty breathing. Asthma may cause chest tightness, wheezing, shortness of breath, and a cough, so you can see how it might make exercise difficult. More and more people are being diagnosed with asthma, yet with certain precautions they can still enjoy aerobic exercise (see the box "Living with Asthma" for more information). Treatment usually includes making healthy lifestyle choices, avoiding triggers for asthma attacks, and taking medications.

Chronic bronchitis and **emphysema,** collectively called chronic obstructive pulmonary disease (COPD), are characterized by chronic, often progressive narrowing of the airways. This makes it difficult for air to move in and out of the lungs. People with emphysema experience a chronic, worsening cough, increased mucus, shortness of breath, and the need to constantly clear their airways. COPD can seriously compromise the cardiorespiratory system and limit a person's CRF. But with the proper medical guidance, someone with COPD can still exercise, although the frequency, intensity, duration, and type of exercise may be restricted.

Q | Is cardio exercise safe after a heart attack?

CARDIOVASCULAR DISEASE. Yes. Many years of research and practice with heart attack survivors has shown not only the safety of regular exercise but also its benefits.[5] Heart attack survivors who engage in regular exercise are much less likely to suffer a second heart attack and don't die quite as young

as those who remain sedentary. Although having a heart attack can kill some heart tissue (part of the muscle pump), exercise can still be performed, sometimes at a relatively high level. Although a physician's clearance is of utmost importance, heart attacks and other forms of heart disease should not be deterrents to physical activity.

There are many forms of heart disease (see Chapter 11 for details), and each creates a different challenge for exercise. Some types of disease affect the heart muscle itself, reducing its pumping ability. Other forms affect the blood vessels and decrease the flow of blood. Still others affect the valves or the electrical conduction system. Whatever form they have, people with heart disease can still perform and enjoy exercise, as long as a physician clears them and they take the needed precautions.

Genetics

Q | Is liking exercise inherited? I don't really like to exercise and neither do my parents.

How much you *like* to exercise doesn't come from your genes. However, the attitudes and beliefs of the family you grew up in probably influenced your likes and dislikes.

Researchers have established that no more than about 50 percent of our ability to *improve* our cardiorespiratory fitness is inherited.[6] The other half is based on what we do—how active we are and what types of activities we engage in. These same researchers also showed that we each have a different ability to adapt to training. If we all did the same amount of training, a few of us would achieve a very high level of fitness, but others would not improve much at all. However, the vast majority of people are between these two extremes and can improve their cardiorespiratory fitness through training and develop a very healthy cardiorespiratory system. Following a reasonable training program enables almost all of us to see noticeable increases in our fitness, which in turn makes us feel more energetic throughout the day, sleep better at night, and be more attentive in class.

Ultimately, regardless of your genetic disposition, regular exercise can benefit you, now and in the future. Don't let your dad's attitude, or your friends', stop you from engaging in one of the healthiest behaviors available to you. And don't compare yourself to others. Focus on the positive changes you experience as you increase fitness rather than how you stack up against others who may have been training much longer, competed in high school, or perhaps even have slightly better fitness genes. Go out, have fun, and get fit!

asthma A medical condition characterized by inflammation and constriction of air passages in the lungs, which makes breathing difficult; in some cases it can be exacerbated by exercise.

chronic bronchitis Persistent inflammation of the bronchi (air passages) in the lungs.

emphysema A condition characterized by progressive destruction of the alveoli, making breathing, especially exhalation, difficult; with chronic bronchitis, known as chronic obstructive pulmonary disease (COPD).

Living with . . .

Asthma

People with asthma can and do exercise regularly. In fact, people with asthma can become elite athletes, including Jackie Joyner-Kersee, Olympic gold medalist in the heptathlon and long jump; marathon world-record holder Paula Radcliffe; and Olympic swimmer Mark Spitz. Appropriate asthma management includes exercise and other physical activities as part of a healthy lifestyle. Check with your doctor before getting started, and he or she will help you use your medications correctly, avoid triggers, and monitor asthma signs and symptoms so that you can achieve all your exercise goals.

People with asthma can participate in a variety of physical actives. Those involving short, intermittent bursts of activity (gymnastics, volleyball, and softball, for example) are generally well tolerated. Activities requiring extended activity (jogging, cycling, soccer, and basketball, for example) may be more difficult but don't need to be avoided. Cold-weather activities (ice hockey, ice-skating, skiing, and so on) may also present some problems because cold, dry air can trigger an asthma attack. Many people with asthma prefer swimming because it is done in warm, moist air.

The general exercise prescription for a person with asthma is not much different from that for any one else. However, exercising with asthma does require some planning and precautions, including the following:

- Always use your pre-exercise asthma inhaler before beginning exercise.
- Perform an extended warm-up and cool-down.
- If the weather is cold, exercise indoors or wear a mask or scarf over your nose and mouth.
- If you have allergic asthma, avoid exercising outdoors when the pollen count or air pollution level is high.
- Limit exercise when you have a cold or other viral infection.
- Don't overdo the exercise.

If you begin to experience asthma symptoms during exercise, stop and repeat your pre-exercise inhaled medication. If your symptoms completely go away, you may slowly restart your workout. If your symptoms return, stop, repeat your quick-relief medication, and call your health care provider.

Asthma is not a reason to avoid exercise. With effective asthma treatment and care, you should be able to enjoy the benefits of an exercise program without experiencing asthma symptoms.

For more information on exercise and asthma, see the American College of Allergy, Asthma, and Immunology at http://www.acaai.org/patients/resources/asthma/Pages/exercising-with-allergies-asthma.aspx.

Finally, a reminder for those lucky few who seem to be naturally fit: Even though you may be relatively fit now without doing anything special, by skipping exercise, you miss out on all the health benefits associated with regular physical activity. And remember that being thin is not the same as being fit! Your current fitness level and body weight may not last, because the process of aging, starting as early as 25 or 30, levels the playing field. It's best to start a lifetime program of exercise now to improve and maintain your fitness level.

Gender

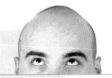

Mind Stretcher
Critical Thinking Exercise

Was exercise part of your life when you were growing up? How much did your parents exercise? Do you think you're influenced by their attitudes and habits? How will you motivate your own children or younger family members to exercise?

Q | Can gender have an effect on cardio fitness?

It can, but it's all relative. Women and men have the same ability to increase their levels of cardiorespiratory fitness, but men can typically achieve a higher absolute level of cardiorespiratory functioning.[7] On average, men have larger hearts and lungs, greater blood capacity (the ability to deliver more oxygenated blood), and more skeletal muscle mass, especially in the upper body. These differences are almost entirely a function of the difference in size between the genders, and they allow men to achieve a higher level of performance. A

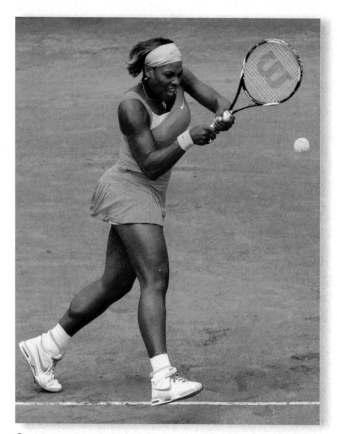

On average, men have larger hearts and lungs and can achieve a higher absolute level of cardiorespiratory fitness. However, women can and do become extremely fit, and both men and women can improve their cardiorespiratory functioning for better health and wellness.

larger heart can pump more blood, bigger lungs can bring in more oxygen, and a greater muscle mass can produce more force—all adding up to better performance. However, on a relative scale or when the difference in body size is taken into account, there is really no difference in fitness between the genders; the differences are only in terms of absolute performance. Women can and do become very fit.

The important message is that whether you're male or female, regular physical activity will improve cardiorespiratory functioning to a level that promotes lifetime wellness, regardless of performance.

Use and Age

Q | My dad is 58 and wants to start exercising. Is he too old?

You're only as old as you feel, and if your dad feels like exercising, he should go for it! A natural result of aging is a steady decline in the functioning of the cardiorespiratory system. However, for people who participate in regular physical activity, the rate of decline is much less than that of their sedentary counterparts. Therefore, a well-conditioned 60-year-old has the same, or better, car-

dioresipratory fitness (CRF) as a sedentary 30-year-old.[8] And it's never to late to start a fitness program, as fitness can increase at any point in the lifespan.[9] Fortunately, there is no evidence that reaching a particular age makes someone too old to exercise.

Most people associate the phrase "use it or lose it" with muscle fitness, but it also holds true for cardiorespiratory fitness. Although it is difficult to see the CR system become less or more fit (at least compared to seeing your muscles change in size or strength), your body is constantly doing what you ask of it. If you ask very little of it, then that is what it will do, making any greater physical effort difficult. Remaining sedentary offsets many of the health benefits associated with physical activity and healthy aging. Your heart doesn't pump as strongly, your lungs don't bring in as much oxygen, your overall blood volume decreases, you have fewer mitochondria, and your arteries stiffen. These deleterious effects all work together to keep your CRF low, which increases your chance of developing heart disease, diabetes, and high blood pressure and dying prematurely (more on this in the next section of the chapter).

If you still aren't convinced that people can exercise at all ages, check out your local Senior Olympics to see runners, jumpers, swimmers, cyclists, and others competing well into their seventies and eighties! But you don't have to be a competitive athlete. Many activities can be enjoyed throughout the lifespan regardless of chronological age, and all bring numerous health and fitness benefits—as well as enjoyment and improved quality of life.

Benefits of Cardiorespiratory Fitness

Increased cardiorespiratory fitness (CRF) may be one of the best investments you can make for your health and wellness. Numerous research studies have established the strong inverse relationship between CRF, chronic disease, and all-cause mortality. Even the most unfit person will reap immediate benefits from just a slight increase in cardiorespiratory fitness. Increasing your fitness requires only a small financial investment and not too much of your time. But the benefits are tremendous!

While attending college, many of you have free access to a campus fitness or wellness center, safe and secure walking paths, personnel (exercise-science faculty, wellness-center staff) who can help you develop an exercise plan, and plenty of friends with a similar interest to help you stay motivated. College offers extra opportunities to be more active; an example of this incidental physical activity is walking across campus several times a day. You don't plan it and probably don't even think of it as activity, yet you reap all the benefits of walking about three miles a day, the typical distance for a residential student.

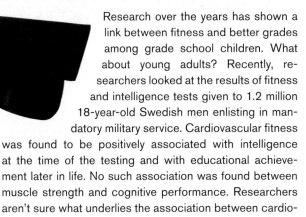

Research Brief

Cardiorespiratory Fitness and Academic Success

Research over the years has shown a link between fitness and better grades among grade school children. What about young adults? Recently, researchers looked at the results of fitness and intelligence tests given to 1.2 million 18-year-old Swedish men enlisting in mandatory military service. Cardiovascular fitness was found to be positively associated with intelligence at the time of the testing and with educational achievement later in life. No such association was found between muscle strength and cognitive performance. Researchers aren't sure what underlies the association between cardio-respiratory fitness and cognition, but they think CRF affects brain function—possibly through improved blood flow to the brain.

What does this mean for you? If you are a young adult, make time for cardiorespiratory exercise even if you are busy—it may boost both your brain power and your grades. And it's just as important for older adults: Other research has found that exercise benefits cognitive function in older adults as well.

Source: Aberg, M. A., and others. (2009). Cardiovascular fitness is associated with cognition in young adulthood. *Proceedings of the National Academy of Sciences, 106*(49), 20906–20911.

Improved Performance

Q | My boyfriend made me do an online fitness survey, and it said my VO_{2max} was 41. What does that mean?

VO_2 is an abbreviation for the volume of oxygen (O_2) consumed over time. This is a measure of your body's ability to take in and utilize oxygen. In fitness magazines and journals, you will see this term or VO_{2max}, which is the absolute maximum amount of oxygen you can consume during peak exercise. VO_{2max} is the term used to refer to a person's peak fitness level—or what was measured on the online fitness survey. To improve cardiorespiratory fitness, you need to increase your body's ability to take in and utilize oxygen.

So, what does your VO_{2max} score of 41 mean? The typical college female has a VO_{2max} in the high 30s, so you're on the high side of average. In comparison, college males are normally in the mid 40s, and very fit aerobic athletes on campus are in the high 60s or even the low 70s. World-class endurance athletes usually have a VO_{2max} in the low to mid 70s.[10]

To perform an aerobic task, the active muscle must have oxygen. How well air is brought into the lungs, delivered to the muscles, and used at the muscle site all contribute to a person's VO_{2max} level. The bigger the lungs, the greater the oxygen intake and the higher the VO_2. The higher the VO_{2max}, the greater the performance potential—such as running faster for a longer time. Because VO_2 is largely determined by the amount of oxygen you can bring into your lungs, the unit of measure for VO_2 is milliliters of oxygen per kilogram of body weight per minute (ml/kg/min.). This measure is a way of correcting for differences in body size. Because men are usually bigger than women, they have a higher absolute VO_2. But if the absolute volume of oxygen is corrected for body size, then we can fairly compare the fitness level of any two people, regardless of size or gender. Later in the chapter you'll learn about techniques for measuring your own VO_{2max}.

VO₂ (volume of oxygen consumed) The absolute amount of oxygen that can be consumed and used by an individual. Usually reported in liters per minute and highly correlated to body size.

VO₂max (maximum volume of oxygen consumed) The maximum amount of oxygen that can be consumed and used by skeletal muscles, typically reported in terms of milliliters of oxygen consumed per minute per kilogram of body weight (ml/kg/min); considered one of the best measures of aerobic fitness.

Q | Every time I start an exercise program I feel worse! Does it ever get better?

Yes, it gets better. For some people, it takes a while before they (and their body) are comfortable with a new exercise routine—anywhere from two weeks to three months. Don't try to go from couch potato to serious jogger in one week. Set realistic short-term goals and ease into it: Start with slow-to-moderate walking. Then gradually mix in some more vigorous activity (brisk walking or slow jogging) during a 20- to 30-minute walk. It takes just two or three spurts, 1–2 minutes long, of more vigorous activity to stimulate and challenge your CR system. Over time, you can add more spurts or make them longer. You'll start feeling comfortable before long, and your newfound cardiorespiratory fitness will have you feeling better throughout the day.

Q | How much do I need to run to be able to do a 5K pretty fast?

It depends. You need to consider many variables when training for and competing in a 5K or any other endurance event. First is the amount of time you have available for training. Second is your current level of fitness. If you have never before even run to catch the bus, then you have a lot of training ahead of you. If you already jog thirty minutes frequently, just a little fine-tuning is needed.

Your training must be based on the overload principle, as described in Chapter 3. Similar to muscle training—in which the more weight you lift or push, the stronger you become—the farther or faster you run, the more aerobically fit you will become. By training both harder and longer, you force your aerobic system (heart, lungs, blood vessels, muscle cells, and so forth) to adapt to a new challenge, thereby increasing their capacity to handle more work.

What actually happens in your body? The changes in response to training include the following:

- Your heart muscle will grow stronger, which allows you to pump more blood to the active muscles.
- Your lungs will become more efficient at bringing in large volumes of oxygen-rich air, which can then be transported around the body by your newly strengthened heart.
- Your blood vessels will become more elastic, meaning they can expand to a greater degree to allow more blood to the active muscles, while at the same time quickly constricting and shunting blood away from noncritical areas during exercise.
- Your cells will develop more mitochondria, which become more efficient at converting pyruvate into ATP, so you have the energy to sustain all of this exercise!

These changes add up to a fit individual, and depending on the specifics of training, someone who can compete in endurance activities.

Q | Since the heart is a muscle, can you bulk it up?

Actually you can. The heart is a muscle, and even though its properties aren't exactly the same as skeletal muscle, the heart can grow in size, known as hypertrophy. The left ventricle is the main pumping chamber, and healthy people engaged in regular aerobic exercise have a thicker left ventricle than sedentary people do. In addition, regular exercise allows the heart muscle to remain flexible or elastic, and the left ventricular cavity remains quite large. Aerobic exercise enables the heart to pump more blood per beat, or have greater **stroke volume.** A higher stroke volume leads to more blood pumped per minute, or higher **cardiac output.**

Both stroke volume and cardiac output are signs of the heart's strength and fitness. One of the main reasons many endurance athletes have an extremely low resting heart rate, sometimes even in the mid 30s, is a very high stroke volume. In essence, their heart can pump as much blood in one beat as a sedentary person's heart can in two

stroke volume The amount of blood pumped by the heart in each beat.

cardiac output The amount of blood pumped by the heart per minute.

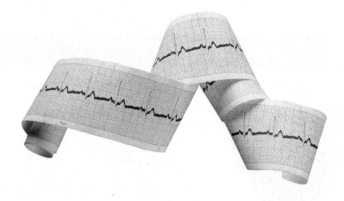

beats; therefore, the highly trained heart doesn't need to beat as often. A low resting heart rate is an indicator of cardiorespiratory fitness and is also linked to a reduced risk of several types of chronic disease.

Reduced Risk of Disease

Q | My mom's doctor told her to walk every day to help lower her blood pressure. Does just walking really work?

Yes, absolutely! Regular physical activity can lower resting blood pressure by as much as 5–7 points in people with high blood pressure,[11] which may be enough to minimize the need for medication. However, anyone with high blood pressure, or hypertension, should check with his or her doctor before starting an exercise program. Daily walks are a great way to start lowering blood pressure. For people whose blood pressure is currently in the healthy range, regular exercise can keep it from rising with age.

According to *2008 Physical Activity Guidelines for Americans,* daily physical activity can also reduce the risk of chronic diseases and improve many other conditions.[12] Although the mechanism affecting each of these conditions is different, here is a brief summary of the positive role physical activity can play:

- *Improved blood pressure:* Physical activity leads to a more efficient heart muscle and more elastic blood vessels.
- *Improved cholesterol levels:* Physical activity increases HDL, or good cholesterol, and lowers LDL, or bad cholesterol.
- *Reduced risk of type 2 diabetes:* Physical activity makes the skeletal muscles more efficient at using blood sugar, helping to keep blood sugar levels in the healthy range.
- *Reduced risk of certain cancers:* Physical activity affects sex hormone levels, cellular metabolism, and the rate of digestion, and it helps control body fat; these changes reduce the risk of cancers of the colon and breast and possibly other sites.
- *Reduced risk of osteoporosis:* Exercise that is weight bearing (such as walking) increases bone density and reduces the risk of fractures.

■ *Reduced risk of cardiovascular disease (CVD):* Elevated blood pressure, unhealthy cholesterol levels, and type 2 diabetes are all major risk factors for CVD, so by improving these, physical activity reduces overall CVD risk.

Figure 4-4 summarizes the benefits and effects of cardiorespiratory fitness. See Chapter 11 for more on preventing chronic diseases.

Q | Will exercise make me live longer?

Although nothing is guaranteed to make you live longer, plenty of evidence suggests that, yes, regular cardiorespiratory exercise may increase longevity and quality of life. Data collected for more than twenty years by the Cooper Institute of Aerobics Research in Dallas, Texas indicates that people who have at least a moderate level of cardiorespiratory fitness (CRF) have almost *half* the rate of premature death from any cause ("all-cause mortality") compared to those who are just barely fit. The Aerobic Center Longitudinal Study (ACLS) has tracked the CRF, disease development, and death rates of more than 30,000 men and women.[13] The ACLS researchers divided participants into five fitness categories, from "least fit" to "most fit" (Figure 4-5). The most dramatic difference in all-cause mortality, almost 50 percent, was between category 1 (least fit) and category 2 (minimally fit). This means that even a small amount of physical activity has huge health benefits, especially compared to remaining sedentary. Therefore, if you want to minimize your risk of dying prematurely, get out and get fit—even just a little fit!

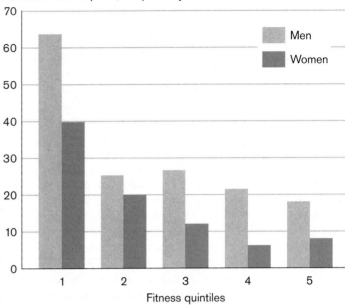

All-cause deaths per 1,000 person years

Figure 4-5 **Cardiorespiratory fitness and all-cause mortality.** Analysis of mortality rates during 10-year follow-up of Aerobics Center Longitudinal Study (ACLS). **Source:** Blair, S. N., & Wei, M. (2000). Sedentary habits, health, and function in older women and men. *American Journal of Health Promotion, 15,* 1–8.

Body Composition

Q | How much exercise do I need to lose some serious weight before spring break?

Well, if spring break is next week, you're out of luck. The healthiest weight loss (that is both safe and sustainable) averages about one or two pounds a week. Do you consider this "serious weight"? Added up over time, it can be significant, but weight loss is difficult to maintain. A one-pound change in body weight represents a change of 3,500 calories through diet or exercise, or both. If you want to lose one pound, you must consume fewer calories or burn more calories, for a net loss of 3,500 calories. (Flip the equation if you want to gain a pound—increase your caloric intake and reduce your caloric expenditure.) Walking and jogging burn around 80–110 calories per mile, so it takes a while to lose weight through exercise alone. For weight loss, many people find it easier initially to make dietary changes. However, weight loss either plateaus quickly or becomes difficult to maintain. Therefore, a combination approach is usually most successful:[14] Including exercise

Increase

Maximal oxygen consumption
Heart muscle strength
Stroke volume
Cardiac output
Lung efficiency
Number of mitochondria
Elasticity of blood vessels
Bone density
Mood
Sleep quality
HDL ("good cholesterol")

LDL ("bad cholesterol")
Resting heart rate
Resting blood pressure
Risk of heart disease
Risk of diabetes
Risk of certain cancers
Risk of osteoporosis
Depression
Stress and anxiety

Decrease

Figure 4-4 **Summary of the effects and benefits of cardiorespiratory exercise**
Source: U.S. Department of Health and Human Services. (2008). *2008 physical activity guidelines for Americans,* Chapter 2 (http://www.health.gov/paguidelines/guidelines/default.aspx#toc).

in your weight loss program burns additional calories and adds many other fitness and health benefits.

Q | What is the best weight-loss exercise?

A former president of the American College of Sports Medicine (ACSM) joked that a dog is the best exercise equipment, because you have to walk it a few times each day![15] If you don't have a dog, you can use a treadmill or an elliptical machine, or just try walking, cycling, jogging, or skating. There is no perfect exercise—the best choice is the one you'll do regularly, whether your goal is weight loss or cardiorespiratory fitness. Any exercise or physical activity will burn more calories than being sedentary, and if you want to lose weight, you need to burn some additional calories. The ACSM recommends that initial weight-loss goals be no more than 10 percent of current body weight and that a healthy diet be combined with regular exercise to achieve this goal.[16] See the discussion of program planning later in this chapter for more information on selecting appropriate exercises for weight loss. For much more on achieving and maintaining a healthy weight, refer to Chapter 9.

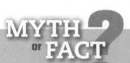

MYTH or **FACT?**

Walking and running burn the same number of calories per mile.

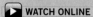 WATCH ONLINE

Stress Management and Improved Emotional Wellness

Q | I feel better after exercising. Why is that?

Exercise or almost any type of physical activity can cause feelings of elation, particularly when it is moderate in duration and intensity. Plenty of research indicates that people who exercise regularly are less prone to depression, have greater self-efficacy and more self-confidence, suffer fewer acute illnesses, and manage stress more effectively.

Although the reasons are difficult to pinpoint, several mechanisms have been proposed to explain how exercise affects emotional wellness:

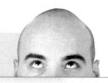

Mind Stretcher
Critical Thinking Exercise

Do you exercise because you like it or because you think you should? Is there any form of exercise that you do just for the love of it? Has exercising ever made you feel elated?

- *Distraction:* Exercise is a distraction from whatever has been making us feel sad, mad, blue, or depressed. By engaging in this healthy, distractive behavior, we forget about our worries and our mood is lifted, at least temporarily.
- *Increased temperature:* Endurance exercise, even at low levels, increases the body's core temperature, thereby allowing our muscles, and in essence our whole being, to relax.
- *Changes in brain chemistry:* Exercise increases the circulation of certain mood-enhancing chemicals (neurotransmitters and endorphins) that make us feel better.

It is likely that a combination of all these factors and others not yet known provide the positive emotional benefits of CR exercise. Benefits have been documented both after a single bout of activity (immediate short-term mood enhancement) and among people who regularly exercise (much lower rates of depression).

Self-efficacy benefits from regular physical activity (see Chapter 1), but it's difficult to determine whether the increase in self-efficacy or the regular exercise behavior comes first. Regardless, being regularly active seems to enhance how people feel about themselves. If you feel overwhelmed when you think about exercise, try adding little bursts of 10–15 minutes of activity at a couple points during your day. The mood-enhancing effects will provide immediate benefits, and you'll likely be more inspired to be active.

Assessing Your Cardiorespiratory Fitness

Assessments for cardiorespiratory fitness come in all shapes and sizes: Some are lengthy, costly, or require extensive equipment and supervision; others are simple to perform, can be done on your own, and are free. Fitness tests can be valuable, but they're not necessary before you start exercising or increasing your CR fitness.

Types of Cardiorespiratory Fitness Tests

Q | How do my friend and I figure out who is more fit?

If you really want to know, both of you can take the same cardiorespiratory fitness (CRF) assessment. Aside from competing with your friends, what is the point of taking one of these tests? Usually to motivate yourself. Maybe you are not as fit as you thought, and the test will motivate you to get more fit. Maybe you are required to have your fitness assessed for a course you are taking. Maybe you just want to know where your fitness level is today, to see if it improves over time as you exer-

Research Brief

Cardiorespiratory Activity and Psychological Health in College Students

Suicide is the third leading cause of death among Americans ages 10–24 years, and about 1,000 college students die by suicide each year. Researchers recently explored the association between physical activity and mental health in college students. They looked at data on over 40,000 students collected from the National College Health Assessment survey and found that physical activity, especially cardiorespiratory fitness activity, was linked to a reduced risk of hopelessness, depression, and suicidal behavior among college students. Students who were not active were

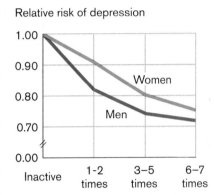

Relative risk of depression

Weekly aerobic activity

Relative risk of depression according to weekly level of aerobic activity

more likely to report feeling hopeless or depressed; rates of depression and thoughts about suicide declined as the amount of time spent in aerobic activity increased.

This study adds to the evidence that cardiorespiratory fitness has many positive psychological health benefits. See Chapter 10 for additional information on depression and suicide.

Source: Taliaferro, L. A., Rienzo, B. A., Pigg, R. M., Jr., Miller, M. D., & Dodd, V. J. (2008). Associations between physical activity and reduced rates of hopelessness, depression, and suicidal behavior among college students. *Journal of American College Health, 57*(4), 427–435.

cise more regularly. Several types of CRF tests are briefly described in this section; details for some common field tests are found in Lab Activity 4-1.

METABOLIC CART MEASUREMENT. Some college exercise-science departments have expensive and specialized equipment that can accurately measure VO_2. The equipment includes a metabolic cart and oxygen and carbon dioxide analyzers. It is a "maximal test" in that the person being tested wears a sealed mouthpiece and runs to exhaustion on a treadmill. The test lasts 8–15 minutes, and both the speed and grade of the treadmill are increased frequently in an attempt to reach the point of exhaustion. Once the person can't go any further, the test ceases. For people who are already fit and active, this can be a fun challenge. But for people who are currently sedentary, it may be a very unpleasant experience, and they would be

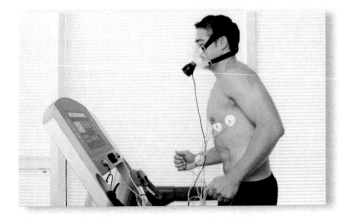

better off with a test that doesn't require working to the point of exhaustion.

FIELD TESTS. Although less accurate than a laboratory test, there are several field tests that are easier and less expensive to administer:

- The Rockport walk test estimates cardiorespiratory fitness (CRF) based on heart rate after walking a mile as quickly as possible. A faster time and a lower heart rate indicate higher fitness. This simple test requires only a timing device and a measured track.
- The 1.5-mile run-walk test is similar to the Rockport test. CRF is estimated based on the time it takes to complete the distance by either running or walking.
- The 3-minute step test involves stepping up and down a 16.25-inch step for 3 minutes at a constant rate. At the completion of the stepping, heart rate is measured for 15 seconds. The lower the heart rate, the better the ability to recover from an aerobic task, which is a sign of better CRF.

See Lab Activity 4-1 for more information on completing one of these field tests.

RESTING HEART RATE. A final method for assessing cardiorespiratory fitness is by measuring true resting heart rate (RHR). Generally speaking, trained people have a much lower RHR than untrained ones, so people with the lowest resting heart rates are likely to be the most fit. For reference, normal RHR is considered to be 60–100 beats per minute (bpm) for both genders, though women's heart rates are typically about 10 bpm higher than men's. Very fit male athletes have an RHR in the low 40s or even the high 30s, and well-trained females are about 10 bpm higher. As you know, genetics play a role in determining fitness, so RHR may not be an extremely accurate assessment of fitness, but it is simple to determine, easy to track, and generally reliable.

To accurately measure true RHR, count your heart rate for one full minute after you've quietly woken in the morning from a restful night's sleep. If you sleep poorly or are awakened suddenly by an alarm clock, your heart rate will be somewhat higher than your true RHR. Heart rates taken at other times of the day, even if you have been inactive, will be noticeably higher than your true resting rate.

Evaluating Assessment Results and Setting Goals

Q | How much can I really improve? How much do I really need to improve?

Improvements in cardiorespiratory fitness (CRF) vary for everyone. The type of training you do, the food you eat, and the genes you were born with are among the variables that determine your rate of improvement and how much improvement you can expect. Aerobic capacity can increase by about 10–30 percent over the course of a fitness program, depending on factors such as the starting level of fitness.[17]

The previous sections have discussed the physiology of CRF and how it improves. In terms of manipulating the FITT equation (see Chapter 3), science tells us that it's best to progress no more than 10 percent per week in frequency, intensity, or time—and probably not all at once.[18] Although 10 percent might not seem like much, it allows you to gradually improve your VO_2 while minimizing your risk of physical and psychological setbacks. Remember the principle of progressive overload discussed in Chapter 3, and think about small achievable steps. Most people don't want to—or can't—improve their VO_2 too much. It takes a lot of work and great genes to have a VO_{2max} of about 60 ml/kg/min. or higher. Therefore, increases of 10–20 percent are realistic for most people. Strive initially for the VO_{2max} of the typical college female (high 30s) or male (mid 40s). If you are already there, try to go 10 percent beyond that. For males this would mean shooting for a VO_{2max} in the upper 40s, and for a female somewhere in the low to mid 40s.

If you have had a recent fitness assessment, you can use it as your personal baseline or compare your results to others like you. Are you a competitive person? If so, you might be motivated by comparing your results to other people's or to national averages for your age and gender (see the tables in Lab Activity 4-1). Or do you just want to know where you stand? However you use it, your fitness score will help you see your improvement along the way, which itself is a great motivator.

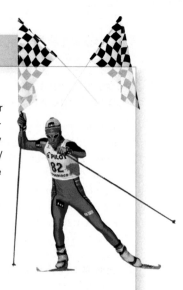

Q | How often should I do an assessment to check for improvement in my cardio fitness?

The rate of progress depends on the individual, the amount of training, and the initial fitness level. Someone who is already at a high level of fitness will not show much improvement, especially in a short time. Conversely, a new exerciser with a low level of fitness may show great gains rather quickly. The longer you stick to your exercise routine and the higher your fitness level becomes, the slower the changes come. For many people, once most fitness goals are met, the purpose of continued training is to maintain all the wonderful gains in fitness and wellness.

So, if you are new to CRF training, you could reassess yourself the first time 4–6 weeks after starting. A relatively short time between assessments will provide positive feedback more quickly and help keep your motivation high. After that, you can push back your assessment schedule to every 8–12 weeks. For accurate results, be sure to use the same fitness test every time.

Q | Can I judge my fitness without taking a test?

Yes. If you haven't had a fitness test or simply don't want one, no problem. You can just use your exercise performance as your guide. If you can currently jog for 10 minutes, then that is your baseline. Can you swim four lengths of the pool? Does it take you 15 minutes to walk a mile? Can you not quite yet cycle to the top of the big hill in town? These are examples of baseline measures of fitness. As you run farther or faster, swim more laps, or cycle farther up the hill, you are improving your cardiorespiratory fitness. Are these baseline measures

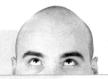

scientific evidence of improvement? No, but you can be sure you are improving; otherwise, you wouldn't be able to do more than before.

Creating a Cardiorespiratory Fitness Program

A successful cardiorespiratory fitness program applies the FITT formula you learned about in Chapter 3. Equally important is that it includes activities you enjoy—and will stick with over time! If you've been sedentary for a while, your first step is to boost your motivation and make a commitment to improve your health and well-being through exercise.

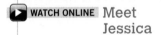
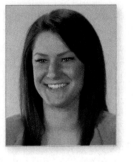
Getting Started

Q How do I learn to like exercise? Right now, I just don't.

Finding some kind of exercise you like precedes everything else concerning improved fitness, because lack of motivation, no matter what the reason, will prevent you from improving your health, including cardiorespiratory fitness (CRF). Increasing CRF is not a typical goal for college students; so many activities are competing for your time—sleep, classes, work, studying, spending time with friends and family—that it may seem there isn't time to get fit or stay fit. Recall, however, the ACLS study that found that higher levels of CRF clearly reduce the risk of disease and death (Figure 4-5). You might be thinking "I'm 20 years old. Disease and death is not my problem, so whatever!" You might think the same at age 40. But you'll feel better right now if you get fitter. And you'll be more attentive in class. And sleep better at night. And think of all the new people you can meet in the wellness center. And how you'll be able to keep up with your kids—today and in the future. There are many physical and emotional reasons to get involved in a fitness routine, but ultimately it is up to you. Only you can decide what your goals are and how motivated you are to reach them. See the box "Getting Started on a Cardiorespiratory Fitness Program" for some strategies you can try.

Although going for a walk or a short bike ride doesn't seem complicated, doing it regularly can be. Many things, both expected and unexpected, can get in your way each day. To reap the health benefits of physical activity, you have to do it most days of the week—so planning and commitment are required. Once you get in the habit, you'll wonder why you didn't start this exercise routine months or years ago!

Applying the FITT Formula

Q How do I know I'm doing all the right things—not going too far, or too fast or too slow?

Use the FITT formula—frequency, intensity, time, and type. As described in Chapter 3, this formula is a simple way of remembering and applying different training variables. Using the basic FITT guidelines will make it easier to plan your program and achieve your fitness goals. The most widely referenced exercise guidelines come from the American College of Sports Medicine, the Surgeon General's report on physical activity and health, the U.S. Department of Health and Human Services' *2008 Physical Activity Guidelines for Adults,* and the U.S. Department of Agriculture's *Dietary Guidelines for Americans.*[19] These public health guidelines all have the same goal—to get Americans moving—although each has a slightly different emphasis.

Wellness Strategies

Getting Started on a Cardiorespiratory Fitness Program

Step I: Set Long- and Short-Term Goals: Your first step is to have a basic goal—such as to feel better about yourself, to improve your health, to lose weight, to meet more people, or to compete in intramurals. Whatever your goal, remember two basic principles to goal setting: KISS and SMART. KISS stands for Keep It Simple and Succeed. SMART is the acronym for the goal criteria you learned in Chapter 2: Specific, Measurable, Achievable, Realistic, and Time-bound. Both of these principles emphasize the importance of small, realistic goals that can be achieved in a short time. Longer-term goals are also important, but getting there is much easier when you have something tangible to keep you going today.

Step II: Choose an Activity: Your next step is to identify types of exercise that you enjoy most and can access easily. Never really liked jogging? Then skip it. Like to swim but your school doesn't have a pool, or the hours don't work for you? Skip it. You always liked bike riding and still have a decent bike. Go for it.

Step III: Plan Ahead: You want to start exercising, you like to ride, and you have a bike. What next? Is your bike in working condition? Do you need a water bottle or comfortable biking clothes and shoes? Can you find your helmet? Taking care of little details like these can take you a long way. If you are all psyched to go riding, only to discover a flat tire, it can be pretty deflating. If you are out riding and get really thirsty and have no water available, it can leave you feeling hot and bothered. Planning for these little things will make that first day out much more pleasant—and make you more likely to do it again soon.

How about a route to ride? You don't want to end up on a dead-end street or a high-traffic road or run out of energy far from home. If you don't know the local streets well, take a peek at MapQuest or Google Maps and pick a good route. Better yet, contact the local bike shop for a riding map or some firsthand advice. Start with a route that isn't too hilly and won't take too long. Sitting on a bike seat for the first time in a while will leave you sore the next day, so don't go too far, and the soreness won't be too bad.

OK, your bike is working, you found your gear, you picked out a route, and you're ready to go. Are you forgetting anything? Think everything through so you can have the best experience possible. What is the weather forecast? Do you have an important appointment early in the day? Think your way through your workout and your day, and address any possible problems.

As you can see, starting and maintaining an exercise program requires planning. The more you do it, the more routine and easier it becomes. Ultimately, when you are done exercising each day, you will feel invigorated and proud—and ready to go at it again tomorrow.

Q | Is it safe to work out every day?

FREQUENCY. Possibly. *Frequency* is the FITT formula term about how often you should exercise. Most exercise guidelines encourage resting one or two days a week to prevent injuries and avoid **burnout.** However, if you vary your routine and exercises and do not regularly exercise at a high intensity, you should be able to work out every day with little if any problem. You can do low-impact activities like walking, swimming, and cycling every day with no real concerns. But you should plan some days off for jogging, step aerobics, and other higher-impact or higher-intensity activities.

Recommendations for exercise frequency range from three days a week to "most" days of the week. The variation among the recommendations is based on exercise intensity, because intensity and frequency need to balance each other. Simply put, the greater the intensity, the less frequent the exercise, and vice versa. The American College of Sports Medicine (ACSM) recommends exercising a minimum of three days a week for vigorous intensity (for at least 20 minutes a day) and five days a week for moderate intensity (for at least 30 minutes a day). The ACSM also notes that additional improvements in cardiorespiratory fitness can be gained by exercising more frequently, but the intensity should be adjusted accordingly. As mentioned earlier, increased frequency, especially at a higher intensity, increases the risk of musculoskeletal injuries. The recommendations in the Department of Health and Human Services (HHS) *2008 Guidelines for Physical Activity for Americans* are very similar to those from ACSM. Instead of daily values, however, the HHS encourages adults to accumulate at least 150 minutes of moderate exercise or 75 minutes of vigorous activity each week.

People with a very low level of fitness might benefit from several short exercise bouts a day, because they often cannot do a lot of exercise at any one time. Bouts of 10 minutes or longer can count toward the daily activity total. Once unfit people increase their level of cardiorespiratory fitness, they find that a single bout of exercise daily is usually more practical and effective. Several short bouts can also be helpful for people with tight schedules.

burnout Physical and emotional exhaustion from exercise.

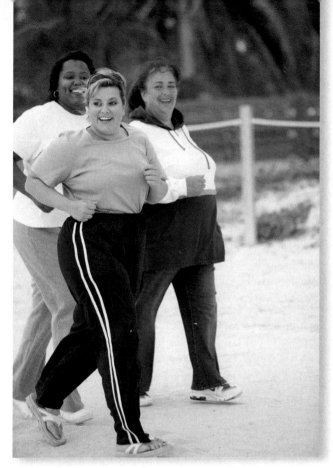

All the public health recommendations for exercise share a common goal: To get Americans moving!

Q | How hard should I exercise?

INTENSITY. You should exercise in your target intensity zone, as described in Chapter 3—hard enough to cause fitness improvements but not so hard that you risk injury. Generally, you can exercise as hard as you want, as long as you are enjoying it! Most people don't enjoy exercising at very high intensities; it's just not as pleasant as more relaxed exercise. Also, the intensity of exercise is very individualized: What may be hard for one person may be easy for another and almost impossible for a third. To avoid the risk of injury and burnout, intensity should be balanced with frequency and duration: The higher the intensity, the shorter the duration and the lower the frequency.

Intensity is closely tied to your personal goals. If enjoyment is at the top of your list, then find an intensity that brings you the most joy. If you are looking to get the most out of your exercise (to get fit or to improve your health, for example), then go for a little higher intensity. And if you are training for a competitive goal, then even higher intensity may be necessary. Remember, if you exercise hard, you don't need to do it as often or for as long as when you exercise at a lower level. If you exercise at a comfortable intensity, you are less likely to run into setbacks.

Exercise guidelines typically differentiate between moderate-intensity activity and vigorous-intensity activity. There are a number of ways to define and calculate target intensity. As a frame of reference, two minutes of moderate activity confers about the same benefit as one minute of vigorous activity. The following section describes different methods of measuring and monitoring intensity.

Q | What's considered moderate activity and vigorous activity?

There are some specific techniques for measuring cardiorespiratory exercise intensity and setting intensity goals. For aerobic activities, intensity, or how hard you exercise, is usually based on your heart rate or on your perception of your level of exertion. Before learning about some common methods of measuring intensity, you should know about the **talk test,** a simple method for judging exercise intensity. This test measures how well you can hold a conversation, or talk, during exercise. The HHS physical activity guidelines describe the talk test this way:[20]

- Moderate intensity exercise: You can talk but not sing.
- Vigorous intensity exercise: You can say only a few words before pausing to take a breath.

The **heart-rate maximum (HR$_{max}$) method** is one of the oldest methods for calculating exercise intensity.

talk test A qualitative assessment of exercise intensity based on the ability to talk during exercise.

heart-rate maximum (HR$_{max}$) method A method of calculating target cardiorespiratory-endurance-exercise intensity based on a percentage range of maximum heart rate.

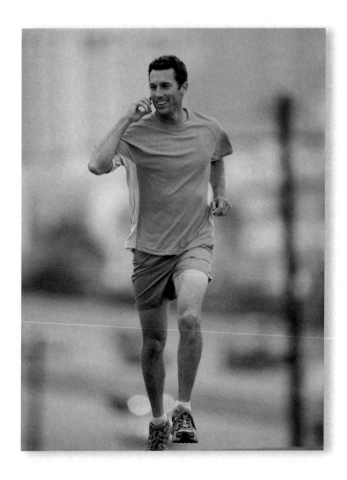

maximum heart rate (MHR) The maximum number of beats per minute of a person's heart, which can be measured directly through laboratory testing or estimated according to age; the value typically starts to decrease at about 20 years of age.

target heart-rate range A range of heart rates that reflects an intensity of exercise that will result in cardiorespiratory fitness improvement.

heart-rate reserve (HRR) method A method of calculating target cardiorespiratory-endurance-exercise intensity based on a percentage range of heart-rate reserve, which is the difference between resting heart rate and maximum heart rate.

Simply put, you exercise at a certain percentage of your **maximum heart rate (MHR)** depending on your current fitness level. The American College of Sports Medicine (ACSM) suggests exercising at 57–94 percent of HR_{max} to ensure increases in cardiorespiratory fitness.[21] Someone who has been sedentary might start at an intensity at the low end of the range, whereas someone who regularly performs vigorous exercise might work out at the top of the range.

Heart-rate maximum (HR_{max}) method:
Target heart rate = MHR × %

How do you find your maximum heart rate? There are two ways. First, you can perform an all-out exercise test that scientifically counts your pulse (with a heart-rate monitor or ECG machine) at the very end of your effort. This would give you your true HR_{max} value. Realistically, not many people want, need, or desire to do this.

The easier second method is to subtract your age from 220 (220 – age = MHR). Even though this classic formula has an error of +/– 15 beats per minute, it is considered generally reliable. Using this method, a 20-year-old who is sporadically active and plans to use 70–90 percent of HR_{max} for her **target heart-rate range** would calculate her range as 140–180 beats per minute (bpm) this way:

Predicted maximum heart rate (MHR) = 220 – 20 = 200 bpm
70% exercise intensity = 0.70 × 200 = 140 bpm
90% exercise intensity = 0.90 × 200 = 180 bpm

The **heart-rate reserve (HRR) method** of calculating intensity is a more accurate means of reflecting energy expenditure during exercise.[22] However, the formula is slightly more complex, and you may find that age-predicted HR_{max} is a more practical method for determining your exercise intensity. To use the HRR method, you need to know both your maximum heart rate (MHR) and your resting heart rate (RHR). You can calculate your MHR according to the formula described above. Your RHR can be determined by counting your pulse for a minute before you get out of bed in the morning—on a day you wake up naturally and are not startled by your alarm. Calculate your HRR by subtracting your resting heart rate from your maximum heart rate. Then multiply that value by the percentage of HRR you are aiming for. Finally, add this result to your resting heart rate (RHR). This will yield a target heart rate for you to use. The American College of Sports Medicine (ACSM) suggests a target heart-rate range based on 30–85 percent of HRR, depending on your initial fitness level.

Heart-rate reserve (HRR) method:
Target heart rate = [(MHR – RHR) × %] + RHR

Using this method, a 20-year-old who has a resting heart rate of 64 and is somewhat active might choose a target range based on 55–80 percent of heart-rate reserve. She would calculate an exercise-intensity target range of 139–173 beats per minute (bpm).

HRR = [(200 – 64) × %] + 64 = exercise heart-rate range
55% exercise intensity: (136 × 0.55) + 64 = 139 bpm
80% exercise intensity: (136 × 0.80) + 64 = 173 bpm

Lab Activity 4-2 will help you work through the appropriate calculations. Table 4-1 shows the ACSM recommendations for intensity based on current fitness levels. These

TABLE 4-1 RECOMMENDED STARTING INTENSITY OF EXERCISE BASED ON CURRENT ACTIVITY LEVEL

ACTIVITY LEVEL	HEART-RATE MAXIMUM (HR_{MAX}) METHOD* (%)	HEART-RATE RESERVE (HRR) METHOD* (%)
SEDENTARY	57–67	30–45
MINIMAL PHYSICAL ACTIVITY	64–74	40–55
SPORADIC PHYSICAL ACTIVITY	74–84	55–70
HABITUAL PHYSICAL ACTIVITY	80–91	65–80
HIGH AMOUNTS OF HABITUAL PHYSICAL ACTIVITY	84–94	70–85

*The percentage values for heart-rate maximum and heart-rate reserve methods of calculating intensity would be multiplied according to the appropriate formula:

   Heart-rate maximum (HR_{max}) = MHR × %
   Heart-rate reserve (HRR) = [(MHR–RHR) × %] + RHR

Source: American College of Sports Medicine. (2009). *Guidelines for exercise testing and prescription* (8th ed.). Baltimore, MD: Lippincott Williams & Wilkins.

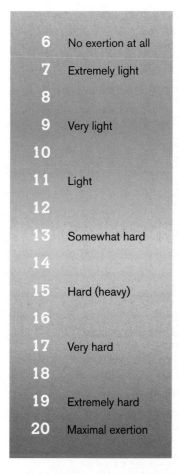

Figure 4-6 Rating of perceived exertion (RPE) scale

Source: Borg, G. (1970). Perceived exertion as an indicator of somatic stress. *Scandinavian Journal of Rehabilitation Medicine, 2*(2), 92–98. © Gunnar Borg, 1970, 1985, 1994, 1998.

are ranges, and there is no need to try to keep your heart rate exactly at one particular level.

The HR_{max} and HRR methods are objective measures of intensity, each requiring certain heart-rate values. **Rating of perceived exertion (RPE),** also called the Borg scale (after its originator, Gunnar Borg), is a subjective measure of exercise intensity that does not require heart-rate information. On a scale of 6 to 20, users rate their level of effort (Figure 4-6). The reason for the unusual range—starting at 6 and ending at 20—is that the levels are meant to loosely correlate to the user's current heart rate. Therefore, if the user rates intensity at 14 on the RPE scale, her or his heart rate is likely to be around 140 bpm. To achieve a moderate intensity on the RPE scale, similar to that calculated by the HR_{max} and HRR methods, the user would strive for an RPE value between 12 and 16. This moderate-exercise intensity should bring about the same increases in cardiorespiratory fitness as HR_{max}, HRR, or the talk test.

Yet another way of measuring exercise intensity is in terms of **metabolic equivalents (METs).** The MET level can be used to estimate the amount of oxygen the body uses during physical activity. It provides a simple method of quantifying activity at different absolute levels. One MET is equal to the energy used by the body when sitting quietly. The harder you work during any activity, the higher the MET requirement. Moderate intensity activity requires 3–6 METs; vigorous intensity activity requires more than 6 METs.[23] Because intensity can vary based on individual effort, the same activity can be classified as light, moderate, or vigorous. Figure 4-7 provides some general intensity classifications of different physical activities.

Beginning exercisers might be in over their heads trying to achieve moderate or vigorous intensities. Instead, beginners should start at a lower intensity, which helps improve retention, avoid injuries, and leave them eager for more. Working slightly below the moderate range will still increase cardiorespiratory fitness and bring about other health-related changes, albeit slower and less profound, for a previously sedentary person. To get started on this plan, calculate target intensity using 40–60 percent HRR or an RPE of 10–12. Once you get comfortable at this intensity and can repeat it over the course of about two weeks, then it is fine to increase the intensity, but never more than 10 percent at a time; more information is provided below on making progress with your cardiorespiratory fitness program.

Lab Activity 4-2 has more information and help for program planning.

Q | What's the best way to take my heart rate when I'm exercising?

The easiest way, but definitely not the cheapest, is with a heart rate (HR) monitor. HR monitors are available with a range of features— and a range of prices. The least expensive HR monitors cost around $50; the most expensive can be more than $400 and will determine calories burned, altitude climbed, distance traveled, the ambient temperature, and more. The most reliable HR monitors are those that come in two parts: a chest strap worn around the torso and a watch or monitor worn on the wrist. A signal is transmitted from the chest strap to the monitor, with the heart rate displayed and updated about every 3–5 seconds. Most brands are relatively reliable, although interference can be a problem for all of them if there are a lot of strong electrical signals nearby or many HR monitor users in a small place (a spinning class, for example).

If you don't want to spend the money on a HR monitor, you don't need to: You can use your fingers to accurately measure your exercise HR. By placing your fingers on the inside of your wrist (thumb side) at the radial artery, or gently on your neck by the carotid artery, you should be able to feel your heart beating. This method is cheap, but it does have some minor drawbacks. First, you probably will need to stop for at least 10 seconds to take your HR. With a HR monitor, you don't need to stop—you just glance at your watch. How long should you count if you taking your own HR? No less than 6 seconds and no more than 15. Whichever you choose (10 and 15 seconds are the most common), you should always use the same system. For example, if your target heart-rate range is 140–170 bpm, and you decide to count your pulse for 10 seconds, you would determine your target 10-second counts by dividing your bpm goal by 6: 23–28 beats.

If you don't want to buy a HR monitor or aren't comfortable taking your pulse, there is always the RPE option.

rating of perceived exertion (RPE) A scale that provides a subjective measure of exercise intensity; widely used when heart-rate monitoring is not available; also known as the Borg scale.

metabolic equivalents (METs) A physiological concept expressing the energy cost of a physical activity relative to resting metabolic rate; the value of sitting at rest is defined as 1.0 MET; more vigorous activities have higher MET requirements.

Moderate Intensity Activity 3.0 to 6.0 METs (3.5 to 7 calories burned per minute)	Vigorous Intensity Activity More than 6.0 METs (more than 7 calories burned per minute)
Walking at a moderate or brisk pace of 3 to 4.5 mph on a level surface (90–110 steps per minute)	Walking at a pace of 5 mph or faster
	Waking or climbing briskly up a hill
Hiking	Jogging or running
	Wheeling a wheelchair
	Mountain climbing or backpacking
Bicycling 5 to 9 mph on level terrain	Bicycling more than 10 mph or on steep terrain
Stationary cycling using moderate effort	Stationary cycling using vigorous effort
Using a stair climber, rowing machine, elliptical, etc., with moderate effort	Using a stair climber, rowing machine, elliptical, etc., with vigorous effort
Dancing with moderate effort	Dancing energetically with vigorous effort
Tennis—doubles	Tennis—singles
	Wheelchair tennis
Swimming–recreational	Swimming—steady paced laps
Basketball—shooting baskets	Basketball—playing a game
Gardening or yard work—moderate (raking the lawn, bagging grass or leaves, digging or light shoveling [less than 10lbs per minute], weeding)	Gardening or yard work—heavy or rapid (shoveling more than 10 lbs per minute, digging ditches, carrying heavy loads)
Pushing a power lawn mower	Pushing a nonmotorized lawn mower
Moderate housework: scrubbing the floor, sweeping outdoor areas, washing windows, general housework tasks	Heavy housework: Moving or pushing heavy furniture (75 lbs or more), carrying household items weighing 25lbs or more up the stairs
Actively playing with children	Energetically/vigorously playing with children

Figure 4-7 Intensity levels of different physical activities

Source: Adapted from Centers for Disease Control and Prevention, National Center for Chronic Disease Prevention and Health Promotion. *General physical activities defined by level of intensity* (http://www.cdc.gov/nccdphp/dnpa/physical/pdf/PA_Intensity_table_2_1.pdf). A complete listing of MET values for many different physical activities can be found at http://prevention.sph.sc.edu/tools/compendium.htm

Simply rate your perception of your effort on the RPE scale. If you use the scale properly, you'll be aware of your effort level every time out.

Q | Doesn't lower intensity exercise burn more fat?

More fat than what? More than sitting on the couch—absolutely. More than jogging or some other higher-intensity activity? No, at least not in absolute terms. When it comes to weight control, what matters is the total calories burned, not whether the body uses fat or carbohydrate for energy.

How does the fuel use compare? Regardless of exercise intensity, both fat and carbohydrate are being used

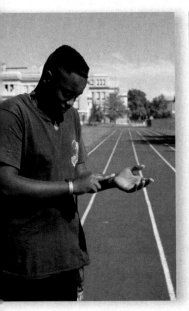
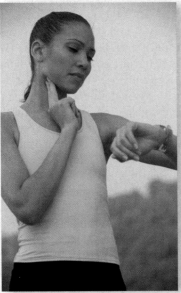

You can monitor your heart rate by taking your pulse at the radial artery in your wrist or the carotid artery in your neck. Use your index and middle fingers and apply light pressure.

("burned"), with very little protein in the mix. For low-intensity exercise, the percentage of fat in the mix is relatively high; at higher intensities, the percentage of fat is relatively low. Although low-intensity exercise uses a higher percentage of fat for fuel, the fat calories are burned at a relatively slow rate (4–5 calories per minute). High-intensity exercise burns a smaller percentage of fat, but the fat is burned at a much higher rate (10–13 calories per minute). Therefore, the total amount of fat burned is greater during high-intensity exercise. In addition, the total calories burned per unit of time are also greater. Walking or running a mile burns roughly 80–100 calories; however, the total caloric expenditure per minute is much higher for jogging, and joggers can cover more distance per minute than walkers, so the total number of calories burned is greater. Higher-intensity exercise burns more total calories and more total fat *per unit of time,* plain and simple.

If your goal is to control body weight, you should exercise at a higher intensity, right? Not necessarily. Even though you burn more calories when you exercise at higher intensities, a high-intensity program is much more difficult to maintain, injuries occur more frequently, and people tend to quit exercising because their program is just too hard. Nobody does 100 percent of their workout at high intensity, but you can intersperse short bouts of higher intensity (30 seconds of fast walking, for example) in your moderate-intensity routine. If you have been going at 50–60 percent of heart-rate reserve (HRR), you can include brief bouts of 70–80 percent HRR. Over time, you will find the lower-intensity pace gets easier and you can maintain the higher intensity even longer—therefore, even more calories are being burned.

Some people find it difficult to do high-intensity exercise. They shouldn't be discouraged; in fact, many people lose weight and successfully keep it off by using moderate-intensity exercise only. It may take a little longer to burn the same amount of calories, but the long-term benefits are the same.

Q | How many hours of cardiovascular activity are necessary to be healthy?

TIME. The amount of time you need to spend on cardiorespiratory exercise depends on a number of factors. In general, *time,* or duration of exercise, refers to how long each exercise session should last. Frequency, intensity, and duration need to be carefully balanced, as they are all dependent on each other. If you work out at a high intensity, you need less time being active in order to achieve health and fitness from exercise, but, as mentioned above, high-intensity exercise is not always best.

The balance between time and intensity applies to individual workouts as well as your weekly exercise plan: For instance, the intensity of a 60-minute exercise session is much lower than that of a 20-minute session. This is not to say that the longer session couldn't include some higher-intensity bouts (see the previous question), but generally speaking, as duration increases, intensity decreases (Figure 4-8). There are, of course, many variations, and as always, some exercise is better than none at all. So, when you are temporarily short on time (during finals week, when a big project is due, or when the boss wants you to work extra hours), shorter bouts of activity are great.

The various exercise guidelines each have somewhat different and specific recommendations for exercise, including duration. The American College of Sports Medicine (ACSM) recommendation for time of exercise is based on intensity: Moderate-intensity exercise should be performed for at least 30 minutes on five or more days per week; vigorous exercise should be done for at least 20 minutes on three or more days per week. Most individuals, according to ACSM, can achieve their fitness related goals with 20–30 minutes of exercise at 75–90 percent of HR_{max}. People who want to promote or maintain weight loss require longer exercise time in order to burn more calories (50–60 minutes per day over the course of a week to total 300 minutes of moderate exercise or 150 minutes of vigorous exercise or an equivalent combination). Bouts of at least 10 minutes count toward the minimum duration recommendations. ACSM also suggests that total caloric expenditure or pedometer step counts can be used as surrogate measures of exercise time: 1,000 or more calories per week in cardiorespiratory fitness activities or the equivalent of walking 3,000 or more steps per day at a moderate to vigorous intensity.

The Surgeon General and the Department of Health and Human Services (HHS) focus on physical activity for achieving health-related benefits, with an accumulation of at least 150 minutes of moderate-intensity activity or 75 minutes of vigorous activity. This recommendation is especially targeted at people who are currently sedentary and emphasizes that *any* physical activity can be accumulated throughout the day to reach health-related goals. For additional and more extensive health benefits, the HHS guidelines suggest that people increase their aerobic physical activity to 300 minutes of moderate-intensity or 150 minutes of vigorous-intensity activity per week.

All the organizations agree that some activity is better than none, more is better than less, and too much may not be good. The law of diminishing returns applies: Doing too much exercise or at too high an intensity may create more problems than benefits. Health and fitness gains are often thought of separately; but in practice it is difficult to separate them. Any improvements in fitness also bring improvements in health: Any improvements in health bring improvements in fitness, with some qualifications. An individual who is currently sedentary will quickly improve in both fitness and health with a minimal amount of physical activity. Maintaining this minimal amount will allow for the maintenance of the associated health benefits, but fitness will quickly plateau. For continued cardiorespiratory fitness improvement, the intensity, duration, and/or frequency of exercise needs to increase. Ultimately, national physical activity recommendations encourage everyone to

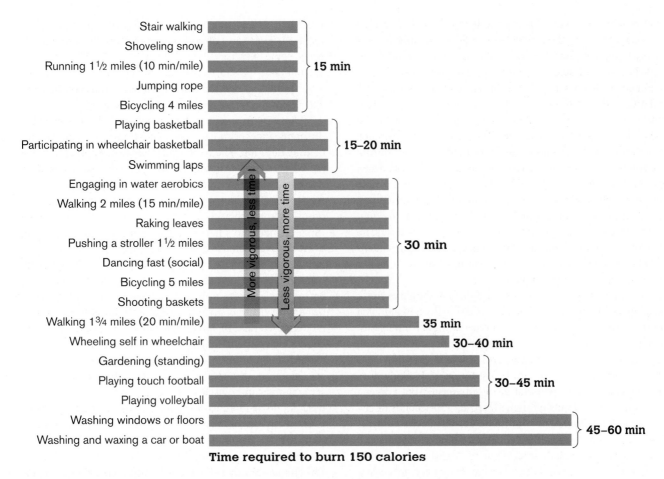

Figure 4-8 Relationship between exercise time and intensity. Each example on the chart is roughly equivalent to physical activity requiring 150 calories. The activities listed near the top require more effort (intensity) and less time to burn 150 calories than those toward the bottom. Therefore, 15 minutes of stair walking is the equivalent of 45–60 minutes of washing or waxing a car.

Source: Adapted from U.S. Department of Health and Human Services. (1996). At a glance. *Physical activity and health: A report of the Surgeon General* (http://www.cdc.gov/nccdphp/sgr/ataglan.htm).

find activities they enjoy and perform them at an intensity and duration that they can sustain on a regular basis. To repeat: *Any exercise is better than none.*

TYPE. Cardiorespiratory fitness (CRF) can be improved through a variety of activities—those that are aerobic, rhythmic, and involve work by large muscle groups. (Anaerobic activities are typically used to develop strength.) What is more important than the particular activity is doing it on a regular basis. The list of aerobic activities is long and includes walking, jogging, cycling, swimming, in-line skating, cross-country skiing, rowing, and dancing in an exercise class or for pleasure. Try different activities, and then focus on the ones you most enjoy.

Q What's the best exercise for me?

There is no one best activity, but some that are more popular than others. You need to consider the specifics of an activity and whether it would work for you—in terms of intensity, necessary equipment and facilities, and whether you enjoy it!

Walking is the main exercise of choice for adults who are regularly active. Most people can walk for exercise, and it requires little specialized equipment—just a sidewalk, shopping mall, park, or country road. Walking is effective at burning calories (about 80–100 per mile), can be a social activity (it is easy to walk in a group and talk), and can be done in several short bouts during the day (10 minutes here and there).

More intense than walking is jogging or even running, which requires specialized footwear and somewhere to change clothes and/or shower in addition to a place to run. Because it is higher intensity than walking, running burns more calories per minute of activity, and the risk of musculoskeletal injury is higher. Running, if it is for you, is a great way to improve fitness and health and control body weight, even with its potential drawbacks.

Research Brief

Short Bout, Long Bout: Which Is Best?

Research indicates that short bouts of exercise may be just as effective as longer bouts for both fitness and weight control. A group of overweight female college students were assigned to one of the following groups:

- Control group, which did no exercise
- Short exercise group, which performed three 10-minute bouts of exercise
- Medium exercise group, which performed two 15-minute bouts of exercise
- Long exercise group, which performed one 30-minute bout of exercise

The primary outcome measures were VO_{2max} and weight loss. With the exception of the control group, the women exercised at about 75 percent of VO_{2max} for a minimum of three days a week. At the end of the study, women in all three exercise groups had improved their VO_{2max} and decreased their body weight, body fat, and body circumference measures. The control group did not show any of these changes.

The conclusion of this study is that exercise duration is not as important as volume. To lose weight or increase fitness, the total volume of work is critical. Whether to do all your exercising at once or in several daily bouts depends on your schedule and preference. And maybe some days you can do one long bout, but on others it is easier to do more than one. Regardless of the number of daily bouts, the main thing is to just do it!

Source: Schmidt, W. D., Biwer, C. J., Kalscheuer, L. K. (2001). Effects of long versus short bout exercise on fitness and weight loss in overweight females. *Journal of the American College of Nutrition, 20*(5), 494–501.

As long as you keep up the intensity, moving to music can be a great cardiorespiratory workout.

Dance, in its many forms, is another popular way to increase cardiorespiratory fitness (CRF). You can dance in an aerobics class, do hip hop or country line dancing, or a use a Dance Dance Revolution machine. Dance can be as intense or as social as you make it. Dancing doesn't require much, other than music (even if it's in your head), floor space, and possibly a partner. Moving to music appeals to lots of people because the music is often a distraction that makes exercise time pass more quickly. Varying the types of music you dance to will encourage you to dance at different intensities.

Cycling, swimming, and in-line skating are other great CRF activities, although their logistics are slightly more complicated. They all require some skill, specialized equipment, good weather, access, and a fair amount of planning. Their advantages are that they are easy on your joints, will increase your fitness, and can be enjoyed throughout adulthood. Cycling and in-line skating require the appropriate equipment, which can range from about $75 for an entry-level pair of skates to more than $3,000 for a top-end road bike. Although you don't need to break the bank to enjoy these exercises, having good equipment makes the activity much more enjoyable. Cycling and skating also are easier in decent weather. If you live somewhere that is often wet, cold, snowy, or icy or somewhere that is extremely hot, your opportunities to enjoy cycling and skating will be limited. Swimming, of course, requires access to a pool, lake, river, or really big puddle. Although many campuses have recreation pools, the hours may be limited to early morning, lunch time, and evening. Student fees usually cover access to the pool, but if you want to swim somewhere off campus, you will probably need to spend at least $20 a month for access.

If you live where winters are long, you have a great excuse to try ice skating, cross-country skiing, or snowshoeing. Although each of these requires special equipment and appropriate conditions, they are all great aerobic activities. As your skill level increases, you can do the activity for a longer time, which should increase your enjoyment. Snowshoeing and cross-county skiing can take you places in the winter you otherwise couldn't go, and the scenery and sounds alone make the venture worthwhile. Ice skating requires fairly

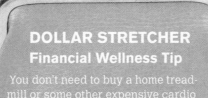

DOLLAR STRETCHER
Financial Wellness Tip

You don't need to buy a home treadmill or some other expensive cardio machine for a home workout. Try a jump rope, an aerobic step, or an exercise DVD or video game.

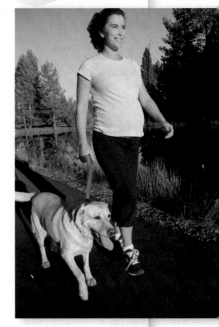

Wellness Strategies

Exercise during Pregnancy

Almost half of all pregnant women in the United States exercise. The exercises of choice for pregnant women include walking, swimming, and other types of low-to-moderate-intensity aerobic activities. As their pregnancy progresses, most women reduce the duration and intensity of exercise because of increasing fatigue, nausea or vomiting, general discomfort, and weight gain.

Regular exercise in healthy pregnant women is safe and often beneficial. Regular moderate exercisers tend to experience fewer pregnancy-related discomforts and benefit from a greater sense of well-being. Women who consume a healthy diet, gain the recommended amount of weight, and avoid activities that are too intense or may cause injury should not worry that exercise will harm them or their baby. However, exercise may not be advised for women who fail to gain weight or have preeclampsia, premature rupture of the membrane, hypertension, heart disease, preterm labor, second- or third-trimester bleeding, or a weak cervix.

Although regular exercise is beneficial for pregnant women, their fetuses can be harmed by overly vigorous activity in the third trimester, activities with a high risk of falling or a high level of contact, and activities in the supine position (lying on the back, face up), especially after the first trimester. Women who continue to exercise after giving birth should notice no adverse effect on lactation in terms of milk composition, milk volume, or their health.

A safe and effective exercise plan for a healthy pregnant woman includes 30–40 minutes of moderate exercise, at least three days a week. Pregnant women should use rate of perceived exertion (RPE) to assess intensity, because it is more reliable than heart rate methods during pregnancy; they should aim for an RPE of 11–13. Women who were sedentary before pregnancy should begin exercising at a low intensity, with low-impact exercises like walking or swimming. Regardless of fitness or activity level pre-pregnancy, all women should consult with their physician prior to exercising during pregnancy.

Source: American College of Obstetricians and Gynecologists. (2002). Exercise during pregnancy and the postpartum period. ACOG Committee Opinion No. 267. *Obstetrics & Gynecology, 99,* 171–173.

smooth ice, but you can be sure that where there is an ice rink, lots of people will be skating.

If you don't want to go outside and like the idea of a consistent routine throughout the year, the aerobic exercise machines in your campus wellness or fitness center may be the choice for you. Treadmills, ellipticals, and stationary and spinning bikes provide an opportunity for a great aerobic workout. The advantages of machines are always knowing what to expect, having a timer close at hand, and usually having the opportunity to let the machine create a workout for you. Machines also provide rough estimates of calories burned, which may be appealing.

Finally, in addition to your likes and dislikes, also think about any health concerns you may have. As discussed earlier, swimming can be an excellent choice for people with asthma. Swimming can also be appropriate, along with cycling and moderate walking, for someone who has joint problems or who is currently overweight and just starting an exercise program. If you are under a physician's care for a condition like diabetes or high blood pressure, check with your health care provider for any special considerations that might apply to you. See the box "Exercise during Pregnancy" for activity guidelines for pregnant women.

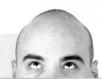

Mind Stretcher
Critical Thinking Exercise

Think carefully about the characteristics of endurance activities you're considering for a fitness program—you'll be more likely to stick with exercise over the long term if you enjoy it!

- What activities are available in your community, at different times of the day or year?
- Do you like working out in a group setting, such as an organized class or a busy fitness center? Or do you prefer exercising with one or two friends or on your own?
- Do you like competitive activities, such as team sports?
- Is your level of fitness currently high enough for full participation in the activities you're considering?

Carefully examine all the pros and cons when you select activities to include in your fitness program.

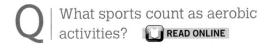

Q What sports count as aerobic activities? **READ ONLINE**

Putting Together a Complete Workout

A complete workout should include a warm-up phase, a conditioning phase, and a cool-down phase.

Q Do I really need a warm-up just to go walking with my friends?

No, you don't need to do a formal warm-up before going for a walk. By definition, a warm-up consists of 5–10 minutes of low-intensity large-muscle activity, such as jogging before running, or slow walking before brisk walking. Because you probably start your walk slow and then gradually increase the tempo, you are in fact warming up even though you don't call it a warm-up.

If you are planning more vigorous exercise or exercise that requires a lot of skill-dependent movement, then you do need a more formal warm-up—for all the reasons described in Chapter 3. You can include stretching exercises at the end of your warm-up, or you can choose to stretch after the more active part of your workout.

The next phase of a complete workout is conditioning. This phase should last 20–60 minutes and be at least moderate intensity. (Exercise bouts of 10 minutes are acceptable if you accumulate at least 20–60 minutes of exercise during the day.) Many beginning exercisers find that maintaining a target heart rate during the conditioning phase is difficult. It is best to come up with a heart-rate range, say 60–70 percent of HR_{max}, and try to stay within that range during most of the conditioning phase. Your heart rate will fluctuate from minute to minute, so don't let that worry you. Instead, try to stay in your target range and expect that your ending heart rate will be a bit higher than your starting heart rate. Over time, you will be able to do the same effort at a lower heart rate, and then you will know it is time to do more (the next section discusses making progress toward your fitness goals).

The final phase of the complete workout is the cool-down, a time of gradual recovery from endurance activity. During the cool-down, you slowly decrease the intensity of what you were doing during the conditioning phase. If you were taking a brisk walk, then you could add several minutes of easier walking at the end, or start slowing down a little before your endpoint. Many people enjoy doing stretching exercises immediately after aerobic activities, so do that too if you'd like. The cool-down helps your body transition to a less active state and facilitates a rapid and effective removal of lactic acid.

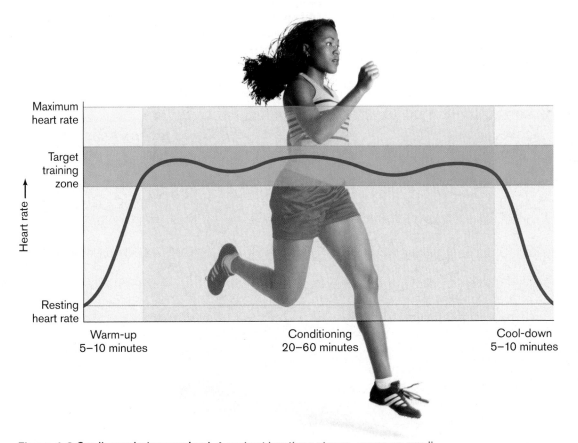

Figure 4-9 **Cardiorespiratory workout.** A workout has three stages—warm-up, conditioning, and cool-down.

Making FITT Work for You

Q | I don't have much time to work out but I still want to get fit. What can I do?

Understanding the FITT guidelines is a first step (Table 4-2). Next, you need to consider your current level of fitness, your schedule, your activity options, your preferences, and your goals. If you're already active, think about how you can adjust your program to meet the recommendations for CRF training—or boost your current program for additional health and fitness benefits. If you are not currently active, consider ways to start adding bouts of moderate activity to your day. The following examples may give you some ideas:

■ *Jenna is very busy—school in the mornings, work in the afternoons—but she has to admit that she isn't very active physically. She doesn't have the time or inclination to go to a gym, so to get started being less sedentary, she's going to add some brisk walking to her daily routine. She timed the walk between the second-closest transit stop and where she works, and walking that distance instead of riding to the closest stop would give her about 20 minutes of brisk walking time, five days per week. She doesn't mind getting a bit winded and sweaty on her way home from work. She arranges with one of her friends to get together for a walk once each weekend, starting with 30 minutes and working up to an hour. They plan to walk outside in good weather and at the mall in bad weather. For added motivation, they'll wear pedometers during their walk to track their steps—trying to increase each week or two. Jenna plans to monitor intensity with the talk test and with her pedometer (tracking steps versus time), but she'll check her heart rate during activity once or twice a week.*

■ *Zach loves to go to the campus fitness center during the week, and he plays about an hour of fast and hard basketball with friends on most Saturdays. At the fitness center, he works out on the strength machines, and he's realized that despite feeling fairly fit, his basketball time doesn't quite add up to the recommended level of cardiorespiratory training. Because he enjoys the campus fitness center, he decides to add some cardio training on the machines there—he'll do two vigorous 10-minute bouts of training three times per week, mixed in with his strength training. He's afraid he'll get bored, so he plans to alternate on different types of cardio training machines. Zach is interested in doing some interval and high-intensity training; he likes to compete with himself, so he'll use a heart-rate monitor to track his intensity.*

Putting Your Personal Fitness Plan into Action

Completing your first workout is a great step, but the key to cardiorespiratory fitness is maintaining your program over time. A successful program is one in which you continue to make progress, exercise safely, and adjust your program to changing goals and conditions.

TABLE 4-2 SUMMARY OF RECOMMENDED EXERCISE GUIDELINES*

	ACSM[a]	HHS[b]	SURGEON GENERAL[c]
FREQUENCY	3–5 days/week	Spread throughout the week, across at least 3 days	Most days of the week
INTENSITY	57–94% HR_{max} 30–85% HRR	Moderate or vigorous	Moderate (3–6 METs)
TIME	20–60 minutes/day, in bouts of 10 or more minutes	150 minutes/week or 75 minutes/week, in bouts of 10 or more minutes	At least 30 minutes a day
CALORIES	≥150/day	N/A	≥150/day
TYPE	Aerobic activities	Aerobic activities	Aerobic activities

*These are minimum guidelines for health/fitness benefits; additional health benefits are obtained by increasing activity over these levels. Additional activity is recommended for people whose goals include losing weight or maintaining weight loss.

Sources: (a) Thompson, W. R., Gordon, N. F., & Pescatello, L. S. (2009). *ACSM guidelines for exercise testing and prescription* (8th ed.). Baltimore, MD: Lippincott Williams & Wilkins.
(b) U.S. Department of Health and Human Services. (2008). *2008 physical activity guidelines for Americans.*
(c) U.S. Department of Health and Human Services. (1966). *Physical activity and health: A report of the Surgeon General.*

Making Progress Toward Your Fitness Goals

Q How long until I can run for 5 miles? The answer depends on your starting level of fitness. If you can't run around the block today, it might be a while. If you can already run for 30 continuous minutes, then it might be much sooner. The aspect of training involved here is **progression,** and each person progresses at a different rate, depending on age, previous training status, training program, goals, and other factors. Aerobic exercise progresses at a different rate for everyone, depending on a variety of factors including baseline fitness and motivation.

The initial phase should include workouts with up to 15 minutes of conditioning—new exercisers may be overwhelmed if they shoot for 20, 30, or more minutes. You don't need to exercise more than three or four days a week during this time, so that you can adapt to the nuances of your new exercise program (Figure 4-10). Increase the duration 5–10 minutes every week or two during the first four to six weeks of training. During this phase, establish individualized, attainable, short-term goals, as well as a reward system to give you positive reinforcement.

After about a month of regular conditioning, increase frequency, intensity, and duration during the following months to slowly and safely achieve your fitness goals. It may be best to increase only one aspect of conditioning each week, so as to avoid doing too much and causing injury. For someone starting in a very deconditioned state, it may take up to eight months to be able to accumulate 30 minutes of cardiorespiratory exercises on most days of the week. For many exercisers, adding a variety of routines, routes, and modes of exercise may help increase adherence and reduce the risk or injury or burnout.

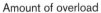
progression Gradual increases in frequency, intensity, and duration of exercise in order to for the body to adapt and increase fitness.

Q My exercise programs usually last about a week. What's the trick to keep from quitting right after I start? Many things can challenge your commitment to an exercise program. Maybe it has been rainy for a few days, or your schoolwork is getting tougher, or you broke up with your sweetheart. For many people, it is harder to keep going than it is to get started. The good news is that it doesn't take long, maybe 6–12 weeks, before a new habit becomes routine. The not-so-good news is that those 6–12 weeks can be a challenge.

Setting goals and knowing some strategies to prevent relapses can help you keep going with an exercise program. You should have both long-term and short-term goals, and they should meet all the criteria described in Chapter 2 and earlier in this chapter. If your goals are realistic, you'll find yourself constantly achieving them, which in turn boosts your confidence and your ability to continue and to achieve even more.

Even with appropriate goals, there may still be bumps in the road—relapses. Having a plan to prevent relapses can help you when the going gets tough. What should you do when finals are coming up and there's no time for exercise? Do half your normal workout—there will be time left for studying and you won't have to feel bad about skipping exercise completely. What if it's been raining for 40 days and 40 nights and you're sick of getting soaked? Try an indoor workout: Do some brisk indoor mall-walking with friends or visit the campus fitness center and enjoy the variety of cardio machines. What if you just started a new job? You may have to alter your routine, but if you plan ahead for change, it should go smoothly. When you are faced with challenges, it's always better to try to do some exercise instead of not exercising at all.

Q Do I need a special diet to increase cardio fitness?

Your diet can't directly increase your CRF, but it can go a long way towards improving your overall health. Fitness gains come from training, and your diet helps determine the quality of training you can sustain. Eating a variety of fruits and vegetables, lean meats, and low-fat dairy will give you

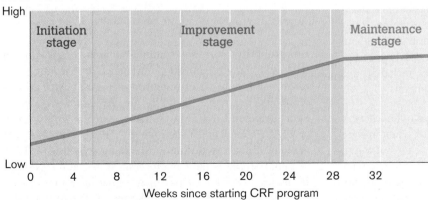

Amount of overload

Figure 4-10 Sample cardiorespiratory-fitness-program progression. The initiation stage, with its short, relatively low-intensity workouts, allows you to develop the habit of exercise without getting too sore or uncomfortable. During the improvement stage, slowly and progressively increase overload until you reach your desired level of fitness (maintenance stage). Don't increase frequency, intensity, and duration during the same week, and don't increase overall exercise volume more than 10 percent a week.

Source: Adapted from American College of Sports Medicine. (2009). *Resource manual to accompany guidelines for exercise testing and prescription* (6th ed.). Baltimore, MD: Lippincott Williams & Wilkins.

Research Brief

How to Choose a Personal Trainer: Experience or Education?

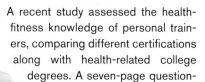

A recent study assessed the health-fitness knowledge of personal trainers, comparing different certifications along with health-related college degrees. A seven-page questionnaire was administered to 115 health-fitness professionals to assess their discipline-specific knowledge, skills, and abilities (KSA). The questionnaire was developed with equal input from the twelve most popular national fitness certifications.

Five topics were covered: nutrition, health screening, testing protocols, exercise prescription, and special populations.

Participants in this study worked in large fitness chains, college wellness centers, and independent gyms, or they were self-employed. Their years of experience ranged from less than one to eighteen.

The participants' KSA scores were unrelated to years of experience. Participants with a bachelor's degree in the field scored higher in all five domains than those without a related degree, and those with certification from ACSM or NSCA scored higher in all domains than those with certification from any other organization. The study concluded that having a health-related bachelor's degree and/or certification through ACSM or NSCA predicted a significantly higher KSA score across the five important health-related domains. So, ask questions about education and certification and choose your personal trainer wisely.

Source: Malek, M. H., Nalbone, D. P., & Berger, D. E. (2002). Importance of health science education for personal fitness trainers. *Journal of Strength and Conditioning Research, 16*(1), 19–24.

the energy you need along with a rich base of vitamins and minerals. This type of diet will allow you to engage in exercise at varying intensities and frequencies without feeling unusually tired or run-down. See Chapters 8 and 9 for more on nutrition.

Making Exercise Safe

Exercise will be fun and enjoyable if you plan ahead for potential problems. To minimize the chances of injury, overuse, boredom, and burnout, take some precautions, listen to your body, and use moderation in your planning. Refer to Chapter 3 for advice on choosing exercise clothing and shoes, guidelines for proper hydration and safety equipment, and additional information on safety, including tips for exercising in hot, cold, and smoggy conditions.

Q | I have a cold. Can I still work out?

You can if you don't have a fever and your symptoms are from the neck up.[24] It might be difficult to maintain intensive exercise with a cold, so put that off for a few days, but otherwise you can work out, maybe at a slower pace or for a shorter duration.

If you think you might have the flu (fever, extreme tiredness, muscle aches, swollen lymph glands), then you should take some time off from your exercise program. Wait about a week before starting back slowly and at least two weeks before you work out at higher intensities.

Personal Training—Online, in Person, or Somewhere in Between?

Personal trainers first came into vogue in the 1950s, after the field of personal fitness was popularized by Jack LaLanne, who opened the first health spa and hosted the first nationally syndicated TV exercise show. Since then, personal training as a profession has grown by leaps and bounds.

Q | How do I know who is a good personal trainer?

Unfortunately, personal training is a loosely regulated field, and many organizations offer personal training certification. A handful of organizations are considered rigorous and creditable, including the American College of Sports Medicine (ACSM), the American Council on Exercise (ACE), the Cooper Institute of Aerobics Research, the National Academy of Sports Medicine (NASM), and the National Strength and Conditioning Association (NSCA). If you are looking for a personal trainer, it is wise to look for certification and a relevant degree. A degree in kinesiology, exercise science, wellness, fitness, or a related field indicates a minimal level of competency. Someone with both a degree in the field and a certification is likely to have the best background. Experience by itself is no guarantee of competency. (For more information, see the box "How to Choose a Personal Trainer.")

Personal trainers can now be found online just as easily as they can be found in your local gym. You should use the same care, if not more, when looking online for a personal trainer. Always ask questions, perform a Web search, and find out as much as you can about a trainer or author of a fitness Web page. If you find a fitness Web site you like but you cannot easily find the author's name or credentials, proceed with caution.

Find out if personal trainers have a fitness-related college degree or even an advanced degree. What certifications, if any, do they have? Do they have references from people they have trained? Don't forget to check their fees—and read all the fine print. Finally, ask them what they expect of you and what you can expect of them; that will give each of you a certain level of accountability in moving towards your goals. A lot of personal trainers are available in most communities, so don't be afraid to switch if you don't like what you have.

If you have a college wellness center, it probably provides some level of personal training, usually from full-time staff or students in fitness-related majors. This service usually costs little, if anything, and a complete baseline evaluation and health screening are often available. If you seek a private trainer, you should expect the same; otherwise, look elsewhere.

Fine-Tuning Your Program to Maintain Success and Enjoyment

Q | Is there anything in particular I should keep track of over time?

What to keep track of depends on your goals and your interests. Some people don't want to feel tied to a fitness log, but others see keeping a diary of their exercise as a motivational tool. Research has found that setting goals and tracking the progress of your fitness routine are good strategies to boost success.

Depending on what type of exercise you do, you can track miles or minutes, days per week, and intensity (heart rate, RPE, and so on). A number of devices in the form of watches, chest straps, and shoe inserts will track almost everything for you. They will track your mileage and speed, and the information can be downloaded onto a computer for later viewing. Some pedometers can also connect to a computer and record, track, and graph your progress.

If you track your exercise, you can really see your progress. And if you are struggling to reach your goal, the information in your log or diary might help you figure out what isn't going well and what adjustments would be most effective. If you don't track your exercise, your adjustments are only guesswork that may not produce results. National bookstore chains and various exercise Web sites are sources for exercise diaries and logs. You can choose to keep your log online or somewhere more personal. With some logs, you can even compare your information with users from around the world, if that's what motivates you.

Q | I get bored easily. Any suggestions?

So many new gadgets are available to make exercise more fun that there is no reason for you to be bored from day to day. While walking, jogging, skating, or biking, you can carry an iPod or MP3 device and listen to music or podcasts of anything from talk radio to your class notes! Just be sure listening won't distract you from hazards while you're on the move. In many wellness centers, you can watch in-house satellite TV while you are on the cardio equipment. Video-game consoles are now available with fitness software, so you can play tennis or dance to get in your workout without ever leaving the house!

If you want to know exactly what your workout accomplished, get a GPS/heart-rate device (they can load in your shoe or be worn as armbands or watches). It will tell you the exact distance you have covered, your exact pace, your heart rate every five seconds of the workout, and even your real-time caloric expenditure! Some of these can even download the information onto your computer, where you can store it, make it into pretty graphs, and compare it over time as your fitness level and goals change.

Need some non-gadget ways to get around boredom? Spice up your workouts by adding faster or higher-intensity spurts, otherwise known as **interval training.** These changes will force you to occasionally break out of your comfort zone, more quickly increase your fitness, burn more calories, and show you how much more you might be capable of—all in the same amount of time you spent exercising yesterday. If your exercise is walking, add three or four bursts of 1–2 minutes of faster walking to your routine. Make sure you are sufficiently warmed up, and do easy walking

interval training Workouts that include periodic higher-intensity bouts of exercise in order to increase maximal oxygen consumption.

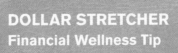

DOLLAR STRETCHER
Financial Wellness Tip

Do you like fitness DVDs? You don't need to buy them—instead, check them out from the library or rent them through Netflix or another service. Save money and enjoy the variation for your exercise routine.

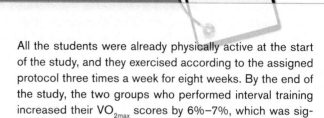

Research Brief

The Interval Advantage

Interval training can add variety to your workout and boost your VO_{2max}. In a recent study, researchers compared VO_{2max} improvements among university students assigned to one of four training protocols:

- Continuous running for 45 minutes at 70% of maximum heart rate
- Continuous running for 25 minutes at 85% of maximum heart rate
- 15/15 interval running (alternating 15 seconds of running at 90%–95% of maximum heart rate and 15 seconds of active rest at 70% of maximum heart rate) for a total of 12 minutes
- 4/4 interval running (four 4-minute runs at 90%–95% of maximum heart rate interspersed with three 3-minute periods of active rest at 70% of maximum heart rate between intervals)

All the students were already physically active at the start of the study, and they exercised according to the assigned protocol three times a week for eight weeks. By the end of the study, the two groups who performed interval training increased their VO_{2max} scores by 6%–7%, which was significantly more than the continuous exercise groups.

What does this mean for you? If increased VO_{2max} is one of your goals, then interval training is a good option. You can perform a training protocol like those described above, or you can just add short periods of more intense exercise to whatever activity you choose.

Source: Helgerud, J., and others. (2007). Aerobic high-intensity intervals improve VO_{2max} more than moderate training. *Medicine and Science in Sports and Exercise, 39*(4), 665–671.

---

cross training A pattern of training that alternates different activities (modes of exercise) that develop the same fitness component; may be done to improve performance or to avoid or rehabilitate injuries.

for at least an equal amount of time between the faster bursts. Over time, you will be able to go faster for longer, and you will quickly start seeing bigger improvements in fitness, calorie expenditure, and the like.

Still want more variety? How about **cross training**? This means that you do a few different activities throughout the week. Walking, yoga, strength training, and salsa dance. Or tennis, basketball, jogging, and strength training. You get the idea. One of the main benefits of cross training is reduced boredom. For some people, it may also reduce injury risk by varying the muscles used; this prevents overuse of a few muscles and provides the opportunity to build fitness in many different muscles. The drawback is that doing many different activities puts you at risk for more different types of injuries. Cross training also requires a lot of planning for the different activities, and buying the appropriate clothing and equipment for all of them may be costly. Many people find cross training rather enjoyable, however, and their activities change with the seasons. They look forward to getting back to an exercise they may haven't done for a few months.

Q | I want to break 20 minutes for 5K. How should I train?

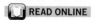

Sticking with Your Program— and Getting It Back on Track After a Lapse

Q | How am I supposed to stick with exercise over time? I've never had much luck.

Careful planning and scheduling can help change your luck. Starting an exercise program is not too hard. Staying with it is much harder. As many as half of the people who join a health club each year never actually use their membership. This is great for the club, but terrible for individual health.

Make a list of all the things you like and dislike about exercise and see which list is longer. Then try to figure out how you can emphasize the items on the "like" side and appropriately deal with the items on the "dislike" side (see the box "Tips for Exercise Motivation and Adherence").

Behavior change is discussed in Chapter 2, where there are many tips and strategies for successful change. There is no one best approach. You have to find what works for you (for example, exercising to music) and not feel obligated to do what others do (for example, exercising outdoors in hot or cold weather). Some people like dancing, but others don't. The same can be said about every form of exercise. When the criterion is sticking to it, what is a good activity for one person can be a bad choice for someone else. Pick an activity and program plan that you think will work for you. If it turns out not to work, change the activity or the schedule. Keep trying.

Wellness Strategies

Tips for Exercise Motivation and Adherence

1. Dedicate a regular time each day for exercise.
2. Do activities you enjoy.
3. Socialize with exercise.
4. Dance whenever you hear music.
5. Do more than one activity (variety is the spice of life).
6. Use quality clothing and equipment.
7. Set realistic short- and long-term goals.

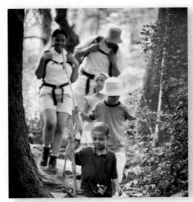

8. Keep a diary or use a pedometer to track your progress.
9. Take walking breaks during the day.
10. Walk or bike when you can.
11. Incorporate exercise into family routines.
12. Listen to your body (don't overdo it).

The most common challenge that keeps people from regular exercise is too little time in the day. People who have successfully integrated exercise into their regular schedule often use early mornings or times just before and after work or meals. This is easier if you have a regular schedule, but more difficult for part-time students, part-time workers, or full-time parents who don't have much "regular" in their life. One technique that can help get you moving in the right direction is to keep a diary of what you do throughout the day. You may be surprised at how much or how little physical activity you accumulate: The average on-campus college student walks two or three miles a day coming and going to class, meals, library, and so on; the typical full-time office worker accumulates very little physical activity.

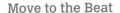

Fast Facts

Move to the Beat

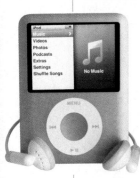

Most research on listening to music while working out has found positive effects. Music provides a pleasant distraction during exercise and, in some cases, a tempo that can help keep you moving. People tend to work out longer when they listen to music and to report less discomfort. A fast tempo of music may be preferable for higher-intensity exercise. Try listening to music during your next workout and see how you feel. Take care, however, if your workout takes you outside; use caution in high-traffic areas or other situations where use of headphones and inattention to your surroundings could risk your safety.

Q | Every semester I start exercising, then my schedule changes the next semester and I have to start all over. Do you have any suggestions?

Changing schedules is one of the biggest challenges to maintaining an exercise program, and college students face this every semester. Here are a few ideas that may help:

- Find a time (morning?) when you know you won't be working or going to class.
- Find a friend or two who can help get you out the door even when you don't feel like it.
- Sign up for an exercise class in the wellness center each semester, so you have some sense of commitment to participate in exercise regularly.
- Use contracts, rewards, and goal setting (all of which are discussed in detail in Chapter 2).

Not to minimize your concerns about your schedule and how little free time you have, but if you can figure out ways to make your schedule work for you now, you will be much better off once you are out of college and face even more demands on your time. It is well documented that parents with children living at home are not likely to get much exercise—and the younger the children, the less exercise their parents get.

Q | I used to exercise but haven't for a while. What would you recommend for me since I'm just getting back into working out?

Restarting an exercise program is a great idea and can do wonders for your physical and emotional health. If your break was due to an injury or illness and has been less than three weeks, then start back slowly, doing about half of what you had been doing. Within a week or two, you should be able to progress back to where you were.

If your break was longer—more than a month—due to injury or other reasons, then you should also start at half of where you were, but you shouldn't expect to catch up as quickly. Instead, focus on the stages of progression and don't exceed the 10-percent rule of increasing duration or intensity.

If your break from exercise has been a long time—more than 6 months—then it will be like starting over again.

Regardless of the cause or length of the exercise break, anyone restarting exercise should be proud and take the proper steps to ensure success. Fitting exercise into a daily routine isn't always easy, but with proper planning, success is just around the corner!

Summary

The benefits of cardiorespiratory fitness (CRF) have been repeated throughout this chapter: increased longevity, reduced risk of chronic disease, more energy, and improved mental health. Being in college is a great time to start an exercise program because you have many resources available. If you already exercise, this is the time to cement your habits, try new activities, and find others to exercise with you. Exercise doesn't have to be hard to do or hard to figure out. Keep it simple and you will likely succeed: Find something you like, be active on most days, accumulating at least 30 minutes each day, and breathe a little heavier during your activity. Once you have developed good exercise habits, you will find a way to keep them throughout life and the benefits will show!

More to Explore

American College of Sports Medicine
http://www.acsm.org
American Council on Exercise: Fit Facts
http://www.acefitness.org/fitfacts
Department of Health and Human Services *2008 Physical Activity Guidelines for Americans*
http://www.health.gov/paguidelines
MedlinePlus: Exercise and Physical Fitness
http://www.nlm.nih.gov/medlineplus/exerciseandphysicalfitness.html
President's Council on Physical Fitness, Sports, and Nutrition
http://www.fitness.gov

SUBMIT ONLINE

NAME   DATE   SECTION

This lab includes three field tests for assessing cardiorespiratory endurance:

1. Rockport 1-mile walk test

2. 1.5-mile run/walk test

3. 3-minute step test

These three tests provide results in terms of VO_{2max}. Choose the test that best fits your current fitness status and the equipment you have available. The 1.5 mile run/walk test is best suited for people who can jog for 15 minutes and have some experience pacing themselves. For people with lower fitness or less running experience, the walk test or the step test is probably a better choice. A partner is helpful to time you, but you can perform the tests on your own, timing yourself. The 3-minute step test is just as reliable when self-administered as it is under the supervision of trained personnel. Refer to the information about safety of exercise in Chapter 3 if you have any questions about whether CRF testing is appropriate for you.

Rockport 1-Mile Walk Test

Equipment:

- A flat track or course that provides a measurement of 1 mile
- Stopwatch, clock, or watch with a second hand
- Weight scale
- Partner to time you (optional)

Preparation:

Perform a general warm-up. Weigh yourself and record the result. Weight: [   ] lbs.

Instructions:

1. **Walk the 1-mile course as fast as possible without breaking into a run.** Record the time it takes you to walk the mile in minutes and seconds.

   Time: [   ] minutes [   ] seconds

2. **As soon as you finish the 1-mile walk, count your pulse for 15 seconds.**

   15-second pulse count: [   ] beats

3. **Cool down after the test.**

Results:

1. **Convert your weight in pounds to kilograms:** [   ] lbs. ÷ 2.2 = [   ] kilograms

2. **Convert your 1-mile walk time in minutes and seconds to a decimal value (the nearest hundredth of a minute).** For example, a time of 13 minutes and 12 seconds would be 13 + (12 ÷ 60), or 13.2.

   Time: [   ] minutes + ([   ] seconds ÷60) = [   ]

3. **Multiply your 15-second pulse count by 4 to determine your 1-minute recovery heart rate.**

   Recovery heart rate (RHH): 15-second pulse count [   ] × 4 = [   ] beats per minute (bpm)

4. Enter your values into the equation below; for gender, enter 1 if you are male and 0 if you are female.

$VO_{2max} = 132.853 - (0.1692 \times$ weight $\boxed{}$ kg$) - (0.3877 \times$ age $\boxed{}$ years$) + (6.315 \times$ gender

$\boxed{}) - (3.2649 \times$ time $\boxed{}$ minutes$) - (0.1565 \times$ RHH $\boxed{}$ bmp$) = \boxed{}$ ml/kg/min.

5. Find the rating for your VO_{2max} value from the table.

Rating: $\boxed{}$

MAXIMAL OXYGEN CONSUMPTION (VO$_{2MAX}$) RATINGS*

Males

AGE (YEARS)	WELL ABOVE AVERAGE	ABOVE AVERAGE	AVERAGE	BELOW AVERAGE	WELL BELOW AVERAGE
20–29	>51.1	45.8–51.1	42.3–45.7	38.1–42.2	<38.1
30–39	>47.5	44.4–47.5	41.0–44.3	36.7–40.9	<36.7
40–49	>46.8	42.4–46.8	38.4–42.3	34.6–38.3	<34.6
50–59	>43.3	38.3–43.3	35.2–38.2	31.1–35.1	<31.1
60+	>39.5	35.0–39.5	31.4–34.9	27.4–31.3	<27.4

Females

AGE (YEARS)	WELL ABOVE AVERAGE	ABOVE AVERAGE	AVERAGE	BELOW AVERAGE	WELL BELOW AVERAGE
20–29	>44.0	39.5–44.0	35.5–39.4	31.6–35.4	<31.6
30–39	>41.0	36.7–41.0	33.8–36.6	29.9–33.7	<29.9
40–49	>38.9	35.1–38.9	31.6–35.0	28.0–31.5	<28.0
50–59	>35.2	31.4–35.2	28.7–31.3	25.5–28.6	<25.5
60+	>32.3	29.1–32.3	26.6–29.0	23.7–26.5	<23.7

*In terms of percentiles, well above average = over the 80th percentile; above average = between 60th and 80th percentiles; average = between 40th and 60th percentiles; below average = between 20th and 40th percentiles; and well below average = below the 20th percentile.

Source: Cooper Institute for Aerobics Research. *Physical fitness assessment and norms.* Dallas, TX: Cooper Institute. For more information: http://www.cooperinstitute.org.

1.5-Mile Run/Walk Test

Equipment:

- A flat track or course that provides a measurement of 1.5 miles
- Stopwatch, clock, or watch with a second hand
- Partner to time you (optional)

Preparation:

Perform a general warm-up that includes brisk walking or slow jogging.

Instructions:

Cover the 1.5-mile course as quickly as possible. Take care to pace yourself, as careful pacing can significantly affect your time; don't overexert yourself at the start. You can alternate walking with jogging or running if needed. Record the time it takes you to complete the 1.5-mile distance in minutes and seconds. Cool down after you complete the test.

Time: [ ] minutes [ ] seconds

Results:

1. **Convert your 1.5-mile run/walk time in minutes and seconds to a decimal value (the nearest hundredth of a minute).** For example, a time of 11 minutes and 12 seconds would be $11 + (12 \div 60)$, or 11.2.

   Time: [ ] minutes + ([ ] seconds $\div$ 60) = [ ]

2. **Enter your time into the equation below:**

   $VO_{2max} = 3.5 + (483 \div \text{time}$ [ ] $\text{minutes}) =$ [ ] ml/kg/min.

3. **Find the rating for your VO_{2max} value from the table in the section on the 1-mile walk test.**

   Rating: [ ]

3-Minute Step Test

Equipment:

- 16.25-inch step
- Stopwatch or clock with a second hand
- Metronome (these can be found at music stores; free versions are also available online)

Preparation:

Warm up before taking the test. Check your equipment: Make sure the step is stable and wide enough to step up and down on comfortably and safely. Set the metronome cadence as follows:

- Women: 88 beats per minute
- Men: 96 beats per minute

Place the metronome close enough so that you can hear it throughout the test, above the sound of your stepping. Take a few practice steps. Start with both feet on the ground and then with each beat, step in this pattern: up-up-down-down. At this pace, women will complete 22 step cycles per minute and men will complete 24 step cycles per minute. You can lead with either foot and can change lead legs at any time during the test.

   Practice your step technique until you are comfortable with it. During the test, you will step for 3 minutes and then stop and take your pulse for 15 seconds. As you practice your stepping technique, also practice taking your pulse; you can take your pulse at the radial artery in your wrist or the carotid artery in your neck.

Instructions:

Once your equipment is set and you are comfortable with the technique, you are ready to begin. Step up and down for a total of 3 minutes. At the end of the test, remain standing and count your pulse for 15 seconds; start counting your pulse 5 seconds into the recovery period (if you keep the stopwatch running, you would count from 3:05 to 3:20). Note your 15-second pulse count. Then cool down for several minutes.

Results:

1. **15-second pulse count:** [ ] beats

2. **Convert your 15-second pulse count into a 1-minute pulse count**

   15-second pulse count [ ] beats $\times$ 4 = [ ] beats per minute (bpm)

3. Enter your 1-minute pulse count into the appropriate formula below.

Women: $VO_{2max} = 65.81 - (0.1847 \times \boxed{}$ bpm$) = \boxed{}$ ml/kg/min

Men: $VO_{2max} = 111.33 - (0.42 \times \boxed{}$ bpm$) = \boxed{}$ ml/kg/min

4. Find the rating for your VO_{2max} value from the table in the section on the 1-mile walk test.

Rating: $\boxed{}$

Reflecting on Your Results:

Copy your results into the chart at the right. Are you surprised with your overall rating? Did your results match what you thought about your own cardiorespiratory fitness?

	VO$_{2MAX}$ (ML/KG/MIN.)	RATING
Rockport 1-mile walk test		
1.5-mile run/walk test		
3-minute step test		

Planning Your Next Steps:

Cardiorespiratory fitness (CRF) is typically a function of training. If your scores were lower than you expected—or want—then it's time to change your activity routine or to start one. If you scored well, then strive to maintain your current level of fitness, or add some new or more advanced activities or training techniques to boost your results and add variety to your program. Set realistic goals for improvement and create a plan to achieve them. Then, in 6–10 weeks, repeat the same CRF tests you completed and note any improvements.

Describe your goals and the specific steps you will take to improve your cardiorespiratory fitness. If needed, refer to Lab Activity 4-2 on program planning.

What effect, if any, did your actions have on your CRF level? Was your plan effective? Why or why not?

Sources: Protocols and formulas for Rockport 1-mile walk test and 1.5-mile run/walk test: American College of Sports Medicine. (2008). *Health-Related Physical Fitness Assessment Manual* (2nd ed.). Philadelphia: Lippincott Williams & Wilkins.

Formula for calculation of VO$_{2max}$ for the 3-minute step test: McArdle, W.D, Katch, F.L., Pechar, G.S., Jacobson, L., & Ruck, S. (1972). Reliability and interrelationships between maximal oxygen intake, physical work capacity, and step-test scores in college women. *Medicine and Science in Sports and Exercise, 4*(4): 182–186.

Liguori, G., & Mozumdar, A. (2009). Reliability of self-assessments for a cardiovascular fitness assessment. *International Journal of Fitness, 5*(1).

LAB ACTIVITY 4-2 Planning a Cardiorespiratory Fitness Program

SUBMIT ONLINE

NAME	DATE	SECTION

Equipment: None required; you may want to develop and track your program using a paper notebook, digital spreadsheet, smart-phone application, or online program.

Preparation: None

Instructions

1. **Set SMART goals:** Set short- and long-term goals for your cardiorespiratory fitness program. Your goals can be about training—number of minutes of cycling or steps on a pedometer—or based on the results of the fitness tests you completed in Lab Activity 4-1, or both.

Current status	Goal	Target date	Notes (rewards, special considerations)

2. **Apply the FITT principal:** Use the chart below to create a program that meets the recommended criteria for success and fitness your schedule and preferences. Use one of the sets of guidelines from the chapter to help structure your program; review Table 4-2 as needed. The basic FITT guidelines from the ACSM are as follows:
   - Frequency: 3–5 days per week
   - Intensity: Target heart rate range based on 57%–94% HR_{max} or 30%–85% HRR
   - Time: 20–60 minutes per day, in bouts lasting 10 or more minutes
   - Type: Aerobic activities (those that are rhythmic, continuous, and involve work by large muscle groups)

To monitor exercise intensity, you may choose to use rating of perceived exercise (RPE) or one of the target heart-rate-range formulas; instructions for the heart-rate calculations appear below the program planning chart. Remember the relationships among frequency, intensity, and time: Higher-intensity activities can be performed for a shorter time and at a lower frequency. So, for example, three 25-minute bouts of high-intensity jogging over the course of a week would be approximately equivalent to five 30-minute bouts of brisk walking.

PROGRAM PLAN

Type of Activity	Frequency (check ✓)							Intensity (bpm or RPE)	Time (min)
	M	T	W	Th	F	Sa	Su		

RECOMMENDED STARTING INTENSITY OF EXERCISE BASED ON CURRENT ACTIVITY LEVEL

ACTIVITY LEVEL	HEART-RATE MAXIMUM (HR_{MAX}) METHOD	HEART-RATE RESERVE (HRR) METHOD
Sedentary	57%–67%	30%–45%
Minimal physical activity	64%–74%	40%–55%
Sporadic physical activity	74%–84%	55%–70%
Habitual physical activity	80%–91%	65%–80%
High amounts of habitual physical activity	84%–94%	70%–85%

SOURCE: American College of Sports Medicine. (2009). *Guidelines for exercise testing and prescription* (8th ed.). Baltimore, MD: Lippincott Williams & Wilkins.

3. **Determine Target Heart Rate Range:** Choose one of the following methods to calculate your range. Use the table to identify appropriate percentages for your level of fitness, and then use those values (in decimal form, e.g., 75% = 0.75) in the appropriate set of formulas below. You'll do the calculations twice to get a bottom and top for your target heart-rate range. You'll also calculate 10-second pulse counts by dividing the total count by 6; these 10-second pulse counts can be more easily used to monitor intensity, because you can count your pulse for 10 seconds rather than a full minute. Both methods require calculation of your maximum heart rate (MHR).

MHR = 220 – age [ ] years = [ ] bpm

Heart-rate maximum (HR_{max}) method: Selected percentage range (from table): [ ]

Bottom of range: MHR [ ] bpm × training % 0.[ ] = [ ] bpm

　　Corresponding 10-second count: [ ] bpm ÷ 6 = [ ] beats

Top of range: MHR [ ] bpm × training % 0.[ ] = [ ] bpm

　　Corresponding 10-second count: [ ] bpm ÷ 6 = [ ] beats

Full target heart-rate range: [ ] to [ ] bpm　10-second counts: [ ] to [ ] beats

Heart-rate reserve (HRR) method: Selected percentage range (from table): [ ]

Resting heart rate (see p. 114): [ ] bpm

Heart-rate reserve (HRR) = MHR [ ] bpm – RHR [ ] bpm = [ ] bpm

Bottom of range: (HRR [ ] bpm × training % 0.[ ]) + RHR [ ] bpm = [ ] bpm

　　Corresponding 10-second count: [ ] bpm ÷ 6 = [ ] beats

Top of range: (HRR [ ] bpm × training % 0.[ ]) + RHR [ ] bpm = [ ] bpm

　　Corresponding 10-second count: [ ] bpm ÷ 6 = [ ] beats

Full target heart-rate range: [ ] to [ ] bpm　10-second counts: [ ] to [ ] beats

Results: Track your progress with a log like the one below or one you create for yourself.

Activity/Date										
1	Intensity									
	Time									
	Distance									
2	Intensity									
	Time									
	Distance									
3	Intensity									
	Time									
	Distance									

Reflecting on Your Results and Planning Your Next Steps

After several weeks of your program, consider your progress. Have you been sticking with your program plan? How have you responded to it? Has your cardiorespiratory fitness increased? How do your workouts make you feel? If you have been keeping up with your program, describe your plans going forward. If you haven't been following your plan, come up with at least three plan changes or strategies to help improve your motivation and adherence.

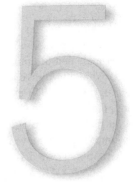

5

Muscle Fitness

>> **COMING UP IN THIS CHAPTER**
Learn how your muscles work and what affects their functioning › Discover the benefits of muscle fitness › Assess your level of muscle fitness › Develop a personalized muscle-fitness program

Wellness Connections

How does muscle fitness relate to your overall wellness? Like many other topics discussed in this text, the physical-wellness dimension of muscle fitness is relatively easy to identify: Either you have the strength and endurance to perform your desired tasks, or you don't. And you can choose to remain as you are, or you can train to increase your muscle fitness. Although this may sound simplistic, it can actually be that easy. Increases in muscle fitness will improve your balance, speed, and agility, while also preventing or reducing musculoskeletal injuries.

But muscle fitness also affects other dimensions of wellness. As you increase your muscle fitness, your self-esteem may also increase, thereby improving social and emotional wellness along with your physical wellness. Once you start improving selected wellness dimensions, you'll become more aware of other areas in your life that you want to improve, and you'll be more likely to try to make positive changes. In this way, improving muscle fitness can have a positive impact on your overall state of wellness.

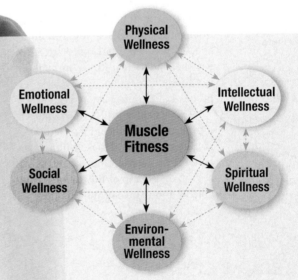

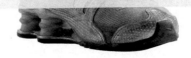

Citius, Altius, Fortius. "Faster, Higher, Stronger." This Latin phrase is the motto of the modern Olympics and of the many amateur and professional athletes who aim to give their best during competition. Muscle fitness isn't their exclusive domain, however. Every person, regardless of age, gender, or ability, can improve through physical training. Training the body to be stronger (or jump higher or move faster) provides numerous physical and emotional benefits throughout the lifespan.[1]

muscle fitness The ability of one or more muscles to perform routine tasks without undue fatigue.

muscle force The speed with which a muscle can move a given object one time. The force of a muscle depends on its size, length, speed, and the joint angle. A muscle develops greater force when it is elongated, and less force when it is shortened.

muscle endurance The ability to sustain an effort for an extended time. This is often measured by determining the maximum number of repetitions of a given resistance.

muscle strength The ability of one or more muscles to exert force by contracting against resistance. This is often measured by determining the most weight lifted during one effort.

muscle power The ability of a muscle to move an object quickly and repeatedly.

Although you may not reach an Olympic pedestal, your prospects of improving your overall wellness through increased muscle fitness are as bright as the Olympic flame. Young or old, male or female, it doesn't take much to improve muscle fitness. And it is important! Muscles make your body function and move. Muscles take fuel from the food you eat and turn it into energy for body processes and purposeful movement. Without muscles, your heart would not beat, your lungs would not inflate, and food would not pass through your digestive tract. Movements large and small—from running up stairs to simply speaking or smiling—are only possible through the precise actions of your muscles. Your muscles will last you a lifetime, and, if you take care of them, they will help you stay strong throughout it. Muscle fitness can significantly improve quality of life at any age.

This chapter will explore muscle fitness in detail, including factors affecting your level of muscle fitness, the benefits of muscle fitness, ways to assess it, and many of the options available to improve your muscle fitness.

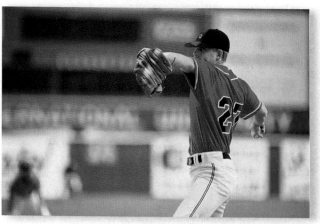

One component of muscle fitness is muscle power, which is the ability to exert force rapidly.

- **Muscle strength:** The ability to generate maximal force against resistance, such as lifting the heaviest weight you can, one time
- **Muscle power:** The ability to exert optimal force rapidly, such as throwing a baseball

Although muscle fitness is not the same as weight lifting, it can be improved through weight lifting. However, gains in muscle fitness are not limited to structured weight-training programs.

Many factors can affect your muscle fitness, including age, gender, injuries, and training. Another key factor is your genetic makeup: Look at your parents and siblings—what you see is usually what you get![2] This doesn't mean you don't have some control of your muscle fitness, because you do. However, if you want to be a champion power lifter, you'll need a set of genes that puts you on that path. If, on the other hand, you simply want to improve your overall health, you don't need any special genes: You simply need a few minutes a week to practice muscle-fitness exercises. The improvement will be quickly noticeable.

skeletal muscle Muscle tissue that is connected to bones and moves them in order to produce body movement.

cardiac muscle A specialized muscle tissue found only in the heart. It has its own electrical conduction system and keeps the heart beating in response to the body's need for oxygen. Cardiac muscle is much less resistant to fatigue than other muscle types.

Factors Affecting Muscle Fitness

Q | What's muscle fitness? Is it the same as weight lifting?

As described in Chapter 3, **muscle fitness**—the ability of muscles to perform routine tasks without undue fatigue—has several components:

- **Muscle force:** The effort required to overcome resistance, such as a barbell or your body weight
- **Muscle endurance:** The ability to sustain an effort for a prolonged period, such as performing multiple sit-ups or holding a bent-arm hang

Types of Muscles

Q | Is it true that there are different kinds of muscles?

Yes, it is true, and we all have some of each kind. The human body has three muscle types:

- **Skeletal muscle,** which is found throughout the body, covering and attached to the skeleton. Skeletal muscles move your bones to produce precise movements.
- **Cardiac muscle,** which is found only in the heart. It has its own electrical conduction system to keep your

smooth muscle Muscle tissue in the walls of body organs such as the stomach and intestines. It controls involuntary movement and makes the organs expand and contract.

tendon The fibrous connective tissue by which a muscle attaches to a bone.

ligament A sheet or band of tough, fibrous tissue connecting bones or cartilage at a joint or supporting an organ.

muscle fiber (muscle cell) Each skeletal muscle consists of hundreds or thousands of tiny fibers bundled together and wrapped in a connective-tissue covering. Muscle fibers coordinate muscle contractions for movement.

myofibrils Microscopic protein filaments that make up muscle cells.

nucleus A structure in a cell that contains most of the cell's genetic material, which controls gene expression.

mitochondria Structures within cells in which most of the chemical reactions in cellular (oxidative) respiration occur; the location for most adenosine triphosphate (ATP) production.

sarcoplasmic reticulum (SER) In muscle cells, a network of vesicles and tubules that store calcium, which is released as one step in the muscle-contraction process.

heart beating at a speed to match your body's need for oxygen.

■ **Smooth muscle,** which is found in the walls of body organs like the stomach and the intestines. It typically acts to make an organ expand or contract.

Cardiac and smooth muscle are involuntary muscles, meaning they contract without any conscious effort on your part. This is a good thing; otherwise, essential activities like respiration, circulation, and digestion would require conscious effort. The action of smooth muscles is controlled by the autonomic nervous system and body chemicals such as hormones, both of which function outside conscious control.

Skeletal muscles, in contrast, are voluntary muscles, meaning they are mostly under your control. Skeletal muscle can be activated with conscious thought, allowing you to decide how, when, and where your body will move. When viewed under a microscope, skeletal muscles appear to have stripes or lines known as striations, which is why skeletal muscles are called striated muscles. Although both cardiac and skeletal muscle can be shaped and strengthened over time through appropriate physical activity, most people are interested in training skeletal muscle, because we can see and feel when these muscles change. This is not to downplay the importance of strengthening cardiac muscle! Chapters 4 and 11 discuss the many risks of not conditioning your heart.

There are over five hundred skeletal muscles in the body, making up 35–45 percent of the body's weight. A typical skeletal muscle stretches from one bone to another, usually crossing a joint. Skeletal muscle attaches to bone via bands of fibrous connective tissue known as **tendons.** (Another type of connective tissue, **ligaments,** connects bone to bone.)

Q How do my muscles actually work?

Skeletal muscle is made up of many tiny **muscle fibers** (muscle cells), which are elongated and typically run the length of the muscle (Figure 5-1). The fibers stay together

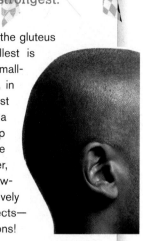

thanks to special connective tissue that also houses blood vessels and nerves. Each muscle fiber contains these parts:

■ **Myofibrils:** Protein filaments making up muscle cells, including thin filaments known as *actin* and thick filaments known as *myosin.*

■ **Nucleus** (plural, *nuclei*): A structure inside a cell that contains the cell's genetic material; muscle cells have multiple nuclei, which enhance their ability to synthesize proteins and to grow.

■ **Mitochondria:** Intracellular structures containing enzymes that convert the energy in food into fuel for the muscle.

■ **Sarcoplasmic reticulum:** A lacy membrane surrounding myofibrils that plays an important role in triggering muscle contraction.

For a skeletal muscle to move or contract, the contractile protein filaments actin and myosin need to slide over each other. This process is explained by the **sliding filament theory.** As described in Chapter 4, in order for a muscle to move, the cellular fuel adenosine triphosphate (ATP) needs to be present. The majority of ATP is produced within the mitochondria from one of the body's energy systems. As you learned in Chapter 4, the aerobic energy system is most important for cardiorespiratory endurance exercise; it can also be important for some muscular endurance activities. However, the aerobic energy system is less important for muscle-fitness training because of the short effort required. Instead, the sources of energy that don't require oxygen—ATP/PC and the anaerobic energy system—are used much more extensively during muscle-fitness training.

sliding filament theory (SFT) An explanation of how muscles shorten, or produce force. According to the SFT, thick and thin filaments within muscle cells slide past one another to shorten the muscle. This process requires the presence of ATP.

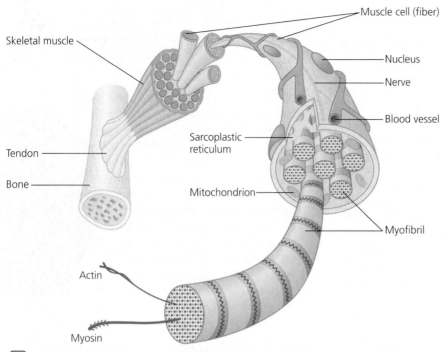

Skeletal muscle

Tendon

Bone

Actin

Myosin

Muscle cell (fiber)

Nucleus

Nerve

Blood vessel

Sarcoplastic reticulum

Mitochondrion

Myofibril

▶ WATCH ONLINE   Figure 5-1 **Basic components of skeletal muscle tissue**

Q | What makes my arms feel "pumped" when I'm lifting?

Your arms feel "pumped" when you lift because of the increase in blood flow to the muscles in your arms. As you engage in any type of exercise, there is a dramatic shift or redistribution of blood flow. The muscles that are being asked to do the work—the arms in this case—receive lots of nourishing blood, while nonessential, nonexercising parts of the body such as the digestive tract receive less blood and tend to shut down and conserve. Maybe this is why your mom told you not to eat right before exercising, because your stomach stops digesting and you are left with food sloshing around!

Types of Muscle Fibers

As discussed earlier in the chapter, there are three main types of muscle: cardiac, smooth, and skeletal. Skeletal muscle—the type that moves our bones, makes us look good, and keeps us strong—is made up of two general fiber types (type I and type II). The percentage of these fibers you are endowed with at birth plays a significant role in determining your muscle-fitness abilities.

Q | Why can my roommate beat me racing to the dining hall even though she never exercises?

Maybe she knows a shortcut? Or more likely, she has a high percentage of the type of skeletal muscle fiber suited for fast sprinting—or at least a higher percentage than you have. There are two

basic types of skeletal muscle fiber: **slow-twitch muscle fibers** (type I) and **fast-twitch muscle fibers**; fast-twitch fibers are categorized as type IIa or type IIx. The fiber types differ in level of endurance, rate of force production, and potential for **hypertrophy** (increase in fiber size). Each of your muscles contains a mix of fiber types.

Our ancestors sometimes needed to travel long distances in search of food, and at other times they needed to run fast or jump high to escape harm. As a result, a typical person has about half fast-twitch and half slow-twitch fibers, although tremendous individual variation exists. Elite athletes are likely to have a lot more of one or the other fiber type, depending on the event in which they excel.[3] Although only a select few are destined for athletic glory, the rest of us have muscle fibers that are well suited for our basic daily needs, which include improving our overall wellness through proper training.

Although there is no difference in the force production of the two muscle-fiber types, the rate at which force can be produced differs. This may be one reason your roommate is faster than you. Her fast-twitch fibers can generate force quickly, whereas your slow-twitch fibers sacrifice quick force production for fatigue resistance—meaning you can run farther rather than faster. Fast-twitch fibers (types IIa and IIx) are much better at generating short bursts of strength or speed by using anaerobic metabolism to create fuel (Table 5-1; see Chapter 4 for more on aerobic and anaerobic energy production). Fast-twitch fibers can

slow-twitch muscle fibers (type I) Muscle fibers that have a slow rate of force generation. Slow-twitch fibers are highly dependent on oxygen and can sustain a given effort indefinitely.

fast-twitch muscle fibers (types IIa and IIx) Muscle fibers that have a fast rate of force production. Fast-twitch fibers can produce force with little, if any, oxygen, but cannot sustain an effort for very long.

hypertrophy An increase in the size of muscle fibers, typically accomplished through resistance training.

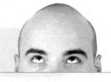

Mind Stretcher
Critical Thinking Exercise

What do you think when you see someone who is especially toned or muscular? Do you associate different personality traits with different levels of muscularity? Where do you think your ideas come from? How have your ideas affected your own goals for strength training?

TABLE 5-1 TYPES OF MUSCLE FIBER

FIBER TYPE	AEROBIC METABOLISM	ANAEROBIC METABOLISM	SPEED OF CONTRACTION	DURATION OF ACTION
Type I	Yes	No	Slow	Indefinite
Type IIa	Yes	Yes	Faster	Limited
Type IIx	No	Yes	Fastest	Brief

generate lots of force in a little time, which is especially important if you want to perform basic strength-related tasks around the house. However, this force production lasts for only a few seconds. Fast-twitch fibers are also more prone to hypertrophy, so the more you have, the bigger your muscles can become with proper training.

Slow-twitch fibers contain more mitochondria and myoglobin than fast-twitch fibers do, making them more efficient at using oxygen, generating ATP, and maintaining muscle contractions for an extended time. This allows us to prolong an activity. Typically, postural muscles tend to be slow-twitch, allowing us to stay erect for long periods.

Ultimately, fiber type plays an important role in who gets to the dining hall first. However, muscle fiber type is largely determined at birth, so if you want to beat your roommate to the dining hall and you can't trade in your parent's genes, you might consider getting a head start!

Gender

Q | As a woman, do I really need to lift?

Yes—but only if you want to maintain your health, weight, and lifelong independence. Multiple studies have confirmed that women benefit from muscle-fitness training just as much as men. Women can see noticeable weight loss and muscle increase in as little as two months of regular strength training. Another benefit is the possibility of delaying or preventing age-related loss of muscle and bone mass, both of which women are highly susceptible to. Women who allow their muscle strength to decrease with age often lose the ability to handle the activities of daily living (such as bathing, cooking, and shopping) and may therefore lose their independence. Women who maintain muscle fitness throughout their lifespan are much less likely to suffer this fate.

Q | Can I get stronger but stay feminine looking? What can I do to get tone instead of looking too muscular?

▶ WATCH ONLINE

Women often fear getting "too big" from strength training. This is perhaps the biggest myth about muscle fitness—because it simply won't happen. There are two main reasons:

muscle-fiber type and hormones. First, remember that type II muscle fibers (fast-twitch) are more prone to hypertrophy than type I muscle fibers are. Compared to men, women have less overall muscle area as type II fibers and thus a decided disadvantage in building big muscles. Second, getting big is highly dependent on **testosterone,** a hormone that helps to increase muscle-fiber size. Women have at least 30 percent less testosterone than

testosterone Derived from cholesterol, this anabolic steroid hormone is the principal male sex hormone and is critical for increasing muscle mass. The average male produces about fifty times more testosterone than a female, thereby allowing men to produce greater muscle mass than women.

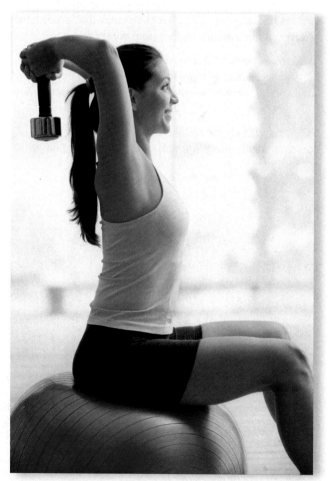

Women can increase strength and muscle size in response to training, but due to fiber-type and hormonal differences, their muscles do not become as large as men's muscles do.

men, so this is another decided disadvantage for women in terms of building big muscles.[4]

Women who lift weights tend to use light weights and a high number of repetitions—this is both good and bad for the "too big" dilemma. A light weight provides a fairly small level of resistance (overload), so gains in strength are fairly small. However, research has established that a high-repetition program (8–15 repetitions) with a lighter weight is more likely to produce hypertrophy than a low-repetition program (1–6 repetitions) with a heavier weight, which is better for building muscular strength. So, ironically, women tend to do the type of program that builds size rather than strength—usually not what they want. To gain strength, a program with fewer repetitions and a heavier weight is more effective.[5] Because of the muscle fiber and hormonal differences between men and women, women will not get big like men from such a program—but they will get stronger.[6]

Q | I heard that weight lifting will make me gain weight. Is that true?

It is possible—but very unlikely. Muscle tissue is denser than fat tissue, meaning the same amount of muscle tissue weighs more than fat tissue.[7] On the flip side, this means that a pound of muscle tissue is smaller than a pound of fat tissue. The typical changes that occur when starting a muscle-training program are these:

1. Loss of body fat due to increased exercise
2. Increased muscle mass (after a few weeks)
3. Loss of inches around the waist, upper arms, and elsewhere

The loss of body fat and the increase in muscle mass may cause a small change in body weight, or they may offset each other. However, if you lose a pound of fat and gain a pound of muscle, there will be a loss of inches because of muscle's greater density (Figure 5-2). The loss of inches, which is the most important change for many people, may not show up on a scale, but you are likely to notice a better fit in your clothes, and possibly a smaller clothes size, along with stronger muscles. A well-rounded exercise program (cardiovascular and muscle training) is most likely to result in a net loss of body weight. Very rarely does anyone accumulate enough muscle to offset the loss of fat unless he or she is involved in bodybuilding or weight-lifting competitions.

Age and Use

Q | Will I get weaker as I get older?

Muscle mass and strength both decrease with age in men as well as women, starting around age 25 or 30.[8] This is largely due to the combination of decreased levels of circulating testosterone and other hormones and decreased physical activity.

Regular strength training, however, is highly effective for maintaining muscle fitness throughout the lifespan. Between the ages of 20 and 60, active and well-trained people can maintain most of their muscle fitness, reaching a peak around the age of 30. In untrained or sedentary people, muscle fitness begins to decline slowly and steadily starting at the age of 30, and by age 40 it is already less than it was at age 20. The typical untrained male loses about 30 percent of his peak strength by the age of 60, whereas a trained male does not lose any noticeable strength by that age. Over age 60, the noticeable reduction in testosterone and growth hormone circulating in the blood causes a more

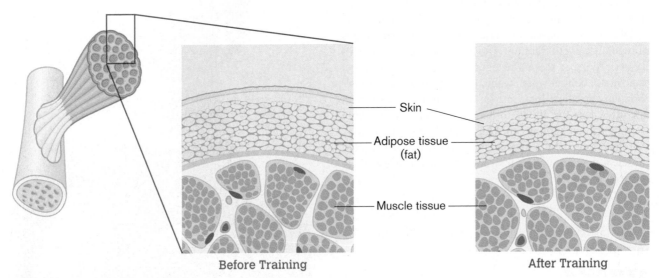

Before Training   After Training

▶ **WATCH ONLINE** Figure 5-2 **Changes in muscle and fat tissue in response to training.** The number of muscle fibers and fat cells does not change, but muscles fibers (especially fast-twitch fibers) increase in size and fat cells decrease in size.

rapid decline in muscle strength—all the more reason to continue with muscle fitness training as you age.[9]

Q | Do my muscles change in any way as I get older?

It depends on how active you are throughout adulthood. If you remain relatively active, there probably won't be many changes. If you are usually sedentary, then yes, your muscles will change, but not in the absolute sense. Muscle-fiber types (slow-twitch, fast-twitch) cannot convert from one to another, nor can muscle change into fat, or vice versa, contrary to popular belief. What does occur with aging or prolonged sedentary behavior is selective atrophy of the fast-twitch muscle fibers, meaning fewer and smaller type II fibers. The fast-twitch fibers do not become slow-twitch fibers; you simply have fewer type II fibers available.[10]

An additional age-related phenomenon is **sarcopenia,** defined as the loss of muscle mass, strength, and function. Because there is a clear relationship between muscle mass and strength, if one decreases, so does the other. Sarcopenia begins in the fourth decade of life and typically accelerates after the age of 75. With aging and inactivity, most atrophy occurs in fast-twitch muscle fibers. Don't be discouraged, because this atrophy can be significantly offset by maintaining a muscle-fitness training program. Without training, however, aging will cause an increase of one tissue (fat) and a decrease of another (muscle).

Q | How long until I start getting big?

Most research shows that muscle size begins to increase after 6–8 weeks of regular training. But an increase in strength is noticeable almost from the beginning of a muscle-training program. This is typically due to improved neuromuscular functioning, however, not to increased muscle size.[11] The neurological change is similar to what you experience when learning how to ride a bike. Your leg muscles don't get stronger right away, but your muscles and nerves get more comfortable with the movement pattern, thereby making the task much easier. This phenomenon is largely responsible for strength gains over the first 6–8 weeks of training. At that point, if the training has included a sufficient amount of overload (progressively more resistance), then muscle-fiber size, or mass, begins to increase. This increase in muscle mass, or muscle hypertrophy, is due to muscle fibers increasing in size, not number. The number of muscle fibers (cells) is largely determined at birth and although increases have been noted in animals, it is yet to be determined if the same is true in humans.[12]

If muscle-fitness training ceases after hypertrophy starts, then **atrophy,** or a decrease in muscle-fiber size, will begin within 4–6 weeks. This is not the same as the age-old myth that muscle turns to fat with disuse. Not true: The size of muscle fibers decreases and, because the person has become sedentary, subcutaneous fat increases, so he or she looks and feels fatter and less "muscley."

Q | Can lifting weights at an early age stunt your growth? **READ ONLINE**

Genetics

Q | Is strength mostly genetic?

Genetics clearly plays a role, but its effects vary. The genetic influence on muscle fitness is difficult to study. Twin and family studies are the best ways to identify the contribution of genes (heritability) in determining muscular strength, power, and endurance. The current evidence seems to indicate that the heritability of muscle differs between genders and also varies for strength, endurance, and power. The role of genes in determining absolute muscle strength appears greater for men than for women.

The overall heritability for hand-grip *strength* is estimated to be about 50 percent. This means your hand-grip strength is half due to your genetic makeup and half due to what you do day to day to get stronger.[13] The genetic contribution to *power,* however, tends to be a bit more than

sarcopenia An age-related loss of muscle fiber, muscle strength, and muscle mass.

atrophy A decrease in the size of muscle fibers, typically as a result of chronic disuse.

Fast Facts

Muscles Lost in Space!

Astronauts face many challenges during long space flights, one of which is maintaining their muscle strength. Although astronauts engage in plenty of physical tasks during the typical space flight, their muscles can suffer greatly due to the lack of gravity and its associated resistance. A zero-gravity environment causes a rapid decrease in muscle fiber size, which can quickly reduce peak muscle power by as much as 50 percent. Spaceships and space stations are outfitted with treadmills and stationary bikes to help astronauts offset the lack of gravity. Although it is not possible to totally counteract the effects of weightlessness, astronauts who regularly exercise in space show only a 13 percent decrease in muscle power compared to a 51 percent decrease for astronauts who do only a little exercise!

50 percent due to the influence of muscle-fiber types: fast-twitch fibers can generate more power by means of faster contraction rates. The heritability of muscle *endurance* seems to be lowest of all. Therefore, your genes are responsible for no more than about 50 percent of any of your muscle functions (strength, power, or endurance). If you want to get bigger, faster, or stronger, you will have to train appropriately and apply the law of specificity!

An aspect of muscle fitness that does have a strong genetic influence is muscle hypertrophy, or the ability of a muscle to increase in size.[14] Type II (fast-twitch) muscle fiber is much more likely to experience hypertrophy than type I (slow-twitch) fiber, and as previously stated, the percentage of type II fibers is largely determined at birth. Type II fibers can get bigger with regular muscle training—through formal strength training, heavy physical labor (through a job such as landscaping), or a recreational pursuit (such as rollerblading). Cardiac muscle can also increase in size, and although less specific, this typically occurs in response to regular aerobic exercise.

Benefits of Muscle Fitness

Muscle fitness is critical to your short- and long-term well-being. If you keep your muscles strong throughout life, you can expect numerous benefits, including improved control of body weight and better-fitting clothes, greater ability to perform work and leisure tasks, a decreased risk of age-related diseases, and better psychological and emotional wellness.

Body Weight Control

Q | Will weight lifting increase my metabolism?

It does seem we read this all the time: Lift weights and your metabolism (the rate at which you burn calories) will increase. But the scientific literature is mixed on this concept.[15] Although the activity of lifting weights does increase metabolism during your workout and for some time afterward, the overall effect may not be substantial. However, muscle is metabolically active, so your metabolism may be affected when your muscle cells grow in size. In other words, as the absolute amount of muscle in your body increases, so does your resting metabolism—and you burn more calories throughout the day. Generally speaking, for each pound of muscle you gain, you burn 35–50 more calories each day. Although that number may seem small, it can add up over time, all the way to the loss of about four pounds of body weight per year—from adding just one pound of muscle!

Q | Which burns more calories—lifting weights or running?

Both types of exercise burn calories, and the number of calories burned is largely dependent on the intensity of the effort. Running is a con-

tinuous activity, and muscle training tends to be discontinuous (you often stop to rest between sets); therefore, running has the potential to burn more calories. However, because of the frequent rests in muscle training, you can work at a consistently higher intensity than you can for a sustained run. The difference is not too significant though, so you should engage in both cardiovascular and muscle-fitness exercises for optimal all-around physical wellness and weight management. If your time for exercise is limited, it is possible to do both types of training together, alternating a few minutes of running with a few minutes of muscle training.

Improved Performance

Q | What can I do to improve my sports performance?

Train, train, and keep on training. Muscle fitness training plays an important role in improving performance in most sports. Skiers ski better, golfers drive the ball farther, and cyclists ride faster for a longer time. Whatever sport you play, muscle training can improve overall performance by boosting speed and intensity and making you more efficient—the results are most dramatic for beginners. Muscle training can also reduce your risk of injury.

The question all budding athletes ask is, How much strength is enough? However, optimal performance depends more on improving individual sports skills (for ex-

---

Behavior Change Challenge
Video Case Study

▶ **WATCH ONLINE** Meet Rhett

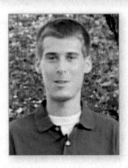

Rhett is a college student attending Georgia Southern University, living off campus. Rhett considers himself on the scrawny side and wants to start working out with weights in order to gain strength and muscle mass. Watch the video to learn more about Rhett, his behavior-change goals and plan, and how successful he is over the initial nine weeks of his program. As you watch the video, think about the following questions:

- How realistic are Rhett's goals and his starting program plan?
- Does Rhett have enough motivation and environmental support for his program? What do you think his key challenges will be?
- What can you learn from Rhett's experience that will help you in your behavior-change efforts?

ample, a swimming stroke or tennis swing) than on simply getting stronger. A swimmer with outstanding muscle strength but poor technique is still going to finish in the back of the pack. The tennis player who has not learned how to hit a decent backhand but has a lot of muscle strength will probably hit the ball over the fence, if and when she does make contact. So overall, strength without skill tends to produce less than optimal results.

The swimmer who has excellent technique but little muscle strength will probably beat the swimmer with poor technique and strong muscles—but he still might not win the race. Ultimately, the swimmer (or tennis, rugby, or judo player) who can combine optimal strength with optimal technique is likely to maximize performance. Athletes, professional or recreational, who can combine strength with stability, power, balance, and skill will be able to perform their sport in a satisfying manner, more easily reach personal goals, and reduce their chance of injury. For most recreational athletes, training at a moderate level of intensity (rather than high intensity) should be sufficient to achieve their personal goals.

Reduced Risk of Injury and Disease

Although it may be asking a lot for any type of exercise to reduce injury and disease, strength training can do both. Muscle fitness can help prevent overuse injuries, improve mobility and balance, and help prevent and manage chronic diseases like diabetes, osteoporosis, and heart disease.

Q | What can I do to keep from spraining my ankle all the time?

Ankle sprains can result from many different activities, so there is no guarantee you can prevent them entirely. However, improved skill efficiency and better balance and mobility will go a long way toward reducing your risk of ankle sprains, tendonitis, bursitis, and other muscle-related injuries.

Although any type of exercise carries a risk of injury, safe and effective training methods minimize this risk. Increasing muscle fitness through strength training has many benefits. For example, tendonitis, a common overuse injury, can be prevented with a moderate level of muscle fitness and can be rehabilitated with appropriate strength-training routines. Good muscle fitness is especially important for older individuals, as it improves balance, making falls and associated injuries much less likely.

Q | I thought walking and jogging were enough to prevent diseases. Do I really need to strength train?

Yes. Strength training is not often the first kind of exercising that comes to mind when people think about disease prevention. However, plenty of evidence supports strength training, or increased muscle fitness, as being quite beneficial for reducing the risk of certain chronic diseases.[16] Osteoporosis, back pain, arthritis, heart disease, and diabetes can all be positively affected by regular muscle-fitness training. Muscle training obviously builds stronger bones and muscles, but did you know it also strengthens connective tissues and increases the stability of joints?

Back pain and osteoarthritis are two major health problems facing adults in the United States. Back pain is usually a result of muscle weakness and poor posture (see Chapter 6). As muscle weakens, it leads to poor posture, and poor posture can in turn lead to further muscle weakness. Strength training is a great way to prevent or reverse this cycle and improve your back's health. Regular muscle training is effective 80 percent of the time in eliminating or reducing symptoms of back pain. You might be thinking, "So what—my back doesn't hurt." But at some point in their lives, 80 percent of all adults miss time from work due to low-back pain, so don't wait until it is too late. Get those muscles fit now!

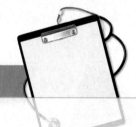

Research Brief

Strength Training and Posture

How's your posture? Thirty-four men and women (average age 45 years) completed a ten-week training program that included about 20 minutes of aerobic activity, 12 strength exercises, and 12 stretching exercises three times a week. The study participants performed one set of 8–12 repetitions of exercises for each major muscle group.

Each study subject was carefully assessed before and after the training program for, among other variables, standing height and head position, which are direct indications of posture. At the end of the study, the standing height of the participants increased by an average of 0.2 inches and their head position improved by 0.4 inches. These changes indicate a significant improvement in posture after only ten weeks of strengthening and stretching exercises.

Source: Westcott, W. (2005). Strength training increases height, improves posture and enhances balance in older adults. *Wellness.MA* (http://www.wellness.ma/senior-fitness/senior-strength-training-posture.htm).

osteoporosis A progressive decrease in bone mineral density that leads to an increased risk of fracture. It is more common in women than in men, especially after menopause.

Osteoporosis is another condition that is noticeably improved with strength training. Osteoporosis is characterized by loss of bone density, which weakens bones, and it can result in hip, wrist, and ankle fractures, especially from falls. Osteoporosis can occur through the effects of aging, inactivity, and poor diet. Well over half of all women will develop this condition, but more men are developing it as well. Strength training is one of the cornerstones for preventing osteoporosis and minimizing its debilitating effects; it helps build and maintain bone density as well as improving balance and reducing falls.

Cardiovascular disease (CVD) and diabetes take many people's lives each year and significantly reduce quality of life for many others (see Chapter 11). People with diabetes typically die of CVD, the number-one cause of death in the United States. Regular strength training can help prevent or improve both of these conditions. Strength training can lower LDL ("bad") cholesterol, raise HDL ("good") cholesterol, and decrease resting blood pressure. Strength training may also improve the body's ability to process sugar, which reduces the risk of diabetes. Therefore, if improving muscle fitness can lessen the risk of CVD and diabetes in these ways, then that is a true health benefit!

Improved Emotional and Psychological Wellness

Although cardiovascular and muscle fitness training has long been accepted as a means of reducing negative emotions, recent evidence indicates that exercise can enhance positive psychological states, particularly increased feelings of energy.[17] Emotional and psychological wellness can also be improved through regular muscle training. Individuals engaged in muscle training or other forms of regular exercise tend to display more positive than negative emotions, more favorable thoughts, more energy and vigor, and less anxiety and depression, all leading to greater levels of emotional wellness, a key component of overall wellness (as noted in the Wellness Connections at the start of the chapter).

Q | Lifting always makes me feel better. Is there a reason for that?

Yes. Muscle-fitness training, like other types of exercise, can elevate mood. The underlying cause isn't entirely understood, but here are some possible explanations for the mood-elevating benefits of physical exercise:

- Distraction—the exercise allows for a time-out from stress and negative emotions
- Release of endorphins, which are hormones linked to pain relief and elevation of mood
- Increased core temperature, which reduces muscle tension and results in a more relaxed psychological state
- Changes in brain chemistry; specifically, alterations in the levels or actions of the neurotransmitters epinephrine, norepinephrine, and dopamine

These changes are typically short-term, occurring after a single session of exercise. Longer-term psychological benefits can also result from regular strength training. Research supports the idea that as little as ten weeks of strength training can reduce clinical depression symptoms more ef-

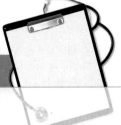

Research Brief

Strength Training for Chronic Neck Pain

Chronic neck pain is an increasingly common problem, as students and workers spend more time in front of computers. A study of women with chronic neck pain found that strength training targeting the shoulder and neck muscles provided long-lasting pain relief. The study assigned the women to one of three groups:

- A group who engaged in supervised, high-intensity strength training of the neck and shoulder muscles

- A group who engaged in general fitness training
- A control group who received general health counseling

After ten weeks, neck pain in the strength-training group decreased by over 70 percent, compared to no significant change in the neck pain for the general fitness-training and health-counseling groups. These findings suggest that strength training of neck and shoulder muscles can be an effective means of treating neck and shoulder pain.

Source: Andersen, L. L., et al. (2008). Effect of two contrasting types of physical exercise on chronic neck muscle pain. *Arthritis Care and Research, 59*(1): 84–91.

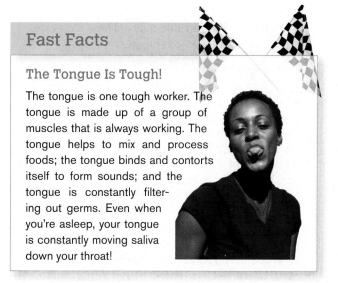

fectively than counseling,[18] and women actively working to improve their muscle fitness commonly report feeling more confident and capable (increased self-esteem and self-efficacy), important factors in fighting depression. Regular exercise positively affects emotional wellness. Conversely, someone suffering from poor emotional wellness is less likely to engage in muscle fitness training or any other type of exercise.

Assessing Your Muscle Fitness

Q | How strong do I need to be?

Your muscle-fitness goals depend on you. You need to be strong enough to complete your daily tasks with energy left over for leisure pursuits. In addition, you want to be strong enough to minimize your risk of injury and disease. This may sound like a lot, but it is really quite achievable.

A better question than "How strong do I need to be?" might be "How do I figure out how strong I am?" As with any fitness component, assessing muscle fitness is important because it allows you to gauge your current fitness level, to design an effective and appropriate training program, and to periodically measure your progress. First, however, you need to determine what component of muscle fitness you want to assess—muscle strength or muscle endurance.

Muscle strength is typically assessed by measuring or estimating the maximum amount of weight you can lift one time, which is referred to as a **one-repetition maximum,** or **1-RM.** When friends brag about how much they can bench press, they are talking about a 1-RM. *Muscle endurance* can be assessed in different ways: For example, you can do as many repetitions as possible of a given exercise, such as push-ups, or you can do a timed test, such as how many curl-ups you can do in one minute. Norms can help you compare your level of muscular strength to others of your age and gender. You can also use strength and endurance tests to assess if your muscle-fitness program is working: Periodically reassess yourself with the same tests to track your progress and to provide feedback so that you can make appropriate adjustments to your program.

Instructions for several strength and endurance tests are found in the labs at the end of the chapter; be sure to pay attention to all the safety guidelines for performing these assessments. If you've been sedentary for a long time or haven't done any muscle-fitness training in a while, don't perform an assessment on your first day of training. Instead, take a few days or weeks to get your muscles used to training and to familiarize yourself with the equipment. Most college-age students in good physical health should have no problem with these assessments. If, however, you have special health concerns or a family history of chronic disease (such as high blood pressure or diabetes), it would be wise to first check with your

1-repetition maximum (1-RM) The maximum amount of weight lifted one time.

TABLE 5-2 CHANGES AND BENEFITS IN RESPONSE TO MUSCLE FITNESS TRAINING

	MALE	FEMALE	YOUNG	OLD
Improved balance, stability, posture	Yes	Yes	Yes	Yes
Increased muscle endurance	Yes	Yes	Yes	Yes
Increased muscle speed, power, strength	Yes	Yes	Yes	Yes
Reduced disease risk	Yes	Yes	Yes	Yes
Weight loss or maintenance	Yes	Yes	Yes	Yes
Muscle gain	Yes	Yes	Yes	Yes
Significant hypertrophy	Yes	Not likely	Yes	Not Likely

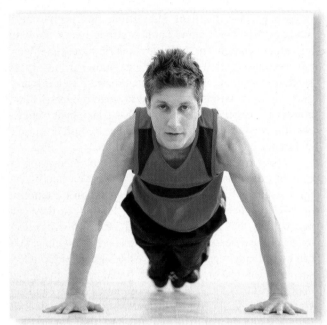

You can assess your muscular endurance by counting the number of times you can complete an exercise like a push-up with good form or the number you can do during a set period of time.

physician before engaging in muscle-fitness training or assessment. (See Chapter 3 for more on exercise safety.)

Q I can bench 130 pounds. What does that mean?

How much weight you can lift, or how many repetitions you can perform, is a measure of your current muscle-fitness level, regardless of what others can do. This value is your baseline, which you can use to evaluate your progress over time.

If you want to know how you compare to others like you (similar age and gender), you can use the established norms presented in the tables in Lab Activities 5-1 and 5-2. If your score ranks you at the 50th percentile, that means half the people in your category can do more and half can do less than you. If you are in the 80th percentile, then 20 percent can do more than you, and 80 percent can do less.

You can assess your fitness and progress in two ways: (1) how you are improving from your own baseline and (2) how your muscle fitness compares to others like you. Remember that genetics plays a role in muscle fitness, so focus first on how you can improve from your own baseline.

Q What is a good goal to set for my strength training?

Goals are important for keeping your program on track, but your goal depends on you! Your goals should be personal, suited to your current fitness level and circumstances. As described in Chapter 2, good goals have a few key characteristics:

- **Specific and measurable goals:** These are necessary so that you can track your progress.
- **Achievable and realistic goals:** Choose goals that will allow you to succeed. Improving strength is a realistic goal, but bench pressing 400 pounds is probably not. In some cases, goals that use relative measures (10 or 20 percent heavier) are more achievable than absolute measures (10 or 20 pounds).
- **Time-bound goals (long- and short-term):** In addition to long-term goals, set goals that you'll be able to achieve within a few weeks or months; short-term milestones are a great motivator. Long-term goals are helpful, but it is easy to lose sight of them or to feel like you'll never get there. Therefore, support your long-term goals with achievable and measurable short-term goals that are no more than one or two months away. This way you are constantly striving for something new, and you also have the flexibility to make changes along the way as circumstances change.

An example of a goal that illustrates these characteristics is "I want to improve my upper-body strength by 10 percent over the next 8–12 weeks." Refer to the box "Motivation for Achieving Goals" for additional advice on getting a program started and keeping it on track.

Putting Together a Muscle-Fitness Program

Now that you are ready to improve your muscle fitness, the next step is deciding what type of exercises to use. Luckily for you, college students often have many options for types of exercises, equipment, and facilities. You can develop a muscle-fitness program that fits your individual goals, schedule, and preferences—a key to keeping strong muscles for life.

Choosing Appropriate Equipment and Facilities

Questions abound as to what type of exercise equipment is best. The key point is that gains in muscle fitness require overload, meaning you have to continuously increase the resistance your muscles are working against. With the overload principle in mind, you can use your creativity—safely, of course—to come up with a variety of ways to create resistance for your muscles. A quick Web search or a scan through a fitness magazine or therapy catalog will reveal free weights, weight machines, elastic bands, rubber balls, bars, bows, ropes, straps, and other equipment—all designed to provide muscle resistance. Which you choose depends on factors such as access, cost, and personal preference. Read on for brief descriptions of some of the more common muscle-fitness training devices.

Wellness Strategies

Motivation for Achieving Goals

Once you have your goals set, you need to use successful techniques to make them happen! There are numerous behavior-change strategies for keeping yourself motivated to reach your goals. However, some work better than others, especially for fitness-related goals.

Find an exercise partner: Having company is a great way to stay motivated and have fun. The best partners are ones with similar daily schedules, similar goals, and similar exercise interests. If your exercise partners (and you can certainly have more than one) like different types of exercise, that is usually a good thing, because switching between activities will help prevent boredom and monotony.

Draw up a behavioral contract: Make a contract with yourself (see Chapter 2), or have your exercise partner make a contract for you. Print the contract on colorful paper, place it in a prominent place, and look at it frequently throughout the week. As you develop your contract, decide what rules you can live with ("I will do my muscle fitness training at least twice each week"), and avoid those that are likely to be impossible ("I will never miss another weight training session"). Make your short-term goal the primary focus of the contract, but also include your long-term goals. Update the contract each time you meet a goal by using a different color paper, displaying it in a different place, and letting those around you know that you have achieved a goal and you are moving on to the next one!

Give yourself a reward: Rewards can be part of your contract, or they can be stand-alone motivators. Reward yourself with some new clothes, a movie, or pampering (like a massage or a manicure)—something you will truly enjoy but might not otherwise do. But be sure your rewards, just like your goals, are realistic and achievable. Don't overspend or do something that gets you off track with your fitness goals. Save the really big reward for when you achieve your ultimate fitness goal.

▶ WATCH ONLINE Specific exercises using a variety of equipment types are described later in the chapter, and there are corresponding video clips online for these and many other exercises.

Q | **Aren't free weights a lot better than machines?**

Although there is an ongoing debate about whether free weights or machines are best for novice weight trainers, the truth is that the best choice comes down to access and personal preference. Free weights (such as dumbbells and barbells) and machines are the most common types of training tools for increasing muscle fitness, but you probably couldn't tell the difference between someone who uses free weights and someone who uses machines. As long as you follow the overload principle, gains in muscle strength and endurance will follow, regardless of the equipment you use.

Free weights are objects or devices that can be moved freely in any direction. Common types of free weights are dumbbells, barbells, medicine balls, and the human body—which may be the ultimate free weight! Research has shown that free weights can promote quicker strength gains than machines, in part due to the greater demand for balance and coordination, which causes more muscle groups to be recruited. Free weights are also considerably less expensive than machines, because you can create an effective muscle-fitness program with a few dumbbells and a little creativity. Free weights, however, require the help of a spotter, and they cause more injuries than machines. Careful instruction and training is necessary to safely and effectively use free weights. (Safety is discussed in greater detail later in the chapter.)

An exercise machine does not move in all directions and is usually tethered to the floor, a wall, or a heavy base. Machines are much safer than free weights and are often preferred by those lifting alone, performing circuit training, or simply looking for a quicker workout.

In short, you should use the muscle-fitness equipment that suits your training needs in terms of accessibility, cost, convenience, and safety. Even world-class athletes use both free weights and machines to train their muscles.

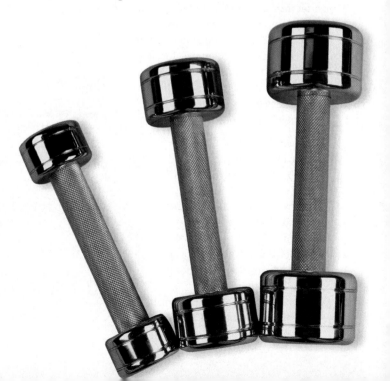

Q I want to work out in my dorm. What do I need?

Not much! When most people visualize training for muscle fitness, they picture a weight room full of machines, dumbbells, and barbells. But one of the most effective strength-training tools is your own body weight, or true resistance training. Body-weight exercises are great if you are just starting muscle-fitness training or whenever you don't have time to make it to the gym. Exercises like push-ups, sit-ups, squats, lunges, and step-ups can make for a great workout. The best part of this workout is that it costs nothing and can be done almost anywhere, any time.

Push-ups, sit-ups, lunges, and squats incorporate most major muscle groups and are challenging enough for most people. The resistance (from your body weight and gravity) can be continuously increased as your muscle fitness increases, so the overload principle is always in play. Adding resistance balls and bands, weight vests, labile (unstable) surfaces, and more will provide a satisfying muscle-fitness workout without your ever stepping in the gym, lifting an actual weight, or going near a machine.

If you need convincing that your own body weight provides enough resistance to increase your muscle fitness, look no further than the world's top gymnasts. These athletes rarely train with conventional weights. Instead, their outstanding muscular fitness is a result of pushing and pulling their bodies through various motions all day long.

Q What's the best gym to join for strength training?

As described in Chapter 3, the best fitness facility for you depends on convenience, cost, available equipment and classes, and the feel of the place. Join a gym that you will use—that's the most important consideration! Don't forget to check out your campus facilities: You may already be paying a student fee to use the campus gym or wellness center.

And don't be intimidated if you are new to strength training; ask for help in setting up an appropriate program and learning safe technique. A little gym etiquette can help improve everyone's experience:

- Remember that you are sharing equipment, so don't sit on a machine after you've finished your set. If you're using a barbell, unload the weight plates after you finish. Return dumbbells, barbells, and weight plates to the racks or floor area designated for storage.
- Keep your sweat to yourself by sitting on a towel you carry with you or by wiping all the parts of the machines you use—or both.
- Don't hog the showers, drinking fountains, or storage lockers.
- Follow the rules of the particular fitness facility.

One of the biggest trends in recent years is women-only gyms. Although the facility may not be dramatically different from a coed gym, there is an emphasis on making women's workouts more pleasant. The machines are designed specifically for women (for example, they are smaller); there are more dumbbells in the range women tend to use; the staff caters to new users; and the entertainment and for-sale products are more women friendly. There even appears to be evidence that women-only workout environments produce better fitness results, as noted in the Research Brief box on gender separation!

Selecting Types of Muscular Training

Q I want to get more fit, but I don't really want muscles. What type of training is right for me?

Everyone has muscles; some are just bigger or stronger than others. To get more fit, the outward appearance of your muscles does not have to noticeably change. It is the inside of your muscles, the muscle fibers, that changes when you apply the overload principle. First you need to decide what equipment to use (such as free weights, machines, body resistance) and then choose a type of muscle-training program. There are three main types of muscle training:

- static
- isokinetic
- dynamic

Static training, also known as *isometric training,* involves a muscle contraction without any change in the length of the muscle because the resistance is too great to move. For example, if you push against a solid brick wall, the wall isn't going to move, but you are generating a great amount of force, though in a small **range of motion (ROM)**. In a short time, your strength will noticeably increase. However, that strength will be limited to the specific ROM you are using, which is not particularly functional—pushing against a brick wall might have results if you were Superman, but it serves no meaningful purpose in a college student's life. Also, the strength gains tend to quickly dissipate if the exercises aren't

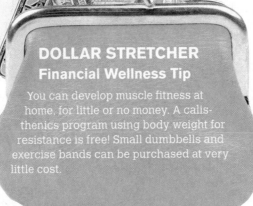

DOLLAR STRETCHER
Financial Wellness Tip

You can develop muscle fitness at home, for little or no money. A calisthenics program using body weight for resistance is free! Small dumbbells and exercise bands can be purchased at very little cost.

Research Brief

Is Gender Separation Best for Physical Activity?

Do women improve their fitness better when there are no men around? A large number of college students were studied in mixed-gender and single-gender fitness environments to compare differences in fitness gains. When women participated in supervised exercise in a mixed-gender setting, their fitness (measured as VO_2) decreased over the course of a semester. Women who participated in self-supervised single-gender activity were able to maintain their fitness level over the same period. Men were unaffected by the exercise environment; they were able to maintain fitness in both mixed- and single-gender settings.

The results of this study indicate that women, at least while in college, may find working out with men to be a deterrent. Men, however, don't seem as influenced as women by their exercise group. Women who are self-conscious about their fitness or abilities might be better off exercising with other women.

Source: Liguori, G., & Stritesky, M. (2005). Oral presentation at the AAHPERD annual meeting, Salt Lake City, UT.

---

static (isometric) training Resistance exercise against a stationary force. During static muscle training, force is applied to an immovable object, so the agonist muscle does not change in length. Strength gains are limited to the range of motion used.

range of motion (ROM) The full range through which a joint can move.

isokinetic training Resistance exercise in which the resistance automatically adjusts throughout the ROM, thereby ensuring a constant rate of speed. This training requires specialized equipment.

dynamic (isotonic) training Exercise in which muscle force is exerted throughout the entire contraction. Resistance may be fixed or variable; the speed of contraction varies because the muscle is weakest at its longest and shortest and strongest in the middle of the ROM.

done daily. For these reasons, static training isn't widely used for general fitness training, although it is effective for rehabilitation.

The second type of training is **isokinetic training,** or exertion of a constant force at a constant speed throughout the entire ROM. Isokinetic training requires special equipment (machines) that controls the speed of contraction so you move at a steady rate and apply a constant force throughout the entire exercise. This equipment is typically used for rehabilitation, such as an isokinetic leg-extension machine used to help people regain strength after knee surgery. The major drawback to isokinetic training is access to the specialized equipment. The advantage, if you have the access, is that you are able to maximize your strength throughout the entire ROM, unlike static training, which has a very limited ROM.

The third type of training is **dynamic** or **isotonic training.** With dynamic training, muscle force is exerted throughout the entire contraction. The amount of resistance may be fixed (free weights, for example) or variable (certain types of weight machines). The speed of the contraction varies because the muscle is weakest when it is longest and shortest and strongest in the middle of the ROM. This is why weight rooms are full of people arching their backs and swinging their arms at the start of a biceps curl, a major safety violation. The biceps is long-

est and weakest when the arm is straight, so the swinging helps to get the weight past the weakest point. When the arm curl moves through the middle of the ROM, the biceps is strongest, so no swinging is needed.

Dynamic training is by far the most common form of muscle training and can be performed with body weight, rubber tubing, machines, free weights, and so on. Although dynamic training doesn't provide quite the strength range of isokinetic training, it is so much more accessible that it is the favored choice of most people. Drawbacks to dynamic strength training are few, especially when done with machines or body weight. Free weights may require a partner to act as a spotter; see p. ** for more on safe training.

Table 5-3 compares the three basic types of training.

Q Is it true that muscles get bigger if you go slow on the way down?

The "way down" in a lift is usually an eccentric muscle contraction. In this context, *contraction* can mean shortening or lengthening. There are two basic contractions a muscle can perform (Figure 5-3):

- **Concentric contraction,** in which the muscle shortens as it contracts
- **Eccentric contraction,** in which the muscle lengthens as it contracts

Thus, muscle contraction can occur during both the shortening and lengthening phases of a lift, and each type of contraction has different benefits.

The absolute amount of force generated during muscle lengthening (eccentric) is greater than the force generated during shortening (concentric). What this means is that you can set down a much heavier object than you can lift

concentric contraction Skeletal muscle movement leading to shortening of the agonist muscle.

eccentric contraction Skeletal muscle movement leading to lengthening of the agonist muscle.

TABLE 5-3 TYPES OF MUSCULAR TRAINING

	STATIC TRAINING	ISOKINETIC TRAINING	DYNAMIC TRAINING
RANGE OF MOTION	Limited	Good	Excellent
RESISTANCE	Static	Adjusting	Fixed or variable
STRENGTH GAINS	Good*	Excellent	Excellent
COST	Inexpensive	Expensive	Inexpensive

* Strength gains are easy to come by in static training, but quick to leave.

up. An example is the biceps curl: It is much more difficult to curl the weight up than it is to let the weight back down.

Eccentric contractions have long been popular for their ability to build strength. Most muscle activity occurs during the lengthening or eccentric phase of a lift, and muscle strengthening appears to be considerably greater when emphasizing the eccentric contraction. One disadvantage of accentuating the eccentric phase is a noticeable increase in muscle soreness, which is due to the greater muscle activity.[19]

If you observe people lifting weights in a gym, you'll notice that they emphasize the concentric, or shortening, phase and let gravity do most of the work on the way down. There may be many reasons (including the pleasure of seeing how much they can lift), but in reality, emphasizing the concentric phase makes the workout much less efficient at building strength, mass, or both compared to a workout focusing on the eccentric, or lengthening, phase.

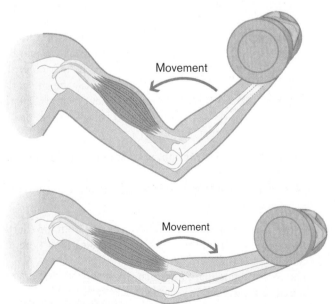

Figure 5-3 Concentric versus eccentric muscle contraction. During a concentric contraction (top), a muscle shortens as it contracts; during an eccentric contraction (bottom), a muscle lengthens as it contracts. Emphasizing the eccentric phase of an exercise usually builds more strength but may cause more muscle soreness.

Applying the FITT Formula: Frequency, Intensity, Time, and Type

As described in earlier chapters, applying the FITT principle may be the best way to optimize your muscle fitness. Just as in cardiovascular training, these four components should form the foundation of your muscle fitness program planning. Through careful planning, improvements in muscle strength and endurance can be achieved in a reasonable amount of time, as long as the balance of intensity, duration, and frequency are set to meet your goals. The type or mode of exercise depends on your needs, preferences, and access to equipment.

Q | Should I lift every day if I want to get really strong?

FREQUENCY. How frequently you perform resistance training depends almost entirely on your personal goals, current fitness status, and access to an appropriate training environment. If your goal is general fitness, the American College of Sports Medicine (ACSM) recommends muscle-fitness training on two or three days per week, with at least 48 hours between workouts. Training on nonconsecutive days—for example, Tuesday and Friday or Monday, Wednesday, and Friday—allows your muscle fibers to recover from each training session and to work effectively. Recall that delayed-onset muscle soreness is likely when you try something new in your muscle-training program—even the most experienced people encounter it occasionally—which is further reason to give your muscles adequate rest.

Once you've moved beyond the beginner level, you can add more frequent training sessions to meet your ever-changing short-term goals. Although you may hear about athletes doing muscle training four to six days a week, it is important to note that they alternate muscle groups to give their muscles adequate rest; they also often have a lot riding on their athletic performance (such as a scholarship or salary). For the typical college student, however, increasing workout frequency increases the risk of injury and fatigue.

Additionally, if you already have a physically demanding job or participate in vigorous leisure activities, increasing your strength training frequency may be ill-advised: You are already doing work- or leisure-related strength training, and adding more would be the same as overtraining.

Finally, there is sufficient evidence that engaging in muscle-fitness training only one day a week may be beneficial for some people.[20] For beginners, strength will almost certainly increase with just one day a week of muscle-fitness training, because this is a lot more than no days a week of training! However, beginners should progress to 2–3 days per week. For all other exercisers, one day a week is enough to maintain muscle fitness for up to six weeks, as long as the resistance or load is held constant. This is especially good news around the start or end of a semester when you are particularly busy and might not have as much time for your preferred exercise program. So if you are new to muscle training, don't feel overwhelmed. One or two days a week along with your aerobic training will have you well on your way to a new, more fit you!

Q | What's the best amount to lift to get stronger?

INTENSITY. You need to lift enough weight to overload your muscles, but the amount depends on your current fitness level and your short-term training goals. As described in Chapter 3, the overload principle means that in order to improve a muscle's fitness, it must be stressed beyond its present capacity. A muscle will adapt to stress by increasing in size, strength, and/or endurance capacity.

The overload principle is applicable to many aspects of training, not just weight training. According to the fable, Milo of Crotona lifted his newborn calf every day. As the calf grew, so did the boy's strength, until one day he was a strapping youth who could lift a full-grown cow. Although it is unlikely you or I will ever lift a cow, if we repeatedly increase the amount of resistance or weight in our training program, our muscle strength will increase accordingly—up to a point of course.

For strength training, *intensity* refers to the amount of weight or resistance required to elicit a training response, or the overload principle. Intensity is often calculated as a percentage of an individual's 1-RM (one-repetition maximum). Similar to frequency and duration, the amount of resistance you should choose depends on your goals and training status. The American College of Sports Medicine (ACSM) recommends the following:[21]

- 60%–70% of 1-RM for deconditioned persons, older adults, or beginners
- 60%–80% of 1-RM for improvement in overall strength, mass, and to some extent endurance
- 70%–100% of 1-RM for advanced-level training

For example, if your 1-RM for the bench press is 125 pounds, a workload of 70 percent means you would be using about 85 pounds of resistance.

Finding your 1-RM is not always practical, so working within a prescribed range of repetitions ("reps") is a useful alternative. The ACSM recommends 8–12 reps for each resistance exercise for general fitness, as this will provide some level of gain in strength, endurance, and hypertrophy. Therefore, if you don't know your maximum strength, or don't want to find out, start with a light weight and see how many reps you can perform while still maintaining good form. (Note: To prevent injury, it is always better to use less weight or do fewer reps with good form than to lift more weight or do more reps with poor form.) If you can easily perform 11 or 12 reps, try a slightly heavier weight next time. Your goal is to use an amount of resistance that is sufficient to fatigue your muscles when you complete 8 to 12 reps with good form.

Recall that many neuromuscular adaptations occur in the first few weeks of training, especially in the first few days. Therefore, you may very well increase your resistance quite a bit over the first few days of training. Take your time, though, and increase slowly so that you decrease the risk of muscle soreness and injury.

Q | So I can just lift the weights ten times and be done?

Yes—although you can also do more. In addition to the intensity and reps of your training, you also need to plan the number of sets. Reps are the number of times you lift the weight up and down. Lifting the weight ten times is one set of ten repetitions. The ACSM recommends performing 2-4 sets to fatigue (with good form!), on two or three days per week, of eight to ten exercises targeting all major muscle groups.

Once you have established some comfort level with your training, met your short-term goals, and reduced the incidence of muscle soreness, you then may want to consider modifications to your program. Changes in intensity, repetitions, sets, or frequency may help keep you challenged and motivated as you work toward your goals.

Remember to start slow, avoid muscle soreness, use good technique, and rest for at least 48 hours between training sessions. One of the beauties of muscle-fitness training is that even the true beginner will notice an almost immediate

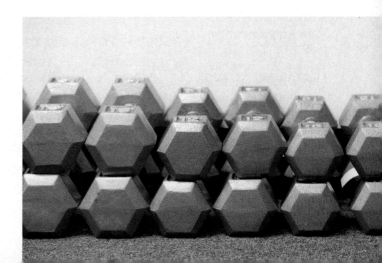

improvement. With some sustained effort, gains in muscle strength, endurance, and fitness will keep coming.

Q | Can I gain muscle by working out for just 15 minutes?

TIME. The amount of time you spend on your muscle-fitness program will be a lot less than the amount of time you might spend in an assisted-living home when you get older if you can't take care of yourself because of poor muscle fitness. More specifically, the time you spend on muscle workouts will depend on—you guessed it—your goals. Doing the minimum workout of one day per week, with eight to ten exercises should take no more than 30 minutes. Using weight machines will probably be a little quicker than using free weights, and using balls, bands, body weight, and so on will be even quicker.

If you don't have 30 minutes, can you still get benefits in half the time? Yes, most likely, but not as many. Although several studies substantiate the efficacy of the "one set" workout, additional sets may result in greater gains in muscle fitness. However, when time is tight, doing one set is better than doing nothing.

The key, however, is making the one set the best you possibly can. This means maintaining good technique throughout the set, yet pushing to the point of fatigue on the set. If you do only one set and don't push yourself, you probably won't see much strength gain. But if you push your muscles to fatigue, you will see sufficient gains.

A question to consider if you are doing multiple sets is how long to rest between sets, which is often referred to as the rest interval. The rest interval depends upon training intensity, goals, and current fitness level (see Table 5-4). A person interested only in strength will typically employ longer rest intervals (2–5 minutes) than someone whose goals include hypertrophy (30–90 seconds) or endurance (less than 30 seconds). A good rule is to allow enough time between sets and exercises to allow you to perform each exercise with proper form.

Time between sets should also be balanced with the muscle groups involved in the exercise. Most experts recommend alternating exercises for opposing muscle groups (for example, biceps on the front of the arm and triceps on the back of the arm) or for the upper and lower body. These alternations will ensure that you don't do consecutive exercises with the same muscle group, allowing for sufficient rest to each muscle group prior to an effort.

The decision on how many sets to do should depend on your goals and the time you have available. Trying to do more but not being able to will only make you feel unsuccessful and less likely to continue. Keep your goals realistic, and chances are you will achieve them!

Q | What can I do to get my arms bigger? And what is the best way to get a six-pack or burn the fat off my belly?

TYPE. Deciding what type of exercises to include in your muscle-fitness program can seem mind-boggling, because there are so many exercises to choose from! Exercises can be classified in two general types: single-joint exercises, which use one major muscle group or joint, and multiple-joint exercises, which stress more than one joint or muscle group. A biceps curl is an example of a single-joint exercise, and a squat is an example of a multiple-joint exercise. Both types of exercises are important to include in your muscle-fitness routine, but multiple-joint exercises are considered to be more effective because of the greater amount of resistance that can be used and because these exercises tend to mimic real-life activities.

Doing tons of crunches might give you strong abdominals, but unless you combine them with aerobic exercise, you might not ever get rid of the belly fat. Also, crunches have limited utility in daily function. A well-rounded plan that includes a variety of core exercises will do more for you; specific examples are included at the end of the chapter.

Doing any one exercise for a single body part (spot training) has limited effects—you may strengthen an individual muscle, but you won't selectively reduce fat in that area and the increased strength may not be particularly functional. For example, doing lots of biceps curls will give you bigger, stronger biceps. However, other than car-

MYTH or **FACT**
Doing lots of sit-ups will make your stomach flatter.
▶ WATCH ONLINE

TABLE 5-4 MUSCLE-FITNESS PROGRAM DESIGN

TRAINING STATUS	FREQUENCY PER WEEK	INTENSITY (% OF 1-RM)	REPETITIONS	REST BETWEEN SETS
BEGINNER/OLDER/ DECONDITIONED	2–3	60%–70%	10–15	1–2 min.
GENERAL STRENGTH	2–3	60%–80%	8–12	2–3 min.
ADVANCED	4–6	70%–100%	1–12*	3+ min.

* The reason for this wide range is that advanced lifters might do only one all-out rep occasionally.

rying groceries, there are very few times in the day when your biceps functions in complete isolation. Therefore, the recommendation is to use "movements, not muscles" to produce the most effective workouts. Biceps typically work with the shoulder muscles, so chin-ups have more overall effect than simple biceps curls. Plus, if you do a chin-up, your biceps performs the same exact movement as in a curl, except that your shoulder is included.

Q | Does it matter how I put exercises together?

For a muscle-fitness program, there are three basic workout structures: (1) total-body workouts, (2) upper- and lower-body split workouts, and (3) muscle-group split routines. All three workout types are effective for improving muscle fitness and can help you achieve your goals within your time constraints.

Total-body workouts typically feature multijoint exercises that work the body's major muscle groups (Figure 5-4). These types of workouts are great for beginners and can be extremely time efficient.

Upper- and lower-body split workouts consist of upper-body exercises on some days and lower-body exercises on other days; for example, you might do upper-body exercises on Monday and Wednesday and lower-body exercises on Tuesday and Thursday. College and professional athletes commonly use upper- and lower-body split workouts because they allow for a greater total amount of work and are more sport specific, although this workout structure is more time consuming.

Muscle-group split routines consist of exercises for specific muscle groups. An example of this type of routine is a chest and triceps workout one day, followed by a back and biceps workout the next session. This workout structure is most commonly used by bodybuilders and people whose sole goal is hypertrophy. Muscle-group split workouts are not the most practical for athletes or those interested in general muscle fitness, because they emphasize single-joint exercises.

Q | I like to bench and do arm curls. Is that enough?

Not really. Those exercises will surely increase your muscle fitness, and depending on how you define *strong,* you may very well get there. However, an exercise program that uses the inherent reciprocity of the skeletal system may better help you reach your goals. For each muscle that controls movement in one direction, or **agonist muscle,** there is an **antagonist muscle** that performs the opposite action. For example, to bend your arm, you need to contract the biceps muscle (agonist) on the front of the arm. In order for this to occur, the triceps muscle, or antagonist on the back of the arm, must lengthen. To straighten your arm, the actions are reversed and the triceps becomes the

agonist muscle The muscle primarily responsible for movement of a bone.

antagonist muscle The muscle opposite the agonist, which must relax and lengthen during contraction of the agonist.

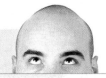

Mind Stretcher
Critical Thinking Exercise

You and your friends strength train several times a week, and you consider yourselves in great shape. Now you are planning a cross-country ski trip—the first time you've skied in several years. One friend wants to ski the toughest and longest trail because you are all in such good shape. Another friend says you should start out with something easier until your muscles get used to the cross-country ski movements. What do you think you should plan for this trip?

agonist while the biceps lengthens and becomes the antagonist. Through this reciprocal coordination of the agonist and antagonist muscles, smooth and complex body movements are made possible, if not simple. Therefore, people in strength-training programs should always perform exercises that allow for equal development of both agonist and antagonist muscles to fully realize their strength potential.

Q | What's the best overall workout?

PUTTING IT ALL TOGETHER. Although the advice is probably getting old by now, the best workout is one that enables you to reach your goals. Balancing the FITT principle with your goals and the time you can commit to exercise is sometimes the hardest part of any exercise program, muscle fitness included. In addition to the actual workout, you still need to include a proper warm-up and cool-down, which are important for minimizing injury and maximizing performance (see Chapter 3):

- Warm up: 5–10 minutes of light physical activity
- Training: Specific strength exercises
- Cool down: 5–10 minutes of light activity; you can stretch while your muscles are warm from your strength workout

Sample workout plans and descriptions of exercises are included at the end of this chapter.

Managing a Safe and Successful Muscle-Fitness Program

Starting a muscle fitness program is great, but for maximum benefits, you must stick with it. A well-designed program based on sound training principles and good technique will not only prevent injuries but also boost both your progress and your motivation.

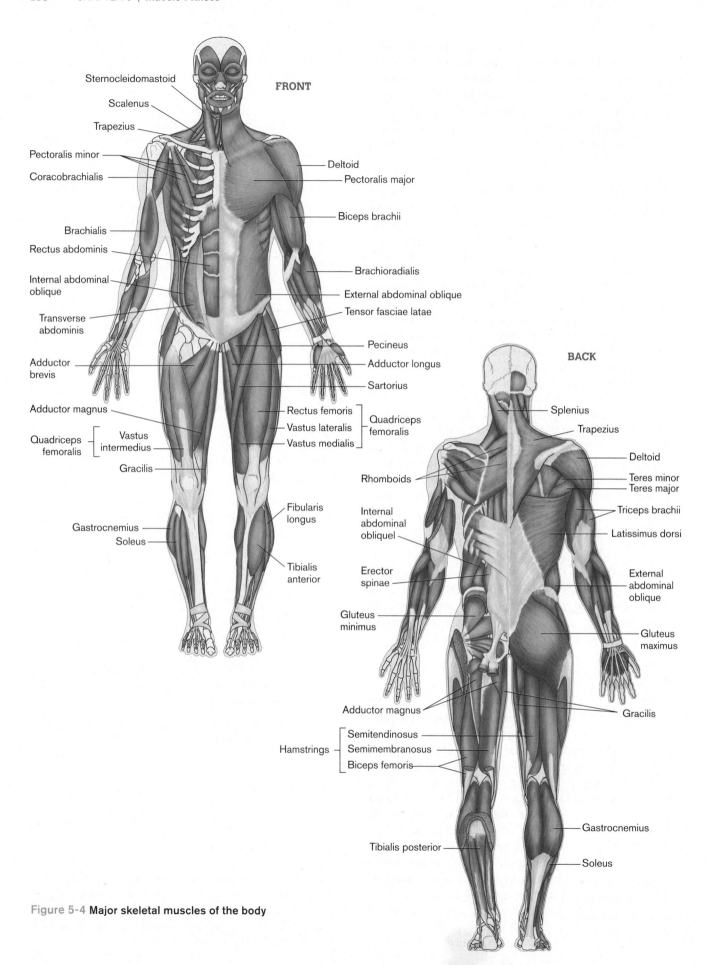

FRONT

Sternocleidomastoid

Scalenus

Trapezius

Pectoralis minor

Coracobrachialis

Deltoid

Pectoralis major

Biceps brachii

Brachialis

Rectus abdominis

Brachioradialis

Internal abdominal oblique

External abdominal oblique

Tensor fasciae latae

Transverse abdominis

Pecineus

Adductor longus

Adductor brevis

Sartorius

Adductor magnus

Rectus femoris

Vastus lateralis

Vastus medialis

Quadriceps femoralis

Quadriceps femoralis

Vastus intermedius

Gracilis

Fibularis longus

Gastrocnemius

Soleus

Tibialis anterior

BACK

Splenius

Trapezius

Deltoid

Teres minor

Teres major

Triceps brachii

Latissimus dorsi

Rhomboids

Internal abdominal obliquel

Erector spinae

External abdominal oblique

Gluteus minimus

Gluteus maximus

Adductor magnus

Gracilis

Hamstrings

Semitendinosus

Semimembranosus

Biceps femoris

Tibialis posterior

Gastrocnemius

Soleus

Figure 5-4 Major skeletal muscles of the body

Weight-Training Safety and Injury Prevention

Q What's the best way to lift weights and not get hurt?

Up to this point, we've focused on the many benefits of strength or resistance training. However, as with any exercise, there are potential risks—for example, using free weights carries the risk of dropping a weight on yourself; lifting too frequently or too heavily can lead to tendonitis or burnout; and using a machine improperly can lead to injury. The risks of muscle-fitness training can be minimized by warming up, using proper technique, following all posted instructions on equipment, getting adequate rest, and eating nutritious foods (see Chapter 8).

WARM-UP. As described in Chapter 3, warming up before exercise is important. If you are engaging in muscle-resistance training and employing the overload principle, then you should begin with an appropriate warm-up:

- Start with five minutes of light aerobic activity to get some blood moving throughout your body.
- Then move your arms and legs through the full range of motion you will be using during your workout routine.
- Finally, use light weights to again move through the range of motion. After that, you should be ready to go.

Q What is "technique"? Don't you just lift the weight up and down?

USE PROPER TECHNIQUE. To a large degree, yes, you just lift a weight up and down. But visit almost any gym, weight room, or fitness club, and you will see many people lifting weights incorrectly. Swinging weights into position, not using a spotter, and holding your breath are all common—and potentially dangerous—practices. See the box "Strength Training Safety" for safety advice.

Q How fast should a repetition be performed?

Every exercise has three general phases:

- **Concentric phase:** The lifting or exertion phase, in which the muscle contracts as it shortens
- **Isometric phase:** The midpoint of the exercise
- **Eccentric phase:** The lowering phase, in which the muscle contracts as it lengthens

Novices to resistance training should use a slow movement in each direction (2–3 seconds) until they are comfortable with the technique. However, resistance-training research shows that intentionally slow movements do not stimulate an increase in muscle-force production. Therefore, a moderate repetition velocity is recommended. For example, for a barbell biceps curl, a properly performed rep should have a 1- to 2-second concentric contraction and a 1- to second controlled lowering, or eccentric action. Some exercises lend themselves to faster speed (for example, a power clean and many multijoint exercises), and some should be performed more slowly (for example, a barbell curl and many single-joint exercises). An advanced lifter may use a slow contraction speed due to an extreme resistance load. This unintentional slow contraction is useful for a heavy load, but it is only for advanced lifters.

Most people who strength train do not pay much attention to the eccentric phase of the exercise. However, eccentric training can lead to much more muscle soreness than usual, so gradually introduce this into your program if you aren't already emphasizing the eccentric. Otherwise you will be so sore you might not come back for more!

Q Why am I sometimes so sore the day after lifting?

GET ADEQUATE REST. Muscles can get sore after a bout of resistance training, usually within twenty-four hours of the exercise session. This is known as **delayed onset muscle soreness,** or **DOMS.** DOMS is a normal response to increased exertion and unfamiliar physical activities.[22] Therefore, if you do an exercise that you've never done or haven't done recently, there is a good chance you will experience some degree of DOMS. Additionally, even for a seasoned weight trainer, DOMS is likely when the effort is dramatically increased. And as the eccentric emphasis of an exercise increases, so does the chance of experiencing DOMS.

The cause of DOMS, although still not entirely understood, appears to be related to the **microtears** and injuries suffered within the muscle cell during new or intensive activity. The process starts with damage to the cell membrane, which is followed by a cascade of inflammatory responses, buildup of waste products, stimulated nerve endings, and the sensation of pain. During DOMS, you experience swelling, stiffness, and loss of strength, though they only last for 24 to 72 hours. It is probably best to give your muscles a rest while you are experiencing DOMS, instead of possibly making yourself more sore and fatigued. If the soreness, stiffness, and swelling don't subside within three or four days, you may want to seek medical advice from a health care professional.

Q How much time do I need between workouts?

Muscle-fitness experts recommend at least one day off between exercises targeting a specific muscle group. In other words, don't strength train the same muscle group on consecutive days.

delayed onset muscle soreness (DOMS) Muscle soreness experienced 12–36 hours after increased exertion. The exact cause of DOMS is unknown, but it may be related to microtears in muscle cells. The discomfort usually subsides within 24 hours.

microtears Tiny tears in muscle fibers that are believed to be at least partly responsible for DOMS.

Wellness Strategies

Strength-Training Safety

Basic exercise-safety recommendations apply to strength training: Warm up before exercise and cool down after, wear appropriate clothing and shoes, tie your hair back if it'll fall in your eyes, and don't chew gum! Specific safety strategies for strength training include the following.

Use proper technique: Common technique mistakes, which can lead to injury, include swinging your back during biceps curls, arching your back during bench press, and poor overall alignment during squats. Lift weights smoothly, in a controlled fashion. Don't lift beyond the limits of your strength, and maintain good form and posture at all times.

Technique is not just a concern for free-weight exercises. Weight machines always have proper technique posted on them in a very user friendly, high visibility spot. It is imperative to follow these instructions; however, it is not uncommon to see people at the local gym using their imagination with creative techniques. This not only violates the machine's warranty and liability of the manufacturer, but it puts the user at greater risk of injury. Why take the chance?

Descriptions of proper technique for many common exercises can be found on pp. 000, and there are corresponding video clips online.

Use a spotter for free weights: Having a spotter will minimize the chances of your dropping weights and getting hurt. A spotter can help you move a weight into the starting position and out of the finishing position. A spotter can also come to your aid if the weight tilts or you cannot complete a lift. Spotters are especially important when you lift heavy weights.

Don't hold your breath: Another key safety issue is breathing. Yes, breathing. Although obviously you breathe while exercising, *when* you breathe can be a safety issue. People often hold their breath during the contraction phase of a lift, especially ones that are more difficult. Although this does provide some core stability, which may improve ability slightly, it also places a large load on your cardiovascular system and often forces your blood pressure to skyrocket. This sudden increase in blood pressure can lead to serious injury—and even death in extreme cases. Instead, it is best to follow the exhale-on-exertion model, which encourages breathing out when the lift is most challenging. Ultimately, breathing is a good thing, and you should strive to do it all the time, especially when exercising!

Check your equipment:

- *Free weights:* Are handles easy to grip? For barbells, are the weight plates secured with collars to keep them from slipping off the ends?
- *Machine weights:* Are you clear of all cables or weight stacks before you begin? Did you reset the machine (resistance, foot or back position, and the like) and lock everything in place?
- *Elastic bands:* Do the bands stretch smoothly? Are there any cracks or other signs of wear and tear?
- *Stability balls:* Is the ball the recommended size for you? Is it inflated to the proper level?

Giving your muscles about 48 hours to recover will help build strength.

A few things happen inside your muscles in the first twenty-four hours after muscle-fitness training. First, the workout itself creates an increase in lactic acid. Contrary to popular belief, lactic acid is not what makes you sore, but it does limit how much exercise you can perform. Rest helps to dissipate the excess lactic acid so that you are ready to go again in forty-eight hours. Second, the workout causes the breakdown of muscle fibers. The microtears in the muscle cells create DOMS, from which you need at least twenty-four hours to recover. Recovery from microtears is key to your program because when the fibers rebuild themselves, they are a little stronger than they were before, thanks to the overload principle. This is all part of the rebuilding process, where the real action is for increasing muscle mass, strength, and endurance. So don't be fooled into believing that lifting every day is twice as good as lifting every other day; instead, you'll find yourself quickly tiring and making little if any gain in your muscle fitness.

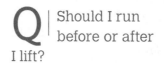

Q | Should I run before or after I lift?

Whichever works best for you. If you are a recreational exerciser, it is not likely to make any difference. If you are a competitive athlete on your college team, then you should do what your coach suggests. Most of us do what is most comfortable and convenient. Some people find it difficult to run after doing muscle training on their legs, but others are not bothered and feel fine. There are many articles in muscle magazines about which order of exercise burns more fat or improves

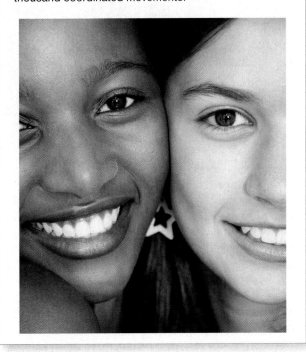

recovery time, frequency of exercise, and so on), the more effective you will be at goal setting—and goal revising—as well as marking improvement and identifying problems.

A sample log is shown in Figure 5-5, but it's best to track whatever factors are most relevant for you and your goals. An online workout tracker is available in your course materials; you can also download other sample logs to use from the same Web site.

Q | **When can I increase the weight I'm lifting?**

If you have been tracking your progress, you will have a good sense of when it is time to increase the resistance. Once you can perform all your sets at the upper end of your desired repetition range (eight to twelve) while still maintaining good technique, it is time for more resistance. For example, when the individual whose program is shown in Figure 5-5 can complete twelve to fourteen bench presses with good form, then it is time to add resistance. Generally, resistance increases of 5–10 percent are best—that would be about 5–10 pounds in the bench press example. Any more than that can lead to injury, and any less won't provide the overload stimulus needed to get stronger. When you are new to muscle fitness training, 5–10 percent won't seem like much of an increase, but eventually it will become quite challenging to attempt an increase of that amount. You can't increase resistance indefinitely; once you reach your strength goal, you can maintain your strength gains by continuing to train at the same intensity.

Q | **Why is my strength barely improving now, when before I could lift more almost every week?**

When you first start resistance training, it is very common to experience dramatic increases in strength. This phase typically lasts six to eight weeks, after which strength gains slow considerably.[23] The reason is not your muscles; instead, it is your nervous system. During the first few weeks, you are teaching your body unfamiliar

performance more, but in truth, there is little if any difference, because you will have done the same amount of work at the end of the day. If you have a routine that you like, stick with it. If you are just starting, try different training schedules until you find what works best for you.

Making Progress

Q | **What parts of my workout should I track?**

Whether you are new to muscle-fitness training or an experienced lifter, you should consider tracking your progress on a regular basis. Tracking can be done in many ways, including writing in a notebook, creating a daily log to fill in, using an electronic spreadsheet, or signing up for a Web site that will store your data for you. The more information you track (sets, reps, resistance,

Exercise	Set 1		Set 2		Set 3		Rest (time between sets)
	Weight	Reps	Weight	Reps	Weight	Reps	
Bench press	110 lbs.	11	110 lbs.	9			2 min.
Lat pull down	45 lbs.	10	45 lbs.	9			2 min.
Crunches	n/a	25	n/a	25	n/a	30	n/a
Side bridges	n/a	20 sec.	n/a	20 sec.	n/a	20 sec.	n/a
Dumbbell squats	5 lb. dumbbells	14	5 lb. dumbbells	11			2 min.

Figure 5-5 **Sample muscle fitness training log**

(and hard!) movements, and the learning curve is steep. These new movements need to be ingrained into your nervous system so they become smooth and efficient. Therefore, your initial gains in strength are due not to muscle changes but to neural adaptations, as your nervous system becomes more familiar with the specific movements.

People who are new to resistance training can usually do more repetitions of a given weight on the second day of training than on the first day. Clearly, one day of training won't make anyone stronger, but it does immediately change the patterns of the nervous system, making it easier to perform the task next time. Think about learning to ride a bike: The first time on it, your motor system had never moved your legs in a pedaling fashion, yet after a few minutes, the pedaling became almost routine (too bad that balance didn't come quite so quickly).

Once this motor-learning process plateaus, after about six to eight weeks of training, strength gains due to neural adaptations are replaced by strength gains due to hypertrophy—your muscles start to get bigger as well as stronger. Therefore, it is a myth that people don't lose weight when they start a muscle-fitness program because they are building muscle. In fact, muscle-mass increases don't occur for two or three months; instead, they are likely eating more calories to compensate for the additional energy expenditure.

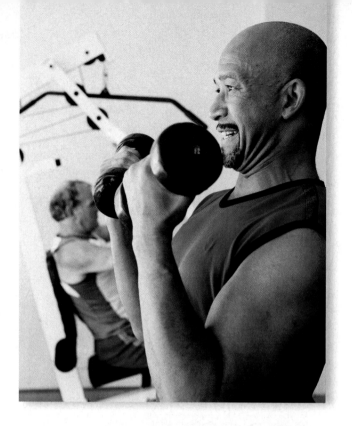

Q | I didn't work out at all during spring break, and then I was busy with finals. How should I start back?

Restarting a muscle-fitness program need not be tricky. If the layoff has been less than about three weeks, you probably haven't lost much strength. In this case, you might want to reduce your FITT by about 10 percent at first, to ease back into your program. For example, reduce the resistance from 110 pounds to 100 pounds; drop the number of reps from ten to nine, and do one less set than you previously did. You may even want to increase the rest period the first week back. These steps will help minimize DOMS, give your nervous system a reminder, and get you back to your pre–spring-break level within a week or two.

If you have had a longer layoff, drop your FITT by about 25 percent to ease the transition back to regular training. Reduce your resistance from 100 pounds to 75 pounds, do only one set, and if you are noticeably sore, take an extra day of rest between workouts. After a long layoff, you will require a bit more time to get back to your previous fitness level, so be patient, keep track of your progress, and stick with it as best you can!

Q | How long do I need to keep lifting?

You should continue muscle-fitness exercises for as long as you want to have fit muscles. Elderly people who have

never performed resistance exercise show dramatic improvement in muscle strength and balance shortly after initiating a resistance-training program.[24] Although older adults typically use much less resistance than someone thirty-five years younger, they too experience significant positive changes in muscle fitness, which makes their daily activities much easier and more enjoyable.

The longer you perform muscle-resistance training, the longer you will reap the benefits. Long-term benefits of muscle training include reduced risk of diabetes, musculoskeletal injury, and osteoporosis; improved control of blood pressure and body weight; and a higher level of self-esteem. This is surely enough good news to keep anyone motivated to start or continue muscle training for many years.

Q | I get bored with the same old workout and lose my motivation. Any ideas?

Boredom can occur with any type of exercise program, and minimizing boredom can go a long way towards keeping your motivation high. Muscle-fitness training programs tend to be very repetitious (do two sets, ten reps, three times a week), so changing your routine frequently can keep you from getting bored. There is considerable interest today in functional muscle training (see the next Question), which relies primarily on body weight for resistance, in stark contrast to the more traditional programs using free weights or machines. Varying your routine, as often as weekly, between traditional training and functional training may help reduce boredom.

Further, frequent changes in your routine will likely increase the number of muscles you are using, vary the way you are using them, and help you reach your goals more effectively. As an example, consider the difference between the bench press and the push-up. Both are primarily chest exercises (pectoralis major), yet compare the muscles involved in each:

- Bench press: pectoralis major, triceps, deltoid
- Push-ups: pectoralis major, triceps, deltoid, abdominals, erector spinae

The push-up not only involves more muscles, but it is also much more accessible and a lot less expensive (just needs floor space)!

The short answer: For much-needed variety, try new exercises frequently, or vary the number of sets, repetitions, and resistance in your usual workout.

Q | I keep hearing about functional training. Does that mean what I've been doing isn't functional? The same goes for core training—what's that?

Core training and **functional training** are nothing new; there has just been a recent increase in awareness of their value in overall fitness and sport performance.

The body's core muscles (abdominals, obliques, and erectors) are the foundation for almost all types of movement and form the core muscular connection between the upper and lower body. Core muscles are located around the torso and stabilize the spine to provide a solid foundation for movement, so "core stability training" is vital to improve fitness and reduce injury. To generate a powerful movement, it is necessary to first contract the core, which provides a solid base in the spine, pelvis, and shoulders. Training the core can also help with posture and injury prevention. Common core exercises include not only traditional abdominal crunches but also exercises designed specifically to build core stability, such as planks, side bridges, and hip extensions. Examples and instructions for popular core exercises appear at the end of this chapter. The biggest benefit of core training may be its ability to develop functional fitness.

Functional fitness is training the body in movement patterns that are needed in daily activity, ranging from sports to just getting around. Traditional training focuses on isolating specific joints or muscle groups. Functional training is more concerned with movement patterns and integrates multiple muscle groups rather than isolating them. Movements that incorporate squatting, lunging, pushing, and pulling develop stability, balance, and other factors than just strength; they require that all muscles be used in a coordinated, functional pattern. When you throw a baseball, kick a soccer ball, or jump high, your muscles are not working in isolation; they are working together to produce the specific movement pattern needed

to complete the task. This is the heart of functional training.

The most basic functional strength exercises are those that require the ability to control your body weight. Exercises such as body-weight squats, lunges, push-ups, and pull-ups are foundation functional exercises. As functional strength is developed, you can try more difficult exercises and progressions. Examples and instructions for popular functional exercises appear at the end of this chapter. Give the basic functional exercises a try—they are more challenging than most people think!

Q | Do I need special equipment for core or functional training?

 WATCH ONLINE

No. Core training and functional training aren't limited to weight rooms or wellness center. All you need is your body weight and some floor space. As previously discussed, your body weight is a simple yet effective source of resistance that allows you to work out in the comfort and privacy of your own room.

Do you think body weight squats are too easy for you? Then don't rest at the top; instead pause for two seconds at the bottom, which will eliminate the recoil effect typical of many gym lifters. Pausing at the bottom means you must recruit more muscles to move your body, instead of letting momentum help you along. You will definitely know which muscles are working! Squats, lunges, and push-ups can all be done in this manner.

Rubber bands and tubing can also take the place of free weights or machines when you choose to work out away from the gym. You are limited only by your imagination in creating exercises to utilize the resistance that bands and tubing provide, ranging from simple curling exercises for the arms to more complex movements of the shoulder joint. It is important to note that exercises utilizing tubing may be challenging at first, but the body will quickly adapt. To apply the overload principle and other tenets of progressive-resistance exercise, you will need to find ways to make the tubing and bands more challenging over time: Try thicker elastic bands or more sets and reps.

Stability balls are another common, commercially available piece of home-exercise equipment. A popular use for these balls is core exercises such as crunches, side crunches, and back extensions. However, with the addition of a pair of dumbbells, the stability ball can take the place of an exercise bench, and movements such as bench press or shoulder press can be done while sitting on the ball, increasing the demands on the core musculature.

core training Training that focuses on the muscles of the abdominal region and lower back. By stabilizing the spine, it can improve posture and decrease risk of falls.

functional training Training that mimics real-life movement patterns and integrates multiple muscle groups.

Q | Can I do Pilates for muscle-fitness training?

Yes, Pilates can build muscle fitness and provide other wellness benefits as well, including increased flexibility, improved body composition and body awareness, and reduced stress.[25] Pilates is named for its creator, German-born gymnast and boxer Joseph Pilates. It's a physical-movement program focused on developing strength and endurance (especially in the core), flexibility, posture, functional spinal alignment, and balance through whole body movements. A Pilates workout involves a small number of repetitions of exercises done with precise form—with careful attention to breathing patterns, coordinated and flowing movement, and body alignment. Some Pilates exercises are done on the floor ("mat work"), and others involve specialized equipment such as the Reformer, an apparatus with cables, pulleys, and a sliding-board seat to provide resistance for exercises.

You can try Pilates at home for just a little money, using a floor workout based on an instructional book or DVD. However, you may learn better by starting with a class or personal session led by an experienced instructor. Many local fitness centers and gyms offer Pilates mat classes, and classes using the Reformer and other equipment are offered at a smaller number of specialized studios. Pilates is effective and, for most people, a safe activity choice. If you are looking for something other than traditional strength training to build muscle fitness—or if you are looking to change your routine—Pilates may be an excellent choice. For more information about Pilates or to locate a certified instructor, visit the Web site of the Pilates Method Alliance (www.pilatesmethodalliance.org).

Q | Is circuit training effective for building strength? 🖥 READ ONLINE

Avoiding Drugs and Supplements

Some people who want to add significant strength or size to their body resort to supplements, drugs, or steroids, many of which are either illegal or have no scientific evidence of effectiveness. Although these substances may be tempting, especially if you are highly competitive, the downside can be severe. Monetary fines, jail time, illness, disease, and death are all possible outcomes of use and abuse of illegal drugs. Supplements that are sold over the counter may be legal, but most have no proof of worthiness, and rely on slick marketing instead of scientific evidence. Ultimately, eating a healthy diet (see Chapters 8 and 9) and following a

DOLLAR STRETCHER
Financial Wellness Tip

Don't waste money on expensive protein supplements or other compounds advertised as muscle builders. A healthy diet with adequate protein is all you need.

well-planned exercise program will help you achieve your goals and leave you with a much better sense of accomplishment than if you had you "supplemented" your progress.

Q | Creatine is a natural substance, so it's safe, right?

CREATINE. Creatine is one of the basic muscle energy stores, typically found in fast-twitch muscle fibers. During exercise, creatine is thought to be an immediate energy source for explosive activities like sprinting or jumping. Creatine is created in the body, usually from eating red meat, and is therefore readily available. The balance of creatine in and creatine out (through the urine) is in perfect harmony for healthy people. Some believe, however, that altering this balance by ingesting additional creatine may allow for greater explosive strength and power. Unfortunately, ingesting extra creatine triggers an internal balance mechanism causing the body to reduce its own creatine synthesis. Human muscle has a capacity of about 150 millimoles of creatine per kilogram of muscle, and once this level is reached, synthesis slows to maintain that level. Therefore, supplementing creatine beyond about 20 grams a day seems fruitless, because you can't store or use any of the excess.

Why bother supplementing creatine in the first place? Well, if your creatine stores are low, supplementation does appear to improve performance in certain explosive activities.[26] The consensus is that creatine supplementation can increase the amount of work done by about 10 percent in the first few seconds of a maximal trial, such as a 1-RM strength trial. However, this amount isn't of practical benefit for most people. In addition, the risks of creatine supplementation have not yet been fully evaluated, especially over the long term.

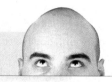

Mind Stretcher
Critical Thinking Exercise

What do you think about the use of drugs and supplements to improve sports performance? Would you use a banned drug if you knew you could get away with it? What would you say about the ethics of drug use? What about potential health risks? How would you distinguish between the performance benefit provided by using drugs and the performance benefit provided by inheriting an above-average muscle mass?

This is similar to the assessment of anabolic steroids a generation ago: They work, but we don't know what long-term effects they have. Well, we now know that anabolic steroids have a host of short- and long-term negative health consequences, some severe. Therefore, anabolic steroids are now a banned substance in sport and illegal for any nonmedical use (see the next section, "Steroids").

People who choose to use creatine supplements should do so with caution. A better choice may be to improve their diet to increase the amount of quality protein they ingest, while not sacrificing other important nutrients.

Q | If steroids are so bad, why are athletes always using them?

STEROIDS. Money is usually the reason why athletes use steroids. Steroids can and do help athletes get stronger and perform better and longer, which typically means more and better paydays.[27] This temptation is too great for some professional athletes, regardless of the physical, emotional, and financial hardships steroid use brings. The desire to outperform others has trickled down to high schools, where some athletes use steroids to improve their performance and therefore their chance of landing a college scholarship. The sport of bodybuilding has long been known for rampant steroid use, to the point where today there is a worldwide bodybuilding competition for "clean" competitors—and those not clean can keep harming themselves all they want. This points out a few things about steroid use: (1) it is difficult to detect, (2) it is problematic to control, and (3) those who engage in it are bound to suffer unfortunate consequences.

How do steroids work? All **anabolic steroids** are derived from testosterone. Steroids help to increase muscle size and strength by increasing protein synthesis. However, taking too much of a steroid increases production of the by-product estradiol, which triggers a feedback mechanism that minimizes the steroid's potency.

Anabolic steroids have been shown to increase weight gain, fat-free mass, and muscle fiber area if they are coupled with an aggressive strength-training program. These effects occur only in people who are already highly trained; in untrained people, steroids have no noticeable benefit.

The point here is that if you are new to muscle-fitness training, the combination of hard work, healthful eating, and plenty of rest is the only way to effectively reach your strength goals. By no means, however, are we advocating the use of steroids for the highly trained, because that is illegal, immoral, unethical, and extremely dangerous.

Most of the side effects of steroids are undesirable, permanent, and quite serious. The additional load on the liver can lead to liver failure.

anabolic steroids Synthetic steroids designed to increase muscle mass. Anabolic steroids, although quite effective in increasing muscle size and strength, have many undesirable side effects, including severe mood swings, decreased libido, decreased testicle size, decreased sperm production, and increased male sexual traits in women.

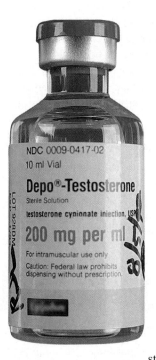

Steroids and related compounds increase muscle-fiber size and fat-free mass. But their use for performance enhancement is illegal, and they have many dangerous side effects, including liver damage, unhealthy cholesterol levels, increased cardiovascular disease risk, and hormonal and behavioral changes.

Increased levels of natural testosterone act negatively on the pituitary gland, decreasing sperm production and levels of testosterone and luteinizing hormone. There is also a noticeable increase in risk for cardiovascular disease, because steroids decrease circulating HDL ("good") cholesterol and increase LDL ("bad") cholesterol. In addition, a number of emotional problems are associated with steroid use: irritability, increased aggressiveness, nervous tension, and frequent mood swings. Women using steroids experience a hoarsening of the voice, excessive hair growth (especially on the face), an enlarged clitoris, and decreased breast size. In men using steroids, their sperm count decreases, their testicles shrink, and they experience frequent mood swings and irritability. None of these side effects seems even remotely appealing, not to mention the legal implications of steroid use, so it makes sense to just say no!

Substances such as steroids, human growth hormone, insulin, and diuretics are all used to create extreme size and boost performance. Regrettably, the use of performance-enhancing drugs is a not-so-secret problem within professional sports. Steroid scandals have shaken virtually every major sport, a sad reminder of how far some athletes will go to increase their performance. These athletes are not only taking giant risks with their honor and credibility but also with their health.

Q | Are protein shakes really worth it?

PROTEIN. If you like their taste and can afford them, there is little risk in protein shakes. On the other hand, if you eat a healthy diet and do regular moderate exercise, you probably won't get any benefit from them either. Recommended daily protein intake for the average adult is 0.36 gram per pound of body weight. Therefore, a 140-pound woman needs about 50 grams of protein a day to meet her basic needs.

Moderate muscle-fitness training does not increase protein needs. Vigorous strength training or competing at a high level of sport (such as college scholarship athletes) may necessitate an increase in daily protein, but there is no need to exceed 1.0 gram per pound of body weight. Further, it is better to get protein from whole sources, especially those low in saturated fat, than to use supplements. Supplements tend to be more expensive than food sources, and their efficacy is not proven.

What about the protein shakes? Shakes might be useful for the high-level athlete needing a lot of protein, since it is easier to drink shakes than eat, say, peanut butter and jelly sandwiches all day long. If you purchase 18-ounce jars of peanut butter and jelly and a loaf of whole-wheat bread, you can have several days of high-protein snacks for about $7.00. A high-protein energy bar sold at a popu-

lar nutrition supplement store goes for about $3.00. That's two bars for the same price as ten PBJ sandwiches. At the same nutritional retailer, you can buy a popular brand of protein powder for $60.00 (yes, sixty), but it yields over eighty servings, for a per-serving price around 75 cents. That isn't a bad value, but a closer look at the label reveals that the main ingredients are soybeans and milk, and there is frequent mention of "naturally occurring" ingredients. It would seem better, then, to consume "natural" foods since they are the source of these protein supplements!

In short, if you are new to muscle-fitness training, you should strive to eat well, have a good exercise plan, and get plenty of rest. Leave the supplements to someone who has lots of money to waste.

Practical Prevention

Supplement Smarts: What's Really Safe?

When it comes to nutritional supplements, "natural" is not necessarily safe. Many supplements can be used safely by most people, but some herbs may cause cancer, some vitamins can be toxic at high doses, and some supplements can cause injury when mixed with medications. Good sources of sound information to help you sort through the hype include the following:

National Center for Complementary and Alternative Medicine

http://nccam.nih.gov

National Institutes of Health Office of Dietary Supplements

http://dietary-supplements.info.nih.gov

Federal Trade Commission: Test Your Supplement Savvy

http://www.ftc.gov/bcp/edu/pubs/consumer/health/hea09.shtm

Summary

Muscle fitness is critical for a long and healthy life. If your muscles are not fit, many mundane tasks become quite challenging, especially as you grow older. During your college years, good muscle fitness allows you to perform all types of tasks with more vigor and enjoyment than if your muscles were not fit. Increasing muscle fitness does not have to take lots of time or be done in a specialized facility. This chapter discusses plans for dorm-room workouts using nothing more than body weight and for more extensive workouts for those with the time, access to equipment, and desire. The key to muscle fitness is to do something, and do it regularly. Although it is possible to maintain your muscle fitness for up to six weeks with very little time and effort, it is much healthier to put in enough effort to ensure that your muscles are regularly stressed according to the overload principle. Muscle-fitness training a few days a week, coupled with regular cardiovas-

cular exercise and a healthy diet will keep you strong, healthy, and happy for many years to come!

More to Explore

American College of Sports Medicine
http://www.acsm.org
American Council on Exercise: Fit Facts
http://www.acefitness.org/fitfacts
National Strength and Conditioning Association
http://www.nsca-lift.org
Strongwomen.com: Fitness Programs
http://www.strongwomen.com/fitness.htm
University of Michigan: Muscles in Action
http://www.med.umich.edu/lrc/Hypermuscle/Hyper.html

Sample Resistance-Training Programs

▶ WATCH ONLINE All the exercises in the Basic Program and Bodyweight Circuit, along with many others, are described in the following section and have corresponding video clips available online.

Program 1: Basic Muscle Fitness Program (Using Machines or Free Weights)

UPPER BODY	LOWER BODY	CORE
Biceps curl (biceps, brachioradialis, brachialis)	Leg press (quadriceps, gluteals)	Curl-up (abdominals, hip flexors)
Triceps extension (triceps)	Leg curl (hamstrings)	Side bridge (abdominals, quadratus lumborum)
Bench press (pectoralis major, triceps, deltoid)	Heel raise (gastrocnemius, soleus)	Prone (forward) plank (anterior and posterior trunk and pelvis)
Lat pulldown (latissimus dorsi, pectoralis major, biceps)		
Shoulder press (triceps, deltoids, pectoralis major)		

Program 2: Upper- and Lower-Body Split Routine

Upper- and lower-body split routines alternate between upper-body exercises on one day and lower-body exercises on another. There are many ways to structure a split routine; in the sample program shown here, days 3 and 6 are rest days, and then the six-day sequence repeats.

DAY 1	DAY 2	DAY 4	DAY 5
Barbell bench press	Front squat	Barbell shoulder press	Step-up
Triceps push-down	Dumbbell lunge	Dip	Deadlift
Dumbbell row	Heel raise	Lat pull-down	Back extension
Barbell biceps curl	Stability-ball curl-up	Dumbbell biceps curl	Cable woodchopper
	Side bridge		Prone (forward) plank

Program 3: Muscle-Group Split Routine

Muscle-group split routines divide workouts by muscle groups; individual muscle groups are typically rested for several days between training sessions. In the example shown here, day 4 is a rest day, and then the four-day sequence repeats.

DAY 1: CHEST, SHOULDERS, TRICEPS	DAY 2: LOWER BODY	DAY 3: BACK, BICEPS
Incline bench press	Back squat	Bent-over row
Dumbbell fly	Lunge	Chin-up
Machine shoulder press	Deadlift	Shrug
Lateral raise	Leg curl	EZ bar biceps curl
Triceps extension	Heel raise	Reverse curl
	Curl-up	
	Reverse crunch	

Program 4: Bodyweight Circuit

This program includes exercises that exclusively use body weight for resistance.

Push-up	Body-weight squat
Pull-up	Curl-up
Prone (forward) bridge	Body-weight lunge
Chair dip	Quadruped hip extension (bird dog)
Inverted row (Australian pull-up)	Body-weight step-up
Side bridge	

STRENGTH-TRAINING EXERCISES

▶ WATCH ONLINE For each major muscle group of the body, several exercise options are presented using different types of equipment (or no equipment). Choose one or more exercises for each muscle group to put together a complete strength-training program that fits your needs. Exercises are organized by the key muscle group they develop, but many exercises work additional muscles; refer to the "Muscles developed" list in each exercise. For best results, pay close attention to the description of correct technique and the training tips. Always use proper body alignment and don't bounce or swing weights. You can make many exercises more challenging by pausing for 1 second at the bottom of each repetition.

MUSCLE GROUP Chest

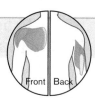
Front | Back

▶ WATCH ONLINE

Barbell Bench Press

Muscles developed: Pectoralis major, triceps brachii, deltoids

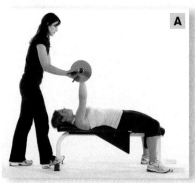
A

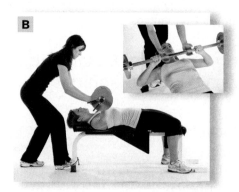
B

Instructions

A. Lie on your back on a bench with your feet flat on the floor. Adjust the bench so that your back is straight and not arched; if your feet don't reach the floor comfortably, place them on the bench with your knees bent. Grasp the bar with your palms upward and hands about shoulder-width apart. Start with the bar over the middle of your chest or slightly above it. Arms should be fully extended, but don't forcefully lock your elbows.

B. Lower the bar slowly to your chest; then press it in a straight line back to the starting position. Each full repetition should take 2–4 seconds.

Training tips

- If the weight is resting on a rack, move it carefully with the help of spotters. If you have one spotter, he or she should stand behind you; if you have two spotters, they should stand at the ends of the bar.
- During the exercise, don't arch your back or bounce the bar off your chest.

Machine Chest Press

Muscles developed: Pectoralis major, triceps, deltoids

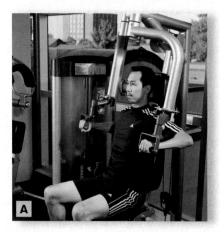
A

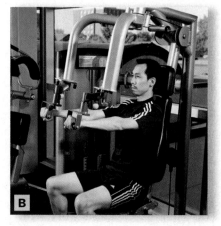
B

Instructions

A. Depending on the type of machine, sit or lie on the seat or bench with your feet flat on the floor or the foot support. Your back and hips should be against the machine pads, and the tops of the handles should be aligned with your armpits. Grasp the handles with your palms facing away from you.

B. Push the bars until your arms are fully extended, but don't forcefully lock your elbows. Return to the starting position. Each full repetition should take 2–4 seconds.

Training tips

- During the exercise, don't arch your back or bounce at the end of the movement.
- If the starting position of the bar is adjustable, set it so that your wrists can remain straight throughout the exercise.

Push-Up and Modified Push-Up
Muscles developed: Pectoralis major, triceps, deltoids

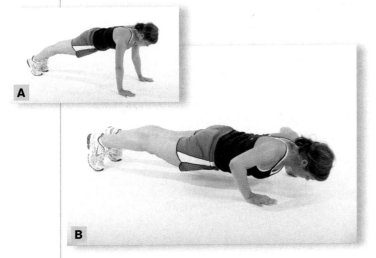

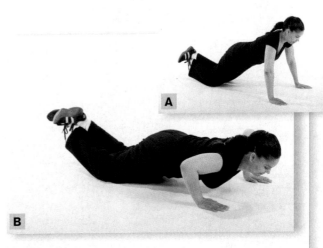

Instructions

A. For push-ups, start with your body in the upright position, supported by your hands and the balls of your feet. For modified push-ups, support your weight with your hands and knees; bend your knees about 90 degrees and keep your ankles together or crossed. Your back should be straight and your neck neutral. Your hands should be about 2–3 inches wider than shoulder-width apart, and your fingers should point forward.

B. Lower your chest to the floor so that your elbows are bent about 90 degrees. Then return to the starting position by fully straightening your arms. Each push-up should take 2–4 seconds.

Training tips

- Use the modified technique if you cannot do more than 8 push-ups; once you can do more than 20–25 modified push-ups, switch to the standard push-up technique.
- Keep your body straight throughout the exercise; don't let your back arch or your hips rise up or sag.
- To ensure that you lower yourself far enough during each repetition, touch your chest on a soft object on the floor, such as a pair of rolled-up socks, a tennis ball, or a friend's fist.
- Push-ups can be made more challenging by raising the level of your feet with a small bench or an exercise ball.

MUSCLE GROUP Shoulders

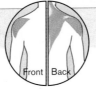

Front | Back

Barbell Shoulder Press
Muscles developed: Anterior deltoid, lateral deltoid, triceps brachii

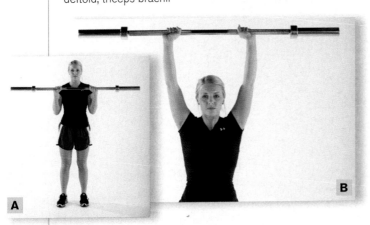

Instructions

A. Stand with your feet about shoulder-width apart. Grasp the bar with your palms facing away from you; the bar should be at the top of the chest.

B. Slowly press the bar straight overhead until your arms are fully extended. Then lower the weight back to the starting position in a controlled manner. Each full repetition should take 2–4 seconds.

Training tip

- Keep your back straight throughout this exercise; don't arch.

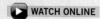 WATCH ONLINE

Machine Shoulder Press

Muscles developed: Anterior deltoid, lateral deltoid, triceps brachii

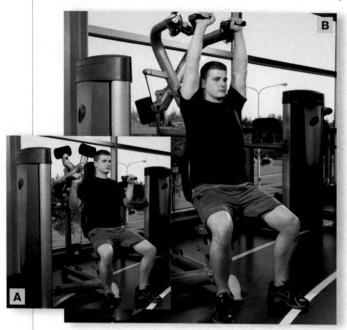

Instructions

A. Adjust the seat so that your feet are flat on the ground or foot bar and the handles or bars are slightly above the level of your shoulders.

B. Slowly press the weight straight overhead until your arms are fully extended. Then lower the weight back to the starting position. Each full repetition should take 2–4 seconds.

Training tips

- Lower the weight in a controlled fashion rather than letting it fall with gravity.
- Not lowering the weight all the way to the weight stack will make this exercise more challenging.

Dumbbell Lateral Raises

Muscles developed: Anterior deltoid, lateral deltoid, trapezius

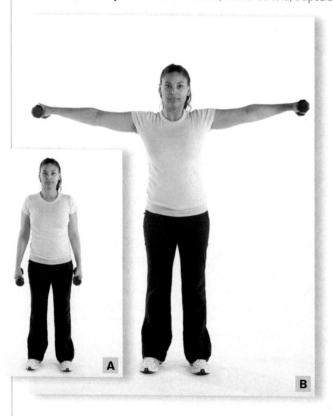

Instructions

A. Stand with feet about shoulder-width apart, holding a dumbbell in each hand by your side.

B. With your palms facing in and wrists held straight, slowly raise the weights out to the sides until your elbows are level with your shoulders. Return to the starting position slowly and in a controlled fashion.

Training tips

- Keep your back straight and your shoulders down throughout this exercise.
- This exercise can be quite challenging, so most people start with a very light weight.

MUSCLE GROUP **Back**

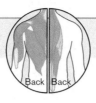

Dumbbell Row

Muscles developed: Posterior deltoid, latissimus dorsi, biceps brachii

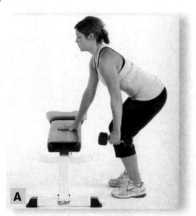 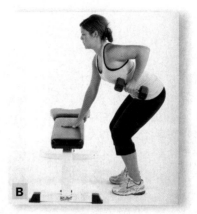

Instructions

A. Stand in front of a bench, grasping a dumbbell in one hand with your feet about shoulder-width apart. With your abdominals tight and your back straight, bend your knees and lean forward at the hips until your support hand is on the bench. The hand with the dumbbell should be directly below your shoulder.

B. Pull the dumbbell up to the side until it makes contact with your ribs or until your upper arm is just beyond horizontal. Lower the weight until your arm is extended and your shoulder is stretched forward. Repeat on the opposite side.

Training tips

- Try to hold your torso in a horizontal plane while pulling the weight upward. Adjust supporting knee and/or arm slightly forward or back as needed.
- The exercise can also be done with one knee and hand on the bench for support. Position the foot of your other leg slightly back and to the side.

Lat Pull-Down

Muscles developed: Posterior deltoid, latissimus dorsi

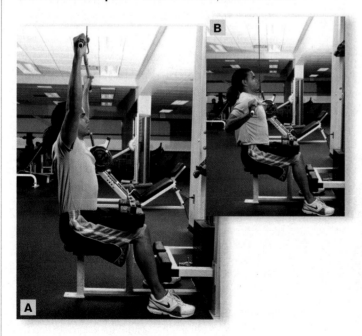

Instructions

A. Grasp the cable bar with a grip slightly wider than your shoulders, palms facing away. Sit with your thighs under the supports and your feet flat on the floor.

B. Pull down on the cable bar until it reaches your upper chest. Move your shoulder blades together and your elbows down. Return the weight to the starting position in a controlled fashion, until your arms and shoulders are extended.

Training tips

- Do not hold too wide a grip; otherwise, your range of motion will be compromised.
- Avoid swinging your body or leaning back to use your weight to pull the bar down; instead, focus on using the muscles of your arms and back to move the weight.

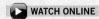 WATCH ONLINE

Chin-Up (Pull-Up)
Muscles developed: Latissimus dorsi, biceps brachii, brachialis

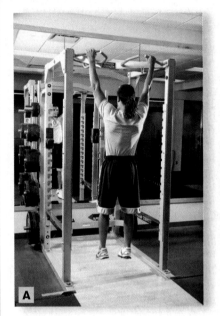

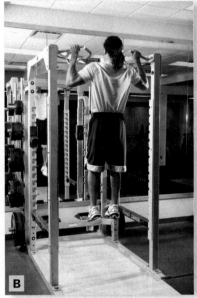

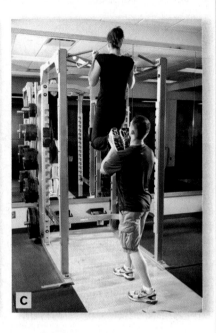

Instructions

A. Using a stable overhead bar, grasp the bar with your palms facing away from you. Ideally, your feet will still be on the ground.

B. Using your arm strength, pull yourself upward until your chin is over the top of the bar, then lower yourself back to the starting position. Don't let your feet rest on the floor until you are completely finished with the movement. Each full repetition should take 2–4 seconds.

Training tips

- Keep your body in a fairly straight position, and don't swing.
- If you can't complete a pull-up, assistance can be provided by a spotter (**C**) or by a weight-lifting band (a rubber-band-like device that supports some of your body weight during the pull-up).
- This exercise can be modified by doing it from a supine position—the "Australian" chin-up, in which you begin lying on your back with a stable bar an arm's length above you.

MUSCLE GROUP Biceps

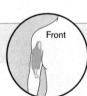

Front

Barbell Biceps Curl
Muscles developed: Biceps brachii, brachialis

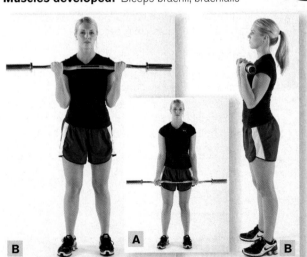

Instructions The exercise can be done with a straight barbell or a curl bar; the curl bar may place less stress on your wrists.

A. Stand with feet about shoulder-width apart, grasping the bar with your palms facing away from you and your hands about shoulder-width apart.

B. Slowly raise the weight until the bar is slightly below the level of your collarbone. Then without pausing, lower the weight back to the starting position. Each full repetition should take 2–4 seconds.

Training tips

- Keep your back straight throughout the exercise; don't let your back arch or your arms to swing through the motion.
- This exercise can also be performed with dumbbells.

Machine Biceps Curl
Muscles developed: Biceps brachii, brachialis

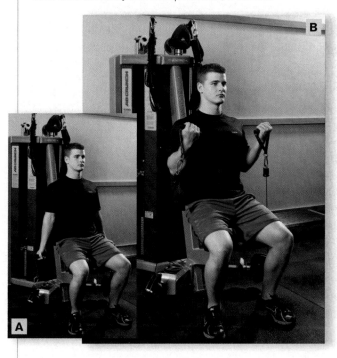

Instructions
A. Adjust the seat so that your feet rest on the ground or foot bar and your back is straight. Grasp the handles or hand grips with your palms facing up.

B. Keep your body still as you bend your elbows until the handles or hand grips are close to your collarbone. Return to the starting position. Each full repetition should take 2–4 seconds.

Training tip
- Keep your back straight throughout the exercise; don't let your back arch or move back during the exercise.

MUSCLE GROUP Triceps

Back

Dumbbell Triceps Extension
Muscles developed: Triceps brachii

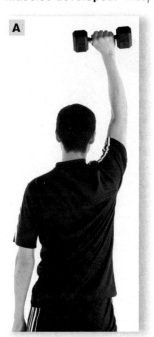
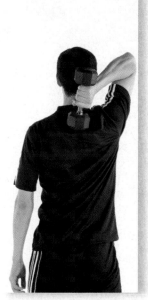

Instructions This exercise can be done seated or standing.
A. Holding one dumbbell, fully extend your arm overhead, palm facing forward.

B. Slowly lower the weight behind your head, keeping your elbow straight up and rotating your palm toward your body, until your arm is fully bent. Slowly raise the weight back to the starting position.

Training tips
- Keep your back straight throughout this exercise.
- Your elbow and upper arm should remain straight up throughout this exercise.

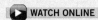

Machine Triceps Push-Down
Muscles developed: Triceps brachii

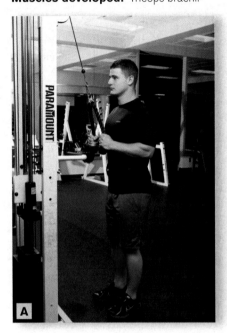
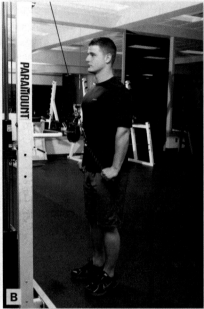

Instructions This exercise requires a lat pull-down machine.

A. Stand facing the machine with your feet about shoulder-width apart. Grasp the bar with your palms facing down. Your elbows should at your sides, bent 90 or more degrees.

B. Keeping your elbows at your side, slowly push the weight down until your arms are almost straight. Then slowly raise the bar back to the starting position.

Training tip

- Keep your back straight throughout this exercise.

Chair Triceps Dip
Muscles developed: Triceps brachii

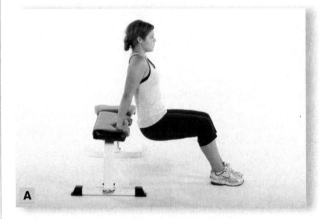
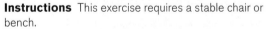
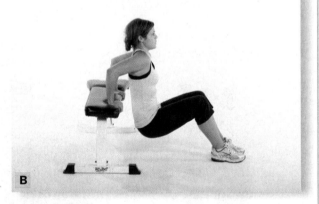

Instructions This exercise requires a stable chair or bench.

A. Start by sitting on the front edge of the chair, with your hands palm-down beside your hips. Use your hands to push your body up (your feet should remain on the floor), and move your hips forward away from the chair.

B. Lower your body in front of the chair by bending your elbows to about a 90-degree angle; then push back up with your arms to the starting position.

Training tips

- Keep your back straight and your elbows close to your body throughout the exercise.

- To make the exercise easier, move your feet closer to the chair. To make the exercise more challenging, move your feet farther from the chair, elevate them on a small bench, or place them on an exercise ball.

MUSCLE GROUP **Quadriceps**

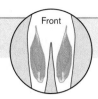
Front

Note: Many of the exercises in this group also develop the gluteal muscles and the hamstrings.

Bodyweight Squat
Muscles developed: Quadriceps, hamstrings, gluteals, erector spinae

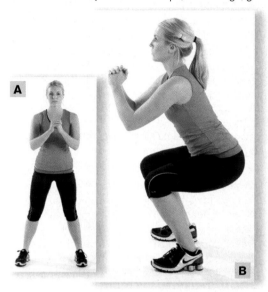

Instructions

A. Stand with your feet just wider than your shoulders and your toes pointed slightly out. For balance, your hands should be together and out in front of you at about shoulder height, with elbows bent.

B. Squat down until your thighs are parallel with the floor; then raise yourself back to the starting position. As you squat, push your hips back and keep your back neutral or slightly arched; don't round your lower back. Each repetition should take 2–5 seconds.

Training tips

- Don't lean forward as you squat down; keep your feet flat on the floor, chest up, and head forward.
- Think of squatting as sitting back on a toilet seat.
- Advanced users can do one-legged squats, which are the same as described above with one leg held up and forward. This exercise can also be done standing on one leg on a slightly elevated, stable surface, while the other leg hangs over the edge.

Barbell Back Squat
Muscles developed: Quadriceps, hamstrings, gluteals, erector spinae

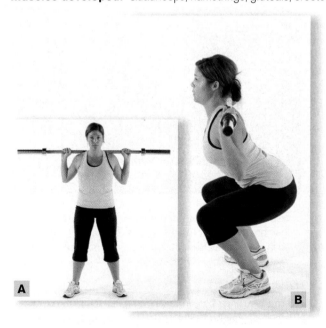

Instructions

A. Stand with your feet just wider than your shoulders and your toes pointing slightly out. The bar should rest on your upper back; grasp it slightly wider than shoulder-width, with your palms facing forward.

B. Squat down until your thighs are parallel with the floor; then raise yourself back to the starting position. As you squat, push your hips back and keep your back neutral or slightly arched; don't round your lower back. Each repetition should take 2–5 seconds.

Training tips

- Keep your head forward, chest up, and feet flat on floor.
- Unless you are using a specialized squat rack, you will need spotters. If you have one spotter, he or she should stand behind you; if you have two spotters, they should stand at the ends of the bar.
- Your knees should point the same direction as your feet throughout the movement.
- Maintain a natural curve (arch) in your back throughout the entire movement.

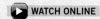
WATCH ONLINE

Dumbbell Lunge

Muscles developed: Quadriceps, gluteus maximus, adductors

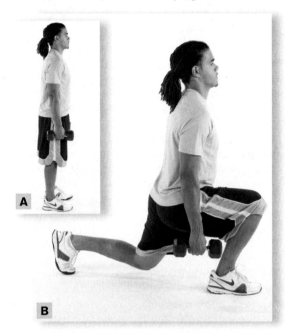

A

B

Instructions

A. Stand with your feet about shoulder-width apart. Hold a small dumbbell in each hand.

B. Take a larger-than-normal step forward, and let your foot land fully on the floor. Bend your forward leg until your thigh is parallel with the floor; make sure your knee is directly above your ankle rather than extending forward in front of your foot. Your back leg should be bent and your heel off the ground. Return to the starting position by pushing off with your forward leg.

Training tips

- Keep your back straight, maintaining its natural curves through the entire movement.
- Beginners can perform lunges without weights to start.
- There are two major variations of this exercise: walking lunges and reverse lunges. To do the walking lunge, once you are in the lunge position, instead of pushing back, simply step forward with the opposing leg, again going in to the lunge position. For a reverse lunge, step backward instead of forward, lowering your back knee towards the floor until your front thigh is parallel with the floor. Push back up to start, and repeat.

Machine Leg Press

Muscles developed: Quadriceps, gluteus maximus, hamstrings

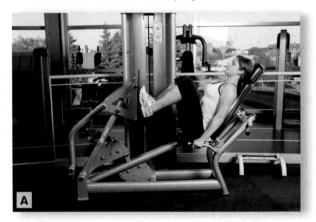

A

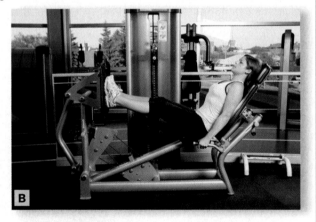

B

Instructions

A. Sit or lie on the seat or bench of the machine; adjust it so that your head, back, and buttocks are against the pads and your hands can grasp the handles. Your feet should be about shoulder-width apart, and your knees comfortably bent and in line with your feet.

B. With your feet flat on the footplate, push to straighten your legs; move through the full range of motion, but don't forcefully lock your knees. Return to the starting position by slowly lowering the weight in a controlled fashion. Keep your head steady and your back pressed against the seat. Each full repetition should take 4–5 seconds.

Training tips

- If the starting position feels cramped, adjust the seat.
- Keep your knees in line with your feet; don't allow them to bow inward or outward.

Machine Leg Extension
Muscles developed: Quadriceps

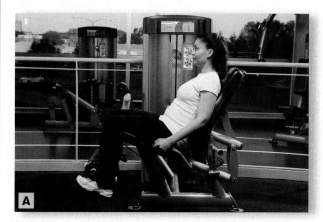

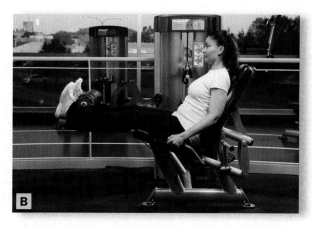

Instructions
A. Sit with your hips and back against the pads. Adjust the seat so that the pads rest comfortably on the top of your shins.

B. Keep your body still as you extend your knees until they are almost but not quite straight. Keep your head steady and your back pressed against the seat. Each full repetition should take 2–4 seconds.

Training tips
- If you feel any knee pain, don't perform this exercise.
- Tightening your abdominal muscles may help you keep your back from arching.

Step-Up
Muscles developed: Quadriceps, gluteus maximus

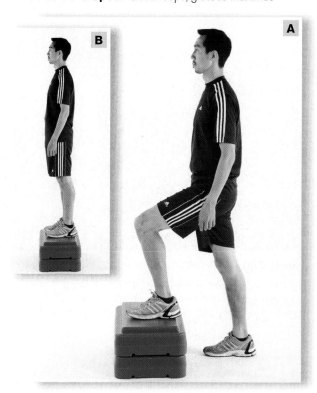

Instructions This exercise requires a stable step or low bench, between 12 and 18 inches high.

A. Start by standing about 2 feet from the bench, with your feet shoulder-width apart, as if you were about to walk up some stairs. Place one foot forward fully onto the step.

B. Step up. Once your forward leg is fully extended, slowly lower back down to the start position. This exercise can be done one leg at a time or alternating lead legs.

Training tips
- Maintain the natural curve (slight arch) in your back through the entire movement.
- This exercise can be made more challenging by holding a dumbbell in each hand or wearing a weighted vest.

MUSCLE GROUP Hamstrings

Back

▶ **WATCH ONLINE**

Stability-Ball Leg Curl
Muscles developed: Hamstrings, gluteals, erector spinae

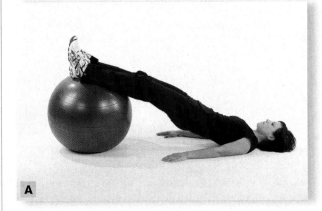

A

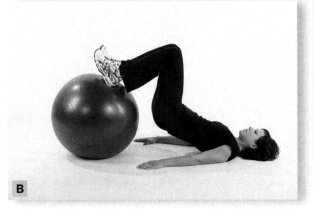

B

Instructions

A. Lie on your back on the ground with your feet up on an exercise ball (at least 15 inches high). Raise your hips so that your back is straight or slightly arched. Keep your arms extended on the floor beside you. You should be able to roll the ball with your feet.

B. Keeping your hips straight, roll the ball toward you until your knees are bent at a 90-degree angle.

Training tips

- Don't do the exercise if it causes low-back pain.
- Keep your hips straight throughout the movement. Bend only your knees and not your hips.
- This exercise can be made more challenging by using a larger ball. It can also be done with a chair or bench in place of the ball, slowly raising your hips up and down.

Machine Leg Curl
Muscles developed: Hamstrings

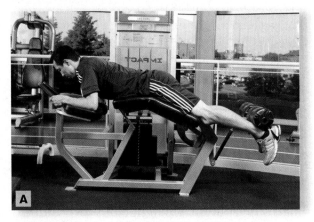

A

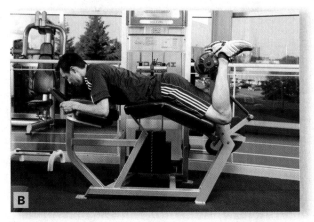

B

Instructions

A. Lie on the front of your body, with hips and forearms aligned with the appropriate pads. The leg pad should rest comfortably against your lower calves. Grasp the hand grips loosely.

B. Keep your body still as you flex your knees until they are bent at a 90-degree angle. Return to the starting position. Keep your head steady and your back straight. Each full repetition should take 2–4 seconds.

Training tip

- Use caution when doing this exercise for the first time. Use a light weight until you are comfortable with the movement, and increase the weight very gradually.

MUSCLE GROUP Core

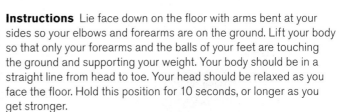

Prone (Forward) Plank

Muscles developed: Obliques, rectus abdominis, deltoids, erector spinae

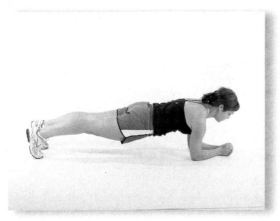

Instructions Lie face down on the floor with arms bent at your sides so your elbows and forearms are on the ground. Lift your body so that only your forearms and the balls of your feet are touching the ground and supporting your weight. Your body should be in a straight line from head to toe. Your head should be relaxed as you face the floor. Hold this position for 10 seconds, or longer as you get stronger.

Training tips

- Keep your body straight throughout the exercise; don't let your lower back arch or sag.
- You can make this exercise easier by spreading your feet wider.
- You can make this exercise more challenging by lifting one arm straight out to the side for 10 to 15 seconds or one leg off the ground for 10 to 15 seconds.

Side Bridge

Muscles developed: Obliques, transverse abdominis

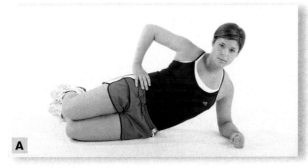

A

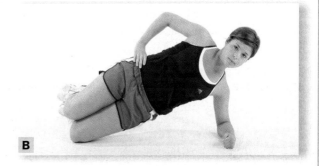

B

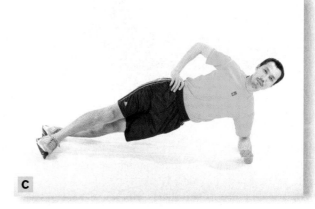

C

Instructions Side bridges can be done in several different positions

A. Lie on the floor on your side, with your knees bent. Your top arm can lie along your side, or you can place your hand on your hip.

B. Lift your hips so that your weight is supported by your forearm and knee. Hold this position for at least 10 seconds, slowly building up to 30 seconds. As you gain strength, you can make the exercise more difficult by supporting your weight with your forearm and your feet (**C**).

Training tips

- Keep your body firm and straight throughout this exercise.
- This exercise can be made more challenging by pointing your top arm straight up.
- An advanced variation involves "rolling" from a side bridge to a forward-plank position with forearms perpendicular to the body and then to a side bridge facing the other direction.

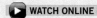

Quadruped Hip Extension (Bird Dog)

Muscles developed: Erector spinae, rectus abdominis, gluteus maximus

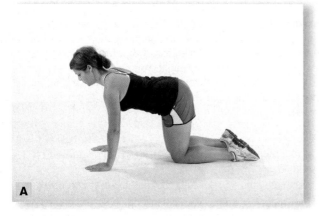

A

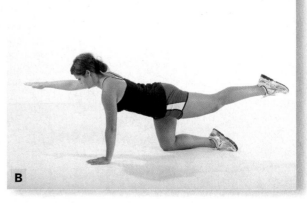

B

Instructions

A. Start on the floor, supporting your weight with your hands and knees. Your knees should be below your hips, and your hands should be below your shoulders and slightly wider.

B. Slowly extend one arm and the opposite leg, keeping your back straight. Hold this position for 5 to 10 seconds. Repeat on the other side.

Training tips

- Use a pad under your hands and knees for more comfort.
- Beginners can start by lifting an arm alone, then lowering it, and then lifting a leg alone.
- Advanced users can hold each pose for 10 to 15 seconds.

Back (Glute) Bridge

Muscles developed: Erector spinae, gluteals, hamstrings

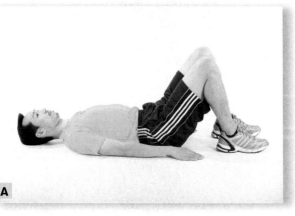

A

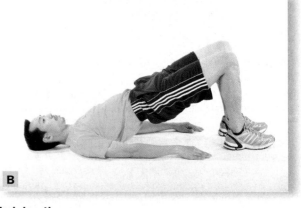

B

Instructions

A. Lie on your back with your arms extended along your sides, legs bent, and feet flat on the floor.

B. Tuck your pelvis under and tighten your gluteal muscles. Raise your hips so that your weight is supported by your head, shoulders, and feet. Hold this position for at least 10 seconds, and slowly build up to 30 seconds.

Training tips

- Keep your back straight throughout this exercise.
- This exercise can be made more difficult by lifting one leg so that the foot is pointing out, in line with the support leg.
- If you feel any pain in your back, don't perform this exercise.

Curl-Up
Muscles developed: Rectus abdominis

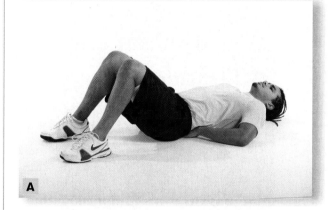

A

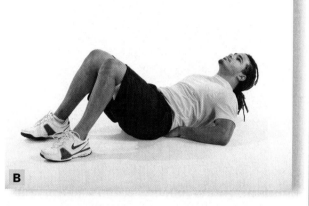

B

Instructions
A. Lie on the floor with your legs bent and your feet flat on the floor. Place your hands under the small of your back; maintain the natural curve of your lower back throughout this exercise.

B. Slowly lift your shoulder blades off the ground, keeping your nose pointed straight upward. Then slowly lower yourself back to the floor.

Training tips
- You can reduce the strain on your back by keeping one leg straight and one leg bent.
- Do not try to lift your entire back off the floor, just your shoulder blades.
- This exercise can be made more challenging with the use of an exercise ball. "Sit" on the ball and slowly lower your back until it is fully extended, and then return to the starting position. Your feet should be firmly on the ground.

MUSCLE GROUP Calf/Soleus

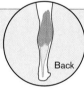

Back

Barbell Standing Heel-Raise
Muscles developed: Gastrocnemius, soleus

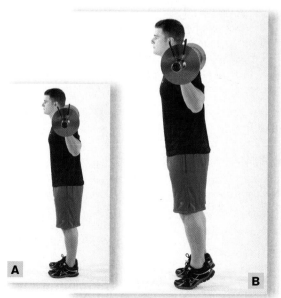

A

B

Instructions
A. Stand with your feet about shoulder-width apart and your toes pointing forward. Grasp the barbell with palms facing forward and rest it comfortably on your upper back.

B. Press down with your toes as you lift your heels. Then slowly lower your heels back to the floor. Don't let your ankles roll in or out during the exercise. Each full repetition should take 2–4 seconds.

Training tips
- Keep your back straight or slightly arched throughout the movement.
- Look forward and keep your neck in a neutral position.
- Don't bounce at the end of the range of motion.

Machine Seated Heel-Raise
Muscles developed: Gastrocnemius, soleus

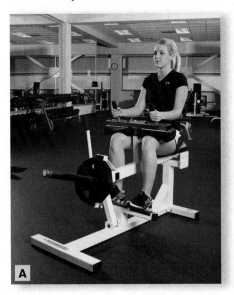

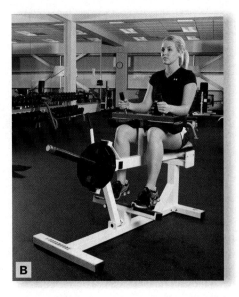

Instructions
A. Sit with the balls of your feet on the platform, your knees bent at 90 degrees, and the pads on top of your lower thighs; your toes should point forward.

B. Press down with your toes as you lift your heels. Then slowly lower your heels back to the starting position. Don't let your ankles roll in or out during the exercise, and keep your back straight. Each full repetition should take 2–4 seconds.

Training tip
■ Don't bounce at the end of the range of motion.

Dumbbell Seated Heel-Raise
Muscles developed: Gastrocnemius, soleus

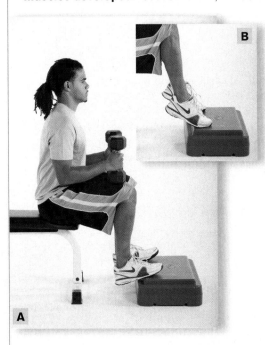

Instructions
A. Sit down on a chair or a bench, with your feet comfortably resting on the ground. Place the balls of your feet on a small block or a low step (2–4 inches high) so that your heels can drop below the level of your toes. Place a dumbbell, barbell, or other small weight on your thighs.

B. Starting with your heels lowered, press onto your toes so that the front of your thighs and knees slightly elevate, as your calves contract. Lower your heels back down to the starting position.

Training tips
■ Keep your back straight or slightly arched throughout the exercise movement.

■ The chair or bench height should allow for a 90-degree angle at the knee.

■ This exercise can be made more challenging by using a heavier weight.

SUBMIT ONLINE

NAME   DATE   SECTION

This lab includes tests for assessing muscular strength of the upper and lower body. The traditional test for strength is a one-repetition maximum (1-RM) test, which measures the greatest resistance that can be moved through one full range of motion with good form. The 1-RM test is the most accurate assessment, but it is not appropriate for people with little or no strength-training experience. For them, there are formulas, although somewhat less accurate, that can convert a multiple-repetitions result to an estimated 1-RM value; in this type of test, you perform multiple repetitions of an exercise just as you would during a strength-training workout. Choose tests that are appropriate for you. Scores and ratings are based on your age, sex, and body weight:

Age: [ ]   Sex (male/female): [ ]   Body weight: [ ] lbs.

Upper-Body Strength: Bench Press

Equipment

- Bench-press machine OR a flat bench, barbell, weight plates, collars, and at least one spotter
- Weight scale (for measuring body weight)

Preparation

Perform a general warm-up; then warm up for the bench press by performing several repetitions using a light weight. If you are using free weights, practice the exercise with your spotter(s).

Instructions

Follow the instructions for the bench-press technique given on p. 168. Keep your feet flat on the floor or bench, and don't arch your back. Push the weight up until your arms are fully extended. Don't hold your breath or bounce the weight on your chest.

For the 1-RM test: Start with a weight that is less than the amount you think you can lift (50%–70% of your estimated 1-RM). Lift that amount of resistance one time with good form. Increase the weight with each attempt, resting 3–5 minutes between attempts. If you lifted the weight easily, add 20 or more pounds; if you are close to your 1-RM, add a smaller amount of resistance (about 5 pounds). Your goal is to reach your 1-RM in 4–5 attempts. Your 1-RM is the final weight you lifted with good form.

Bench press 1-RM: [ ] lbs.

For estimating 1-RM from multiple repetitions: Choose a weight that is an amount you think you can lift about 10 times. Using correct form, perform as many repetitions as you can. Estimate your 1-RM for the bench press with the following formula:

$$\text{Bench press 1-RM} = \frac{\text{resistance } \boxed{} \text{ lbs.}}{1.0278 - (0.0278 \times \text{repetitions } \boxed{})} = \boxed{} \text{ lbs.}$$

Results

Divide your 1-RM score by your body weight:

1-RM [ ] lbs. ÷ body weight [ ] lbs. = [ ] bench-press weight ratio

Find the rating for your bench-press weight ratio on the table below: [ ]

183

BENCH-PRESS WEIGHT-RATIO RATINGS*

Males

AGE (YEARS)	WELL ABOVE AVERAGE	ABOVE AVERAGE	AVERAGE	BELOW AVERAGE	WELL BELOW AVERAGE
<20	>1.34	1.19–1.34	1.06–1.18	0.89–1.05	<0.89
20–29	>1.32	1.14–1.32	0.99–1.13	0.88–0.98	<0.88
30–39	>1.12	0.98–1.12	0.88–0.97	0.78–0.87	<0.78
40–49	>1.00	0.88–1.00	0.80–0.87	0.72–0.79	<0.72
50–59	>0.90	0.79–0.90	0.71–0.78	0.63–0.70	<0.63
60+	>0.82	0.72–0.82	0.66–0.71	0.57–0.65	<0.57

Females

AGE (YEARS)	WELL ABOVE AVERAGE	ABOVE AVERAGE	AVERAGE	BELOW AVERAGE	WELL BELOW AVERAGE
<20	>0.77	0.65–0.77	0.58–0.64	0.53–0.57	<0.53
20–29	>0.80	0.70–0.80	0.59–0.69	0.51–0.58	<0.51
30–39	>0.70	0.60–0.70	0.53–0.59	0.47–0.52	<0.47
40–49	>0.62	0.54–0.62	0.50–0.53	0.43–0.49	<0.43
50–59	>0.55	0.48–0.55	0.44–0.47	0.39–0.43	<0.39
60+	>0.54	0.47–0.54	0.43–0.46	0.38–0.42	<0.38

*In terms of percentiles, *well above average* = over the 80th percentile; *above average* = between 60th and 80th percentiles; *average* = between 40th and 60th percentiles; *below average* = between 20th and 40th percentiles; and *well below average* = below the 20th percentile.

Source: Cooper Institute for Aerobics Research. (2009). *Physical fitness assessment and norms for adults and law enforcement.* Dallas, TX: Cooper Institute.

Lower-Body Strength: Leg Press

Equipment

- Leg-press machine
- Weight scale (for measuring body weight)

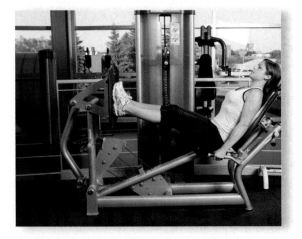

Preparation

Perform a general warm-up; then warm up for the leg press by performing several repetitions using a light weight.

Instructions

Follow the instructions for the leg-press technique given on p. 176. Keep your feet flat on the footplate about shoulder-width apart. Push the weight up until your legs are fully extended, but don't forcefully lock your knees. Don't hold your breath.

For the 1-RM test: Start with a weight that is less than the amount you think you can press (50%–70% of your estimated 1-RM). Press that amount of resistance one time with good form. Increase the weight with each attempt, resting 3–5 minutes between attempts. If you lifted the weight easily, add 25 or more pounds; if you are close to your 1-RM, add a smaller amount of resistance. Your goal is to reach your 1-RM in 4–5 attempts. Your 1-RM is the final weight you pressed with good form.

Leg press 1-RM: [ ] lbs.

For estimating 1-RM from multiple repetitions: Choose a weight that is an amount you think you can press about 10 times. Using correct form, perform as many repetitions as you can. Estimate your 1-RM for the leg press with the following formula:

$$\text{Leg press 1-RM} = \frac{\text{resistance} \boxed{} \text{ lbs.}}{1.0278 - (0.0278 \times \text{repetitions} \boxed{})} = \boxed{} \text{ lbs.}$$

Results

Divide your 1-RM score by your body weight:

1-RM $\boxed{}$ lbs. ÷ body weight $\boxed{}$ lbs. = $\boxed{}$ leg-press weight ratio

Find the rating for your leg-press weight ratio on the table below: $\boxed{}$

LEG-PRESS WEIGHT-RATIO RATINGS*

Males

AGE (YEARS)	WELL ABOVE AVERAGE	ABOVE AVERAGE	AVERAGE	BELOW AVERAGE	WELL BELOW AVERAGE
20–29	>2.12	1.97–2.12	1.83–1.96	1.63–1.82	<1.63
30–39	>1.92	1.77–1.92	1.65–1.76	1.52–1.65	<1.52
40–49	>1.81	1.68–1.81	1.57–1.67	1.44–1.56	<1.44
50–59	>1.70	1.58–1.70	1.46–1.57	1.32–1.45	<1.32
60+	>1.61	1.49–1.61	1.38–1.48	1.25–1.37	<1.25

Females

AGE (YEARS)	WELL ABOVE AVERAGE	ABOVE AVERAGE	AVERAGE	BELOW AVERAGE	WELL BELOW AVERAGE
20–29	>1.67	1.50–1.67	1.37–1.49	1.22–1.36	<1.22
30–39	>1.46	1.33–1.46	1.21–1.32	1.09–1.20	<1.09
40–49	>1.36	1.23–1.36	1.13–1.22	1.02–1.12	<1.02
50–59	>1.24	1.10–1.24	0.99–1.09	0.88–0.98	<0.88
60+	>1.17	1.04–1.17	0.93–1.03	0.85–0.92	<0.85

*In terms of percentiles, *well above average* = over the 80th percentile; *above average* = between 60th and 80th percentiles; *average* = between 40th and 60th percentiles; *below average* = between 20th and 40th percentiles; and *well below average* = below the 20th percentile.

Source: Cooper Institute for Aerobics Research. (1994). *Physical fitness assessment and norms.* Dallas, TX: Cooper Institute.

Summary of Results

Fill in the scores and ratings for the tests you performed

TEST	ACTUAL 1-RM	ESTIMATED 1-RM	RATING OF RATIO
Bench press			
Leg press			

Reflecting on Your Results

Are you surprised by your test results and ratings? Did your results match what you thought about your own muscle fitness?

Planning Your Next Steps

Muscle strength is typically a function of training. If your scores were lower than you expected, then it may be time to start or change your muscle fitness routine. If you scored well, then strive to maintain your current level of fitness, or add some new or more advanced exercises or training techniques to boost your results. Set realistic goals for improvement and create a plan to achieve them. Then repeat these tests in several weeks and note any improvements.

Describe your goals and the specific steps you will take to improve your muscular strength. If needed, refer to Lab 5-3 on program planning.

What effect, if any, did your plan have on your muscular strength?

Source: Conversion formula for multiple reps to 1-RM from Brzycki, M. (1993). Strength testing: Predicting a one-rep max from reps to fatigue. *JOPERD 64*: 88–90.

SUBMIT ONLINE

NAME	DATE	SECTION

Muscle endurance can be assessed by performing multiple repetitions of push-ups and curl-ups.

Upper-Body Endurance: Push-Up/Modified Push-Up

Most people can perform push-ups, and they require little training. For this test, the ratings are based on males performing standard push-ups and females performing modified push-ups.

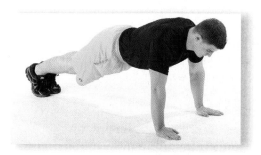

Equipment

- A mat or similar firm, padded surface

Preparation

If you haven't performed push-ups or modified push-ups in the past, practice to familiarize yourself with the movement. Do a general warm-up before the test.

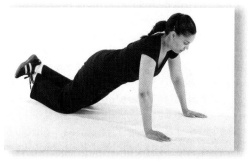

Instructions

The push-up test starts with hands shoulder-width apart, arms extended straight out under the shoulders, back and legs in a straight line, and toes curled under. For the modified push-up's starting position, the weight is supported by the knees and hands; the hands should be slightly ahead of the shoulders so that the hands are in the proper position for the downward motion.

For both versions of the test, the objective is to lower your body in a straight line, keeping your back straight, until your chin touches the mat. Your stomach should not touch the mat at any time. Once your chin touches the mat, you push back up to the start position, or until your arms are straight again. Continue this for as many repetitions as possible until (1) no more push-ups can be completed, (2) your technique is no longer appropriate (back and/or legs not straight), or (3) there is a pause in the cadence.

Results

Your score is the number of push-ups or modified push-ups completed with good form. You can use the chart below to compare your push-up score to others of your age and sex.

Number of push-ups or modified push-ups [　　] Rating [　　　　　]

PUSH-UP/MODIFIED PUSH-UP RATINGS BY AGE AND GENDER

	Age and Gender											
	15–19		20–29		30–39		40–49		50–59		60–69	
RATING	M	F	M	F	M	F	M	F	M	F	M	F
Excellent	≥39	≥33	≥36	≥30	≥30	≥27	≥25	≥24	≥21	≥21	≥18	≥17
Very good	29–38	25–32	29–35	21–29	22–29	20–26	17–24	15–23	13–20	11–20	11–17	12–16
Good	23–28	18–24	22–28	15–20	17–21	13–19	13–16	11–14	10–12	7–10	8–10	5–11
Fair	18–22	12–17	17–21	10–14	12–16	8–12	10–12	5–10	7–9	2–6	5–7	2–4
Needs improvement	≤17	≤11	≤16	≤9	≤11	≤7	≤9	≤4	≤6	≤1	≤4	≤1

Source: Canadian Society for Exercise Physiology. (2003). *The Canadian physical activity, fitness & lifestyle approach: CSEP-Health & Fitness Program's health-related appraisal and counseling strategy* (3rd ed.). Reprinted with permission from the Canadian Society for Exercise Physiology.

Abdominal Endurance: Curl-Up
Curl-ups measure strength and endurance of the abdominal muscles

Equipment

- A mat or similar firm, padded surface
- Metronome or other way to keep time (the cadence for the test is 50 beats per minute)
- Two strips of tape about 8–10 inches (20–25 cm) in length; these should be placed 4 inches (10 cm) apart
- Partner to observe your technique and count the number of curl-ups you complete

Preparation

If you haven't performed curl-ups in the past, practice to familiarize yourself with the movement. Do a general warm-up before the test.

Instructions

Lie on your back on a mat with knees bent 90 degrees. Arms should be at your sides, palms facing down with the middle fingers touching a piece of masking tape. A second piece of tape is placed 10 cm away. Keep your shoes on during the test.

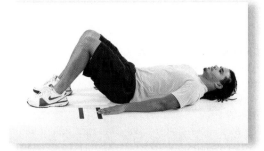

Set the metronome to a pace of 50 beats per minute. Do slow, controlled curl-ups as you lift your shoulder blades off the mat in time with the metronome. You will curl up on one beat and lower down on the next beat, for a rate of 25 curl-ups per minute. As you curl up, slide your fingers forward until they reach the second piece of tape. Your trunk should make a 30-degree angle with the mat at the top of the curl-up. Your low back should be flattened before curling up. The test continues for 1 minute. Complete as many curl-ups as possible in time with the metronome without pausing or using poor technique. The maximum number is 25 curl-ups completed during the 1-minute test time. Make sure that the fingertips start behind the first line of tape and reach the second line of tape during each curl-up.

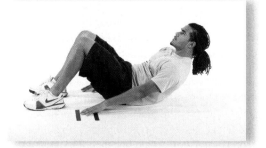

Results

One repetition is counted each time the shoulder blades touch the floor. After determining the total number of curl-ups, you can use the chart below to determine your abdominal endurance compared to others of the same age and gender.

Number of curl-ups [____] Rating [____]

CURL-UP RATINGS BY AGE AND GENDER

	Age and Gender											
	15–19		20–29		30–39		40–49		50–59		60–69	
RATING	M	F	M	F	M	F	M	F	M	F	M	F
Excellent	25	25	25	25	25	25	25	25	25	25	25	25
Very good	23–24	22–24	21–24	18–24	18–24	19–24	18–24	19–24	17–24	19–24	16–24	17–24
Good	21–22	17–21	16–20	14–17	15–17	10–18	13–17	11–18	11–16	10–18	11–15	8–16
Fair	16–20	12–16	11–15	5–13	11–14	6–9	6–12	4–10	8–10	6–9	6–10	3–7
Needs improvement	≤15	≤11	≤10	≤4	≤10	≤5	≤5	≤3	≤7	≤5	≤5	≤2

Source: Canadian Society for Exercise Physiology. (2003). *The Canadian physical activity, fitness & lifestyle approach: CSEP-Health & Fitness Program's health-related appraisal and counseling strategy,* 3rd ed. Reprinted with permission from the Canadian Society for Exercise Physiology.

Reflecting on Your Results

Are you surprised by your test results and ratings? Did your results match what you thought about your own muscle fitness?

Planning Your Next Steps

Muscle fitness is typically a function of training. If your scores were lower than you expected, then it may be time to start or change your muscle fitness routine. If you scored well, then strive to maintain your current level of fitness, or add some new or more advanced exercises or training techniques to boost your results. Set realistic goals for improvement and create a plan to achieve them. Then repeat these tests in several weeks and note any improvements.

Describe your goals and the specific steps you will take to improve your muscular fitness. If needed, refer to Lab 5-3 on program planning.

What effect, if any, did your plan have on your muscular fitness?

SUBMIT ONLINE

NAME	DATE	SECTION

Equipment None required; you may want to develop and track your program using a paper notebook, digital spreadsheet, smart-phone application, or online program.

Preparation None

Instructions

1. **Set SMART goals:** Set goals for your muscle fitness program. Your goal could be something about training—number of workouts per week—or it could be based on one of the tests in Lab Activities 5-1 and 5-2.

Current status	Goal	Target date	Notes (rewards, special considerations)

2. **Apply the FITT principal:** Create a program that meets the recommended criteria for success and fits your schedule and preferences. Fill in the exercises for your starting program below.

- *Frequency:* 2–3 days per week, with muscle groups rested at least 48 hours between workouts
- *Intensity:* A resistance that allows 8–12 repetitions of each exercise to be performed to fatigue with good technique; usually 60%–80% of 1-RM
- *Time:* 2–4 sets of 8–12 repetitions of each exercise
- *Type:* Perform exercises to train each major muscle group

MUSCLE GROUP	EXERCISE	Starting		
		RESISTANCE	SETS	REPS
Chest				
Shoulders				
Back				
Core				
Quadriceps				
Hamstrings				
Lower legs				
Arms: Biceps				
Arms: Triceps				
Additional exercises:				

Results Track your progress with a log like the one on the next page or one you create for yourself. Make as many copies as you need.

STRENGTH TRAINING LOG

Date: _____

Exercise	Set 1		Set 2		Set 3		Set 4	
	Wt	Reps	Wt	Reps	Wt	Reps	Wt	Reps

Date: _____

	Set 1		Set 2		Set 3		Set 4	
	Wt	Reps	Wt	Reps	Wt	Reps	Wt	Reps

Date: _____

Exercise	Set 1		Set 2		Set 3		Set 4	
	Wt	Reps	Wt	Reps	Wt	Reps	Wt	Reps

Date: _____

	Set 1		Set 2		Set 3		Set 4	
	Wt	Reps	Wt	Reps	Wt	Reps	Wt	Reps

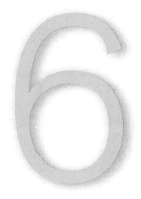

6

Flexibility and Low-Back Fitness

>> **COMING UP IN THIS CHAPTER**

Learn what factors affect your flexibility › Identify the benefits of flexibility › Assess your flexibility › Create a successful flexibility program › Identify ways to protect and care for your back

Wellness Connections

How does flexibility affect wellness? The physical dimension of wellness is the most directly affected. An adequate range of motion in your joints lets you perform daily tasks easily and efficiently, and over time, it helps prevent stiffness, soreness, and falls and their associated injuries. In addition to maintaining good flexibility, stretching exercises promote relaxation and reduce stress.

Low-back pain is often a result of poor flexibility, muscle fitness, and posture. It can, like any other physical health problem, have a negative impact on the other wellness dimensions. Pain and the inability to engage in normal activities with ease can lead to stress and depression, undermining emotional well-being. These in turn can affect your intellectual wellness by reducing your ability to think clearly. Your social wellness may be affected if you withdraw from others due to depression or physical limitations. On a larger scale, social as well as environmental wellness may be harmed by the high costs associated

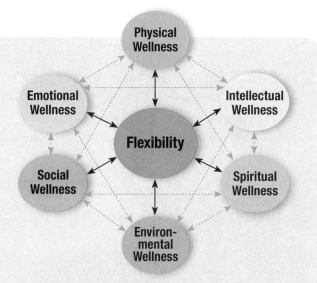

with chronic low-back pain, which is a common cause of missed workdays and reduced productivity. Any of these erosions of the other dimensions of wellness may affect your spiritual wellness. Fortunately, the converse is true also. A sufficient amount of physical flexibility boosts your overall physical functioning and enhances all the dimensions of your life.

Flexibility is a key component of health-related fitness, but in spite of the recent popularity of activities like Pilates and yoga, flexibility is often neglected. You can easily find information about aerobic or strength-training activities, but you'll rarely see an article about flexibility or hear from a friend regarding their stretching routine. This is unfortunate because, just like the other components of fitness, flexibility affects all the dimensions of wellness and your day-to-day living.

Factors Affecting Flexibility

Q | Why are some people more flexible than others?

As discussed in Chapter 3, **flexibility** is the ability of a joint to move through its full range of motion. You don't need an extremely high level of flexibility for good fitness and wellness. The goal of flexibility training is to be able to move a joint through its normal range of motion without experiencing pain or being limited in the performance of activities of daily living. Both too little and too much flexibility can be detrimental.

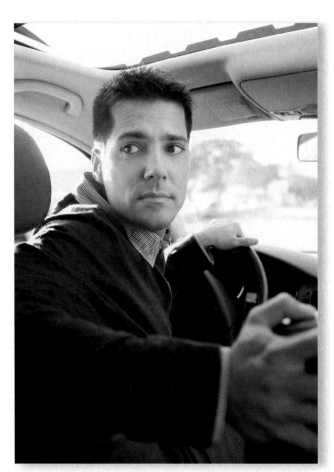

An extremely high level of flexibility isn't necessary for most people—your goal should be a range of motion in your joints that allows you to perform daily activities easily and without pain.

Flexibility is highly variable: It differs from person to person and joint to joint. A number of factors contribute to your level of flexibility—some of these are under your control, but others cannot be affected by training.

Joint Structure

Q | Why are some of my joints more flexible than others?

Some of your joints are designed to have a greater range of motion than others; in addition, your flexibility varies from joint to joint due to other factors.

A joint is a place where two or more bones meet. The structure of a joint plays a role in its range of motion. Some joints are designed to move very little, such as the ones where the bones of your skull come together. Others, like those in your spine, allow small movements. Joints such as those in your hips, shoulders, and limbs are called *synovial joints* and move much more freely. Figure 6-1 illustrates the main components of synovial joints:

- **Cartilage** covers and cushions the ends of the bones that meet in the joint, reducing friction as the joint moves and serving as a shock absorber.
- A fibrous **joint capsule** surrounds the joint; the inner layer of the capsule, known as the *synovial membrane,* surrounds the joint cavity and secretes **synovial fluid,** which lubricates and nourishes the tissues inside the cavity.

flexibility The ability of a joint to move through its full range of motion.

cartilage A type of stiff but flexible tissue in various areas of the body, including joints, the ears and nose, and parts of the rib cage; it is not as hard as bone but stiffer than muscle.

joint capsule A sac or envelope enclosing a synovial joint, with an inner layer (the synovial membrane), which secretes synovial fluid, and a fibrous outer layer.

synovial fluid Fluid that lubricates and nourishes the tissues in the cavity of a synovial joint.

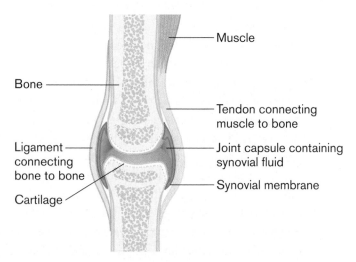

Figure 6-1 **Basic structure of a joint.** Inside the joint capsule, the ends of the bones are covered by cartilage that absorbs shock and reduces friction; the synovial fluid inside the joint cavity lubricates the tissues and helps the joint move smoothly and easily.

- **Ligaments** inside and around the joint connect the bones and provide stability.
- Muscles connected to tendons around the joint contract and move the bones.

Problems with any of these components, including injury, inflammation, or stiffness, can limit a joint's range of motion.

The shape of the cartilage-covered surfaces and the way in which bones come together determine how—and how much—a joint can move. For example, elbow joints function somewhat like a hinge and primarily bend up and down in one direction. The hips and shoulders are ball-and-socket joints, in which the rounded end of one bone fits into a cup-shaped depression in the other bone. This type of joint allows for the widest range of motion but it is less stable and has a greater risk of injury.

Because each joint has a different structure, your relative flexibility varies from joint to joint—reflecting the principle of *specificity* (see Chapter 3). For example, you may have normal range of motion in your hips but limited mobility in your shoulders. For this reason, no single test can measure overall flexibility.

Connective Tissues and Nervous System Action

Q | How does someone become more flexible?

You become more flexible by increasing the range of motion in a joint. The precise mechanisms are still being studied, but it is thought that increases in range of motion occur through changes in the **connective tissues** in muscles, tendons, and ligaments. (Muscle fibers themselves aren't connective tissue, but they are held together in bundles by sheaths of connective tissues.) All the connective tissues affect your flexibility, but the tissues in your tendons and muscles probably play the largest role.

Both the length of tissues and their tolerance of stretching may affect flexibility.[1] **Collagen** is the key component of tendons, ligaments, and the connective tissue within muscle. It typically has a wavy structure when relaxed, but when stretched, the fibers first straighten and align and then may elongate as additional stretching force is applied. The overlapping fibers in muscle tissue shift to decrease the amount of overlap, also allowing tissues to elongate. Because connective tissues have elastic properties, they snap back to almost their resting length. Over time, however, the elasticity and resting length of some tissues may increase as they are repeatedly stretched, which increases the joint's range of motion.

ligament Fibrous tissue that connects bone to bone.

connective tissue A type of fibrous tissue in many body organs and systems, often providing support and structure; it may be soft and flexible or hard and rigid. Cartilage and bone are both types of connective tissue.

collagen Key protein in bone, cartilage, ligaments, tendons, skin, and connective tissue.

osteoarthritis Inflammation of the joint, usually involving damage to the cartilage-covered surfaces in the joint.

Tolerance of stretching has an important role in increasing flexibility.[2] When you hold a stretch for a period of time and then repeat the stretch, you will begin to feel less pain when you apply the same force of stretch. Although the exact mechanism isn't entirely clear, this increase in stretch tolerance increases range of motion. Changes in the activities of sensors and nerves in and around the joint and its associated muscles and tendons may reduce the pain felt during the stretch and allow for greater flexibility.[3]

Injury and Disease

Q | I recently recovered from a knee injury and don't have the same movement. Will I get it back?

Probably. Immobilization of bones and joints by casts or braces can lead to a loss in range of motion, but this is usually temporary. Loss of flexibility from the injury itself depends on the type and extent of your injury. In many cases, flexibility and strength exercises will help you maintain as much of your normal movement and strength as possible as you recover.

Some injuries can have longer-term effects on flexibility. For example, the condition known as "frozen shoulder," in which the joint capsule thickens and contracts, causing pain and stiffness, can take six months to two years to resolve. Frozen shoulder affects about 10 percent of the general population and 30 percent of people with diabetes at some time in their lives.[4]

Osteoarthritis, which occurs when the cartilage inside a joint breaks down, is a common disease that affects flexibility. More than 20 million Americans have osteoarthritis; risk factors include obesity, age, injury, and overuse. Loss of range of motion in people with arthritis is associated with increased disability.[5] Treatment for osteoarthritis often includes strengthening and stretching exercises to help stabilize joints and improve range of motion and overall physical functioning.

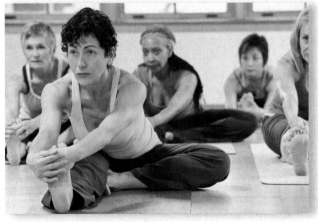

Although aging and osteoarthritis decrease range of motion, exercises to maintain flexibility can reduce pain and disability and prevent injuries.

Genetics

Q | Do people who are double-jointed have a higher flexibility level?

Some people are more flexible than others—and genetics is one reason for individual differences in flexibility, for being a little or a lot more flexible than average.[6] Some people have extreme levels of flexibility: **Hypermobility** in a joint, or being double-jointed, runs in families and is thought to have a genetic basis. The prefix *hyper-* means "over" or "beyond." So people who are hypermobile are too flexible; their joints move beyond the normal range of motion. Specific examples of hypermobility include being able to bend your thumb to your forearm, bend your little finger backward to a 90-degree angle, bend forward with your knees straight and place your hands flat on the floor, or hyperextend your knees or elbows 10 degrees beyond their natural, straight position.

For some people, hypermobility causes no problems. However, hypermobile joints are less stable and can be more prone to injury and arthritis. Muscles have to work harder to stabilize a hypermobile joint during activity, potentially causing muscle fatigue and reduced performance. Showing off hypermobile joints may have been a way to amuse your friends when you were young, but it can be much less amusing as you age if your joints do not return to their proper position as easily. People with joint hypermobility should check with their health care provider; recommendations include developing and maintaining strong muscles to help stabilize joints.

Gender

Q | Are women more flexible than men?

Although there is a wide range of flexibility within each gender, in general, yes, females are more flexible than males. This is primarily due to differences in anatomical structure and hormone levels. Larger muscles are less flexible and can block free movement at a joint, and men tend to have larger muscles than women. Women's wider hips contribute to their greater flexibility in the pelvic region and lower body. (Women have a wider pelvis to allow for childbirth.) Researchers have found that hormone levels also affect flexibility: Women have greater range of motion during certain points in the menstrual cycle.[7] Hormones released during pregnancy also substantially increase looseness of women's joints.

Use and Age

Q | Why are people less flexible as they get older?

As with other areas of fitness, the "use it or lose it" adage is true. When considering flexibility, it's difficult to separate the effects of disuse from the effects of aging because the two often go together.

Once you have passed that magical time in your life known as puberty, the only way to maintain your flexibility is through activity that utilizes the full range of motion of your joints. In your teens and twenties, you are likely to participate in recreational or competitive activities that do this. As we age, however, we're less likely to include these activities in our regular routine. The problems that result from this decrease in activity are sometimes compounded by occupations or daily routines that require long hours of sitting or poor postural positions. In addition, the direct effects of aging and wear and tear over time—resulting in degeneration of collagen fibers and joint structures—adversely affect joints' flexibility.[8] Also, people tend to gain weight as they age, and body-fat deposits can impair flexibility by physically blocking a joint from moving through its full range of motion.

Without regular full-range-of-motion activities, tissues may begin to shorten and tighten. In most instances, activities designed to improve flexibility are necessary to prevent significant declines in flexibility. Our tendency to become less flexible as we age is primarily a result of inactivity rather than of the aging process itself. Studies have shown that, unless people have an injury-related trauma or disease, a regular routine of flexibility exercises can preserve sufficient flexibility throughout the lifespan—people's range of motion may decrease but it will remain

hypermobility Excessive range of motion in a joint, making it less stable and more susceptible to injury.

Fast Facts

Stretch and Bend

Ever wonder if you could be an acrobat or a contortionist?

- Most contortionists have an unusually high degree of natural flexibility, enhanced through significant training.
- Most contortionists excel at one particular skill—such as front-bending, back-bending, over-splitting, or squeezing into a small container—depending on which way their spine is most flexible.
- Most contortionists do not dislocate their joints when they flex or extend them very far.
- Studies have shown that contortionists have very high degrees of flexibility, but they also can develop joint problems, including fractures.

Source: Peoples, R. R., Perkins, T. G., Powell, J. W., Hanson, E. H., Snyder, T. H., Mueller, T. L., & Orrison, W. W. (2008). Whole-spine dynamic magnetic resonance study of contortionists: Anatomy and pathology. *Journal of Neurosurgery: Spine, 8*(6), 501–509.

at a level that allows safe and effective movement. Studies also tell us that people of any age can benefit from beginning an appropriate flexibility-exercise routine.[9]

Benefits of Flexibility

Q | Why should I bother with stretching?

Like the other components of fitness, flexibility is needed in order to perform daily functions easily and efficiently and to reduce the likelihood of injury. Other benefits of flexibility and stretching exercises are improved posture and reduced stress.

Improved Performance

Q | Will flexibility help me play basketball better?

Possibly. As we learned in earlier chapters, performing stretching exercises right before an activity that requires a high degree of muscle power can harm performance in the short term because stretching can temporarily decrease peak muscle force.[10] On the other hand, for gymnastics, diving, and other sports in which joints move through extreme ranges of motion, stretching exercises beforehand may improve performance.

Over time, flexibility training has the potential to improve performance in these sports and other skilled activities. Most athletes develop an optimal range of motion required for their particular sport as a result of regular participation in it. An optimal level of flexibility will afford you greater efficiency in the movements required for your sport—in your case, basketball.

Different sports require different amounts of flexibility for optimal performance. For example, gymnasts, ice skaters, and divers need greater flexibility than runners, but runners need enough flexibility in their legs and hips to achieve good running mechanics.[11] However, as discussed earlier, too much flexibility can hurt performance: Hypermobility can increase the risk of injury and reduce speed, strength, and power needed for a sport.

Although you may think first of sports when you hear the word *performance,* flexibility is also important for the performance of routine daily activities. You need flexibility to climb stairs, put on your shoes, back up your car, get clothes out of the dryer, feed your pets, lift your backpack or your kids, put away the groceries, and hang pictures on the wall. Unfortunately, many of us don't think in these terms until we have trouble with some of these activities. Maintaining a normal range of motion in your joints through flexibility training will allow you to go about your day-to-day tasks with ease and efficiency. For non-athletes, a stretching program can, over time, improve exercise performance and measures of muscle strength.[12] See the box "Stretch for Strength Gains" for more information.

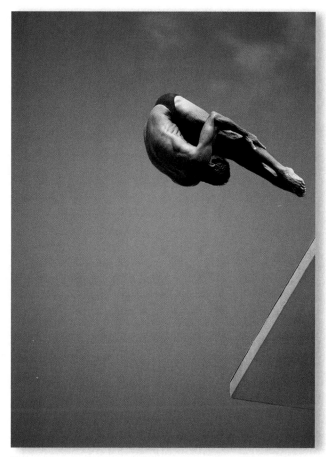

Only a few sports and activities—such as gymnastics, diving, dancing, and ice skating—require an extremely high level of flexibility for optimal performance.

Reduced Risk of Injury

Q | Does stretching prevent injuries?

It depends. The relationship between stretching, flexibility, and injury is complex, controversial, and still under investigation.[13] The answer to this question will depend on whether you're considering stretching's immediate effects on sport-injury risk or its longer-term effects on all types of injuries.

For many years, it was believed that stretching as part of a warm-up before an exercise session or competition would reduce muscle soreness and the risk of injury. Recent research has not supported this idea, finding no reduction in sport injuries associated with stretching. A review of over 360 articles and research projects comparing stretching with other injury-prevention methods concluded the evidence is not sufficient to either support or oppose routine stretching before or after activity.[14] Findings differ, however, depending on the type and intensity of the activity, the type of stretching, and other factors. When stretching is done as part of a warm-up, it can be difficult to distinguish the effects of stretching from the effects of the warm-up; warm-ups have been shown to

Research Brief

Stretch for Strength Gains

Are you new to strength training? If so, research indicates that you may become stronger faster if you also engage in regular stretching.

In a study of college students who were novice lifters, researchers paired students who had comparable starting strength. They assigned one student from each pair to a strength-training group, and the other student to a strength-training-plus-stretching group. All the students did three sets of strength-training exercises three days a week; the stretching group also stretched twice a week for thirty minutes. After eight weeks of progressive strength-training with knee-flexion, knee-extension, and leg-press exercises, the two groups were compared. Both groups significantly improved, but the strength-training-plus-stretching group had significantly greater gains in strength.

What does this mean for you? If you're just starting a strength-training program, also engaging in regular flexibility training may boost your strength gains.

	Increase in 1-RM	
	Strength-training group	Strength-training-plus-stretching group
Knee flexion	12%	16%
Knee extension	14%	27%
Leg press	9%	31%

Source: Kokkonen, J., Nelson, A. G., Tarawhiti, T., Buckingham, P., & Winchester, J. B. (2010). Early-phase resistance training strength gains in novice lifters are enhanced by doing static stretching. *Journal of Strength and Conditioning Research, 24*(2), 502–506.

reduce sport-injury risk. More research is needed, especially about different activities and stretching techniques. It may be that for each sport, a different combination of warm-up, stretches, and other pre-exercise activities will enhance performance and reduce injury risk.

What about the effects of stretching for non-athletes? Research findings have been mixed, but evidence suggests that routine stretching may reduce the rate of certain types of muscle and tendon injuries as well as some types of soreness from physical activity.[15] Stretching can also be a key component of rehabilitation of injuries—to return joints to a normal and healthy range of motion.[16]

Flexibility, along with muscular fitness, is also important for good posture, which in turn helps reduce joint strain and may decrease risk of certain types of injuries. Abnormal posture can strain ligaments and muscles and contribute to musculoskeletal problems, including low-back pain. For example, if the muscles and tendons in the front of your thighs and hips are tight, your back may be pulled into a more arched position. Posture will be discussed in greater detail later in this chapter.

Finally, maintaining flexibility in joints is critical as you age; if you don't stretch, your joints will stiffen—and having less than the normal range of motion in a joint increases your risk of injury. Loss of flexibility in the hips and ankles, for example, increases the risk of falls. Regular stretching will improve your flexibility and walking mechanics and reduce the risk of falls and associated injuries.[17]

Other Benefits of Flexibility and Stretching Exercises

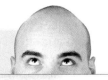

Mind Stretcher
Critical Thinking Exercise

Do you include flexibility training in your fitness program? If not, why not? If you do, is it a complete stretching routine or just a few quick stretches? If you are doing less than a complete stretching routine in your fitness program, review the benefits of stretching described in the chapter and identify the ones that are important to you. How does stretching make you feel, beyond just its fitness benefits? What else can you do to increase your motivation to engage in flexibility training?

Q | I feel better when I stretch after a workout. Does stretching help me relax?

Yes, it does. Stretching exercises have benefits beyond maintaining joint range of motion. As you have experienced, stretching can reduce muscle tension, blood pressure, and breathing rate—all indicative of a more relaxed physical state.[18] After stretching, people also report improved mood, reduced stress, and subjective feelings of relaxation. You can also use stretching to treat exercise-associated muscle cramps—painful muscle contractions that occur during or just after exercise.[19] If you experience muscle cramps with exercise, try rest and stretching.

Research Brief

Flexible Body, Flexible Arteries?

Healthy arteries are elastic, meaning they can expand to accommodate increased blood volume and then snap back to their original size. Stiff arteries are a risk factor for high blood pressure, heart disease, and death. Arteries become stiffer as we age, and physical activity has been shown to delay the process. But how does flexibility affect your arteries?

Researchers recently looked for an association between body flexibility and arterial flexibility in a group of healthy adults ranging in age from 20 to 83. They measured flexibility using the sit-and-reach test, and they measured blood pressure and blood flow. For participants age 40 and older, there was a strong association between trunk flexibility and arterial stiffening: The more flexible people had more elastic arteries; they also had lower blood pressure, another sign of a healthy cardiorespiratory system. The findings were independent of cardiorespiratory fitness and muscular strength.

Why are body flexibility and arterial flexibility linked? The researchers aren't sure, but they considered several possibilities. Arteries are made of many of the same types of tissues as muscles and tendons and so may be affected by some of the same factors, including stretching. In addition, stretching exercises cause short-term activation of the nervous system, which may reduce nervous-system activity at rest. (This is similar to the relationship of aerobic exercise and blood pressure—the short-term effect of exercise is to raise blood pressure, but in the long term, exercise reduces resting blood pressure.) Lower resting nervous-system activity may reduce both arterial stiffness and blood pressure.

More research is needed to determine the underlying mechanisms, but in the meantime, this study provides more evidence that a lifetime of stretching exercises will help you maintain good flexibility—in more ways than one.

Source: Yamamoto, K., Kawano, H., Gando, Y., and others. (2009). Poor trunk flexibility is associated with arterial stiffening. *American Journal of Physiology—Heart and Circulatory Physiology, 297,* H1314–H1318.

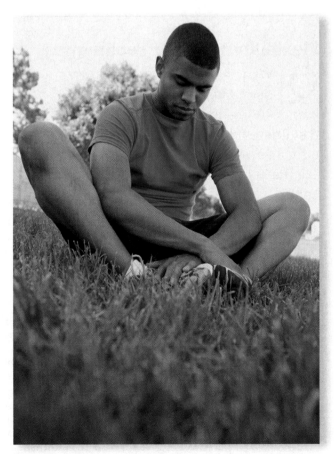

Stretching exercises can relieve stress by reducing muscle tension, blood pressure, and breathing rate.

Assessing Your Flexibility

Flexibility is assessed in several ways; there is no single test to assess flexibility because it is specific to each joint. Remember that more flexibility isn't necessarily better; your goal should be a normal range of motion in all your major joints.

Q | How is flexibility rated? The most common test for flexibility is the sit-and-reach test, which reflects the range of motion of the hamstrings, hips, and lower back; these joints are especially important for the prevention of low-back problems.[20] Lab Activity 6-1 includes instructions and norms for the sit-and-reach test. For other joints, range of motion is measured with other tests. Lab Activity 6-1 also includes assessments for shoulder, hamstring, and hip flexor range of motion. There are no precise flexibility measures associated with peak performance or wellness, but averages can provide points of reference to help you determine if any of your joints have a range of motion that is significantly below normal.

The most important preparation for flexibility assessments is to warm up beforehand; you can stretch farther and more safely after a warm-up. Before you complete the flexibility tests in the lab activities, read through the list in Table 6-1 of factors that can affect your scores. You'll also want to take several of these factors into account when you plan and carry out your regular stretching program.

TABLE 6-1 FACTORS THAT AFFECT FLEXIBILITY TESTS

FACTOR	CONSIDER THIS:
TIME OF DAY	Most people are more flexible in the afternoon.
TEMPERATURE OF THE ROOM AND YOUR MUSCLES	Most people can stretch farther in a warm room and after they've completed a warm-up consisting of 5–10 minutes of light aerobic activity.
YOUR CLOTHING	Nonrestrictive clothing allows for easier stretching.
SORENESS OR INJURIES	Because soreness or an injury can limit flexibility, try to delay testing until you are pain-free. Always take care not to aggravate an existing problem.
YOUR LEVEL OF COMPETITIVENESS	Will you be in a group setting for testing? Do you have a competitive nature or a high pain tolerance that might cause you to push yourself too far?
YOUR ABILITY TO RELAX	Being tense during testing is likely if the situation is new to you. Try your best to relax and follow the specific guidelines for each test.
HUMAN ERROR	Will your testers know how to administer the tests? You may not have a choice, but keep this factor in mind when evaluating your scores.

Q | How flexible should I be?

Unless you participate in a sport or activity that requires significant flexibility, a good goal for a flexibility program is to achieve and maintain a normal range of motion in all your major joints. How did you score on the flexibility assessments in the lab activities? If you are significantly less flexible in one joint than the others, you might want to give special attention to it in your stretching program—but you should continue to stretch all your joints regularly. If you don't currently do any flexibility training, then a good goal is to start now!

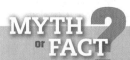

Static stretching before activities like sprinting or jumping decreases performance.

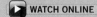
▶ WATCH ONLINE

Putting Together a Flexibility Program

As with any other component of fitness, flexibility must be purposely addressed. Exercises specifically designed to build and maintain flexibility should be a regular part of your routine. Although you may not feel like you need flexibility exercises at this point in your life, incorporating them into your regular routine will help you to maintain your flexibility so it doesn't become a problem in the future. To reduce your likelihood of injuries later, develop good habits now. To put together a safe and effective program, consider the types of training and then apply the FITT formula.

Flexibility Training Techniques

Q | What is the best way to stretch? What are the different kinds of stretches, and what are the benefits of each?

Though you have already read that stretching is a type of exercise that affects your flexibility, you may not be aware of the different types of stretching you can use to increase or maintain flexibility. Stretching techniques include static stretching, ballistic stretching, dynamic stretching, and proprioceptive neuromuscular facilitation (PNF).

STATIC STRETCHING. In **static stretching,** you stretch each muscle group using a slow, steady stretch with a hold at the end of the range of motion. You relax the muscle being stretched as it lengthens. Because you hold the stretch for a while and then repeat it, you can usually stretch a little farther as your tissues adjust to the stretch.

Static stretching may be performed either actively or passively. In **active stretching,** you take an *active* role by contracting the muscles opposite those being stretched; the force for the stretch comes from your own mus-

static stretching A stretching technique that involves a slow, steady stretch with a hold at the end of the range of motion.

active stretching A stretching technique in which the force for the stretch comes from a contraction of the muscles opposite those being stretched.

passive stretching A stretching technique in which the force for a stretch comes from an object, a partner, or another body part.

ballistic stretching A stretching technique that involves quick jerks or bounces to move joints to the ends of their range of motion; momentum provides the force for this stretch.

cle contraction. In **passive stretching,** you allow an outside force, rather than the contraction of a muscle group, to assist in the stretching. The external force for a passive stretch can be provided by another person, an object, gravity, or another body part. For example, to actively stretch your calves, you could sit on the ground with your legs out in front of you and contract the muscles in your shins to pull your toes back. To passively stretch the same muscle group, you could perform the exercise in the same seated position—but with a partner providing the force to gently move your toes back rather than using your own muscles. You could also do a passive stretch of the calf in a standing position by using the floor for resistance to move your toes closer to your shins without contracting the opposing muscle group (Figure 6-2). Static stretching is a widely recommended technique because it is safe, easy to learn, may be done without a partner or special equipment, and can be done fairly quickly.

BALLISTIC STRETCHING. In **ballistic stretching,** you use quick jerky or bouncing movements to stretch your joints and move them to the ends of their typical range of motion—and beyond it. Ballistic stretching uses the momentum of body movement to produce the force required to lengthen the muscles and other tissues; the endpoint of the stretch is not held. This type of stretching is effective for increasing flexibility, but because it is less controlled than other types of stretching, there is greater potential for

overstretching, soreness, and injury. Ballistic stretching is generally not recommended for most people, but athletes in certain sports use it, especially if the activity involves ballistic movements such as throwing, kicking, running, or batting.

DYNAMIC STRETCHING. Like ballistic stretching, **dynamic stretching** involves movement. However, dynamic stretching uses controlled movement through the active range of motion for a joint rather than bouncing movement at the endpoints of the range of motion. For example, a lunge position stretches the hamstrings and the front of the hip. In a static stretch, you would slowly and gently move into the lunge position and hold it. In a ballistic stretch, you would repeatedly bounce in the lunge position at the end of the range of motion. In a dynamic stretch, you would do a series of lunges, moving through the full range of motion of a lunge in a controlled manner.

Many dynamic stretches require muscular strength and endurance to complete safely with good form. Some athletes like to use dynamic stretching in conjunction with a warm-up before an event because it helps elevate body and muscle temperature and may help prepare the body for optimum performance.[21]

PROPRIOCEPTIVE NEUROMUSCULAR FACILITATION. **Proprioceptive neuromuscular facilitation (PNF)** is group of techniques originally developed for rehabilitation; it has become a popular form of stretching in recent

dynamic stretching A stretching technique that involves controlled movement through the active range of motion of a joint.

proprioceptive neuromuscular facilitation (PNF) A group of stretching techniques that combine stretching and muscle contraction; the most common PNF techniques combine passive stretching and isometric contraction.

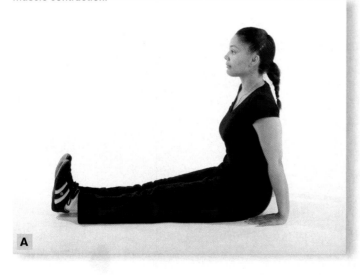

Figure 6-2 **Active vs. passive stretching. A.** In an active stretch, the force for the stretch is provided by contraction of the opposing muscle group. **B.** In a passive stretch, the force comes from an outside source—another person, an object, gravity, or another body part—rather than from one's own muscle contraction.

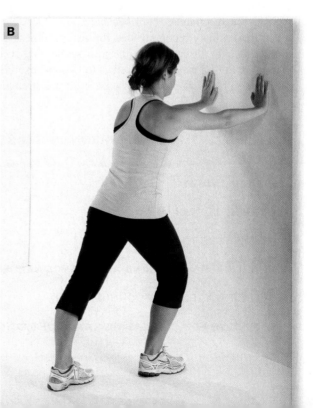

years. PNF techniques are designed to affect both connective tissues and nerves in order to increase flexibility; they typically combine muscle contraction and stretching. Some PNF stretches require a partner or another source of resistance. Here are two basic PNF techniques applied to a hamstring stretch:

- *Contract-relax:* After an initial stretch, you contract the muscle being stretched isometrically (6 seconds) against resistance. Then relax and stretch again. You should be able to stretch farther during the second and subsequent stretches. An example is an assisted stretch of the hamstring, in which a partner aids in a static stretch of the hamstring and provides resistance for the isometric contraction (Figure 6-3).
- *Contract-relax-opposite contract:* You perform a contract-relax stretch as described above, but during the second stretch of the targeted muscle, you assist with the static stretch by actively contracting the opposing muscle group. During the second static hamstring stretch, you would contract the muscles on the front of your leg (quadriceps) and hip to extend the stretch. This additional contraction is thought to elicit a reaction and stretching of the target muscle group.

Although they are an effective means of increasing flexibility, PNF techniques not often used for regular stretching routines because they require more time and often the use of partner. Like other stretching techniques, it isn't entirely clear why PNF stretching works—whether through changes to tissue length or changes to stretch tolerance, or both—but it does increase flexibility.[22]

Table 6-2 compares the three stretching techniques. Among the techniques described here, static stretching is the most widely recommended for general fitness. For this reason, the discussion in the next section about applying the FITT formula—as well as the sample exercises at the end of the chapter—are based on static stretching

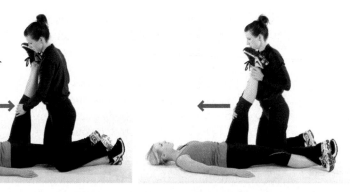

Figure 6-3 Contract-relax PNF stretch of the hamstring. After a passive static stretch of the hamstring, you push against a partner for a 6-second isometric contraction of the hamstring, and then you do another passive static stretch. You could also use a towel or strap around your foot or ankle to provide resistance for the isometric stretch and force for the passive stretch.

techniques. If you are an athlete involved in specialized activities or high-performance events, talk to your coach or trainer about the best stretching techniques for you.

Applying the FITT Formula

Q | Can stretching hurt my muscles?

If done incorrectly, stretching can cause soreness and other problems. As with other components of fitness, the best way to avoid injury is to plan your exercise routine carefully. Applying the FITT formula (frequency, intensity, time, and type) to your flexibility training can help you come up with a sensible plan.

Q | How often should I stretch?

FREQUENCY. Opinions vary on the number of times per week you should perform stretching exercises but most agree on a minimum of two or three times per week.[23] Stretching every day isn't harmful

TABLE 6-2 COMPARISON OF STRETCHING TECHNIQUES

FACTOR	SLOW STATIC	BALLISTIC	PNF
RISK OF INJURY	Low	High	Medium
DEGREE OF PAIN	Low	Medium	High
RESISTANCE TO STRETCH	Low	High	Medium
PRACTICALITY (TIME AND ASSISTANCE NEEDED)	Excellent	Good	Poor
EFFICIENCY (ENERGY CONSUMPTION)	Excellent	Poor	Poor
EFFECTIVE FOR INCREASING RANGE OF MOTION	Good	Good	Excellent

Source: Heyward, V. (2010). *Advanced fitness assessment and exercise prescription* (6th ed.). Champaign, IL: Human Kinetics.

and won't hurt the development of flexibility. As with all types of exercise, start with a relatively low frequency if you are a beginner. Then work your way up to as many days per week as your comfort and schedule allow. Stretching can be incorporated into training sessions for cardiorespiratory or muscular fitness; you don't have to schedule separate stretching workouts.

Q | How do I determine the right amount of stretch?

INTENSITY. Because flexibility is specific to each joint, you will have a different threshold and target zone for each exercise. You can't quantify these concepts as you can in other areas; you have to use your own abilities and perceptions to determine the appropriate levels of stretching.

As you perform each movement, stretch to the point you feel *slight tension* or *mild tightness* but not discomfort or pain. This point of slight tension is your threshold. Once you reach the threshold, move slowly and carefully just *slightly* beyond it into your target zone. If you need to quantify this effort in your mind, imagine your threshold to be 75 percent of your maximum and your desired target zone to be 85 percent (or slightly above the threshold) of your maximum.

Q | How long should I stretch?

TIME. The total time for your flexibility training depends on the type of stretches you do. A workout based on static stretches will typically require the shortest amount of time. The American College of Sports Medicine (ACSM) recommends that for static stretches, each stretch be performed four or more times and held for 15–60 seconds each time.[24] Because you should do stretches for all major joints (muscle/tendon groups), the minimum time for a complete flexibility-training cycle is about 10–15 minutes. A longer time would be required for a larger number of stretches or for different training techniques. If you haven't been stretching recently, you might start out with a small number of repetitions and short "holds," and then work your way up as your body adjusts to the training.

Q | Should I stretch before or after exercise? If I jog first, then weight lift, do I need to stretch before both?

It depends on your goals and how much flexibility training you want to do. The best time to stretch is when your muscles are warm and therefore more pliable and can better respond to changes in range of motion. You can do a separate warm-up for your stretching exercises, or you can combine flexibility training with another workout. You can stretch after the active part of a warm-up or after the conditioning phase of a cardiorespiratory- or muscular-fitness workout;

if you enjoy stretching, you can stretch both before and after your workouts. If you jog and then lift weights in one conditioning phase, you can choose to stretch after your initial warm-up, between your cardiorespiratory training and your weight training, or after your strength workout; you don't need to stretch before or after both.

As described earlier, if you plan to engage in a high-performance sport or activity where muscular strength and power are important, it might be better to stretch after the activity. Many people prefer to stretch after a cardiorespiratory- or muscle-fitness workout, as part of the cool-down and for relaxation. Experiment to learn the stretching timing that works best for you and the other activities you've included in your overall fitness program.

Q | Is stretching considered physical activity?

Yes, stretching is physical activity. However, time spent stretching doesn't count toward total daily or weekly aerobic or muscle fitness time if you are measuring your activity time against the Department of Health and Human Services physical activity guidelines.[25] An exception is dynamic stretches performed at an intensity high enough to be considered at least moderate—in terms of elevating your heart and breathing rates. Stretching to maintain good flexibility is considered an important part of an overall fitness program, for all the reasons outlined in this chapter.

Q | What are the best stretches?

TYPE. Your program should include a stretch for each major muscle/tendon group or joint: neck, shoulders, upper and lower back, pelvis, hips, and legs. As described in Table 6-3, one of the principles for flexibility training is the principle of specificity. The sample exercises on pp. 213–219 include choices for each, and Lab Activity 6-2 can guide you in setting up a flexibility program that fits your needs. You may want to do additional exercises for joints or areas where tests show your range of motion is below average. The exercises at the end of this chapter are not the only choices for flexibility training; if you'd like to try dynamic or PNF stretches, check with your instructor or a trainer at a fitness facility.

Q | Are there any stretches that are unsafe?

Yes. Certain stretches can place too much strain on your joints. Avoid stretches involving full bends of the

Wellness Strategies

Flexibility Program Planning: FITT

The ACSM recommends the following basic program:

- **Frequency:** 2–3 days per week or more.
- **Intensity:** Stretch to the point of slight tension or mild tightness.
- **Time:** Hold the stretch for 15–60 seconds, and do four or more repetitions of each stretch.

- **Type:** Perform a stretch for each major muscle/tendon group or joint: neck, shoulders, upper and lower back, pelvis, hips, and legs.

Always warm up before you stretch.

---

knee, significant arching or rounding of the lower back, or pressure on the neck, especially when bent. Some widely known stretches aren't the best choices; see Figure 6-4 for alternatives.

Q | Is yoga a way to do flexibility training?

Yes, many types of yoga include stretches—and more. The focus of hatha yoga, the most popular type practiced in the United States, is postures or poses called **asanas**. These asanas promote flexibility, strength, good posture, and focused breathing; yoga practice may also include meditation, which can reduce stress and increase concentration. Yoga's slow, concentrated stretches encourage you to move your muscles through a complete range of motion. Regardless of your age or fitness level, you do only the yoga stretches that you are able to, so there is no need to worry that you "can't do yoga." If your yoga practice includes stretches for all the major muscle/tendon groups, then it can count as a complete flexibility workout.

Increased strength, particularly in the core, is another benefit of yoga. Although some types of yoga (ashtanga and power yoga) focus on more vigorous movements, the most basic type of yoga also has many strength benefits. Many yoga asanas (plank, downward dog, upward dog, and chair pose) can build upper-body and core strength. Increasing both flexibility and core strength has the added benefit of improving posture.

Having a stronger and more flexible body, more focused breathing, and better concentration are good goals for everyone. The potential benefits of yoga extend beyond this list, however. Research suggests yoga may reduce blood pressure, increase lung capacity, and help treat insomnia. Studies are ongoing on the use of yoga for specific health conditions; for up-to-date information, visit the Web site for the National Center for Complementary and Alternative Medicine (http://nccam.nih.gov/health/yoga).

TABLE 6-3 FLEXIBILITY AND TRAINING PRINCIPLES

WARM-UP AND COOL-DOWN	Warm muscles stretch farther. If you have not already warmed up, begin with a few minutes of light aerobic activity. Because most flexibility training isn't done at a heart-rate-raising intensity, cool-down is not as critical as with some other types of exercise. If you tend to push yourself too hard or go too quickly through your stretches, playing soothing music can help you maintain a slower pace. You can also follow your routine with a few deep-breathing exercises to help your body further relax.
SPECIFICITY	Choose exercises that will allow you to work specifically on each major muscle/tendon group. If you tested below average in a specific area, you may want to add additional exercises for it.
PROGRESSIVE OVERLOAD	Progressive overload happens naturally during static stretching exercises. You may be stretching farther (overloading) before you even realize it. Don't focus on stretching farther; instead, concentrate on the point of slight tension. If you're motivated by fitness-test results, you can repeat the assessment procedures after several weeks of training to see changes in your flexibility.
REVERSIBILITY	Although loss of flexibility is rarely as noticeable when you are young as decreases in other fitness components, don't forget the factors discussed at the beginning of the chapter. Age and use play a big role in maintaining or increasing your flexibility.

Avoid	Try Instead

Stretches that hyperextend or forcefully flex the neck.

Example: Back head tilts

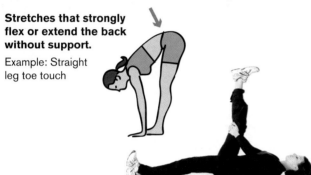

Example: Plow

Lateral head tilt

Standing cat stretch

Stretches that strongly flex or extend the back without support.

Example: Straight leg toe touch

Leg extension

Stretches that twist the knee, involve deep knee bends, or push the knee out in front of the supporting ankle.

Example: Hurdler stretch

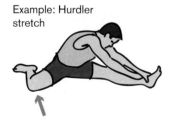

Modified hurdler stretch

Example: Deep forward lunge

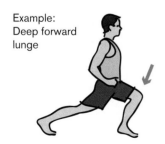

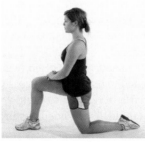

Kneeling hip flexor

Figure 6-4 **Types of stretches to avoid and safer alternatives**

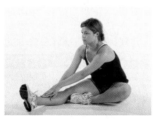

There are many types of yoga classes. Some focus on strength, some on relaxation, and some on posture. Ultimately, like with any other physical activity, choose the one you are most likely to do regularly, and then start doing it and enjoy the benefits!

Low-Back Fitness

Q | Why did my mother always nag me to sit up straight? Other than looking a little better, what difference does it make?

Once again your mother was right! Poor posture not only gives the appearance of low self-esteem and apathy, but it can also have negative effects on your health. In order to better understand why, you must first understand a little about the structure and function of your spine and about body mechanics.

Structure and Function of the Spine

Q | I hear some people say "spinal cord" and some say "spinal column." Are they the same thing?

No. The *spinal cord* is a long, thin bundle of nerves, fluid, and support cells that extends from the brain down the back. The spinal cord is enclosed in the bony *spinal column,* also called the backbone or spine (Figure 6-5). A healthy spine appears straight if you look at it from the back, but it has natural curves when viewed from the side. The human spine is made up of five sections of thirty-three individual bones called **vertebrae**:

- The cervical, or neck, section of the spine has seven vertebrae.
- The thoracic, or upper back, section has twelve vertebrae.
- The lumbar, or lower back, section has five vertebrae.
- The sacrum is formed by five fused vertebrae.
- The coccyx or tailbone is formed by four fused vertebrae.

Ligaments and muscles surround the spine to provide support and to aid movement.

Though they vary slightly in size and structure, the vertebrae in the top three sections of the spine have a similar design and characteristics; the vertebrae in the lower two sections are smaller and shaped differently. The vertebrae in the upper three sections of the spinal column have a large, flat, cylindrical body that allows them to stack on top of each

vertebra One of the thirty-three ring-like bones that make up the spine; together, they provide structural support, help protect the spinal cord, and aid in movement.

Wellness Strategies

Tips for Safe Yoga Practice

Yoga is an effective way to build flexibility as well as to improve muscle fitness, balance, and coordination and to reduce stress.

- You can learn yoga at home from a book or DVD, but beginners will likely find it helpful to learn with an instructor.
- Ask about the physical demands of the type of yoga in which you are interested, as well as the training and experience of the yoga teacher you are considering.
- Ask the instructor about any concerns you have, such as whether a class is aimed at your goal (such as increased flexibility) and what you should bring to class (a mat or towel, for example).
- If you have a medical condition, consult with your healthcare provider before starting yoga. Yoga is generally safe, but people with certain medical conditions should not use some yoga practices. For example, people with disk or inflammatory disease of the spine, extremely high or low blood pressure, glaucoma, fragile arteries, a risk of blood clots, ear problems, or severe osteoporosis should avoid some inverted poses.
- Although yoga during pregnancy is safe if practiced under expert guidance, after about the twentieth week of

pregnancy, pregnant women should avoid poses that involve lying flat on the back.
- Always warm up to prepare your body for activity.
- Don't push yourself beyond the limits of your strength or flexibility in order to perform a specific pose. Don't force your body into a position that is difficult for you. Yoga is not a competitive sport; listen to your body and use common sense and self-awareness.
- Review the guidelines in this chapter regarding the intensity of stretches (see the section "Intensity"). Ask the instructor about alternative poses or methods. Your instructor should provide modifications appropriate for people at different levels of flexibility and yoga experience.

Sources: Adapted from National Center for Complementary and Alternative Medicine. (2008). *Yoga for health: An introduction* (http://nccam.nih.gov/health/yoga/introduction .htm). Crews, L. (2006, February). Injury prevention: Yoga. *IDEA Fitness Journal* (http://www.ideafit.com/ fitness-library/injury-prevention-yoga).

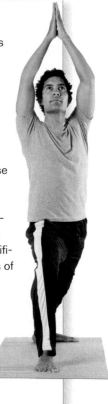

---

intervertebral disk Fibrous, gel-filled disk between vertebrae that acts as a shock absorber and allows the spine to move.

body mechanics Application of basic mechanical principles to the human body.

posture Position of body parts in relation to each other.

other. Between the vertebra are flat, elastic, gel-filled disks (Figure 6-6). These **intervertebral disks** act as shock absorbers and permit spinal column movement. Protruding from the back of the body of the vertebrae is a horseshoe-shaped piece of bone with projections called *processes*. Like the body of the vertebra, this section of bone and its processes are sized and shaped differently in different locations in the spine. The special shapes of the processes form small synovial joints—the rounded end of a process on one vertebra fits into a matching hollow in a process on the neighboring vertebra. These joints both provide stability and allow for movement. The shapes of the vertebrae and processes create protected passageways for the spinal cord and for nerves that branch off the spinal cord and extend through the body.

The spinal column has many important functions, most of which you can probably guess from its structure:

- Provides structural support for the body
- Allows the upper body to bend and twist
- Protects the spinal cord and the roots of nerves
- Serves as an attachment site for muscles, tendons, and ligaments

- Supports and distributes much of the body's weight
- Absorbs impact and helps maintain balance

A healthy spine is essential for living an active life.

Understanding Body Mechanics and Good Posture

Q | I've never even heard of body mechanics. What does it mean?

Simply put, **body mechanics** is the application of basic mechanical principles to the human body. As a system made up primarily of levers, your body is designed to function optimally—that is, to perform activities in the most safe, efficient, and energy-conserving manner. Unfortunately, our habits and lifestyles tend to encourage poor mechanics more often than proper mechanics. Closely related to body mechanics is **posture,** or the position of body parts in relation to each other. Just as your mother always reminded you, good posture is important.

Q | I think I have pretty good posture. Is there a way to tell?

Good posture is essential for optimal body function; good posture means the body is properly aligned. In order to examine the condition of your posture, have a friend observe you from the side and from behind. From the side, your friend should look at your ear, shoulder, elbow, hip, knee, and mid-foot. Are these points in a straight line? From the back, your friend should observe the same points. Are they level? For example, are both shoulders and both hips even? When observing your feet, your friend should look for balance. Is your weight equally distributed, and is it balanced on the same part of each foot? To further evaluate your posture, complete Lab Activity 6-3.

Q I've been told my headaches are probably caused by bad posture. Could this be true?

Poor posture or holding your head in one position for a long time (while working on the computer without a break, for example) can lead to headaches as well as other health problems. Too much forward head tilt as well as lack of endurance of the cervical muscles has been associated with tension headaches.[26] Irregular head and neck posture, especially in combination with many hours of computer use, is linked to neck and shoulder pain.[27]

Over time, poor posture can cause abnormal wear and tear on the joints and stress muscles and ligaments. For example, if the spine is misaligned, there may be pressure on the spinal nerves, resulting in pain. If the neck is tilted or

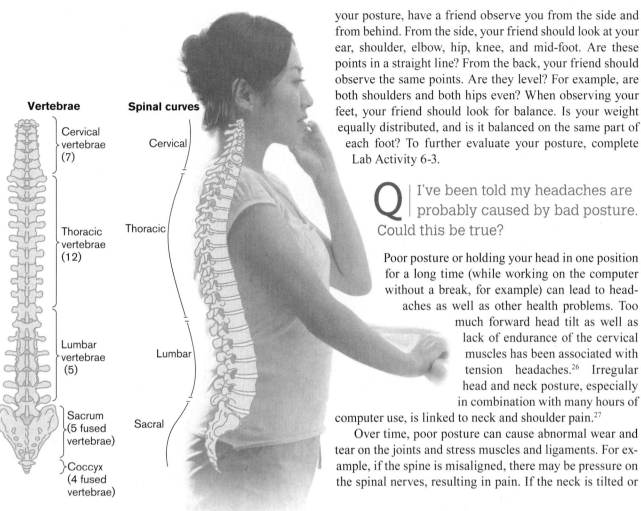

Vertebrae

Cervical vertebrae (7)

Thoracic vertebrae (12)

Lumbar vertebrae (5)

Sacrum (5 fused vertebrae)

Coccyx (4 fused vertebrae)

Spinal curves

Cervical

Thoracic

Lumbar

Sacral

Figure 6-5 **The spine.** The spinal column is made up of five sections with a total of thirty-three individual bones called *vertebrae.* The spine is straight when viewed from the back but has natural curves when viewed from the side.

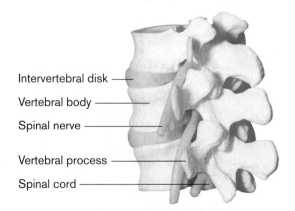

Intervertebral disk

Vertebral body

Spinal nerve

Vertebral process

Spinal cord

Figure 6-6 **Vertebrae and intervertebral disks.** The vertebrae are separated by flat, elastic, gel-filled disks. The processes that extend from the body of the vertebrae form small synovial joints, and the shapes of the vertebrae and processes create passageways for spinal nerves.

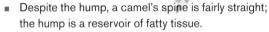

Fast Facts

A Spine Is a Spine . . .

- Despite the hump, a camel's spine is fairly straight; the hump is a reservoir of fatty tissue.
- The necks of giraffes and humans contain the same number of vertebrae (seven), but each of the giraffe's cervical vertebrae can be over 10 inches long, more than a third of the length of the entire human spine.
- Owls have fourteen vertebrae in their neck, giving them a huge range of motion (up to 270 degrees compared to 150–180 degrees in humans)—this is important because their eyes are fixed in the sockets so they can look to the side only by turning their heads.
- Certain squid species are the largest creatures without a backbone; they can grow to be over 40 feet long and weigh more than a ton.

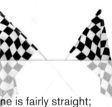

Practical Prevention

Good Posture for Good Health

Factors important for good posture:

- Good muscle flexibility
- Normal motion in the joints
- Strong postural muscles
- A balance of the muscles on both sides of the spine
- Awareness of differences between your posture and proper posture, leading to conscious correction

Practicing good posture isn't difficult. Try the "wall test." With your heels about 4 inches from the wall, stand so that the back of your head, your shoulder blades, and your buttocks lightly touch the wall. You should be

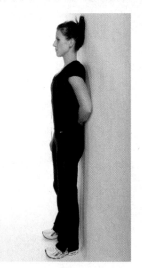

able to slide one hand into the curve of your lower back with your palm against the wall. Arch your back a little if you need more room in order to slide your hand behind you. If you need to decrease the arch in your back to bring your posture into alignment, try tightening your abdominal muscles. Maintain this posture as you step away from the wall.

Sources: Adapted from MayoClinic.com. (2009). *Prevent back pain with good posture* (http://www .mayoclinic.com/health/back-pain/LB00002_D&slide =4). Cleveland Clinic. (2009). *Posture for a healthy back* (http://my.clevelandclinic.org/healthy_living/ Back_health/hic_Posture_for_a_Healthy_Back.aspx).

the shoulders hunched over, muscles become fatigued and weak, leading to muscle and joint pain and increasing the risk of injury. Proper posture, on the other hand, can help prevent fatigue because the body can move with good body mechanics.

Poor posture has many causes. Postural problems can result from hereditary or congenital conditions, disease, or injuries that are beyond our control. The majority of postural problems, however, are within our control. Ill-fitting clothing and inappropriate furniture can lead to poor posture, as can fatigue, excess weight, weak muscles, and emotional issues such as low self-esteem. There are many actions you can take to improve your posture and avoid the problems associated with poor posture.

Q | **How can I improve my posture?**

One of the most important things you can do is think about your posture. Become more aware of your posture, and correct it when you notice that you are slouching or arching your back. Improving muscular endurance and flexibility can also improve your posture.

Contrary to what many think, the cause of poor posture for most of us is the muscles surrounding the spine rather than the spine itself. The muscles of the neck, trunk, and legs work together to support proper alignment and posture. These muscles must have both sufficient strength and flexibility to support proper alignment during our many movements.

Good posture is not just about standing straight or sitting straight. That's only one kind of posture, and it's typically referred to as *static posture*. *Dynamic posture* is the alignment of your body when in motion. As with static posture, the proper dynamic posture involves using the

stance and movements that are most mechanically efficient and least stressful on your body. See the box "Maintaining Good Posture and Body Mechanics" for specific strategies. Later in the chapter, you'll learn more tips for improving posture and body mechanics while using a computer.

Prevention and Management of Low-Back Pain

Q | **My dad has bad problems with low-back pain. His doctor always says it is a common problem. How common is it?**

Very common. At some point in our lives, nearly all of us will have back pain that is severe enough to interfere with work, school, recreation, or daily activities. According to the National Institutes of Health, back pain is the most common cause of job-related disability and second only to headaches as a neurological problem; Americans spend at least $50 billion each year on low-back pain.[28] Back pain can occur at any time during adulthood, with pain varying from mild to severe and from short- to long-term.

Q | **What causes back pain?**

CAUSES OF BACK PAIN. There are many potential causes of back pain. Because the lower back bears the majority of the body's weight, it is the most frequent site of pain or injury. The lower back provides the core from which the body generates power and mobility along with the strength to stand, walk, and lift, all while allowing for turning, twisting, and bending movements. Proper low-back function is critical for almost all activities of daily

Research Brief

Adjustable Tables and Chairs Improve Students' Posture and More

Do you ever get tired of just sitting at a desk? In Finland, a group of thirty high school students were subjects for research to compare the effects of adjustable tables and chairs on posture, pain and tension levels, and learning success. Half the students were a control group, and the other half received tables and chairs that were personally adjusted for their size and shape.

At the onset of the study, students who used the new adjustable tables and chairs reported immediate reduction in lower-back and neck tension. Additional improvements were observed at the end of the two-year research period, including improved posture while sitting and standing, less frequent headaches, continued decrease in tension in the lower back and neck—and significantly better grades!

This study shows the influence of posture on many aspects of wellness. How can you benefit from its findings? Adjust your chair height, desk height, or any other factor you can control to help yourself maintain good posture. If you have a nonadjustable chair or desk at work or school, ask if alternatives are available. It's worth the time and effort to improve your posture.

Source: Koskelo, R., Vuorikari, K., & Hänninen, O. (2007). Sitting and standing postures are corrected by adjustable furniture with lowered muscle tension in high-school students. *Ergonomics, 50*(10), 1643–1656.

---

living. Without smooth low-back function, people begin to experience pain, discomfort, and restriction of typical activities. If left untreated for too long, disability can occur.

Pain may come from muscle strains, spasms, or soreness or from the compression of nerves. Short-term (acute) back pain lasts from a few days to a few weeks; it may be the result of trauma, overuse, or an underlying condition such as arthritis. Acute back pain often resolves with time and self-help measures, although it can return if the underlying causes, such as weak core muscles and poor posture, are not addressed. If pain persists for three months or more, it is considered chronic back pain, which can be difficult to treat successfully.

Triggers for back pain include lifting or moving something too heavy, overstretching while lifting, or engaging in more than usual physical activity—for example, being sedentary during the week and then engaging in heavy yard work or high-intensity recreational activities during the weekend. Back pain can also develop slowly over time, from frequent but less intense stresses—for example, sitting every day for long periods with poor posture. Whether you develop back pain from your activities depends on other factors, including some you can't control (such as age and heredity) and many that you can.

Degeneration of the intervertebral disks is a relatively normal part of the aging process and is a contributor to back problems. As people age, the disks begin to wear away, lose water content, and shrink; in some cases, a disk may collapse completely and no longer provide a cushion between the vertebrae. In other cases, a disk may bulge out from between vertebrae and put pressure on one of the spinal nerves, causing pain. Compression of a sciatic nerve, which is a large nerve that extends from the lower back down the leg, can lead to severe and debilitating leg or foot pain known as *sciatica*. It's important to note, however, that not everyone with back pain has a bulging disk, and not everyone with a bulging disk has back pain. Other risk factors for back pain include heredity and a family or personal history of degenerative diseases such as arthritis or osteoporosis.

Many other important risk factors for back pain are controllable, including the following:

- Poor physical fitness—especially limited muscular strength, endurance, and flexibility in and around the core
- Poor posture, especially if you sit for long periods
- Overweight, especially excess weight around the middle
- A job that involves frequent heavy lifting, twisting, or bending or activities that vibrate the spine (such as operating machinery or driving a truck)
- Smoking—past or current[29]
- Stress and fatigue

The link between smoking and back pain may seem surprising, but smoking can damage arteries and restrict the flow of blood and nutrients to the disks and joints in the back; it also increases the risk of osteoporosis and slows healing from injuries.

Q What helps prevent back pain? Are there special exercises?

PREVENTION OF BACK PAIN. If you look at the list of risk factors for low-back pain in the previous section, you'll probably think of many steps you can take to reduce your risk. Being physically active and building strength and flexibility in the core muscles helps prevent overweight and aids in the maintenance of good posture and good body mechanics. Eating a moderate diet will help you maintain a healthy weight and get enough calcium and vitamin D to keep your bones strong (see Chapter 8). In addition, don't smoke, and manage stress effectively. See pp. 218–219 in this chapter for descriptions of specific exercises designed to help prevent and manage low-back pain.

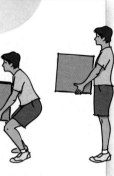

Wellness Strategies

Maintaining Good Posture and Body Mechanics

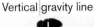

Vertical gravity line

Ear

Shoulder

Hip

Knee

Ankle

Standing

- Hold your head up with your neck straight and your chin neutral, making sure your earlobes are in line with the middle of your shoulders.
- Keep your shoulder blades back and your chest forward; tuck your stomach in.
- Keep your pelvis straight (not tilted forward or backward) and maintain the natural curves in your back without excessive rounding or arching.
- Be sure the arches in your feet are supported. Wear low-heeled shoes.
- If possible, adjust the height of your work table to a comfortable level to avoid bending.
- When standing for an extended period, elevate one foot by resting it on a stool or box; change feet every 5 to 15 minutes.

Walking

- Maintain your good standing posture when walking.
- Keep your head up and eyes looking 10-20 feet ahead.
- Keep your arms bent, and swing your arms from the shoulder.
- With each step, your heel should strike first, then you should roll through the step from heel to toe, followed with a push-off from the toe.
- Your stride should be longer in back of your body than in front of your body.

Sitting

- Sit up with your back straight, your shoulders back, and your buttocks touching the back of your chair.
- Distribute your body weight evenly on both hips. Don't cross your legs, and keep your feet flat on the floor.
- Bend your knees at a right angle, keeping them even with or slightly lower than your hips. Use a foot rest (such as your backpack) if necessary.
- Avoid sitting for a long time whenever possible.
- It is OK to assume other sitting positions for short periods of time, but most of your sitting time should be spent as described above to minimize stress on your spine.

Lifting

- Don't lift beyond the limits of your strength; don't try to lift awkward or especially heavy objects by yourself.
- To pick up an object that is lower than the level of your waist, make sure you have firm footing and use a wide stance. Stand close to the object to be lifted. Keep your back straight and bend at your knees and hips. Do not bend forward at the waist with your knees straight. Tighten your stomach muscles and lift the object using your leg muscles. Straighten your knees in a steady motion. Don't jerk the object up to your body. Stand completely upright

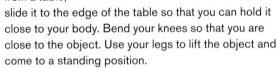

without twisting. Always move your feet forward when lifting an object. Use the reverse action to place the object down, focusing on bending the legs, not the waist.

- To lift an object from a table, slide it to the edge of the table so that you can hold it close to your body. Bend your knees so that you are close to the object. Use your legs to lift the object and come to a standing position.
- Carry items close to your body.

Carrying a backpack or computer bag

- Packs on wheels are the best solution for reducing strain on your back. If this is impractical for you, choose a lightweight pack that doesn't add a lot of weight to your load. It should have two wide, padded shoulder straps and a padded back; a waist belt; and multiple compartments to help distribute the weight evenly.
- If you must use a tote or similar bag, choose one with a long shoulder strap. Slip it over your head onto the opposite shoulder (across the body like a seatbelt) to help distribute the weight more evenly.
- Work on maintaining good walking and standing posture while carrying your load.

Sleeping

- Sleep in a position that allows you to maintain the natural curve in your back. If you sleep on your side, bend your knees slightly and try placing a pillow between your knees; don't pull your knees too far up toward your chest. If you sleep on your back, try placing a pillow under your knees or a lumbar roll under your lower back. Avoid sleeping on your stomach, especially if your mattress sags in the middle.
- Regardless of your sleeping position, your pillow should be under your head (not your shoulders) and should be a thickness that allows your neck to be at a neutral angle.
- Your mattress and box spring should not be too soft. For people with back pain, a medium firm mattress is recommended.

Sources: Adapted from Cleveland Clinic. (2009). *Posture for a healthy back* (http://my.clevelandclinic.org/healthy_living/Back_health/hic_Posture_for_a_Healthy_Back.aspx). Maurer, E., & Spinasanta, S. (2005, June 27). *A head's up on posture: Don't be a slouch!* (http://www.spineuniverse.com/displayarticle.php/article1290.html). Kovacs, F. M., Abraira, V., Peña, A., and others. (2003). Effect of firmness of mattress on chronic non-specific low-back pain: Randomised, double-blind, controlled, multicentre trial. *Lancet, 362*(9396), 1599–1604.

It's also important to follow the suggestions earlier in the chapter (the box "Maintaining Good Posture and Body Mechanics") for appropriate posture and bio-mechanics while sitting, standing, walking, and lifting. If you spend many hours every day on a computer, pay special attention to your posture and the placement of your computer and related equipment (Figure 6-7):

■ The monitor should be directly in front of you, about arm's length away, with the top of the monitor tilted back about 10–20 degrees. The top of the viewing screen should be at or slightly below eye level when you sit up straight.

■ Sit in the position suggested earlier in the chapter, with your back against the backrest and the backrest (or a lumbar pad) adjusted to fit the curve of your lower back. Your feet should be flat on the floor or on a footrest, your thighs parallel to the floor, and your knees at about the same level as your hips.

■ The keyboard should be placed at about the level of your elbows so that you can hold your forearms and wrists relatively straight and parallel to the floor.

■ Take a break every thirty minutes. Stand up and walk around. Stretch your neck, shrug your shoulders, and place your hands gently behind your head and pull your shoulders back. Hold your arms straight out in front of you and stretch your wrists by pulling your hands backwards and then pressing them down; alternate between making a fist and extending your fingers.

Laptops are designed for short-term mobile use and usually require you to hold your neck, arm, and wrist at stressful angles. Pay particular attention to your posture when you use a laptop. Whenever possible, dock your laptop at a desktop computer station or hook it up to a separate monitor, keyboard, and/or mouse. If you aren't already keyboard literate, set that as a goal: Looking down at the laptop keyboard while you type puts a lot of stress on your neck.

Q | If you have back problems, what can you do to help them improve?

MANAGEMENT OF BACK PAIN. Most cases of back pain improve within a short time. Typically, a few days of rest along with a safe dose of acetaminophen or a nonsteroidal anti-inflammatory drug such as ibuprofen can be helpful in managing discomfort. Hot or cold packs (or both) can reduce muscle spasms, pain, and swelling. Stronger medications, such as muscle relaxants and prescrip-

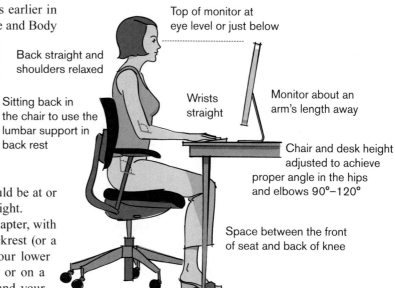

Top of monitor at eye level or just below

Back straight and shoulders relaxed

Sitting back in the chair to use the lumbar support in back rest

Wrists straight

Monitor about an arm's length away

Chair and desk height adjusted to achieve proper angle in the hips and elbows 90°–120°

Space between the front of seat and back of knee

Feet flat on the floor or on foot rest

Figure 6-7 Recommended sitting posture and computer placement

tion painkillers, should be reserved for severe pain and be used only under a doctor's supervision. Prolonged bed rest (more than two or three days) is no longer recommended for managing low-back pain. Gradually getting back to your usual activities will help prevent stiffness and weakness that can worsen back problems over time. Once your pain is improved, you should address any underlying risk factors, such as poor posture or body mechanics.

If your pain is severe or accompanied by other symptoms—weakness, numbness, or tingling; fever; trouble urinating; or unexpected weight loss—see a physician. Back pain is usually diagnosed through a physical exam, a history of your symptoms, and possibly diagnostic tests such as X-rays or magnetic resonance imaging (MRI). It is not unusual for the cause of back pain to remain undetermined. In addition to the self-help measures described above, a doctor may prescribe stronger medications or recommend treatments such as electrical stimulation, physical therapy, spinal manipulation, or acupuncture.[30] A physician can inject a local anesthetic or steroids (to reduce pain and inflammation) or both, but such injections are usually a last resort after more conservative treatments have failed to provide relief. Most people with back pain do not need surgery.

Chronic low-back pain is difficult to treat and may recur. See the box "Living with . . . Low-Back Pain" for more information on treatment and management.

DOLLAR STRETCHER
Financial Wellness Tip

If the chairs you typically sit in don't have adjustable lumbar support, create your own inexpensive version. Roll up a small towel or shirt and place it to maintain the natural curve of your lower back. Try this at home, work, and school, and in your car.

Living with . . .

Low-Back Pain

Although medication and injections can be effective for decreasing pain in the short term, they don't address the root causes or help prevent or reduce the severity of future episodes of low-back pain. Among the most successful methods for minimizing the risk of low-back pain or reducing its reoccurrence are physical exercise and proper body mechanics. Approaches include many of the strategies described in this chapter, including safe lifting and carrying techniques, adequate lumbar support on seats and chairs, and avoiding stationary upright posture for long periods. Pay attention to your posture throughout the day.

Exercise to restore motion and strength to the lower back and core can be very helpful. An appropriate program should include activities to boost overall fitness, including aerobic activities such as walking, swimming, and so on; resistance training with machines, free weights, bands, or body resistance; and whole-body flexibility. Some of the most effective low-back exercises strengthen the core. Three core exercises that help low-back pain are the following (see instructions on pp. 218–219):

- side bridge
- curl-up
- quadruped hip extension (bird dog)

Performing these core exercises along with aerobic, resistance, and flexibility exercises to promote overall fitness will go a long way towards maintaining good back health. In addition, regular exercise helps maintain a healthy body weight, which is also important for reducing low-back pain. Although exercise won't absolutely prevent low-back pain, people who exercise regularly suffer much less from low-back pain throughout their lifetime. If some exercises and activities cause you pain, check with your health care provider for advice on which ones are safe and beneficial for your condition. Avoid any exercise that strains your back; see the exercises at the end of this chapter recommended for low-back health.

For those with chronic back pain, relaxation techniques to reduce stress can also help. The causes of back pain are usually physical, but emotional stress influences how severe the pain is and how long it lasts.

Sources: McGill, S. (2007). *Low back disorders: Evidenced-based prevention and rehabilitation.* Champaign, IL: Human Kinetics. American Academy of Orthopaedic Surgeons. (2008). *Your orthopaedic connection* (http://orthoinfo.aaos.org/main.cfm). National Institute of Arthritis and Musculoskeletal and Skin Diseases. (2009). *Handout on health: Back pain* (http://www.niams.nih.gov/health_info/back_pain/default.asp).

Summary

Flexibility—the ability of joints to move through their full range of motion—is an often overlooked component of health-related fitness, ignored until later in life when problems develop. Your level of flexibility in a particular joint is affected by the structure of the joint, genetics, age, gender, history of injuries and disease, and whether you engage in some form of stretching exercises. Benefits of flexibility include fewer of certain types of injuries and less muscle soreness as well as maintenance of the ability to easily perform daily activities. By initiating a regular stretching program now, utilizing FITT principles, you may be able to avoid many problems in the future. Stretching exercises also promote relaxation.

Flexibility, along with muscle strength and endurance, will reduce the risk of low-back pain. Good posture, along with a program of regular exercise, helps prevent and manage many types of low-back problems. Flexibility training and improvement of posture through small changes in your day-to-day routine can make a big difference in the long run.

More to Explore

American Academy of Orthopaedic Surgeons:
Your Orthopaedic Connection
  http://orthoinfo.aaos.org
Cornell University Ergonomics Web
  http://ergo.human.cornell.edu
MayoClinic.com
Slideshow: How to Stretch Your Major Muscle Groups
  http://www.mayoclinic.com/health/stretching/SM00043
Slideshow: Prevent Back Pain with Good Posture
  http://www.mayoclinic.com/health/back-pain/
  LB00002_D
Slideshow: Core Exercises
  http://www.mayoclinic.com/health/core-strength/
  SM00047
MedlinePlus: Back Pain
  http://www.nlm.nih.gov/medlineplus/backpain.html
Spine Universe
  http://www.spineuniverse.com

Flexibility Exercises

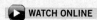

Head Tilt and Turn
Muscles stretched: Splenius muscles, sternocleidomastoid, medial layer of erector spinae

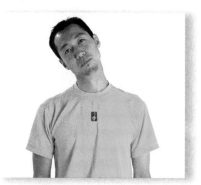 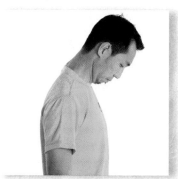 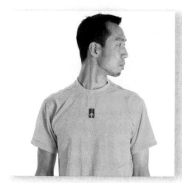

Instructions
Head tilts: Stand or sit comfortably. Begin by leaning your head to one side, moving your ear toward your shoulder. Keep your shoulders relaxed. Hold the stretch. Then gently roll your neck so that your chin moves forward and downward toward your chest. Hold. Then continue the movement until your other ear and shoulder are aligned. Hold. Repeat in the opposite direction.

Head turns: Keeping your shoulders relaxed, turn your head to the right and hold the stretch. Repeat on the left side.

Training tip
- Keep your shoulders relaxed and in a neutral position. Don't perform full neck circles, and take care not to extend your neck back

Triceps Stretch
Muscles stretched: Triceps brachii

Instructions
In a sitting or standing position, raise one arm directly overhead, bending the arm at the elbow to reach toward your back, in the middle of your shoulders. With the opposite arm, reach across the back of your head and grasp the elbow of the first arm. Gently push up and back on your elbow and hold the stretch. Repeat on the other side.

Training tip
- Keep your neck straight, and hold the stretched arm directly beside your head.

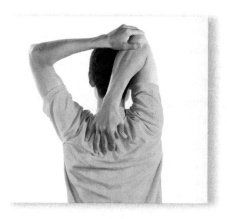

Across-the-Body Shoulder Stretch
Muscles stretched: Deltoid

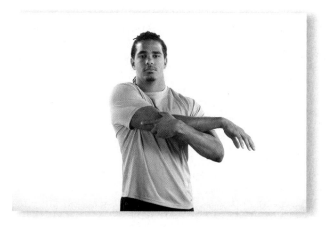

Instructions
Keep your back straight and your torso forward as you cross your right arm in front of your body and grab your elbow or back of the upper arm with your left hand. Gently pull your right arm toward your body. Hold the stretch. Repeat on the other side.

Training tip
- Keep your shoulders relaxed and down. Look forward and keep your neck neutral.

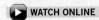 **WATCH ONLINE**

Wall Stretch for Chest

Muscles stretched: Pectoralis major, pectoralis minor, subscapularis

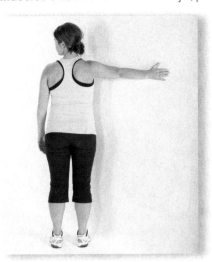

Instructions

Stand in front of a wall and extend one arm out against the wall, palm facing away from you. Turn away from the wall until you feel a stretch in your chest and upper arm. Hold the stretch. Repeat on the other side.

Training tip

- Keep your arm parallel to the floor.

Standing Cat Stretch

Muscles stretched: Deltoid, latissimus dorsi, teres major, erector spinae

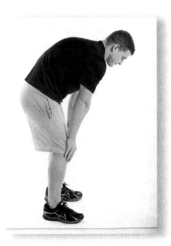

Instructions

Stand with your feet about shoulder-width apart. Bend forward, and place your hands on your knees or lower thighs. Keep your head stationary as you round your back. Hold the stretch and then straighten your back to return to the starting position. Repeat.

Training tip

- Don't bend your neck excessively; this is a stretch of the upper back and not the neck.

Overhead Reach and Lateral Stretch

Muscles stretched: Latissimus dorsi, internal and external obliques, erector spinae

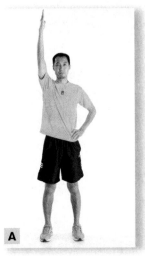
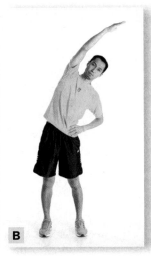

Instructions

Stand comfortably, with your feet about shoulder-width apart and knees slightly bent.

A. With one hand on your hip, reach straight up with the other arm. Hold the stretch. Repeat on the other side.

B. If you can perform this exercise comfortably, try a more advanced lateral stretch. From the same position, bend sideways from the waist as you support your trunk with your opposite hand on your hip or thigh for support. Keep your pelvis tucked in. Hold the stretch, and then repeat on the other side.

Training tips

- Keep the movement directly to the side—don't lean forward or backward.
- Bend at the waist, keeping the lower body stable.

Hip and Trunk Rotation

Muscles stretched: Internal and external obliques, piriformis, erector spinae, gluteal muscles

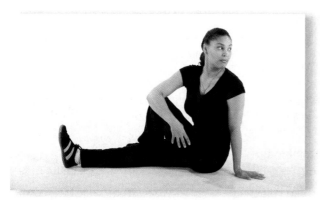

Instructions

Sit comfortably on the floor with your right leg straight out in front of you. Bend your left knee and cross it over your right leg, placing your left ankle against the outside of your right knee. Place your left hand on the floor next to your left hip. Rotate your trunk to the left, using your right elbow to aid in the stretch by placing it on the outside of your left knee. Hold the stretch. Repeat on the other side.

Training tip

- Turn with your trunk, not your neck. Don't let your lower back round excessively

Lying Trunk Twist

Muscles stretched: External and internal obliques

Instructions

Lie on your left side with your left leg straight, right knee bent, right lower leg resting on the ground, and left arm extending out on the floor perpendicular to your body. Leading with your right shoulder, twist your trunk to the right as you push down with your right knee. If needed, you can use your left hand to gently hold your right leg in place. The goal is to get both your shoulders and your upper body flat on the floor while keeping your right knee on the ground. Hold the stretch. Repeat on the other side.

Training tip

- Move your neck in line with your torso; look toward the ceiling rather than over one shoulder.

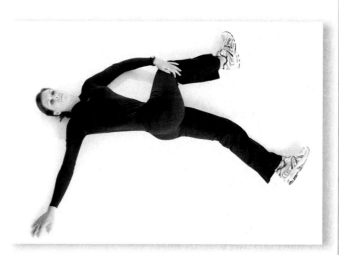

Modified Hurdler's Stretch

Muscles stretched: Hamstrings, erector spinae, gastrocnemius

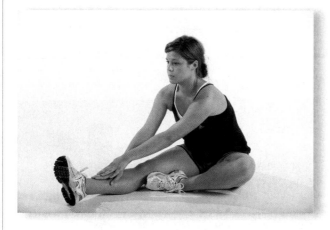

Instructions

Sit on the floor with your right leg extended and the sole of the left foot pressed against the inner right thigh or knee. Keeping your back straight, lean forward at the hips and reach toward your right foot. Hold the stretch. Repeat on the other side. If you are very flexible, grab the toes of the extended leg.

Training tips

- Don't round your shoulders or flex your upper back; keep your back straight.
- Keep your extended leg straight and don't roll your leg out.

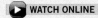 **WATCH ONLINE**

Knee-to-Chest and Leg Extension Stretch

Muscles stretched: Hamstrings, gluteus maximus, erector spinae

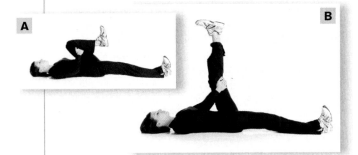

Instructions

Lie on your back with your knees extended.

A. Bend your right leg and grasp it behind your knee, at the back of your thigh. Keeping your left leg flat on the ground, pull your right leg toward your chest. Hold the stretch.

B. Then extend your right leg toward the ceiling; your hands can rest at the back of the thigh. Hold the stretch. Repeat on the other side.

Training tip

- Take care not to flex your neck or arch your back. Keep the straight leg flat on the ground throughout the stretch.

Gluteal Stretch

Muscles stretched: Gluteus maximus

Instructions

Lie on your back with your knees bent and feet flat on the floor. Place your right ankle just above your left knee, with your hip turned out. Reach through with both hands to get a hold of the back of your left knee. (Your right arm will reach through between your legs, your left arm will be outside your left leg.) Gently pull your left knee toward your chest. Your head and torso should be resting on the floor. Hold the stretch. Repeat on the other side.

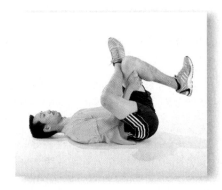

Training tip

- Don't force the movement or arch or strain your back. For an easier variation, place your right foot on your left knee and gently pull your right knee toward your chest with your hands.

Standing Quad Stretch

Muscles stretched: Quadriceps

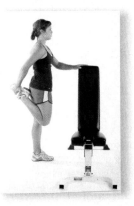

Instructions

Stand comfortably. Begin the stretch by bending one knee, raising your foot to the rear. Grasp the raised ankle with the same hand and pull gently toward your buttocks. Rest the opposite hand on the back of a chair or other support to help maintain your balance. Hold the stretch. Repeat on the other side.

Training tips

- Take care not to arch your back or lean forward.
- Keep your knees together and don't let the bent knee move out to the side. If you feel pain in your knee, stop the stretch.

Kneeling Hip Flexor Stretch

Muscles stretched: Quadriceps, iliopsoas, sartorius, tensor fasciae latae

Instructions

Start in a half kneeling position, with your left knee and your right foot on the ground. Your right knee should be directly above your right ankle. Rest both hands on your right knee. Keeping your abdominals and gluteals tight, shift your entire body forward until you feel a stretch at the front of the hip and in the upper thigh. Your right knee should not extend out in front of your right foot. Hold the stretch, and repeat on the other side.

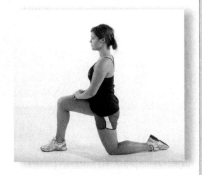

Training tip

- Don't let your lower back arch. Tuck your pelvis under and tighten your abdominals if you feel your back start to arch.

Standing Side Lunge Stretch
Muscles stretched: Hip adductors

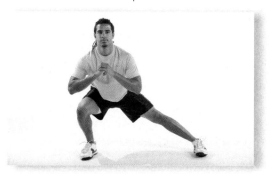

Instructions
Stand in a wide straddle with legs turned slightly out. With your hands clasped in front (or on your thighs for more balance), lunge to the side by bending one knee. Keep the knee directly over the ankle and don't let it extend out in front of your foot. Hold the stretch and repeat on the other side.

Training tip
- Don't lean forward or to the side with your torso; the movement comes from the lower body.

Groin Stretch (Butterfly)
Muscles stretched: Hip adductors

Instructions
Sit on the floor with your torso upright. Bend your knees and rotate your thighs out to bring the soles of your feet together in front of you. Place your hands around your feet or ankles and gently pull your feet toward your body. Keeping your back straight, lean slightly forward. If you can, gently push your knees down with your forearms or elbows. Hold the stretch.

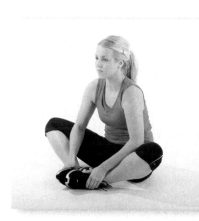

Training tips
- Be sure to use slow, smooth motions and go only to the point of a comfortable stretch.
- Keep your back straight and don't round your shoulders or upper back.

Calf, Soleus, and Shin Stretch
Muscles stretched: Gastrocnemius, soleus, tibialis anterior

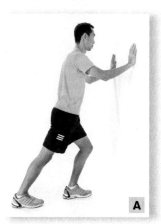 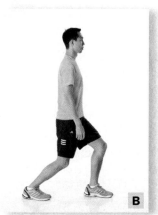 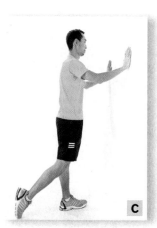

Instructions
A. Stand facing a wall with your toes about 12 inches from the wall. Lean forward and place both hands on the wall. Step back with your right leg about 2 feet as you bend your left leg. Extend your right leg and keep your foot flat on the floor. If you don't feel a stretch in the right calf, bend your elbows slightly and move your hips and torso toward the wall until you feel a stretch. Hold the stretch.

B. Pull your right foot in, bend your right knee, and shift your weight as you remove your hands from the wall. Support your weight with your right leg. Hold the stretch.

C. Straighten your legs, shift your weight forward onto your left leg, and rest your hands lightly on the wall. Place the top of your right foot on the ground; try to point your toenails toward the floor. Push down gently to stretch the front of your shin. Repeat on the other side.

Training tip
- Push only to the point of a comfortable stretch.
- Keep your toes pointed forward throughout parts A and B.

Exercises for the Lower Back

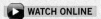 WATCH ONLINE

Cat and Camel

Purpose: Reduces joint friction and resistance to movement

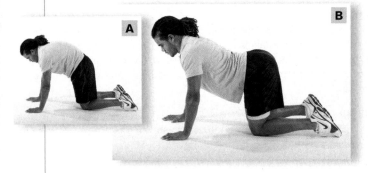

Instructions

A. Kneel on your hands and knees, with your hands directly below your shoulders and your knees directly below your hips. Begin by pushing up your back, pulling in your abdomen, dropping your head slightly, and tucking your pelvis down and under.

B. Next, slowly lower your back, shift your pelvis up, and lift your chin slightly until your back is flexed. Stop if you feel any pain. Complete 5–10 cycles of flexion and extension.

Training tips

- This is a movement and not a stretch—move gently through the entire range of motion and don't press at the ends of the range of motion.
- Keep your hands and hips facing directly forward for both positions.

Curl-up

Purpose: Builds endurance in the rectus abdominis

Instructions

A. Lie on your back with one leg straight and the other knee bent. Place both hands under your lumbar spine to help keep your spine neutral during the exercise. Your elbows should touch the floor.

B. To perform the curl, raise your head and upper shoulders off the floor. Alternate the bent leg midway through your repetitions.

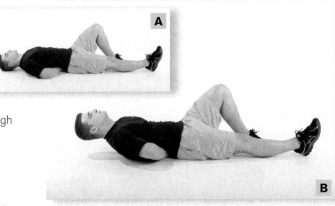

Training tips

- Don't curl up with your head; the movement should come from your thoracic region.
- You can make the exercise more challenging by raising your elbows off the floor.

Side Bridge

Purpose: Builds endurance in the quadratus lumborum, abdominal obliques

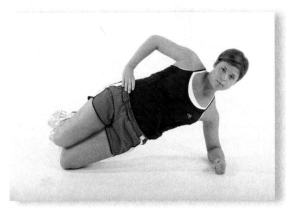

Instructions

Start by lying on the floor on your side, with your knees bent. Your top arm can lie along your side or across your chest, or you can place your hand on your hip. Lift your hips so that your weight is supported by your forearm and knees. Hold this position for 7–8 seconds. Return to the starting position. Repeat. As you gain strength, you can make the exercise more difficult by supporting your weight with your forearm and your feet.

Training tips

- Keep your body firm and straight throughout this exercise.
- This exercise can be made more challenging by pointing your top arm straight up.

Quadruped Hip Extension (Bird Dog)

Purpose: Builds endurance in the erector spinae, multifidus spinae, and rectus abdominis

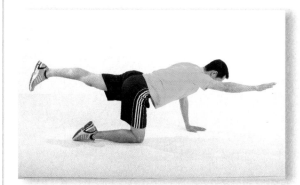

Instructions

Start on the floor on your hands and knees. Knees should be below the hips and hands should be below the shoulders and slightly wider. Slowly extend one arm and the opposite leg, keeping your back straight. Hold this position for 7–8 seconds, then lower your hand and knee and "sweep" the floor with them before raising them for the next repetition. Alternate to the opposite arm and leg.

Training tips

- Use a pad under your hands and knees for more comfort.
- Beginners can start by lifting an arm alone, then lowering it, and then lifting a leg alone.

Back (Glute) Bridge

Purpose: Builds strength and endurance in the gluteus maximus, erector spinae, hamstrings

Instructions

Start by lying on your back with your arms extended along your side. Tuck your pelvis under and tighten your gluteal muscles. Raise your hips so that your weight is supported by your head, shoulders, and feet (flat on the floor). Hold this position for at least 10 seconds, slowly building up to 30 seconds.

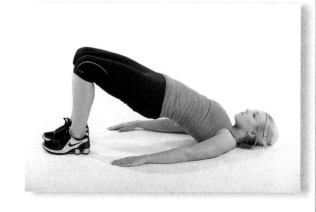

Training tips

- Keep your back straight throughout this exercise. Don't push your hips up, forcing your back to arch and straining your neck.
- This exercise can be made more difficult by lifting one leg so the foot is pointing out, in line with the support leg.
- If you feel pain in your back, don't perform this exercise.

Wall Sit (Squat)

Purpose: Builds endurance of the quadriceps, hamstrings, gluteus maximus, and rectus abdominis

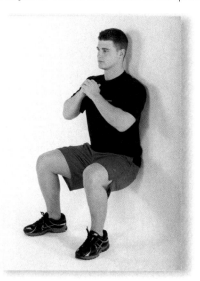

Instructions

Stand in front of a wall and lean against it with your back. Walk your feet out and then bend your knees and slide down the wall until you are in a squat position. Imagine you are sitting in a chair; focus on using the muscles in your thighs, buttocks, and abdomen. Begin by holding the position for 10–15 seconds and work your way up to a 1-minute hold.

Training tip

- Make sure that your knees don't extend out in front of your toes; stop if you feel any pain in your knees.

NAME	**DATE**	**SECTION**

Complete one or more of the tests for flexibility described in this lab activity and then answer the questions in the "Reflecting on Your Results" section at the end.

- Sit-and-reach test (flexibility of the lower back and hamstrings)
- Shoulder flexibility test
- Hip range of motion and hamstring flexibility test
- Hip-flexor flexibility test (Thomas Test)

Sit-and-Reach Test

Equipment

- Sit-and-reach box with the footline set at 26 centimeters (cm). You can also create your own measuring device from a firm box or pieces of wood and a metric ruler. The ruler should be set so that the 26-cm mark is aligned with the end of the box or board. (If you can reach past your feet, your score will be higher than 26 cm; if you can't reach as far as your feet, your score will be below 26 cm.)
- Partner to check measurement

Preparation

Warm up for 5–10 minutes, using low-intensity aerobic activity. Stretch your hamstrings and lower back.

Instructions

Remove your shoes and sit with your feet flat against the sit-and-reach box. As described, your feet should be at the 26-cm mark of the metric ruler or measuring device. The inner edges of your feet should be within 2 cm of the ruler or scale. With your hands parallel and in contact with the measuring portion of the sit-and-reach box or the ruler, slowly reach forward as far as possible. Your fingertips can be overlapped, but do not lead with one hand. Your knees should be extended but not pressed down. Don't hold your breath; to aid in your performance on the test, exhale and drop your head between your arms as you reach forward. Hold the position of farthest reach for about 2 seconds. Your partner should note this measurement. Repeat the test.

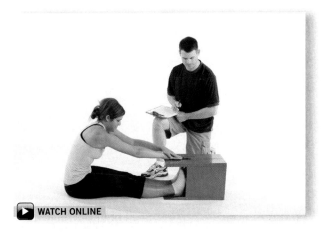

WATCH ONLINE

Results

Your score is the most distant point (in centimeters) you reached with your fingertips. Find the rating that corresponds to your score. (Note: If the sit-and-reach box has a different footline or zero point, adjust the score accordingly. For example, if the footline of your box is 23 cm, you would add 3 cm to your score.)

Trial 1: _____ cm   Trial 2: _____ cm   Best trial: _____ cm   Rating (from table): _____

RATINGS FOR THE SIT-AND-REACH TEST (IN CENTIMETERS)*

Age (years)

	15–19	20–29	30–39	40–49	50–59	60–69
MEN						
Excellent	≥39	≥40	≥38	≥35	≥35	≥33
Very good	34–38	34–39	33–37	29–34	28–34	25–32
Good	29–33	30–33	28–32	24–28	24–27	20–24
Fair	24–28	25–29	23–27	18–23	16–23	15–19
Needs improvement	≤23	≤24	≤22	≤17	≤15	≤14
WOMEN						
Excellent	≥43	≥41	≥41	≥38	≥39	≥35
Very good	38–42	37–40	36–40	34–37	33–38	31–34
Good	34–37	33–36	32–35	30–33	30–32	27–30
Fair	29–33	28–32	27–31	25–29	25–29	23–26
Needs improvement	≤28	≤27	≤26	≤24	≤24	≤22

*Footline of box set at 26 cm.

Source: Canadian Society for Exercise Physiology. (2003). *The Canadian physical activity, fitness and lifestyle approach: CSEP health and fitness program's health-related appraisal and counselling strategy* (3rd ed.). Ottawa, ON: CSEP.

Shoulder Flexibility Test

Equipment

- Small ruler or tape measure
- Partner to check measurement

Preparation

Warm up for 5–10 minutes, using low-intensity aerobic activity. Stretch your shoulders.

Instructions

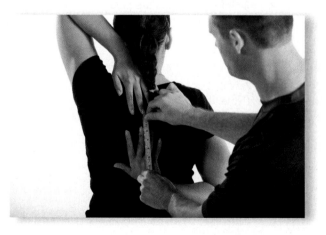

1. Raise your right arm straight over your head, bend your elbow, and reach between your shoulders as far as possible, palm against your back (see the Triceps Stretch in this chapter).

2. At the same time, extend your left arm down toward the ground, bend at the elbow and reach up behind your back, trying to touch or overlap the fingers of both hands.

3. Your partner should measure the distance of finger overlap or the distance between your fingers to the nearest quarter inch. If your fingers overlap, the score is a positive number. If your fingers fail to meet, the score is a negative number.

4. Repeat with the left arm up and right arm down.

Results

Your score is the average of the two measurements: The distance between your fingertips (negative number) or the distance of overlap of your fingers (positive number). Find your rating in the table.

Right elbow up: [_____] in.

Left elbow up: [_____] in.

Average of two measurements: [_____] in.

Rating: [_____]

RATINGS FOR SHOULDER FLEXIBILITY TEST

RATING	AVERAGE OF TWO SIDES IN INCHES
Excellent	≥5
Above average	2 to 4.75
Average	0 to 1.75
Below average	−1 to −0.25
Poor	< −1

Source: Nieman, D. (2003). *Exercise Testing and Prescription: A Health-Related Approach* (5th ed., pp. 185, 197). New York: McGraw-Hill.

Hip Range of Motion and Hamstring Flexibility Test

Equipment

- Partner to check range of motion
- Goniometer or other joint measurement tool (optional)

Preparation

Warm up for 5–10 minutes, using low-intensity aerobic activity. Stretch your hamstrings and lower back.

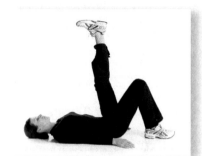

Instructions

Lie on your back with your arms at your sides. Bend one knee and place your foot flat on the floor. Keeping your other leg straight, raise it. Compare the range of motion in the raised straight leg relative to a 90-degree position perpendicular to the floor. If a partner and a measuring instrument such as a goniometer are available, you can obtain a more precise measurement of the joint angle. Repeat the test on the other leg.

Results

Average flexibility for this test is about 90 degrees. If you cannot raise your leg so that it is at least perpendicular to the floor, then your hamstring flexibility is below average. Note for each leg whether hamstring flexibility is below average, average, or above average:

Right leg: [_____]   Left leg: [_____]

If you used a goniometer for joint angle measurement, record the results below:

Right leg: [_____] degrees   Left leg: [_____] degrees

Hip-Flexor Flexibility Test (Thomas Test)

Equipment

- Partner to check range of motion
- Training table or bench (optional)

Preparation

Warm up for 5–10 minutes, using low-intensity aerobic activity. Stretch your hip flexors, quadriceps, and hamstrings.

Instructions

If you are performing the test on the floor: Lie on your back and bring both knees to your chest. Grab your right leg behind the knee and hold your knee at your chest. Let your left leg straighten and lower it toward the floor or mat by relaxing your hip. Have your partner note whether the straight leg is flat on the floor or the knee and lower thigh are "floating" above the floor. Repeat the test on the other leg.

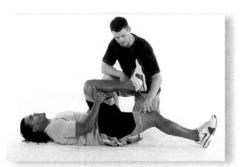

If you are performing the test on a training table or bench: Sit so that your tailbone is at the edge of the table. Lie back on the table, pulling your knees to your chest. Grab your right leg behind the knee and hold it to your chest. Gently lower your left leg beyond the edge of the table or bench. The table or bench should be tall enough that your leg can hang freely. Your lower back should maintain its natural curve throughout the movement by touching the table or bench at all times. Have your partner note the angle of your thigh on the extended leg. If your leg is lifted above the level of the table, this indicates poor hip-flexor flexibility; if your leg extends below the level of the table, this indicates good hip-flexor flexibility. Repeat the test with the other leg.

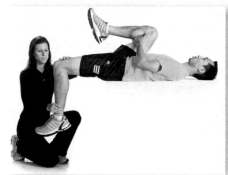

Rating

For each side, note the position of the test leg. If your leg does not lower all the way—if your knee and lower thigh float above the ground or come off the table—then your hip flexors are tight and their range of motion is below average.

Right leg: ☐ (flat / floating)   Rating: ☐ (OK / below average)

Left leg: ☐ (flat / floating)   Rating: ☐ (OK / below average)

Reflecting on Your Results

Record the results of the tests you completed.

	SCORE	RATING
Sit-and-reach test		
Shoulder flexibility test		
Hip range of motion and hamstring flexibility test	Right: Left:	Right: Left:
Hip-flexor flexibility test	Right: Left:	Right: Left:

Are you surprised by your ratings? Did your results match what you thought about your level of flexibility?

☐

Planning Your Next Steps

If the results of the tests indicate that the flexibility in some of your joints is below average, consider starting or expanding your flexibility training. Set realistic goals for improvement and create a plan to achieve them. Then repeat these tests in several weeks and note any improvements.

Describe the specific steps you will take to improve your flexibility:

☐

What effect, if any, did your plan have on your flexibility?

☐

📷 **SUBMIT ONLINE**

NAME   DATE   SECTION

Equipment

None required, but you may want to develop and track your program in a paper notebook, digital spreadsheet, smartphone application, or online program.

Preparation: None

Instructions

1. **Set SMART goals** (specific, measurable, achievable, realistic, time-bound): The goals for your flexibility program can be about training—such as number of stretching workouts per week—or they can be based on one of the flexibility tests you completed in Lab Activity 6-1.

Current status	Goal	Target date	Notes (rewards, special considerations)

2. **Apply the FITT principle:** Create a program that meets the recommended criteria for success and fits your schedule and preferences.
   - *Frequency:* 2–3 days per week or more
   - *Intensity:* Stretch to the point of slight tension or mild tightness.
   - *Time:* Hold the stretch for 15–60 seconds, and do four or more repetitions of each stretch.
   - *Type:* Perform a stretch for each major muscle/tendon group or joint: neck, shoulders, upper and lower back, pelvis, hips, and legs. Fill in the exercises for your starting program below.

EXERCISE	MUSCLE/TENDON GROUP OR JOINT STRETCHED

Results

Track your progress with a log like the one below or one you create for yourself.

FLEXIBILITY TRAINING LOG

DATE	DURATION/TIME	WORKOUT (IF DIFFERENT FROM STARTING PROGRAM)	NOTES (E.G., CHANGES IN FLEXIBILITY, HOW STRETCHING PROGRAM MAKES YOU FEEL)

Reflecting on Your Results and Planning Your Next Steps

Have you been sticking with your program plan for flexibility training? How have you responded to the program? Has your flexibility increased? How does your stretching routine make you feel? Do you plan to change your program going forward? If so, describe the changes. How do you plan to stick with your program going forward?

[ ] **SUBMIT ONLINE**

NAME	DATE	SECTION

Standing Posture

Equipment

Partner

Preparation

None. The assessment is easier to complete if you wear clothing that allows your posture and body lines to be easily seen. Remove your shoes.

Instructions

Have a partner compare your *typical* standing posture to the illustrations and key points listed below. Your partner should describe any differences between your posture and the recommended posture.

From the side:

____ Yes ____ No   Straight line between the ear, shoulder, hip, knee, and ankle.

____ Yes ____ No   Back relatively straight while showing natural curves, without too much rounding in shoulders, too much arch in lower back, and so on.

____ Yes ____ No   Neck straight and chin neutral (not pushed forward or pulled in).

____ Yes ____ No   Shoulder blades back and chest forward.

____ Yes ____ No   Knees straight but relaxed (not locked).

From the back:

____ Yes ____ No   Ears level.

____ Yes ____ No   Shoulders level.

____ Yes ____ No   Hips level.

____ Yes ____ No   Feet parallel, with weight evenly balanced on both feet; ankles tilted neither inward nor outward.

Description of potential posture problems:

Desk/Computer Posture

Equipment

- Partner
- Computer and desk/chair where you typically use your computer

Preparation

None. The assessment is easier to complete if you wear clothing that allows your posture and body angles to be easily seen.

Instructions

Have a partner compare your *typical* sitting posture when you use your computer to the illustration below. Your partner should note and describe any problems.

___ Yes ___ No   Eyes level or just above top of monitor.

___ Yes ___ No   Eyes about arm's length away from monitor.

___ Yes ___ No   Elbows bent and close to body, angle of 90–120°.

___ Yes ___ No   Wrists straight (not angled upward, downward or to either side).

___ Yes ___ No   Upper back relatively straight while showing natural curves, without rounding of the shoulders.

___ Yes ___ No   Shoulders down and relaxed, directly over hips (not lifted or pulled forward).

___ Yes ___ No   Lower back relatively straight while showing natural curves, without too much arch or rounding.

___ Yes ___ No   Sitting all the way back in the chair, with a backrest supporting lower back.

___ Yes ___ No   Hips bent to achieve angle of 90–120°.

___ Yes ___ No   Knees out in front of the edge of the chair.

___ Yes ___ No   Feet even and flat on the floor or resting on a footrest.

Top of monitor at eye level or just below

Back straight and shoulders relaxed

Sitting back in the chair to use the lumbar support in back rest

Wrists straight

Monitor about an arm's length away

Chair and desk height adjusted to achieve proper angle in the hips and elbows 90°–120°

Space between the front of seat and back of knee

Feet flat on the floor or on foot rest

Description of potential posture problems:

Reflecting on Your Results

How did you do? How close or far is your typical posture from the recommendations? Do you ever think about your posture or have problems that might be attributed to your posture (such as a sore neck or back)?

Planning Your Next Steps

Practice using correct posture. First, for standing posture, practice realigning your body to match the recommendations; you can use the checklist in the lab and also try the wall test on p. 208. If you need to pull your shoulders back and open your chest, try the following: With your arms hanging loosely in front, place your palms toward your body and point your thumbs inward at each other. Then rotate your arms (at the shoulder joint) so you're your thumbs are pointing outward. After you try correct standing posture a few times, describe what you did to achieve it and how it feels. What can you use as a reminder to periodically check and correct your posture until the recommended posture becomes habit?

For your desk/computer posture, determine what steps are needed to improve your posture so that it matches the guidelines. You may need to adjust your chair and desk in addition to your body positions. List and describe the changes needed in your work area and include a plan for each. (If you make significant changes to your work area, you may need to reevaluate your desk/computer posture.) Next, list and describe the changes needed in your posture. What specific steps can you take to work on improving your desk/computer posture?

NAME	DATE	SECTION

This lab activity includes three muscle-endurance tests that focus on different muscles that are important for low-back stability.

Side-Bridge Endurance Test

Equipment

- Floor mat
- Stopwatch, watch, or clock with a second hand
- Partner

Preparation

Warm up for 5–10 minutes, using low-intensity aerobic activity. If you haven't performed side bridges before, practice.

Instructions

Lie on your side with your legs extended. Place your top foot slightly in front of your lower foot for support. Lift your hips off the mat so that your weight is supported by your forearm and your feet. Your body should form a straight line. Keep your neck neutral and don't hold your breath. Hold the position as long as possible. Your score will be the total time you maintain the position with good form. A partner can monitor the time and watch your form. Rest for several minutes and then repeat the test on the other side.

Results

Your score is the total number of seconds you held the side bridge position. Compare your score to the average score in the table at the end of this lab activity.

Right side: [＿＿＿] seconds   Left side: [＿＿＿] seconds

Back-Extensors Endurance Test

Equipment

- Padded bench
- Partner
- Stopwatch, watch, or clock with a second hand

Preparation

Warm up for 5–10 minutes, using low-intensity aerobic activity.

▶ WATCH ONLINE

Instructions

Lie face down on the test bench. Your hips, pelvis, and knees should be flat on the bench while your upper body extends out over the end of the bench. Fold your arms across your chest, placing each hand on the opposite shoulder. Your feet can be secured by a strap or a partner can hold them. Lift your upper body to form a straight horizontal line with your lower body. Your score will be the total time you are able to hold the horizontal position. Keep your neck neutral and don't hold your breath or arch your back. Stop if you feel pain in your neck or lower back.

Results

Your score is the total number of seconds you held the extended position: [＿＿＿] seconds. Compare your score to the average score in the table at the end of this lab activity.

Trunk-Flexors Endurance Test

Equipment

- Mat or padded bench
- Strap or partner to hold feet
- Backrest, bench, or spotter to support back
- Stopwatch, watch, or clock with a second hand

▶ WATCH ONLINE

Preparation

Warm up for 5–10 minutes using low-intensity aerobic activity.

Instructions

The position for this endurance test is a modified sit-up position. Your feet should be flat on the floor or bench, held down by a partner or secured under a strap. Bend your knees at a 90-degree angle, and flex your hips 90 degrees. Cross your arms on your chest. Your back should be at a 60-degree angle to the floor, supported by a partner, a support, or an adjustable bench. At the start of the test, the support is moved away about 4 inches, and you hold the position for as long as possible. Don't hold your breath or arch your back. Your score is the total time you hold the position with correct form. The support should be ready to catch your weight as soon as you can no longer hold the position.

Results

Your score is the total number of seconds you held the sit-up position: [   ] seconds. Compare your score to the average score in the table below of average endurance times.

Reflecting on Your Results

Record a summary of the scores of the tests you completed. Find your rating by comparing your scores to the average scores in the table below.

	SCORE (IN SECONDS)	RATING (ABOVE AVERAGE, AVERAGE, BELOW AVERAGE)
Side-bridge endurance test	Right: Left:	Right: Left:
Back-extensors endurance test		
Trunk-flexors endurance test		

Average Endurance Times (in seconds)

TEST	MEN	WOMEN
Right side bridge	95	75
Left side bridge	99	78
Back extensors	161	185
Trunk flexors	136	134

Source: McGill, S. M. (2003). *Low back disorders: Evidence-based prevention and rehabilitation.* Champaign, IL: Human Kinetics.

Are you surprised by your ratings? Did your results match what you thought about your own level of muscle endurance and low-back health?

Planning Your Next Steps

If the results of the lab indicate your muscle endurance in any of the areas tested is below average, consider incorporating some specific exercises to build endurance in the muscles that help support back health. Set realistic goals for improvement and create a plan to achieve them. Then repeat these tests in several weeks and note improvements.

Describe the specific steps you will take to improve your muscle endurance for low-back health:

What effect, if any, did your plan have on your muscle endurance?

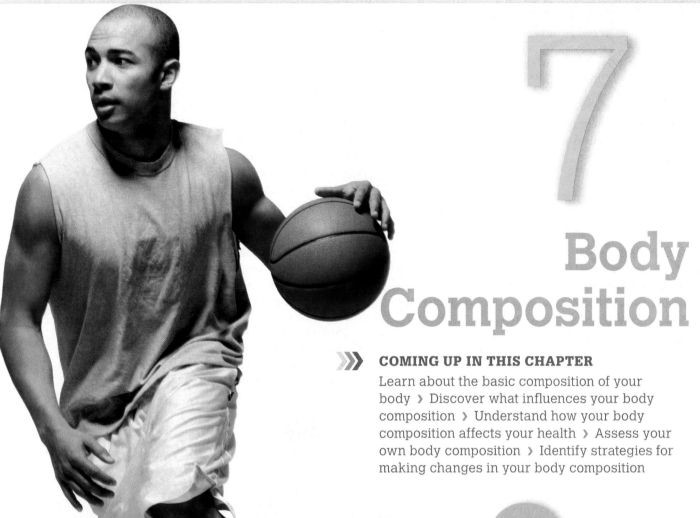

7

Body Composition

≫ **COMING UP IN THIS CHAPTER**
Learn about the basic composition of your body ❯ Discover what influences your body composition ❯ Understand how your body composition affects your health ❯ Assess your own body composition ❯ Identify strategies for making changes in your body composition

Wellness Connections

How does body composition relate to your overall wellness? The impact on physical wellness is fairly clear, especially if you have significantly too much or too little body fat. Either one can cause serious short-term and long-term health problems and severely limit your day-to-day activities. But body composition also affects other wellness dimensions. Your perceptions of your body weight and shape influence your emotional, spiritual, and social wellness. Do you experience positive or negative emotions when you think about your body? Does your body image affect your decisions about recreational or social activities? Do you feel like you are missing out on anything because of your body image?

The planning and critical thinking skills of intellectual wellness can help you make good decisions about lifestyle choices that affect your body composition. These skills can also help you evaluate media messages that may hurt your body image and emotional wellness. Your environment plays a large role in determining your body composition—it can provide many opportunities for healthy food choices and physical activity, or it can limit your ability to incorporate healthy changes into your daily life. You can also influence your environment in positive ways—campaign for streets that are safe for walking and bicycling, for grocery stores and restaurants with healthful food, and for a positive focus on healthy body image.

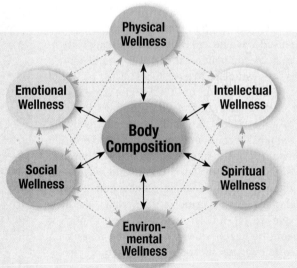

This chapter presents basic information about body composition. You'll learn more about the body's makeup and how it affects your health, the factors that affect your body composition, methods of assessing your body composition, and basic steps for making changes in body composition.

Basics of Body Composition

There are different ways to think about the makeup of the body—its joints, muscle groups, limbs, organs, and so on. In this chapter, we'll look at how the proportion of muscle, fat, and other body tissues affects your health and well-being in both the short and long term.

Q | What is body composition?

Body composition is exactly what it sounds like—the makeup of the body. It is typically defined as the relative proportions of different types of body tissues:

- muscle
- bone
- fat
- other vital tissues

For adults of all ages, the proportion of body weight that is fat—**percent body fat**—is the measure most often used to define and evaluate body composition. For example, an individual who weighs 150 pounds and who is estimated to have 30 pounds of fat would have percent body fat of 20 percent. As described later in the chapter, too much or too little body fat has adverse effects on health, so percent body fat is an important consideration and body composition is one of the health-related components of physical fitness. Percent body fat is one of the ways—but not the only way—of defining underweight, overweight, and obesity. Among older adults, the density and weight of bone tissue is also an important measure of health since loss of bone mass with aging (known as osteoporosis) can lead to fractures.

Q | Is there such a thing as good body fat?

Yes. Your body needs fat in order to function—and body fat is much more than just a reservoir of energy. You can think of body fat in two categories: essential fat and storage fat.

Essential fat is the fat found in the central nervous system, in bone marrow, and in various organs throughout

the body. Fat is a key component of cell membranes and of the sheath that surrounds nerve fibers in the brain and enables transmission of messages. Fat is necessary for normal physiological functioning—to maintain life and for reproductive functioning. Women typically have more essential fat than men due to hormonal and reproductive demands—essential fat is about 8–12 percent of women's body weight and about 3–5 percent of men's body weight (Figure 7-1). Women have more fat tissue in the breasts and pelvic area. And both women and men need a certain amount of fat for healthy hormone production.

Storage fat, also called adipose tissue, can be further divided into two subcategories. The first type is found

percent body fat The proportion (percentage) of total body weight that is fat; the measure most often used to evaluate body composition.

essential fat Fat necessary for normal body functioning; found in nerves, cell membranes, bone marrow, the central nervous system, and other organs.

storage fat Fat stored under the skin (subcutaneous fat) and surrounding internal organs (visceral fat); provides insulation, protects organs, serves as an energy store, and releases hormones and other chemical messengers.

body composition Relative proportions of muscle, fat, bone, and other vital tissues; often expressed in terms of fat and fat-free body mass.

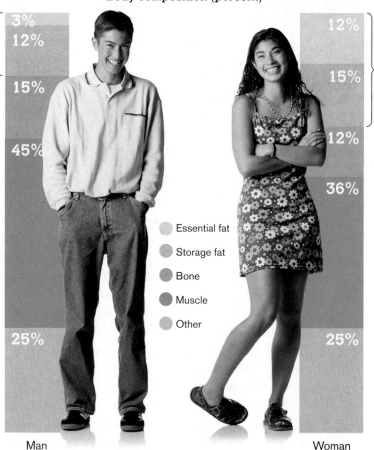

Body composition (percent)

15%

3%
12%
15%
45%
25%

27%

12%
15%
12%
36%
25%

Essential fat
Storage fat
Bone
Muscle
Other

Man

Woman

Figure 7-1 Body composition of young adults (ages 20–24). The values here are not goals or averages; they only provide a basis for comparison. Note the larger percentage of essential fat for women compared to men.

Source: Behnke, A. R., & Wilmore, J. H. (1974). *Evaluation and regulation of body build and composition* (p. 123). Englewood Cliffs, NJ: Prentice Hall.

deep within the abdominal cavity surrounding internal organs. This fat is known as internal storage fat or **visceral fat,** and it provides a cushiony protection for organs such as the kidneys and intestines. The other type, known as **subcutaneous fat,** is storage fat found just beneath the skin; this is the fat you can see and pinch with your fingers (Figure 7-2). Subcutaneous fat helps to insulate the body and regulate temperature. It can be found in many parts of the body, but the largest deposits are typically in the abdomen, hips, buttocks, and thighs. You need a certain amount of each type of storage fat, but too much storage fat, especially visceral fat, has negative health effects.

As indicated by its name, storage fat is a site for the storage of energy. As described in Chapter 4, the body can used stored fat as fuel to produce ATP for energy. Fat tissue also serves other functions: It releases many different kinds of molecules and hormones that affect appetite, blood pressure, immune system function, insulin and glucose levels, and many other body systems and processes.[1]

Q | My friends and I look about the same but most of them weigh around 15 pounds less than I do. How is that possible?

Body weight and body size are obviously related, but they don't tell the entire story. Different types of tissue vary in density, so two people who are the same size can have different weights and different body compositions. Muscle is denser than fat, so a pound of muscle takes up less space—about 18 percent less space—than a pound of fat. Fat is even less dense than water, which means that it floats, whereas muscle is denser than water; this difference is the reason underwater weighing is used to estimate body composition (see p. 248). If an exercise program causes you to gain muscle mass and lose body fat, your weight on a scale may not change, but you are likely to notice your clothes getting looser because your new muscle takes up less space than the fat you lost.

If two people are about the same size, the heavier of the two likely has more muscle and less fat. Similarly, two people of the same weight can look very different and have different body compositions. Consider two people who both weigh 150 pounds: One might have

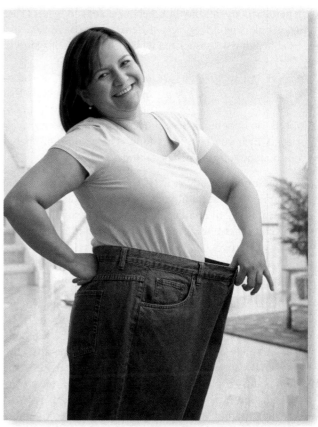

Muscle is more dense than fat, so a pound of muscle takes up less space than a pound of fat. If you lose a pound of fat and add a pound of muscle, your body weight won't change but your body size will.

visceral fat Storage fat found around and between organs in the abdominal cavity.

subcutaneous fat Storage fat found just under the skin.

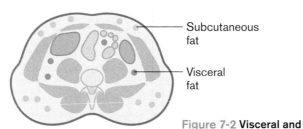

Lean (low percent body fat)

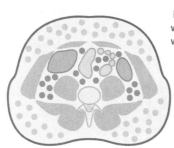

Excess body fat

Figure 7-2 **Visceral and subcutaneous fat in the abdomen.** Visceral fat is located around organs within the abdominal cavity, whereas subcutaneous fat is located just beneath the skin. Excess body fat of any kind carries health risks, but excess visceral fat is particularly unhealthy.
Source: Adapted from Stehno-Bittel, L. (2008). Intricacies of fat. *Physical Therapy: Diabetes Special Issue, 88*(11), 1265–1278.

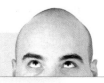

Mind Stretcher
Critical Thinking Exercise

How do you feel about your own body weight, size, and shape? Do you have strong feelings about what an ideal male or female body should look like? Where do you think you learned these ideals? Are they realistic?

20 percent body fat, and the other 40 percent body fat. These two people would look very different—and have very different health risks associated with their body compositions.

Q | What is metabolism?

In technical terms, **metabolism** is all the processes that occur in your body to maintain its functioning. These processes require energy (calories), which you take in as food. The amount of energy your body requires depends on three criteria:

- **Resting metabolic rate (RMR):** The energy required to maintain essential body processes at rest, including respiration, circulation, and temperature regulation
- Dietary thermogenesis: The energy required for digesting and processing the foods you eat
- Physical activity: The energy required for activities of daily living as well as formal exercise sessions

People with a higher resting metabolic rate and higher level of physical activity require more calories. Your RMR depends on a number of factors, including genetics, body size, and body composition. Larger people generally have a higher RMR simply because their body has more tissue to maintain. People with a higher proportion of muscle tissue and a lower percent body fat also have a higher RMR: Muscle is more metabolically active than fat, so the more pounds of muscle in your body, the more calories you require. Resistance training also increases RMR; research suggests that the microtears in muscle tissue caused by training (see Chapter 5) require energy to repair, and this tissue-remodeling process increases RMR for several days following a workout.[2]

The connection between metabolism and body composition is energy balance—the number of calories you take in versus the number of calories your body burns (see p. 251 for more information).

Q | How do we get fat—literally? What causes the body to retain fat and where does it go?

The body produces and stores fat when more energy is consumed than is used to maintain body functions and fuel activities, including regular daily activities plus exercise. Stored body fat is an adaptation that protects humans from starvation when food is scarce or infrequent—something that is rare in modern life in many parts of the world. Stored body fat can also be used as a source of energy when energy demands increase—for example, dur-

ing times of significant body growth or during pregnancy.

Calories from any source—fat, protein, carbohydrate, alcohol—can cause increases in body fat if consumed in excess. You'll learn more about this delicate balance of energy later in the chapter. For now, consider that 3,500 calories is the equivalent of a pound of body weight, so if you consume 3,500 calories more than your body uses, you will gain a pound. Over the course of a year, consuming just 150 extra calories a day—the number of calories in one can of beer or regular soda—can add up to 15 pounds.

Most fat is stored in fat deposits, which are about 80 percent fat and 20 percent support cells, immune cells, and blood vessels. Droplets of fat are stored in specialized fat cells in these deposits. The number of fat cells stays fairly constant throughout adulthood. If you gain weight as fat, these fat cells enlarge, storing more fat. And if you lose body fat, your fat cells shrink. Some evidence suggests that significant fat gain may also increase the number of fat cells.[3]

It is possible to gain weight as muscle rather than fat, but it requires a careful program of increased energy intake combined with resistance training; see Chapter 9 for specific strategies for healthy weight gain.

Q | Do *overweight* and *obese* mean the same thing?

No. Although there are several ways to assess and define overweight and obesity, obesity is considered a more extreme and serious condition. **Overweight** generally means a body weight above a recommended range, based on large-scale population surveys or studies. **Obesity** is a more serious degree of overweight, characterized by excessive body fat; obesity may also be defined by body weight or a related measure. In addition to body weight and percent body fat, height and waist circumference may be considered in evaluating the health risks associated with a particular body weight or shape. More about specific fat percentage ranges as well as other means of defining overweight and obesity are discussed later in the chapter, in the section "Assessing Body Composition."

Q | Have Americans really gotten fatter?

On average, yes. Twenty years ago, the average weight for Ameri-

metabolism All the processes within the body required to maintain its functioning.

resting metabolic rate (RMR) The energy required to maintain essential body processes at rest, including breathing, blood circulation, and temperature regulation.

overweight Body weight above the recommended range for good health.

obesity A serious degree of overweight characterized by an excessive amount of body fat.

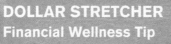

DOLLAR STRETCHER
Financial Wellness Tip

Don't waste money on gadgets or supplements promising fat loss. There's no way to burn calories effortlessly or reduce body fat in a specific spot. Physical activity is free, and consuming fewer calories can also save you money. Visit the Web site of the Federal Trade Commission for additional tips: http://www.ftc.gov/bcp/menus/consumer/health.shtm.

can men and women in their twenties was about 15 pounds less than the average weight for adults in their twenties today. Going back further, fifty years of tracking body mass index, a measure related to body weight and body composition (see p. 246), shows that the prevalence of obesity among Americans has increased significantly, particularly in the 1980s (Figure 7-3).

Factors Affecting Body Composition

Q | Do shorter people have a higher body fat percentage?

No, shorter people don't necessarily have a higher percentage of body fat. Your body composition depends on a combination of factors and, although height may be related to some of them, it doesn't directly predict the amount of fat within your body. Like height, some of the factors that determine body composition are beyond your control. But there are other influences on body composition that you can do something about.

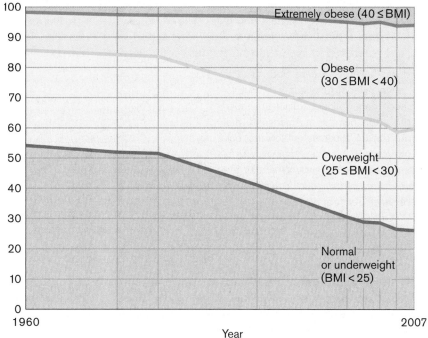

Percent of American adults

Figure 7-3 Prevalence of overweight, obesity, and extreme obesity among U.S. adults

Source: Ogden, C. L., & Carroll, M. D. (2010). Prevalence of overweight, obesity, and extreme obesity among American adults, June 2010. *National Center for Health Statistics Health E-Stat* (http://www.cdc.gov/nchs/data/hestat/obesity_adult_07_08/obesity_adult_07_08.htm).

Fast Facts

The Amazing Human Body Available in All Shapes and Sizes

Height

Average American man:	5 ft. 9 in. tall	Average American woman:	5 ft. 4 in. tall
Tallest man on record:	8 ft. 11 in.	Tallest woman on record:	8 ft. 2 in.
Shortest man on record:	22 in.	Shortest woman on record:	23 in.

Weight

Average American man:	195 lb.	Average American woman:	165 lb.
Heaviest man on record:	1,235 lb.	Heaviest woman on record:	1,189 lb.

Sources: Guinness World Records; World Records Academy; CDC National Center for Health Statistics.

Genetics

Q | Is my body composition going to be similar to that of my parents? Is body composition based at all on genetics?

Yes. Genes influence body size, amount and distribution of body fat, resting metabolic rate, response to exercise and overeating, and other factors related to energy balance. Depending on the factor, the contribution of heredity will be between 25 and 75 percent.[4] However, it can be difficult to separate the effects of genetic inheritance from the eating and activity habits that you "inherit" from the family you grow up in.

Scientists have identified hundreds of genes that appear to have an effect on the levels of fat in the body. For example, the INSIG2 gene controls insulin and slows the synthesis of cholesterol and fatty acids, but about 10 percent of people carry a gene variation that makes them less able to inhibit this synthesis and more likely to build up excess body fat.[5] The fat-mass-and-obesity-related (FTO) gene—dubbed the "Fatso" gene—is associated with increased size and body fat. Researchers found that people with one copy (from one parent) of a particular variant in the FTO gene are likely to be fatter than those with no copies, and people

Research Brief

Beating the "Fatso" Gene

Researchers have identified many genes linked to excess body fat and unhealthy body fat distribution. But do these genes alone explain the rapid rise in the number of Americans who are obese? It seems unlikely that our genes have changed dramatically in the past 20–30 years. What can researchers tell us about the relationship between genes and other factors?

One recent study looked at the effect of variations of the FTO gene, a gene that is clearly associated with obesity. Researchers tested adults to identify which variants of FTO they carried and then compared their body mass index values (body mass index is a method of classifying and evaluating body weight). They also had the study participants wear a device called an accelerometer for a week to track their physical activity.

The researchers found that the FTO gene has a significant effect on whether people are overweight—but only people who are not physically active. Among the study participants who were physically active, body fatness was about the same regardless of the version of the gene they

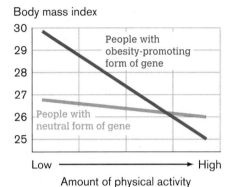

Body mass index

People with obesity-promoting form of gene

People with neutral form of gene

Low ———————→ High
Amount of physical activity

Body fatness versus physical activity for two variations of the FTO gene

carried. Physical activity overcomes the effects of the obesity-promoting variations of the FTO gene.

The results of this study highlight the interaction between genes and environment. Humans have long carried genes that can potentially promote obesity, but these genes came into play only in recent centuries, when a sedentary lifestyle and an abundance of food became possible for many people. It may seem unfair that some of us are born with genes that predispose us to gain body fat and others are not, but the results of this research are good news! A genetic predisposition for obesity is rarely destiny—those of us with obesity-promoting genes may have to work harder to prevent unhealthy fat gain, but we do have some control over our genes through the food and activity choices we make.

Source: Rampersaud, E., Mitchell, B. D., Pollin, T. I., and others. (2008). Physical activity and the association of common FTO gene variants with body mass index and obesity. *Archives of Internal Medicine, 168*(16), 1791–1797.

---

with two copies (from both parents) are likely to be fatter than those with one copy.[6] About one in six adults carries two copies of the FTO gene variant. Other genes influence where fat is most likely to be stored in the body—in the abdomen or in the hips, for example, or as visceral fat versus subcutaneous fat.

Genes do not tell the full story, however. Body composition is a complex trait, influenced by many environmental factors as well as many genes. Some genes that influence body composition come into play only under conditions of excess energy intake or inactivity. For example, researchers have found that for people who are physically active, having a variant of the FTO gene that predisposes them to obesity has no effect;[7] see the box "Beating the 'Fatso' Gene" for more information.

Q | Why is it so hard for skinny guys to gain muscle mass?

As described in Chapter 5, people are born with different numbers of muscle cells and a different proportion of muscle-cell types. Some people are also less likely to gain body weight of any kind—fat or muscle—because

their resting metabolic rates are high and their bodies simply aren't designed for weight or muscle gain. Although "skinny guys" can certainly build muscle, they won't be able to radically change their body type. See Chapter 5 for more about muscle tissue and strength training; see Chapter 9 for strategies for gaining weight.

The same is true for all general body types: We can't change our genetic structure or, in most cases, radically alter our body shape. But we don't all have to be shaped the same in order to have healthy bodies.

Gender

Q | I know men and women's bodies are different, but when my boyfriend and I eat together, it seems like I am more susceptible to weight gain than he is. Why is this?

It's hard to compare any two people—even when they are similar in age or genetic makeup—because so many factors contribute to each person's body composition. As described in the earlier section "Basics of Body Metabolism," if your boyfriend is larger, weighs more, and has more muscle mass than you do, then he can eat more than you without gaining weight because his resting metabolic rate is likely to be higher. Even if they are the same weight, a man will likely have a higher metabolic rate than a woman due to differences in their proportion of muscle and fat; women have a higher proportion of essential body fat. But other gender differences are related to body composition as well—differences that change with age.

On average, male babies are heavier at birth and in the first few months of life than female babies. However, male and female babies often have a similar amount of fat mass. This means girl babies typically are proportionally fatter than boy babies (a higher percent of their total weight is fat). Between ages 1 and 6, both boys and girls tend to lose body fat. After that point, girls' fat levels typically begin to increase, while boys' lean mass increases. As boys and girls move into puberty and adolescence, the differences become even greater—with girls gaining fat mass but very little lean mass, and boys gaining lean mass but very little fat. By early adulthood, males and females are often similar in weight-height ratios, but males tend to have less body fat (Figure 7-4). Female reproductive maturity and childbirth can further contribute to the disparities in body-fat mass.[8]

In midlife, both men and women tend to begin to lose muscle mass—leaving a higher proportion of fat mass. For men, this typically begins in their fifties. For women, it often begins in their forties and is frequently accompanied by increases in fat mass.[9] These declines typically continue for both males and females as they grow older, though by the time they hit their seventies and eighties, both men and women may begin to lose total mass.[10]

Q | Why do men gain fat in their belly, and women in their hips?

Although there is a great deal of individual variation, on average, men are more likely to store excess fat in the abdomen, and women are more likely to store it in the hips and thighs (Figure 7-5).

- *Android,* or apple-shaped, fat distribution is more common in men and postmenopausal women.
- *Gynoid,* or pear-shaped, fat distribution is more common in premenopausal women.

The gender difference is due at least in part to the effects of estrogen in premenopausal women. After menopause, women's estrogen levels drop, and their body shape tends to change to an apple shape. As we'll see later in the chapter, the apple-shaped pattern of fat distribution is associated with more health risks than the pear-shaped pattern of fat distribution. People with an apple shape tend to have a higher proportion of unhealthy visceral fat. You'll have a chance to evaluate your own shape in Lab Activity 7-1.

Age

Q | Does body composition always get worse as we get older?

It's hard to separate the effects of age from use, because we tend to become less active as we age. With each decade they don't strength train, adults lose about 4–6 pounds of muscle mass, and their resting metabolic rate also declines.[11] If calorie intake is not decreased, the energy that had been used to maintain the lost muscle tissue will be stored as fat, thereby increasing percent body fat.

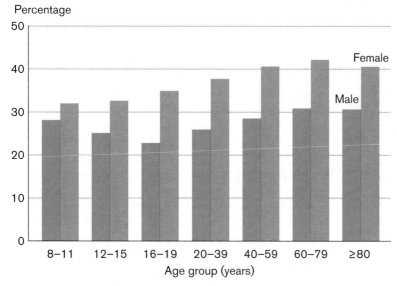

Percentage

Figure 7-4 Average percent body fat by age and gender
Source: U.S. Department of Health and Human Services. (2009). Mean percentage body fat by age group and sex—National Health and Nutrition Examination Survey, United States, 1999–2004. *MMWR Weekly, 57*(552), 1383 (http://www.cdc.gov/mmwr/preview/mmwrhtml/mm5751a4.htm).

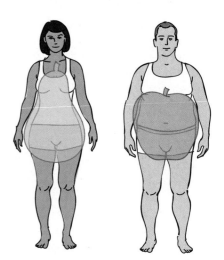

Figure 7-5 Body-fat distribution. Are you an apple or a pear? A pear shape is healthier because it typically means less visceral fat.

Studies have found that older adults usually have a higher percent body fat than younger adults.[12] Excess body fat in young adults is a serious concern because we typically gain fat and lose muscle as we age; an unhealthy amount of body fat in young adulthood makes achieving and maintaining a healthy body composition over time more challenging. The good news is that physical activity, especially resistance training, can maintain muscle mass as you age; strength training can help build muscle and reduce fat at any age.

Ethnicity

Q | Do different ethnicities have different body compositions?

Research tells us the body composition patterns related to gender and age are true across all ethnic groups.[13] However, ethnic differences have been found in average height, weight, and body composition. The extent of the differences can be affected by lifestyle and environmental factors related to culture and ethnicity. More research is needed, especially about how these differences may affect the health and fitness risks and benefits associated with different body compositions. Findings from one study involving detailed body scans of nearly 2,000 adults are shown in Table 7-1. General trends don't apply to every individual in an ethnic group, but findings from this and other research may be relevant when you assess your body composition:

- At a given body weight, Asian Americans and Latinos have a higher percent body fat and a higher percent of abdominal fat than whites and African Americans.
- At a given body weight, African Americans have a lower percent body fat and lower percent of abdominal fat than other ethnic groups, indicating greater relative bone density and muscle mass.

It's important to be aware of these trends when evaluating your body weight and body composition. It also reinforces the fact that each of us is different—and there is no single body size or body composition that is best or even possible for everyone.

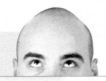

Mind Stretcher
Critical Thinking Exercise

What do you think when you see someone who is especially thin or heavy? Short or tall? Do you associate particular personality traits with different body types? Where do you think your ideas come from? Do you think they are fair and accurate?

Lifestyle and Environment

Q | Some of my cousins are really fat, but my brothers and I are skinny. Why aren't we more alike since we have many of the same genes?

Genetics is one factor in body composition, but there are other influences as well, including age and gender. Different lifestyles and environments may also play a role in your different body compositions, including these four factors:

- **Energy intake:** The amount of energy you take in as food obviously affects body composition. If you consume more calories than you burn, then you will gain weight and possibly fat. If you consume fewer calories than you burn, then you will lose weight and possibly fat. Whether you gain or lose weight as muscle or fat depends on factors such as your genes and activity level.
- **Physical activity:** The amount of energy you burn during daily activity and purposeful exercise also obviously affects energy balance and body composition.
- **Sleep:** Consistent short sleep duration is associated with increased overall body fat and increased abdominal body fat. Lack of sleep may interfere with the regulation of appetite—causing people to eat more—and with the balance of glucose and insulin, possibly increasing the risk of diabetes.[14]
- **Stress:** Excess psychological stress is linked to increased energy intake, weight gain, and excess abdominal fat.[15] During the stress response, the liver produces more glucose to provide energy. If you don't use all the extra glucose, your body reabsorbs it. But if you are frequently or chronically stressed, the extra blood sugar can contribute to glucose intolerance, insulin resistance, and type 2 diabetes. Excess insulin in the blood also encourages the body to store fat.

The good news about lifestyle factors affecting body composition is that you can control or at least influence many of them. However, some environmental factors linked to your body composition, such as the socioeconomic status of the household where you grew up and your parents' educational attainment, may be beyond your control. The characteristics of your neighborhood can also influence your body composition. Is it walkable, so that you have many easy opportunities for daily physical activity? Are there healthy grocery options? How many fast-food restaurants are there? Living in a neighborhood with limited opportunities for physical activity and poor access to healthy foods is a risk factor for unhealthy body composition.[16] These neighborhood characteristics are most often associated with socioeconomically disadvantaged populations and ethnic minorities.

Finally, it's important to remember that overall body size isn't necessarily an indicator of a higher percent of

TABLE 7-1 COMPARISON OF AVERAGE HEIGHT, WEIGHT, BODY MASS INDEX, AND TOTAL AND ABDOMINAL FAT AMONG ADULTS FROM FOUR ETHNIC GROUPS*

	WHITE	AFRICAN AMERICAN	LATINO	ASIAN AMERICAN
MEN				
HEIGHT	69 in.	69 in.	67 in.	67 in.
WEIGHT	176 lb.	177 lb.	173 lb.	152 lb.
BODY MASS INDEX	25.7	26.0	27.1	23.6
ABDOMINAL FAT	9.3 lb.	7.9 lb.	9.1 lb.	9.9 lb.
PERCENT BODY FAT	20.4%	18.6%	20.9%	22.5%
WOMEN				
HEIGHT	64 in.	64 in.	61 in.	62 in.
WEIGHT	156 lb.	174 lb.	150 lb.	120 lb.
BODY MASS INDEX	27.0	29.2	28.4	22.2
ABDOMINAL FAT	12.7 lb.	12.2 lb.	12.7 lb.	13.3 lb.
PERCENT BODY FAT	35.6%	35.3%	37.4%	36.8%

*Based on measurement and dual-energy X-ray absorptiometry of 604 men and 1,192 women ages 18–96 years.
**Body mass index, described on p. 246, is a measure of relative body weight.

Source: Adapted from Wu, C-G., Heshka, S., Wang, J., Pierson, R. N., Heymsfield, S. B., Laferrère, B., Wang, Z., Albu, J. B., Pi-Sunyer, X., & Gallagher, D. (2007). Truncal fat in relation to total body fat: Influences of age, sex, ethnicity and fatness. *International Journal of Obesity, 31(9)*, 1384–1391.

body fat. Just because your cousins are larger doesn't mean they are automatically fatter. You would have to assess their body composition in order to determine their degree of fatness or overfatness.

Body Composition and Wellness

Q | Why is it important to know how much fat is in your body? What can one statistic like percent body fat tell you about health?

Body composition is just one component of health-related fitness. However, as with the other components, there is a desired range for easy performance of daily activities and long-term health maintenance. Maintaining an appropriate level of body fat is vital to a healthy, longer life.

Your body composition can tell you a lot, but as will be described in the section "Assessing Body Composition,"

you will need to consider more than just a single number (percent body fat). A certain amount of fat is healthy and necessary, but too much fat, or too little, can harm your health. As the next two sections discuss, an extremely low or high percent body fat can significantly compromise your quality of life and reduce your life expectancy.

Problems Associated with Excess Body Fat

Q | My dad is really big (I don't like to say "fat") and I worry about him. What are the biggest health risks for him?

The biggest problem for people who are overweight and have a high percent body fat is the increased risk for a number of deadly chronic diseases, leading to reduced life expectancy.

- *Cardiovascular disease:* Obesity is linked to high blood pressure, unhealthy blood fat levels, and increased risk of developing and dying from cardiovascular disease.

Research Brief

Screen Time and Waistlines

Many studies conducted over the past few decades have demonstrated an increase in the average number of hours of television people watch each day. Studies have also shown a connection between hours of television and obesity, especially in children. What about for adults?

Researchers recently looked at the number of reported hours of screen time (television and computer) among nearly 100,000 adults to determine if there was a relation-

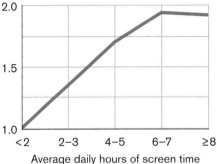

Screen time and relative risk of obesity

ship among screen time, physical activity, obesity, and other factors. They found that the risk of obesity increased for both men and women with increasing amounts of screen time, no matter what their physical-activity level was. Adults who averaged six or more hours of screen time per day had almost double the

rate of obesity risk of adults who averaged less than two hours of daily screen time.

What does this research mean for you? Limiting screen time is a good strategy for reducing your risk for unhealthy body composition. You may have a job—now or in the future—that requires a lot of screen time, so it's important to note that this study found that physical activity could reduce the risk of obesity due to too much screen time. So if you can't reduce the number of hours you spend in front of screens for work or school, cut back on your leisure screen time and engage in regular physical activity instead. For parents, it's important to limit children's screen time, because other research has shown that childhood television viewing habits often persist into adulthood.

Source: Banks, E., Jorm, L., Rogers, K., Clements, M., & Bauman, A. (2010, April 22). Screen time, obesity, aging, and disability. *Public Health Nutrition*, epub ahead of print.

- *Type 2 diabetes:* Excess body fat is the main risk factor for type 2 diabetes, and rates of diabetes among Americans have increased along with the rates of overweight and obesity.
- *Cancer:* Excess body fat increases the risk for cancer of the breast, prostate, colon, pancreas, esophagus, endometrium (part of the uterus), kidney, and other sites. One recent report estimated that obesity causes 100,000 cases of cancer in the United States each year.[17]

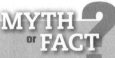

MYTH or FACT?

It's healthier to be 25 pounds overweight and physically active than to be at an optimal weight and sedentary.

▶ WATCH ONLINE

Other health problems associated with overweight and obesity include osteoarthritis, sleep apnea, asthma and other respiratory problems, gallbladder and liver diseases, and reproductive problems.

As described earlier, the risk for some health problems is greater if the excess fat is in their abdomen instead of the hips. Visceral fat is closely linked to unhealthy cholesterol levels, problems with insulin regulation, and increased blood pressure. Researchers are still investigating the exact mechanisms by which visceral fat harms health. One idea relates to its

proximity to the liver; substances released by visceral-fat stores may influence the liver's production of cholesterol in unhealthy ways.

So although subcutaneous fat may be what most people have in mind when they think about losing excess body fat, it's visceral fat that can do more damage to your health. Removal of subcutaneous fat through liposuction doesn't improve metabolic measures such as insulin sensitivity, whereas weight loss through diet and exercise does. Losing body fat through changes in diet and physical activity reduces the amount of dangerous visceral fat in the body.[18]

In addition to shortening life expectancy, obesity can also reduce years of healthy life. Obese people spend a greater portion of their life with disabilities that interfere with day-to-day living. Obesity has many serious consequences, but obesity can be reversed. It is never too late to start making changes that can lead to a longer and healthier life.

Q | Can you be sort of overweight or over-fat and healthy at the same time?

Maybe. The health consequences of a moderate degree of excess body fat and weight are controversial and the subject of ongoing research. The following factors can make a difference:

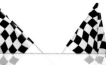
- *Age and weight history:* Overweight in someone young is of extra concern because his or her body will be exposed to the effects of overweight for a longer period. Also, we usually gain weight and fat as we age, so someone who is moderately overweight as a young adult is at increased risk of becoming dangerously obese in later life. Has your weight remained stable, or has it gone up as you've gotten older?

- *Body fat distribution:* As described earlier in the chapter, health risks from body fat are greater if the excess fat is stored in the abdomen rather than in the hips and thighs.

- *Other health risk factors:* Someone who is overweight and who has, for example, high blood pressure and elevated glucose levels is at greater risk for health problems than someone who is overweight but doesn't have additional risk factors.

- *Lifestyle:* Even if it doesn't significantly lower your weight, regular exercise can improve body composition and reduce some of the risks associated with overweight, including high blood pressure and unhealthy cholesterol levels.

Once gained, excess fat is difficult to shed. If you have a slightly or moderately elevated percent body fat, strive to adopt a healthy diet and physical activity habits that will help prevent weight and fat gain and reduce other risk factors.[19] One of the biggest concerns about a small degree of overweight is that it won't stay small.

Problems Associated with Too Little Body Fat

Q What is the lowest body fat percentage you can have and still maintain a healthy lifestyle? Is it even possible for a woman to have absolutely no body fat?

No, it's not possible for a woman (or a man) to have zero body fat—and you wouldn't want to. As noted earlier, a certain amount of fat is essential for the body to function properly and to sustain life. Underweight people with low body fat are often malnourished. As a result they may have fluid imbalances, vitamin and mineral deficiencies, and kidney problems; they are more likely to lose bone mass and develop osteoporosis. Women may also experience reproductive disorders. Appropriate body fat ranges are presented in the section "Assessing Body Composition."

Q If I exercise a lot and my period stops, is that a good thing or a bad thing?

Usually that is a bad thing. Some women develop a condition known as the **female athlete triad.** It is most common in those participating in sports that emphasize

female athlete triad
A condition in active females that develops because excess exercise or insufficient energy intake or both results in insufficient available energy; characterized by amenorrhea and loss of bone density.

leanness, such as gymnastics, diving, ice skating, and cross-country running, but it can occur in any sport or with any form of regular strenuous exercise.[20] The disorder is called a triad because it has three components, each of which can occur on a continuum between optimal/healthy and unhealthy (Figure 7-6):

- **Energy availability:** A healthy level of available energy supports physical activity, bone health, and menstruation. Insufficient energy intake leads to loss of bone density and menstrual disorders. Low energy availability is usually the result of insufficient calorie intake or increased energy expenditure through exercise without increasing calorie intake. The Triad can be caused by disordered eating patterns or full-blown eating disorders.
- **Menstruation:** Healthy energy availability supports hormonal function and regular menstruation. Low energy availability leads to menstrual disorders and eventually to amenorrhea (absence of menstruation for more than 90 days), which can reduce bone density. Amenorrhea and other types of menstrual dysfunction are associated with a state of estrogen deficiency similar to menopause. Menstrual irregularities and low bone mass increase the risk of stress fractures.
- **Bone health:** Low energy availability reduces bone density in two ways—by suppressing hormones that promote bone formation and by causing amenorrhea. The loss of bone density may not be fully reversible even if the issues underlying the Triad are addressed.

If you experience any of the signs of developing the Triad, you should consult a medical professional and be assessed for all the components. Many athletes can continue with their regular training and deal with Triad-related health problems with adequate nutrition and energy intake.

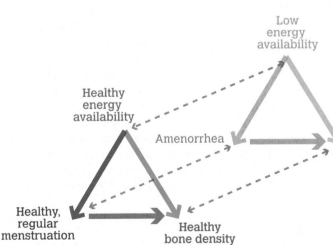

Figure 7-6 The female athlete triad. The disorder includes three components, each of which occurs on a continuum between healthy and unhealthy.

Source: Adapted from American College of Sports Medicine. (2007). Position stand: The female athlete triad. *Medicine and Science in Sports and Exercise, 39*(10), 1867–1882.

Body Composition and Athletic Performance

Q | I'm a runner. Will decreasing my body fat help make me faster?

That's a difficult question because many factors beyond body composition determine your running speed. Other factors being equal though, a decreased level of body fat (that is still in the healthy range) might improve your performance and reduce your susceptibility to performance-related injuries.[21]

Most athletes rely on two things for good performance: the ability to sustain both aerobic and anaerobic power and the ability to overcome resistance, or what is often referred to as "drag." This presents a dilemma for athletes who associate overcoming drag with eating less and losing weight—which they may think equates to losing body fat. However, most of them also know they need to eat more in order to increase energy and sustain their activity.

With the intention of losing weight and decreasing fat, some athletes fall into a bad cycle of eating too little, burning a lot of calories through activity, losing lean muscle mass (and thus increasing percent body fat), decreasing performance, eating even less, and so on. This spiral can sometimes lead to eating disorders that pose serious risks to health (see Chapter 9) as well as to the female athlete triad in women.

Decreased body fat can improve performance in some athletes, but only if it's still at a healthy level. Athletes must consume enough calories to fuel their efforts and maintain lean body mass and a healthy level of body fat. Too little energy intake and body fat harm both health and athletic performance.

There is not an ideal percent body fat for each sport, but your coach, trainer, or doctor can help you find an appropriate range for your sport.

Body Composition, Body Image, and Emotional Wellness

"I'm too fat." "I'm too skinny." "I'd be happy if I were taller / shorter / had bigger muscles / longer legs . . ." Do any of these statements sound familiar? Many of us have difficulty accepting our bodies, and this dissatisfaction can hurt our self-esteem and emotional wellness.

Q | What exactly is body image?

Body image is your mental picture of your body and how you feel about it. Body image includes thoughts, attitudes, emotions, and perceptions.

body image An individual's subjective mental representation of his or her body, including thoughts, attitudes, emotions, and perceptions.

Mind Stretcher
Critical Thinking Exercise

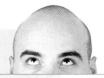

Think about your work, play, home, and school activities. How might a body fat percentage that is too low or too high be negatively affecting your daily activities? What about your friends and family members? Use the behavior change technique of self-reevaluation (Chapter 2) to imagine how various body compositions would change your day-to-day life.

It is subjective, so what you "see" in the mirror may not be the same as what others see. Your body image may be realistic or unrealistic, just like your goals for your body shape or size. Many of us have internalized cultural ideals of appearance that are far removed from what is possible, or even healthy, for us to achieve.

A negative body image can cause stress, anxiety, and depression; in some cases, it can lead to disordered patterns of eating and other negative health habits (see Chapter 9 for more on eating disorders). A positive body image supports emotional wellness and healthy attitudes, behaviors, and self-esteem.

Many of us have small or moderate body-image issues, but a few people develop an extremely negative and unrealistic body image. **Body dysmorphic disorder (BDD)** is characterized by extreme preoccupation with an imagined defect in appearance—the focus might be on a particular feature, such as the skin or nose, or on body shape in general. People with BDD typically isolate themselves from others out of fear of being judged for their "defect," and they have very low self-esteem. They may engage in compulsive behaviors such as mirror checking, use cosmetics or clothing to camouflage the imaged defect, and seek multiple plastic surgeries. Although more common in women, BDD can also affect men. A form of BDD more common in men is **muscle dysmorphia,** or becoming obsessed with the idea of not being big or muscular enough. People with muscle dysmorphia may spend all of their time at the gym while ignoring other parts of their life; they use exercise compulsively to feel better about themselves and may also take supplements or even steroids in an effort to fix the perceived problem. BDD is different from eating disorders, but like them, it is considered a psychological disorder that requires professional treatment.

body dysmorphic disorder (BDD) A psychological disorder characterized by extreme preoccupation with an imagined defect in appearance.

muscle dysmorphia A form of BDD more common in males, characterized by preoccupation with perceived lack of muscularity.

Q | Where does body image come from?

Two key sources of body image (and self-esteem) are family and the media. Parents who criticize their children and the way they look, rather than praising them, create a negative self-image and lower self-esteem. These family influences are often subtle and are often dismissed ("It's no big deal; my mom says that about everyone"), but over time they have a cumulative effect on body image and self-esteem. Peers and

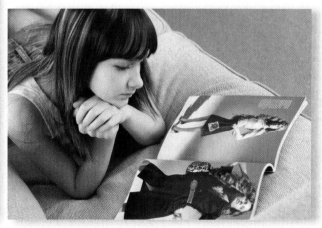

Body image is our subjective mental picture of how our body looks and how we feel about it. A negative body image can cause stress and impair emotional wellness.

teachers can also influence our attitudes about body image through their comments and how they treat people of different body shapes and sizes.

The media is a major influence on body image. The pressure to look a certain way, male or female, is everywhere. All forms of media contain messages about how we should look, and they imply that if we don't conform, something is terribly wrong. These daily messages have an impact, especially on young people already predisposed toward a negative body image. Here are some sobering statistics:

- In surveys, the biggest wish of girls 10–14 is to lose weight.
- For adolescent girls, the media tends to be the main source of information about women's health issues; the majority of middle school girls read at least one fashion magazine regularly.
- Women's magazines have more than ten times more advertisements and articles promoting weight loss than men's magazines.
- A study of over four thousand network television commercials revealed that 1 of every 3.8 commercials sends some sort of "attractiveness message," telling viewers what is or is not attractive; the average adolescent sees over 5,260 "attractiveness messages" per year.[22]

Barbie dolls are a classic example of body image distortion promoted by the media. We all know that Barbie and Ken's body proportions are absurdly unreal, yet they continue to be regarded as having ideal, albeit unattainable, bodies. Similarly, male action figures have grown increasing large and muscular over the years and now have a degree of muscularity not found in even bodybuilders. Another example is fashion models and the winners of the Miss America pageant, who have gotten significantly thinner since the 1920s and many of whom now would be classified as underweight (Figure 7-7). The growing gap between actual and idealized body type can contribute to a negative body image.

Fast Facts

If Barbie and Ken Were Real

If Barbie and Ken were blown up to life size,

- Barbie would be 7 feet 5 inches tall, with a 40-inch chest and a 22-inch waist.
- Ken would be 7 feet 8 inches tall, with a 50-inch chest and a 43-inch waist.

Typical American adults are quite different:

- The average American woman is 5 feet 4 inches tall and has a 35-inch waist.
- The average American man is 5 feet 10 inches tall and has a 37-inch waist.

Sources: National Center for Health Statistics. (2008). Anthropometric reference data for children and adults. *National Health Statistics Reports*, No. 10. Brownell, K. D., & Napolitano, M. A. (1995). Distorting reality for children: Body size proportions of Barbie and Ken dolls. *International Journal of Eating Disorders, 18*(3), 295–298.

Q So we're supposed to worry about how we look for health reasons, but not worry about how we look. How does that work?

For body composition and body image, what's important is what is healthy for you. Assess your body com-

Figure 7-7 Average young women vs. fashion models and Miss America (1920s–2000s). In the 1920s, the idealized body type represented by Miss America and fashion models was very close to the typical body type of young women. During the twentieth century, however, the gap widened between real and idealized young women.
Sources: Byrd-Bredbenner, C., Murray, J., & Schlussel, Y. R. (2005). Temporal changes in anthropometric measurements of idealized females and young women in general. *Women & Health, 41*(2), 13–30. National Center for Health Statistics. (2008). Anthropometric reference data for children and adults. *National Health Statistics Reports, 10.*

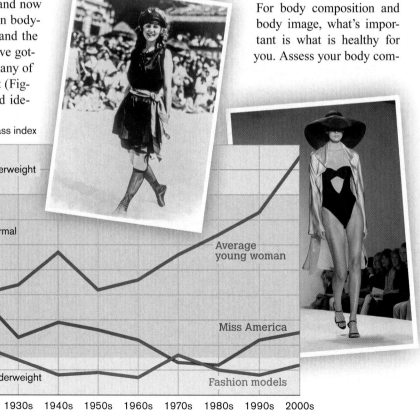

Wellness Strategies

Accepting Your Body

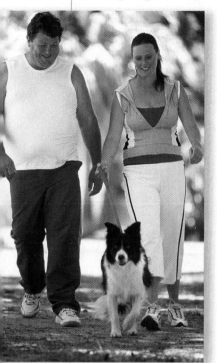

To avoid body image problems and boost your self-esteem, focus on good physical and emotional health and engage in some body acceptance.

- **Focus on the positives—** your body's unique beauty and functionality. Remember, too, that body composition, weight, and shape are just one aspect of wellness. Your self-esteem and self-image should be based on all the things you think and do.

- **Focus on health and healthy habits.** Evaluate your body composition based on health criteria. Engage in healthy eating and physical activity habits—and feel good about yourself for making positive wellness choices. For many people, exercise improves body image even if it doesn't change their weight or body shape; regular exercise can provide feelings of competency and mastery that boost self-esteem and body image.

- **Realistically evaluate which aspects of your body you can change.** Everyone has things they can't change and need to accept—your height and your shoe size, for example. Look around at your family; if most of

them have narrow shoulders or broad hips, or are "small-muscled" or "big-boned," then those are likely inherited characteristics of your body too. Some people are genetically designed to be bigger or smaller than others. Accept that and move on.

- **Set goals that are small and attainable.** Unrealistic goals can undermine your efforts at behavior change and damage your self-esteem. This is especially true for people who have a negative body image. Focus on behavior-oriented goals—such as engaging in regular strength training workouts—rather than on goals related to specific aspects of your body.

- **Avoid negative self-talk about your body.** Don't compare yourself to other people or to media ideals. Remember that the models you see in the media typically have atypical body types supported by expensive cosmetics and clothing as well as photographic touch-ups. Focus on the good things you do and the positive aspects of your life.

- **Recognize advertisements from the fitness and beauty industries as what they are**—attempts to make you dissatisfied with yourself and your life so that you will buy their products. Be a media-literate consumer.

- **Just as you don't judge yourself by appearance, don't judge others.** Body size and shape are just one external characteristic. Judge the people in your life based on what they say and do, not on how they look.

Sources: Wood-Barcalow, N. L, Tylka, T. L., & Augustus-Horvath, C. L. (2010). "But I like my body": Positive body image characteristics and a holistic model for young-adult women. *Body Image, 7*(2), 106–116. Vocks, S., Hechler, T., Rohrig, S., & Legenbauer, T. (2009). Effects of a physical exercise session on state body image. *Psychological Health, 24*(6), 713–728.

position according to health criteria (see the next section), and avoid comparing yourself to unachievable cultural and media ideals. Instead of trying to change the way you look, which isn't always easy, change the way you think about your body. Recognize that, regardless of its size and shape, your body is a gift to you. Treat it as such, and you will begin to appreciate the marvel your body is. See the box "Accepting Your Body" for ideas to improve your body image.

Assessing Body Composition

Q | What's my ideal weight?

That's a tough question to answer. As you've learned in this chapter, body weight

and even percent body fat don't provide a full picture of how your body composition might affect your health and wellness. A healthy body composition for you also depends on other health risk factors including fat distribution, blood pressure, and your exercise habits.

Percent body fat is a better indicator of health status than overall body weight—a scale can't distinguish between fat, muscle, and bone—but it is difficult to measure. In fact, even high-tech tests for percent body fat yield only estimates because exact body composition can be determined only after death.

This section will review various techniques for evaluating body weight, percent body fat, and body fat distribution. Lab Activity 7-1 walks you through the steps of calculating and evaluating your own BMI, percent body fat, and body fat distribution.

Wellness Strategies

Calculating Body Mass Index

Visit the book's Web site for an online BMI calculator. To perform the calculations by hand, use the formulas below or in Lab Activity 7-1. Measure your height with shoes off and your weight with minimal clothing. To measure waist circumference, place a measuring tape flat against your skin, above the iliac crest (hip bone) at the narrowest point of your waist; keep the tape horizontal as you measure. Look up your BMI and waist circumference in Table 7-2.

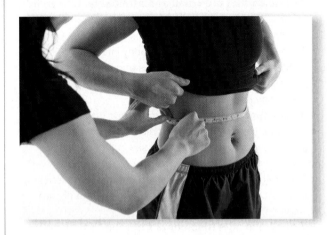

If you know your body weight in kilograms and your height in meters:

Formula	Example	
$\dfrac{\text{Weight (kg)}}{(\text{Height [m]})^2}$	$\dfrac{70 \text{ kg}}{(1.7 \text{ m})^2}$	$= 24.2 \text{ kg/m}^2$

If you only know your body weight in pounds and your height in inches:

Formula	Example	
$\dfrac{\text{Weight (lb.)}}{(\text{Height [in.]})^2} \times 703$	$\dfrac{165 \text{ lb.}}{(68 \text{ in.})^2} \times 703$	$= 25.1 \text{ kg/m}^2$

Note: 1 pound = 0.4536 kilograms; 1 inch = 0.0254 meters; in the second formula, the multiplier 703 converts the units to kg/m^2.

Body Mass Index: An Indirect Measure of Body Fat

Q How do I determine my BMI?

Body mass index (BMI) is one of the most common techniques for assessing body fatness, and it is useful if you don't have access to equipment for estimating percent body fat. Many research studies have compared BMI against the risk of developing health problems, so BMI can provide guidance in determining if your weight places you at risk. Although, like the old insurance company tables, BMI is based on height and weight, it is a more accurate indicator.

BMI is calculated by dividing your weight (in kilograms) by the square of your height (in meters); see the box "Calculating Body Mass Index" or refer to Figure 7-8. According to guidelines from the National Institutes of Health, a person is classified as underweight if his or her BMI is below 18.5, overweight if it is 25 or above, and obese if it is 30 or above (Table 7-2). Because BMI doesn't distinguish between weight from fat and weight from lean tissue, measurement of waist circumference is used to help classify the health risks associated with different BMI values. As described earlier, excess fat in the abdomen is linked to greater health risks than fat stored in other regions of the body.

body mass index (BMI) An indirect measure of body fatness calculated by dividing body weight (in kilograms) by the square of height (in meters); for non-athletic populations, BMI correlates closely with more precise measures of body composition.

Q Is BMI relevant and accurate for both athletes and people who are out of shape?

Not entirely, no. BMI is only an indirect measure of body composition. BMI is most accurate for non-athletes and people who don't do a lot of strength training; for them, BMI measures have been highly correlated with more precise measures of body fat. However, athletes and people with an above-average amount of muscle mass are likely to have a BMI in the overweight range when they actually have a healthy body composition. If you are athletic or heavily muscled, one of the methods of estimating percent body fat is probably a more accurate assessment for you. Look as well at waist circumference and some of the other measures of body fat distribution described in the next section.

BMI may also be less accurate for older adults, who tend to have more fat mass and less muscle mass than younger people of the same weight. Older adults may be classified in the normal BMI range when they actually have excess body fat. In addition, there has been a significant amount of debate about whether there should be different cutoffs for people in different ethnic groups. As mentioned earlier in the chapter, Asian Americans tend to have a higher percent body fat and African Americans a lower percent body fat at a given weight. For Asian Americans, researchers have proposed lower BMI cutoff points for the classification of overweight and obesity; however, there is no universally agreed upon standard.[23]

Figure 7-8 **Body mass index.** Find your height in the left column and then your weight in the appropriate row. Your BMI will be in the top row of the table above your weight. For example, if you are 5′ 7″ and weigh 160 pounds, your BMI is 25.

Source: Ratings from the National Heart, Lung, and Blood Institute. (1998). *Clinical guidelines on the identification, evaluation, and treatment of overweight and obesity in adults.* Bethesda, MD: National Institutes of Health.

	<18.5 Underweight		18.5–24.9 Normal						25–29.9 Overweight					30–34.9 Obesity (class I)					35–39.9 Obesity (class II)					>40 Extremely obese
BMI	17	18	19	20	21	22	23	24	25	26	27	28	29	30	31	32	33	34	35	36	37	38	39	40
Height (inches)												Body weight (pounds)												
58	81	86	91	96	101	105	110	115	120	124	129	134	139	144	148	153	158	162	168	172	177	182	187	192
59	84	89	94	99	104	109	114	119	124	129	134	139	144	149	154	159	163	168	173	178	183	188	193	198
60	87	92	97	102	108	113	118	123	128	133	138	143	149	154	159	164	168	174	179	184	190	195	200	205
61	90	95	101	106	111	117	122	127	132	138	143	148	154	159	164	169	174	180	185	191	196	201	207	212
62	93	98	104	109	115	120	126	131	137	142	148	153	159	164	170	175	180	186	191	197	202	208	213	219
63	96	102	107	113	119	124	130	136	141	147	153	158	164	169	175	181	186	191	198	203	209	215	220	226
64	99	105	111	117	122	128	134	140	146	152	157	163	169	175	181	186	192	197	204	210	215	222	227	233
65	102	108	114	120	126	132	138	144	150	156	162	168	174	180	186	192	198	204	210	216	222	229	235	241
66	105	112	118	124	130	136	143	149	155	161	167	174	180	186	192	198	204	210	217	223	229	236	242	248
67	109	115	121	128	134	141	147	153	160	166	173	179	185	192	198	205	211	217	224	230	236	243	249	256
68	112	118	125	132	138	145	151	158	165	171	178	184	191	197	204	211	216	223	230	237	244	250	257	263
69	115	122	129	136	142	149	156	163	169	176	183	190	197	203	210	217	224	230	237	244	251	258	264	271
70	119	126	133	139	146	153	160	167	174	181	188	195	202	209	216	223	230	237	244	251	258	265	272	279
71	122	129	136	143	151	158	165	172	179	187	194	201	208	215	222	230	237	244	251	258	265	273	280	287
72	125	133	140	148	155	162	170	177	184	192	199	207	214	221	229	236	243	251	258	266	273	280	288	295
73	129	137	144	152	159	167	174	182	190	197	205	212	220	228	235	243	250	258	265	273	281	288	296	303
74	132	140	148	155	164	171	179	187	195	203	210	218	226	234	242	249	257	265	273	281	288	296	304	312
75	136	144	152	160	168	176	184	192	200	208	216	224	232	240	248	256	264	272	280	288	296	304	312	320
76	140	148	156	164	173	181	189	197	206	214	222	230	238	247	255	263	271	280	288	296	304	312	321	329

TABLE 7-2 BODY MASS INDEX (BMI) CLASSIFICATION AND DISEASE RISK*

	BMI (kg/m²)	DISEASE RISK RELATIVE TO NORMAL WEIGHT AND WAIST CIRCUMFERENCE*	
		MEN: WAIST ≤40 in. (102 cm) WOMEN: WAIST ≤35 in. (88 cm)	MEN: WAIST >40 in. (102 cm) WOMEN: WAIST >35 in. (88 cm)
UNDERWEIGHT	<18.5		
NORMAL	18.5–24.9		
OVERWEIGHT	25.0–29.9	Increased	High
OBESITY (CLASS I)	30.0–34.9	High	Very high
OBESITY (CLASS II)	35.0–39.9	Very high	Very high
EXTREME OBESITY (CLASS III)	≥40.0	Extremely high	Extremely high

*Disease risk for type 2 diabetes, hypertension, and CVD; increased waist circumference can be a marker for increased risk even in persons of normal weight.

Source: National Heart, Lung, and Blood Institute. (1998). *Clinical guidelines on the identification, evaluation, and treatment of overweight and obesity in adults.* Bethesda, MD: National Institutes of Health.

Despite its limitations, BMI can be relatively accurate for the average adult. Although it's not the most accurate way to estimate body composition, it is a good place to start if you don't have access to more direct methods of assessment.

Methods for Estimating Percent Body Fat

Q How can you determine body-fat percentages?

There are a number of different ways to estimate percent body fat. Some methods require expensive medical equipment, but others can be done in a gym or classroom. Check with your instructor or your campus or community health center to find out what methods are available to you.

Table 7-3 gives an overview of some of the more common methods for estimating percent body fat, along with information about each method's accuracy. The margin of error refers to how close the estimate is likely to be to your actual percent body fat; if you have 20 percent body fat, then a method with a 2.5 percent margin of error may yield a result between 17.5 percent and 22.5 percent body fat.

For best results, follow the directions given by the professional helping you with the test. Follow his or her instructions about the type of clothing you should wear and

TABLE 7-3 PERCENT-BODY-FAT ASSESSMENT METHODS

METHOD	MARGIN OF ERROR	DESCRIPTION
SKINFOLD MEASUREMENTS	±3.5%	Folds of skin and subcutaneous fat at specific body locations are measured with an instrument called a *caliper*. These measurements are used in equations that link the thickness of skinfolds to percent-body-fat calculations made from more precise assessment methods. The accuracy of skinfold calculations depends on the skill of the person taking the measurements as well as the quality of the calipers. Spring-loaded metal calipers with parallel surfaces are generally best.
UNDERWATER (HYDROSTATIC) WEIGHING	±2.5%	The person is weighed under typical conditions and then submerged and weighed under water. Percentages of body fat and fat-free weight are calculated from the results. This method is based on the differing densities of fat and muscle (see p. 233). A person with a greater proportion of body fat will weigh relatively less under water.
BIOELECTRICAL IMPEDANCE ANALYSIS (BIA)	±3.5–5.0%	The person stands on or holds a specialized scale, or electrodes are attached to the skin, or both. A small electrical current is sent through the body, and the body's resistance ("impedance") to the current is recorded. The signal is impeded most in fatty areas of the body because there is less water in body fat. The amount of resistance relates to the amount of water in the body, and the measurement is used in calculations that estimate percent body fat.
AIR DISPLACEMENT PLETHYSMOGRAPHY	±2.2–3.7%	The person sits in a small sealed chamber; the best-known is the BodPod. Computer sensors measure the amount of air the person displaces, and percent body fat is calculated from the results. The BodPod is an expensive piece of equipment and not widely available.
DUAL X-RAY ABSORPTIOMETRY (DXA)	±1.8%	A specialized medical scanner aims two X-ray beams with differing energy levels at the person. DXA scans were initially developed to measure bone density, but the results can also be used to estimate body fat content. DXA has a small margin of error and is a noninvasive procedure; however, the scanners are not widely available outside medical settings or for routine use.

Source: Margin of error data from American College of Sports Medicine. (2009). *ACSM's resource manual for guidelines for exercise testing and prescription* (6th ed.). Baltimore, MD: Lippincott Williams & Wilkins.

whether you should refrain from eating, drinking, or exercising for any period of time prior to the test. If you repeat the assessment method in the future to compare results, try to replicate the conditions as closely as possible—for example, the same time of day—for more accurate results.

Q | What's the right percent body fat for me?

There are no universally accepted standards for percent body fat for either health or athletic performance; Figure 7-9 shows the standards published by the American College of Sports Medicine. The appropriate, right, or ideal level of body fat for you depends on your age, gender, current body composition and health status, and, to some extent, your goals. For example, women have and need more fat than men, and the level of fat typically increases with age. Therefore, an appropriate, healthy level of fat for a 20-year-old-man is not the same as what is appropriate and healthy for a 45-year-old woman, which is not the same as what is appropriate and healthy for a 60-year-old woman.

If you are an athlete whose performance may be affected by body fat, you may choose to work to maintain a lower level of fat than the average person. Of course, you should always maintain a sufficient level of energy and nutrient intake to support performance and good long-term health.

Methods for Assessing Body-Fat Distribution

Q | Does body shape make any difference when assessing weight and percent body fat?

Yes, it does. As described earlier in the chapter, fat in the abdomen is a greater risk to health than fat stored in other areas. DXA scans can estimate the amount of fat in the abdomen, but other simpler methods provide information about whether your body fat distribution is healthy.[24] Instructions for each of these methods appear in Lab Activity 7-1.

- **Waist circumference:** As discussed in the section on BMI, simply measuring your waist can provide an estimate of body fat distribution. Women with waist measurements over 35 inches and men with waist measurements over 40 inches are at higher risk for health problems; see Lab Activity 7-1 for a more detailed set of waist circumference standards.
  - **Waist-to-hip ratio:** Comparing your waist measurement and your hip measurement is another means of assessing abdominal obesity. Divide your waist measurement by your hip measurement; your waist should be measured at its narrowest point and your hips at the widest point. Women with waist-to-hip ratios over 0.71 and men with waist-to-hip ratios over 0.83 are at higher risk for health problems; see Lab Activity 7-1 for a more detailed set of standards for waist-to-hip ratio.
  - **Waist-to-height ratio:** A third way to judge abdominal obesity is to compare your waist measurement to your height (both measured in either inches or centimeters). A healthy ratio is less than 0.5, meaning your waist is no larger than half your height.[25] Waist-to-height ratio reflects your overall body shape.

These three tests provide some estimate of the risks associated with abdominal fat. However, they cannot distinguish between subcutaneous fat and visceral fat. Tests based on waist circumference may not identify people who have little subcutaneous fat in their abdomen but an unhealthy amount of visceral fat. In most cases, though, people with significant visceral fat have enough combined subcutaneous and visceral abdominal fat that the tests described in this section—

Women

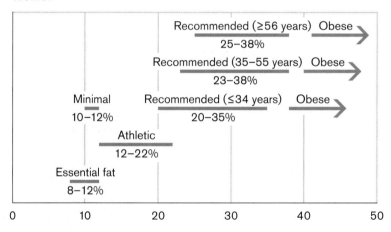

Men

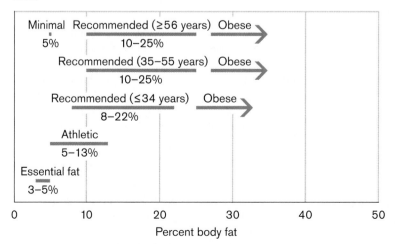

Percent body fat

Figure 7-9 Percent body-fat standards for men and women

Source: American College of Sports Medicine. (2009). *ACSM's resource manual for guidelines for exercise testing and prescription* (6th ed.). Baltimore, MD: Lippincott Williams & Wilkins.

waist circumference, waist-to-hip ratio, and waist-to-height ratio—will identify them as at risk.

Making Changes in Body Composition

Achieving and maintaining a healthy body composition is a huge challenge in our society—most people have sedentary jobs and are surrounded by tempting, high-calorie foods. But you can take control, set goals, and develop strategies that will work for you. Your eating choices and activity patterns are the two main factors determining body composition that are under your control. You've learned a lot about exercise and physical activity in Chapters 3–6; healthy foods and dietary patterns are described in detail in Chapters 8 and 9. This section introduces the energy balance equation (Figure 7-10).

Setting Appropriate Goals

Q | What's a good goal for body weight and body fat?

Before setting any type of goal, review the results of your assessment tests and any related health-risk factors. Do the assessments indicate that your body composition is a potential risk factor for you? If so, choose a goal based on BMI, percent body fat, or body fat distribution. If you are close to the healthy range for body composition, you might want to set a goal based on lifestyle—such as increasing daily physical activity or starting a strength-training program. Exercise can improve measures of health even if it doesn't significantly change your body composition or body weight. Exercise is also extremely helpful for preventing future increases in body fat and weight.

Apply the SMART criteria to your goal. Remember that your goal needs to be realistic and achievable. Genetics limit your capacity to change—whether your goal is to lose body fat or gain muscle—and any goal you set should be consistent with overall good physical and emotional wellness. BMI and percent body fat can guide you in setting a goal, but consider your individual health and lifestyle factors as well. Set a goal that you will be able to maintain over the long term.

If you are significantly overweight or overfat, or if you have risk factors such as high blood pressure or diabetes, consult a physician in order to set a body-composition goal that is appropriate for you. For people who are obese, even modest fat loss, especially if combined with increased exercise, is likely to bring significant health improvements. It is better to maintain a modest amount of fat loss than to lose much more and then quickly gain it all back.

To track progress toward your goal, you can periodically weigh yourself even though weight isn't a precise measure of your body composition. If you are losing pounds

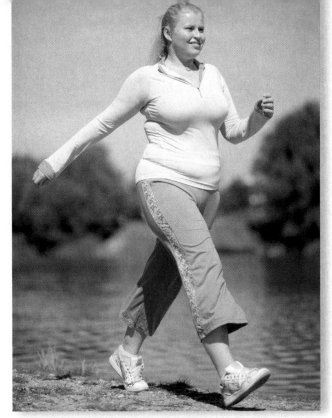

For people with excess body fat, even a small amount of weight loss can significantly improve health—especially if exercise is part of the plan!

Behavior Change Challenge
Video Case Study

▶ WATCH ONLINE   Meet Oscar

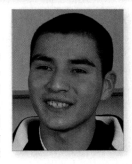

Oscar attends a community college and has just been accepted to a four-year school in the architectural program. He is physically active and currently has a percent body fat in the healthy range, but he is concerned about his family history of diabetes and what will happen when he goes away to college and is no longer eating at home. Oscar has set a specific goal for lowering his percent body fat. Watch the video to learn more about Oscar, his behavior-change goals and plan, and how successful he is over the initial weeks of his program. As you watch the video, think about the following questions:

- How realistic are Oscar's goals and his starting program plan?
- Does Oscar have enough motivation and environmental support for his program? What are likely to be his biggest challenges? What do you think of the strategies he's chosen?
- What can you learn from Oscar's experience that will help you in your behavior-change efforts?

at a slow rate while maintaining an exercise program, it is likely that you are losing body fat. For some people, checking their weight can be a motivation to keep their behavior-change program on track; for others, checking their weight is stressful and actually decreases motivation. Pick a monitoring strategy that works best for you.

You can repeat percent-body-fat tests periodically as well. Don't get too hung up on any particular measure—body weight, BMI, or body fat—none are precise, and as you've learned in this chapter, they don't tell the full story about your particular body composition. Also consider how you feel—your energy level, the fit of your clothes, and how well you are sticking with the lifestyle strategies you planned for improving your body composition.

Focusing on Energy Balance

Q | What's the best way to lose body fat?

There's no one best way to lose body fat, and it's important to look at both sides of the energy balance equation (Figure 7-10). You can choose strategies that affect both the "Energy In" side of the balance (calories consumed) as well as the "Energy Out" side. If your weight is currently stable, then the two sides of the equation are balanced. If you're currently gaining or losing weight—or would like to—then the balance is tipped in one direction or the other.

Q | Why do I lose weight but not body fat?

Weight loss doesn't automatically equal fat loss. Any weight decrease can be in the form of fat, water, or muscle, and if you lose weight as muscle, your body composition will not improve. Losing more muscle than fat is most likely if you focus only on the "energy in" side of the balance—especially if you lose weight quickly through large cuts in energy intake. Depending on other factors, your body may respond by slowing resting metabolism and preserving its fat stores—definitely not your goal. Dieting can lead to weight loss, but dieting alone is not the best way to decrease body fat and improve body composition. Exercise during a weight loss program helps preserve muscle so that the weight lost is in the form of fat. The best programs for fat loss include increased exercise and modest reductions in energy intake. Chapters 8 and 9 provide much more information about healthy food choices, including recommended strategies for adjusting your diet to lose or gain weight safely.

Q | What's the best kind of exercise to lose body fat?

Just as the intake side of the balance scale shouldn't be tackled alone, neither should the energy-output side. On the "Energy Out" side of the scale, body composition is best improved by a combination of activity types. Aerobic activities are essential for burning calories and fat. Research tells us that high-intensity exercise works best for improving body composition, and as we get progressively better at aerobic exercise, we begin to burn body fat better and more efficiently.[26] However, as described in Chapter 4, moderate-intensity exercise may be easier for people to maintain over the long term. The best endurance activities are those you stick with, regardless of intensity. In addition, you'll definitely want to incorporate resistance training into your program. It increases muscle mass, thereby improving body composition directly, and it also helps

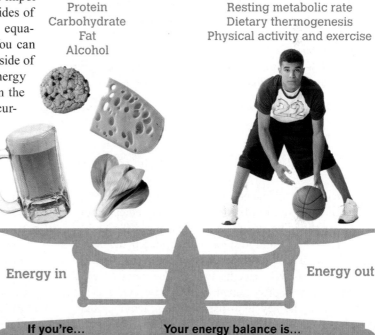

If you're...	Your energy balance is...
Maintaining your weight	**In balance.** You're eating roughly the same number of calories that your body is using. Your weight will remain **stable**.
Gaining weight	**In caloric excess or positive energy balance.** You're eating more calories than your body is using. You will **gain** weight and store these extra calories as fat (unless you are incorporating exercise specifically to gain muscle).
Losing weight	**In caloric deficit or negative energy balance.** You're eating fewer calories than your body is using. Your body is pulling from its fat storage cells for energy, so your weight will **decrease**.

Figure 7-10 **Energy balance**
Source: Adapted from Centers for Disease Control and Prevention. (2009). *Balancing calories* (http://www.cdc.gov/healthyweight/calories/index.html).

Wellness Strategies

"Snack Packing" for Your Body . . . Your Brain . . . and Your Bank Balance

Our bodies need to refuel every few hours, but hectic class schedules—along with work and home schedules—don't always allow time for regular sit-down meals. Taking a little extra time in the morning (or at the beginning of the week) to pack a few healthy take-along snacks will pay off in the long run. Healthy, regular snacks not only give you energy and needed nutrients, they help to control total calorie, fat, and sugar intake; regulate blood glucose levels; and fend off hunger and fatigue. Additionally, studies have shown that well-timed snacks can improve cognitive abilities including memory, attention span, reading speed, reasoning skills, and math skills. Finally, having your snacks readily available helps you avoid the convenient temptation of vending machines and drive-through windows—also saving you money.

For those times when meals are more than four hours apart, satisfy yourself with a snack from your pack. What works well? Try small whole-grain bagels, fruits, raw vegetables, whole-wheat crackers with peanut butter or cheese, nuts and seeds, low-fat granola, flavored rice cakes, pretzels, bran muffins, string cheese, tuna, popcorn or low-fat yogurt. And, don't forget water. (If you don't want the extra weight in your pack, you can always carry a re-fillable bottle.)

Of course, some of your choices will be limited by the season or your location (always err on the side of food safety), but with a little creativity, you may be surprised to discover what travels well. Also, remember to choose snacks that fit your schedule—both prep time and eating time. You won't continue to make the effort if the packing becomes cumbersome or the snacks aren't enjoyable.

Sources: AARP. (2007). *Healthy snacking* (http://www-static-w2-md.aarp.org/health/healthyliving/articles/snacking.html). Mayo Clinic. (2009, December 10). *Snacks: How they fit into your weight loss plan* (http://www.mayoclinic.com/health/healthy-diet/HQ01396). Family Education. (2010). *Stocking up on smart snacks* (http://life.familyeducation.com/snacks/nutrition-and-diet/48798.html). Women Fitness. (n.d.). *Top 10 healthiest snacks: You can just keep on eating* (http://www.womenfitness.net/top10_healthiest_snacks.htm).

to increase metabolism and utilize the body's fat more efficiently.

If the thought of engaging in multiple types of exercise or intense exercise in order to address body composition seems overwhelming, keep in mind these types of exercise also increase your cardiorespiratory and muscular fitness. You will get multiple gains for your efforts. Also, keep in mind that intensity is specific to you. You don't have to be an athlete or highly trained in order to exercise at an intense level. The key is to participate in activities that are safe and appropriate for your needs—and that you can stick with throughout your life.

Q | How much exercise do I need to do to maintain my weight range over time?

The answer to this question is different for each person due to genetic differences and other factors. The U.S. Department of Health & Human Services provides the following estimates for the amount of exercise needed for weight management.[27]

- **To prevent weight gain:** Engage in a minimum of 150 minutes per week of moderate-intensity aerobic exercise or 75 minutes of high-intensity exercise. Some people may need to engage in more exercise in order to prevent increases in weight and fat over time.

- **To lose a modest amount of weight or to maintain weight loss:** The general advice might be "more is better," but more research is needed to determine exactly how much. Based on current evidence, about 50 minutes a day of moderate-intensity exercise or 25 minutes a day of high-intensity exercise will help you lose a modest amount of weight and keep it off.

- **To lose a more significant amount of weight:** To lose more than 5 percent of body weight, engage in more than 300 minutes of moderate-intensity exercise or 150 minutes of high-intensity exercise per week.

In studies of people who lost a significant amount of weight and maintained the loss over the long term, physical activity levels averaged about 60 minutes per day.[28]

See Chapters 3–6 for more information on creating a fitness program that is right for you. Be sure to include strength training in your program—although it doesn't burn many calories directly, it helps maintain your muscle mass and, as described earlier in the chapter, your body's response to strength training (repair of muscle microtears) raises your resting metabolic rate for several days after your workouts. If you want to increase your "Energy Out"

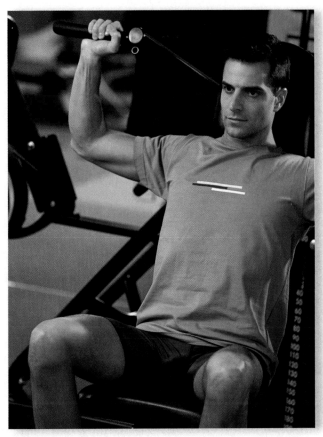

Strength training is a cornerstone of any program to improve body composition. Strength training helps maintain muscle mass as you lose weight, and it can help boost your resting metabolism.

TABLE 7-4 APPROXIMATE CALORIE COSTS OF SELECTED PHYSICAL ACTIVITIES

ACTIVITY	CALORIES PER POUND PER MINUTE*
Sitting in class or at computer	0.014
Child care (dressing, bathing)	0.023
Vacuuming or heavy cleaning	0.026
Shoveling snow	0.045
Walking, brisk (3.5 mph)	0.029
Walking, very brisk (4.5 mph)	0.048
Jogging, moderate (5 mph, 12 min./mile)	0.060
Jogging (7.5 mph, 8 min./mile)	0.095
Cycling, light effort	0.045
Cycling, moderate	0.060
Cycling, vigorous	0.076
Swimming laps, moderate effort	0.053
Basketball, game (moderate/vigorous)	0.060
Roller blading, vigorous	0.091
Tennis, singles	0.060
Frisbee, ultimate (vigorous effort)	0.060
Weight lifting	0.045
Circuit training	0.060

*To determine the approximate number of calories burned, multiply the value in the right column by your total body weight and the number of minutes you engage in the activity. For example, if you weigh 150 pounds and walk briskly for 30 minutes, you will burn about $0.29 \times 150 \times 30 = 130$ calories. The values given here are estimates; due to metabolic differences, some people will burn more or fewer calories than indicated by this table.

Source: Adapted from Centers for Disease Control and Prevention, National Center for Chronic Disease Prevention and Health Promotion. (1999). *General physical activities defined by level of intensity* (www.cdc.gov/nccdphp/dnpa/physical/pdf/PA_Intensity_table_2_1 .pdf); a complete listing of MET values for many different physical activities can be found in *The Compendium for Physical Activities* at http://prevention.sph.sc.edu/tools/compendium.htm

by a particular number of calories, refer to Table 7-4 for approximate calorie costs of some common activities.

Q | Why can't I just focus on improving one part of my body, such as getting rid of unwanted fat in one area?

As described in Chapter 5, it is impossible to target one area for fat burning (so-called spot reduction). You can strengthen the muscles in a particular area of your body through exercise, but such workouts will not reduce fat from that specific area. When you exercise, fat is burned from the body generally—the exact areas where the body will mobilize fat for fuel depend on a number of factors, including genetics. Many people find this frustrating, but it is true. The good news in terms of health and wellness is that research has shown that exercise will reduce dangerous visceral fat.

Don't focus too much of your attention on aspects of your body that you can't change. Strive to make healthy changes in your body composition and accept that healthy bodies come in many shapes and sizes.

Summary

Body composition includes the relative amounts of muscle, fat, bone, and other tissues that make up the body. It is typically assessed in terms of the percent of total body weight that is fat. A number of factors contribute to your body composition—including genetics, gender, age, ethnicity, lifestyle, and environment. A certain percentage of body fat is necessary and healthy; however, high fat levels can contribute to functional problems as well as deadly chronic diseases. Too little body fat is also dangerous and can affect athletic performance, bone density, and hormonal balance. Along with a healthy body composition, people should strive to develop a positive and realistic body image.

Body mass index (BMI) is a common method of indirectly measuring body fat and classifying the health risks associated with body weight, but it is not accurate for all body types. There are several methods of estimating percent body fat, including skinfold measurement, underwater weighing, and bioelectrical impedance analysis.

A program to change body composition should include realistic goals and attention to both sides of the energy balance equation—energy in as food and energy out as physical activity. Both aerobic exercise and resistance training contribute to positive changes in body composition.

More to Explore

Centers for Disease Control and Prevention: Assessing Your Weight
http://www.cdc.gov/healthyweight/assessing/index.html

MedlinePlus: Obesity
http://www.nlm.nih.gov/medlineplus/obesity.html

Department of Nutrition and Food Science, University of Vermont: Methods of Body Composition Analysis Tutorials
http://nutrition.uvm.edu/bodycomp

National Heart, Lung and Blood Institute: What Are Overweight and Obesity?
http://www.nhlbi.nih.gov/health/dci/Diseases/obe/obe_whatare.html

The Surgeon General's Call to Action to Prevent and Decrease Overweight and Obesity
http://www.surgeongeneral.gov/topics/obesity

womenshealth.gov: Body Image
http://www.womenshealth.gov/bodyimage/

SUBMIT ONLINE

NAME   **DATE**   **SECTION**

This lab includes several tests for measuring and evaluating factors related to body composition:

- Body mass index, with waist circumference
- Percent body fat using skinfold measurement
- Body fat distribution, using waist circumference, waist-to-hip ratio, waist-to-height ratio

Standards for evaluating percent body fat are also included in the lab activity, and these can be applied to any method of measuring percent body fat that you complete.

Calculating and Evaluating Body Mass Index

Equipment

- Weight scale
- Tape measure or other means of measuring height and waist circumference
- Partner (optional)

Preparation

None

Instructions

Measure your height, weight, and waist circumference, and record the results. Be sure to record the units of measurement. Measure your waist at the smallest point. For best results, have a partner measure your waist while standing at your side; be sure to keep the measuring tape flat against your skin and parallel to the ground. Measure your height with shoes off and your weight with minimal clothing.

Height: [   ] in./m   Weight: [   ] lbs./kg   Waist circumference: [   ] in./cm

Calculate your BMI using the following formulas. You need to complete steps 1 and 2, which convert the units of measurement, only if your height was measured in inches or your weight in pounds.

1. **Convert your body weight to kilograms by dividing your weight in pounds by 2.2.**

   Body weight [   ] lbs. ÷ 2.2 lb./kg = body weight [   ] kg

2. **Convert your height measurement to meters by multiplying your height in inches by 0.0254.**

   Height [   ] in. × 0.0254 in./m = height [   ] m

3. **Square your height measurement (in meters, from step 2).**

   Height [   ] m × height [   ] m = height [   ] m²

4. **BMI equals body weight in kilograms (from step 1) divided by height in meters squared (from step 3).**

   BMI = body weight [   ] kg ÷ height squared [   ] m² = [   ] kg/m²

Results

Refer to the table for a rating of your BMI. Use your waist circumference to further classify your level of risk. Record the results below and on the final page of this lab.

BMI classification: [_____]   Disease risk from waist circumference (if any): [_____]

BODY MASS INDEX (BMI) CLASSIFICATION AND DISEASE RISK

	BMI (KG/M²)	Disease risk relative to normal weight and waist circumference	
		MEN: WAIST ≤ 40 IN. (102 CM) WOMEN: WAIST ≤ 35 IN. (88 CM)	MEN: WAIST > 40 IN. (102 CM) WOMEN: WAIST > 35 IN. (88 CM)
Underweight	< 18.5		
Normal	18.5–24.9		
Overweight	25.0–29.9	Increased	High
Obesity (Class I)	30.0–34.9	High	Very high
Obesity (Class II)	35.0–39.9	Very high	Very high
Extreme obesity (Class III)	≥40.0	Extremely high	Extremely high

Source: National Heart, Lung, and Blood Institute. (1998). *Clinical guidelines on the identification, evaluation, and treatment of overweight and obesity in adults.* Bethesda, MD: National Institutes of Health.

Calculating Percent Body Fat: Skinfold Measurements

Equipment

- Skinfold calipers
- Partner to take measurements (Note: results are most accurate if the person measuring the skinfolds is experienced)
- Water-soluble marking pen (optional)
- Tape measure (optional)

Preparation

- Wear clothing that allows easy access to the skinfold sites being measured. The skinfold sites for males are chest, abdomen, and thigh; for females, triceps, suprailiac, and thigh.
- If needed, the person taking measurements should practice. Grasp the skin with the thumb and forefinger about 3 inches apart; the pinched skinfold should contain two layers of skin with just fat in between. If it feels like there may be any muscle tissue in the skinfold, the person being measured should contract the muscle to allow the measurer to more easily distinguish muscle from skin and fat.

Instructions

1. ***Locate the correct sites for measurement.*** All measurements should be taken on the right side of the body as you stand. If the person taking skinfold measurements is inexperienced, it may be helpful to measure and mark the correct sites with a water-soluble pen.
   - *Chest.* Pinch a diagonal fold halfway between the nipple and the shoulder crease.
   - *Abdomen.* Pinch a vertical fold about 2 cm to the right of the umbilicus (navel).
   - *Thigh.* Pinch a vertical fold midway between the top of the kneecap and the inguinal crease (hip).
   - *Triceps.* Pinch a vertical skinfold on the back of the right arm midway between the shoulder and elbow. The arm should be held freely at the side of the body.
   - *Suprailiac.* Pinch a fold at the top front of the right hipbone. The skinfold will be slightly diagonal in line with the natural angle of the top of the hipbone.

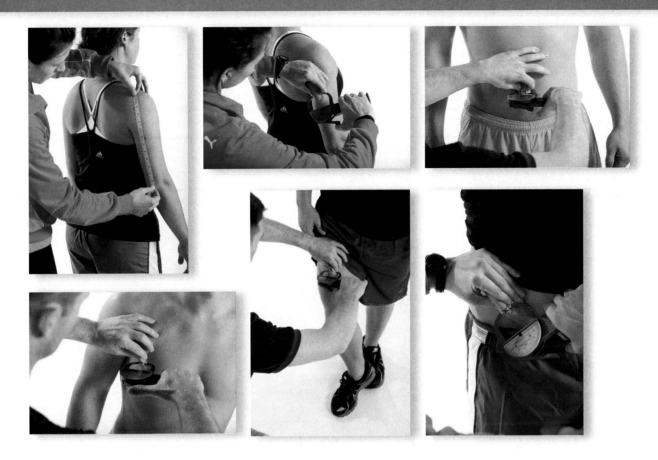

2. ***Measure the appropriate skinfolds and record the values.*** Pinch a fold of skin between your thumb and fore-finger. Pull the fold up so that no muscular tissue is included; don't pinch too hard. Place the calipers directly on the skin surface perpendicular to the fold, and measure the skinfold about 1 cm away from your fingers. Wait 1–2 seconds before reading the caliper. Take readings to the nearest half millimeter. Don't let go of the skinfold until you've removed the caliper from the skin. Take at least two measurements at each site, and retest if the measurements are not within 1–2 millimeters. Allow the skin to regain its normal position and appearance before repinching a fold. Make a note of the final measurements for each site.

Results

To determine percent body fat, average the measurements for each site and then add the three average measurements together for a sum of the three skinfolds. Then refer to the appropriate table on pp. 258–259 and the figure on p. 260 to determine your estimated percent body fat and rating. Record the result below and in the chart at the end of the lab.

	TRIAL 1	TRIAL 2	AVERAGE OF TWO TRIALS
MEN			
Chest	mm	mm	mm
Abdomen	mm	mm	mm
Thigh	mm	mm	mm
Sum of three skinfolds			**mm**
WOMEN			
Triceps	mm	mm	mm
Suprailiac	mm	mm	mm
Thigh	mm	mm	mm
Sum of three skinfolds			**mm**

Percent body fat (from table): [   ] %   Rating of percent body fat (from figure): [   ]

PERCENT BODY FAT ESTIMATE FOR MEN: SUM OF CHEST, ABDOMEN, AND THIGH SKINFOLDS

SUM OF SKINFOLDS (MM)	AGE								
	UNDER 22	23–27	28–32	33–37	38–42	43–47	48–52	53–57	OVER 57
8–10	1.3	1.8	2.3	2.9	3.4	3.9	4.5	5.0	5.5
11–13	2.2	2.8	3.3	3.9	4.4	4.9	5.5	6.0	6.5
14–16	3.2	3.8	4.3	4.8	5.4	5.9	6.4	7.0	7.5
17–19	4.2	4.7	5.3	5.8	6.3	6.9	7.4	8.0	8.5
20–22	5.1	5.7	6.2	6.8	7.3	7.9	8.4	8.9	9.5
23–25	6.1	6.6	7.2	7.7	8.3	8.8	9.4	9.9	10.5
26–28	7.0	7.6	8.1	8.7	9.2	9.8	10.3	10.9	11.4
29–31	8.0	8.5	9.1	9.6	10.2	10.7	11.3	11.8	12.4
32–34	8.9	9.4	10.0	10.5	11.1	11.6	12.2	12.8	13.3
35–37	9.8	10.4	10.9	11.5	12.0	12.6	13.1	13.7	14.3
38–40	10.7	11.3	11.8	12.4	12.9	13.5	14.1	14.6	15.2
41–43	11.6	12.2	12.7	13.3	13.8	14.4	15.0	15.5	16.1
44–46	12.5	13.1	13.6	14.2	14.7	15.3	15.9	16.4	17.0
47–49	13.4	13.9	14.5	15.1	15.6	16.2	16.8	17.3	17.9
50–52	14.3	14.8	15.4	15.9	16.5	17.1	17.6	18.2	18.8
53–55	15.1	15.7	16.2	16.8	17.4	17.9	18.5	19.1	19.7
56–58	16.0	16.5	17.1	17.7	18.2	18.8	19.4	20.0	20.5
59–61	16.9	17.4	17.9	18.5	19.1	19.7	20.2	20.8	21.4
62–64	17.6	18.2	18.8	19.4	19.9	20.5	21.1	21.7	22.2
65–67	18.5	19.0	19.6	20.2	20.8	21.3	21.9	22.5	23.1
68–70	19.3	19.9	20.4	21.0	21.6	22.2	22.7	23.3	23.9
71–73	20.1	20.7	21.2	21.8	22.4	23.0	23.6	24.1	24.7
74–76	20.9	21.5	22.0	22.6	23.2	23.8	24.4	25.0	25.5
77–79	21.7	22.2	22.8	23.4	24.0	24.6	25.2	25.8	26.3
80–82	22.4	23.0	23.6	24.2	24.8	25.4	25.9	26.5	27.1
83–85	23.2	23.8	24.4	25.0	25.5	26.1	26.7	27.3	27.9
86–88	24.0	24.5	25.1	25.7	26.3	26.9	27.5	28.1	28.7
89–91	24.7	25.3	25.9	26.5	27.1	27.6	28.2	28.8	29.4
92–94	25.4	26.0	26.6	27.2	27.8	28.4	29.0	29.6	30.2
95–97	26.1	26.7	27.3	27.9	28.5	29.1	29.7	30.3	30.9
98–100	26.9	27.4	28.0	28.6	29.2	29.8	30.4	31.0	31.6
101–103	27.5	28.1	28.7	29.3	29.9	30.5	31.1	31.7	32.3
104–106	28.2	28.8	29.4	30.0	30.6	31.2	31.8	32.4	33.0
107–109	28.9	29.5	30.1	30.7	31.3	31.9	32.5	33.1	33.7
110–112	29.6	30.2	30.8	31.4	32.0	32.6	33.2	33.8	34.4
113–115	30.2	30.8	31.4	32.0	32.6	33.2	33.8	34.5	35.1
116–118	30.9	31.5	32.1	32.7	33.3	33.9	34.5	35.1	35.7
119–121	31.5	32.1	32.7	33.3	33.9	34.5	35.1	35.7	36.4
122–124	32.1	32.7	33.3	33.9	34.5	35.1	35.8	36.4	37.0
125–127	32.7	33.3	33.9	34.5	35.1	35.8	36.4	37.0	37.6

PERCENT BODY FAT ESTIMATE FOR WOMEN: SUM OF TRICEPS, SUPRAILIUM, AND THIGH SKINFOLDS

SUM OF SKINFOLDS (MM)	UNDER 22	23–27	28–32	33–37	38–42	43–47	48–52	53–57	OVER 57
				AGE					
23–25	9.7	9.9	10.2	10.4	10.7	10.9	11.2	11.4	11.7
26–28	11.0	11.2	11.5	11.7	12.0	12.3	12.5	12.7	13.0
29–31	12.3	12.5	12.8	13.0	13.3	13.5	13.8	14.0	14.3
32–34	13.6	13.8	14.0	14.3	14.5	14.8	15.0	15.3	15.5
35–37	14.8	15.0	15.3	15.5	15.8	16.0	16.3	16.5	16.8
38–40	16.0	16.3	16.5	16.7	17.0	17.2	17.5	17.7	18.0
41–43	17.2	17.4	17.7	17.9	18.2	18.4	18.7	18.9	19.2
44–46	18.3	18.6	18.8	19.1	19.3	19.6	19.8	20.1	20.3
47–49	19.5	19.7	20.0	20.2	20.5	20.7	21.0	21.2	21.5
50–52	20.6	20.8	21.1	21.3	21.6	21.8	22.1	22.3	22.6
53–55	21.7	21.9	22.1	22.4	22.6	22.9	23.1	23.4	23.6
56–58	22.7	23.0	23.2	23.4	23.7	23.9	24.2	24.4	24.7
59–61	23.7	24.0	24.2	24.5	24.7	25.0	25.2	25.5	25.7
62–64	24.7	25.0	25.2	25.5	25.7	26.0	26.7	26.4	26.7
65–67	25.7	25.9	26.2	26.4	26.7	26.9	27.2	27.4	27.7
68–70	26.6	26.9	27.1	27.4	27.6	27.9	28.1	28.4	28.6
71–73	27.5	27.8	28.0	28.3	28.5	28.8	29.0	29.3	29.5
74–76	28.4	28.7	28.9	29.2	29.4	29.7	29.9	30.2	30.4
77–79	29.3	29.5	29.8	30.0	30.3	30.5	30.8	31.0	31.3
80–82	30.1	30.4	30.6	30.9	31.1	31.4	31.6	31.9	32.1
83–85	30.9	31.2	31.4	31.7	31.9	32.2	32.4	32.7	32.9
86–88	31.7	32.0	32.2	32.5	32.7	32.9	33.2	33.4	33.7
89–91	32.5	32.7	33.0	33.2	33.5	33.7	33.9	34.2	34.4
92–94	33.2	33.4	33.7	33.9	34.2	34.4	34.7	34.9	35.2
95–97	33.9	34.1	34.4	34.6	34.9	35.1	35.4	35.6	35.9
98–100	34.6	34.8	35.1	35.3	35.5	35.8	36.0	36.3	36.5
101–103	35.3	35.4	35.7	35.9	36.2	36.4	36.7	36.9	37.2
104–106	35.8	36.1	36.3	36.6	36.8	37.1	37.3	37.5	37.8
107–109	36.4	36.7	36.9	37.1	37.4	37.6	37.9	38.1	38.4
110–112	37.0	37.2	37.5	37.7	38.0	38.2	38.5	38.7	38.9
113–115	37.5	37.8	38.0	38.2	38.5	38.7	39.0	39.2	39.5
116–118	38.0	38.3	38.5	38.8	39.0	39.3	39.5	39.7	40.0
119–121	38.5	38.7	39.0	39.2	39.5	39.7	40.0	40.2	40.5
122–124	39.0	39.2	39.4	39.7	39.9	40.2	40.4	40.7	40.9
125–127	39.4	39.6	39.9	40.1	40.4	40.6	40.9	41.1	41.4
128–130	39.8	40.0	40.3	40.5	40.8	41.0	41.3	41.5	41.8

Source: Jackson, A. S., & Pollock, M. L. (1985). Practical assessment of body composition. *The Physician and Sportsmedicine, 13*(5), 76–90, Tables 6 & 7.

PERCENT BODY FAT STANDARDS FOR MEN AND WOMEN

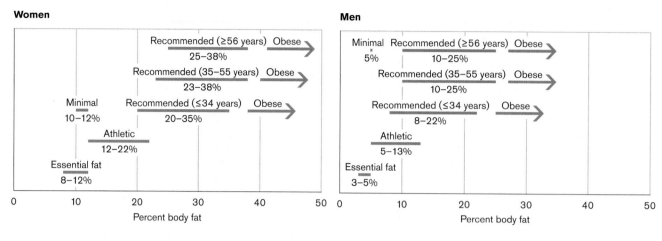

Source: American College of Sports Medicine. (2009). *ACSM's resource manual for guidelines for exercise testing and prescription* (6th ed.). Baltimore, MD: Lippincott Williams & Wilkins.

Percent Body Fat: Other Techniques

If you use a different method for estimating percent body fat, record the type of assessment and the result below and in the chart at the end of the lab activity. Find your body composition rating on the table.

Method used: ☐   Percent body fat: ☐ %

Rating of percent body fat (from figure): ☐

Evaluating Body Fat Distribution

To evaluate your body fat distribution, complete one or more of the assessments in this section:

- Waist circumference
- Waist-to-hip ratio
- Waist-to-height ratio

Equipment

- Tape measure or other means of measuring waist and hip circumferences and height
- Partner (optional)

Preparation

None

Instructions and Results

For ease of calculation, use the same units (inches or centimeters) for all measurements.

For waist circumference:

1. Measure your waist at the smallest point. For best results, have a partner measure your waist while standing at your side; be sure to keep the measuring tape flat against your skin and parallel to the ground. Record the measurement and the units:

   Waist circumference: ☐ in./cm

2. Find your rating in the appropriate table. Record it here and in the chart at the end of the lab:

Waist circumference rating: ☐

For waist-to-hip ratio:

1. Measure your waist (see instructions above). Waist circumference: ☐ in./cm

2. Measure your hips at the widest point. For best results, have a partner measure your hip circumference while standing at your side; keep the measuring tape flat against your skin and parallel to the ground.

Hip circumference: ☐ in./cm

3. Calculate your ratio by dividing your waist circumference by your hip circumference; make sure both measurements are in the same units:

Waist-to-hip ratio = waist circumference ☐ ÷ hip circumference ☐ = ☐

4. Find your rating in the appropriate table. Record it here and in the chart at the end of the lab:

Waist-to-hip ratio rating: ☐

For waist-to-height ratio:

1. Measure your waist (see instructions above). Waist circumference: ☐ in./cm

2. Measure your height with shoes off and record the results:

Height: ☐ in./cm

3. Calculate your ratio by dividing your waist circumference by your height; make sure both measurements are in the same units:

Waist-to-height ratio = waist circumference ☐ ÷ height ☐ = ☐

4. If your ratio is 0.5 or less, record a rating of "OK"; if your ratio is above 0.5, record a rating of "increased risk":

Waist-to-height ratio rating: ☐

WAIST CIRCUMFERENCE AND HEALTH RISK

Waist circumference (inches, centimeters)

RISK CATEGORY	WOMEN	MEN
Very low	<27.5 in. (70 cm)	<31.5 in. (80 cm)
Low	28.5–35.0 in. (70–89 cm)	31.5–39.0 in. (80–99 cm)
High	35.5–43.0 in. (90–109 cm)	39.5–47.0 in. (100–120 cm)
Very high	>43.5 in. (110 cm)	>47.0 in. (120 cm)

Source: Adapted from Bray, G. A. (2004). Don't throw the baby out with the bath water. *American Journal of Clinical Nutrition*, 79(3), 347–349.

WAIST-TO-HIP RATIO AND HEALTH RISK

	AGE	RISK			
		LOW	MODERATE	HIGH	VERY HIGH
MEN	20–29	<0.83	0.83–0.88	0.89–0.94	>0.94
	30–39	<0.84	0.84–0.91	0.92–0.96	>0.96
	40–49	<0.88	0.88–0.95	0.96–1.00	>1.00
	50–59	<0.90	0.90–0.96	0.97–1.02	>1.02
	60–69	<0.91	0.91–0.98	0.99–1.03	>1.03
WOMEN	20–29	<0.71	0.71–0.77	0.78–0.82	>0.82
	30–39	<0.72	0.72–0.78	0.79–0.84	>0.84
	40–49	<0.73	0.73–0.79	0.80–0.87	>0.87
	50–59	<0.74	0.74–0.81	0.82–0.88	>0.88
	60–69	<0.76	0.76–0.83	0.84–0.90	>0.90

Source: Heyward, V. (2010). *Advanced fitness assessment and exercise prescription* (6th ed.; p. 222, table 8.8). Champaign, IL: Human Kinetics.

Summary of Results

Fill in the scores and ratings for the tests you performed.

	RESULT	RATING
BMI	kg/m²	
[WAIST CIRCUMFERENCE]	in./cm	OK / increased risk
SKINFOLDS	% body fat	
OTHER METHOD: _____	% body fat	
WAIST CIRCUMFERENCE	in./cm	
WAIST-TO-HIP RATIO		
WAIST-TO-HEIGHT RATIO		OK / increased risk

Reflecting on Your Results

Are you surprised with your test results and ratings? Did your results match what you thought about your own body composition?

Planning Your Next Steps

Body composition is a function of your individual energy balance. If your body composition rates as healthy, then strive to maintain it. If the results of your assessment indicate that your body composition places you at elevated risk, then it may be time to make changes in your exercise or eating habits. Set realistic goals for improvement and create a plan to achieve them. As a first step here, describe the type of goal you'd like to set for body composition and the lifestyle parameters you plan to focus your efforts on. For assistance in setting a more precise goal, complete Lab Activity 7-2.

[icon] SUBMIT ONLINE

NAME   DATE   SECTION

If the results of the assessment tests in Lab Activity 7-1 indicate that your body composition is a health risk for you, then you can use this lab activity to set a goal for weight based on BMI or percent body fat. (As described in the chapter, if you lose weight slowly and incorporate exercise into your program, then your weight loss will likely be fat loss.) Alternatively, you might want to set a lifestyle goal, such as starting a strength-training program or increasing physical activity, instead of a specific body-composition goal.

Equipment

None required, although a calculator is helpful for doing the calculations. You'll also need the data and results from Lab Activity 7-1.

Height: [   ] in./cm/m   Weight: [   ] lb./kg

Current BMI: [   ] kg/m²   Current percent body fat: [   ] %

Preparation

None

Instructions and Results

Body weight goal based on BMI:

Based on the BMI ratings and your current BMI, select a BMI goal:

Current BMI: [   ] kg/m²   Goal BMI [   ] kg/m²

To calculate a target body weight based on your BMI goal, use the following steps:

1. If needed, convert your height measurement to meters by multiplying your height in inches by 0.0254.

   Height [   ] in. × 0.0254 m/in. = height [   ] m

2. Square your height measurement (in meters, from step 1).

   Height [   ] m × height [   ] m = height [   ] m²

3. Multiply your target BMI (from above) by the square of your height (from step 2) to get your body weight goal (in kilograms).

   Body weight goal = Target BMI [   ] kg/m² × height squared [   ] m² = [   ] kg

4. If needed, convert your body weight goal (in kilograms) to pounds by multiplying your weight in kilograms by 2.2.

   Body weight goal = [   ] kg × 2.2 lb./kg = [   ] lb.

Body weight goal based on estimated percent body fat:

Based on the percent body fat ratings and your current percent body fat, select a goal for percent body fat:

Current percent body fat: [   ] %   Goal percent body fat [   ] %

To calculate a target body weight based on your percent body fat goal, use the following steps. You can do the calculations for either pounds or kilograms as long as you are consistent.

1. Multiply your current weight by your percent body fat to obtain your current body fat weight; express percent body fat as a decimal (20% would be 0.20).

   Current weight [＿＿＿] lb./kg × current percent body fat [0.＿＿＿] = current fat weight [＿＿＿] lb./kg

2. Subtract your current fat weight (from step 1) from your total weight to get your current fat free weight.

   Current weight [＿＿＿] lb./kg − current fat weight [＿＿＿] lb./kg = current fat-free weight [＿＿＿] lb./kg

3. Subtract your target percent body fat (expressed as a decimal) from 1 to calculate your goal fat-free percent of body weight.

   1 − Goal percent body fat [0.＿＿＿] = Goal percent fat-free weight [0.＿＿＿]

4. Divide your current fat-free weight (from step 2) by your goal percent fat-free weight (from step 3).

   Body weight goal = Current fat-free weight [＿＿＿] lb./kg ÷ Goal percent fat-free weight [0.＿＿＿] =

   [＿＿＿] lb./kg

Reflecting on Your Results and Planning Your Next Steps

BMI goal: [＿＿＿] kg/m^2 or Percent body fat goal: [＿＿＿] %

Body weight goal (calculated from BMI or percent body fat): [＿＿＿] lb./kg

Check your goal against the SMART criteria described in Chapter 2 (specific, measurable, achievable, realistic, and time-bound). Describe why you think this goal is a good one for you, or revise your goal to make it a better fit for your situation. Consider your current body composition and body type, heredity, health status, and personal preferences in setting your goal.

[＿＿＿＿＿＿＿＿＿＿＿＿＿＿＿＿＿＿＿＿＿＿＿＿]

Based on what you've learned so far, list several specific strategies you could use to help achieve your body composition goal; additional advice and strategies related to food choices are found in Chapters 8 and 9.

[＿＿＿＿＿＿＿＿＿＿＿＿＿＿＿＿＿＿＿＿＿＿＿＿]

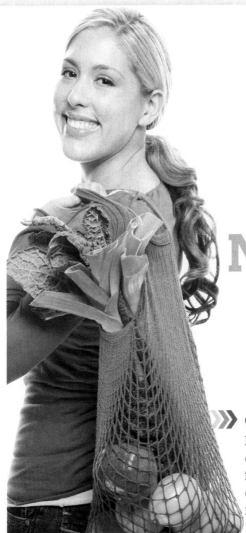

8

Nutrition Basics: Energy and Nutrients

>> **COMING UP IN THIS CHAPTER**

Learn about the sources of energy in your diet > Discover essential nutrients for your health and wellness > Use food labels to compare the energy and nutrients in food choices > Measure your energy and nutrient intake against recommended intakes—and identify areas of concern for you

Wellness Connections

How does healthy eating relate to your overall wellness? Food provides the nutrients and energy you need to realize your full wellness potential. Proper nutrition starts during fetal development and continues throughout the lifespan—"from cradle to grave." In the short term, healthy eating is needed for optimal physical functioning every day; in the long term, it affects your risk for chronic diseases.

Following a healthy eating plan gives you confidence and satisfaction, boosting your self-esteem and emotional wellness. Having positive ways to deal with difficult emotions and spiritual challenges can also help keep you from using unhealthy food choices as a coping mechanism. Intellectual and social wellness also influence your eating habits—are you thinking critically about your food choices? Can you stay committed to a dietary plan and personal nutrition goals? Can you avoid being overly influenced by unhealthy food choices of those around you?

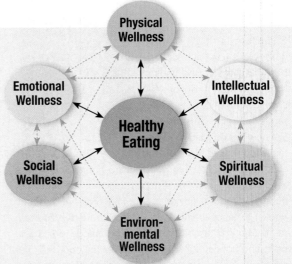

Finally, consider your environment. Be aware of whether the foods easily available to you include healthy choices. And pay attention to how your food choices affect the environment. What resources were used to grow and ship the foods you eat? How much food packaging do you dispose of? Your food choices can affect environmental wellness on both a local and a global scale.

This is the first of two chapters on healthy eating. It describes the basic nutrients—the components of foods—that you need to be healthy and to meet your energy (calorie) needs. Chapter 9 describes how to combine foods into healthy eating patterns that prevent chronic diseases and don't lead to unhealthy weight gain or loss; it also addresses the problems of overweight and obesity in our society today.

Americans today consume more calories than we have in the past, but many of us do not get all the nutrients we need. We are both overfed and undernourished.[1] Learning about nutrients—where they come from, what they do in the body, and how much of each you need—can help you put together a diet that is right for you.

Dietary Components and Concepts

Q | I'm healthy. Does it really matter what I eat?

Yes. If you are like most Americans, you consume too much of some nutrients and not enough of others to support health and wellness. In the short term, unbalanced energy and nutrient intakes can reduce energy levels and impair body processes; in the long term, they increase your risks of becoming obese and of developing chronic diseases and conditions such as high blood pressure, type 2 diabetes, heart disease, and certain forms of cancer. Appropriate energy and nutrient intakes are keys to the optimal functioning of your body, today and throughout your life.

nutrients Carbohydrates, fats, proteins, vitamins, minerals, and water—the compounds required for growth and survival that must be obtained from food.

macronutrients Nutrients such as carbohydrates, fats, and proteins that must be consumed in large amounts and that provide calories.

To reap the full benefits offered by food, you have to eat an appropriate mix of nutrients from a variety of foods, all within an appropriate energy intake. **Nutrients** are substances you must obtain from foods because your body can't produce them on its own—or at least not in sufficient quantities to maintain its structure and function. Nutrients are typically divided into six classes:

- Carbohydrates
- Fats
- Proteins
- Vitamins
- Minerals
- Water

Your body obtains nutrients through the process of digestion, in which mechanical and chemical processes break down the foods you eat into small compounds (Figure 8-1). Food is chewed, mixed with digestive enzymes, and moved through the digestive tract. Nutrients are broken down into molecules that can be absorbed into the bloodstream and then circulated and used throughout the body.

Most foods contain a mix of nutrients. For example, whole milk contains carbohydrate, fat, protein, calcium (a mineral), and water. However, some foods are particularly good choices for specific nutrients—one large orange contains a full day's supply of vitamin C, and half a cup of cooked sweet potato has a full day's supply of vitamin A.[2] Your daily food choices must work together to provide all the nutrients and energy you need.

Behavior Change Challenge

Video Case Study

▶ WATCH ONLINE   Meet Sharnita

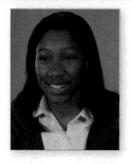

Sharnita is a fit 20-year-old who plays on her college basketball team. She doesn't have a weight problem, but she very much wants to improve her diet. She doesn't like how eating fried food and fast food makes her feel, and she wants to establish good eating habits now. She's a little unsure how to get started, and she finds her schedule and her environment—including her mother's cooking—to be challenges. Watch the video to learn more about Sharnita, her behavior-change goals and plan, and how successful she is over the course of her program. As you watch the video, think about the following questions:

- Do you think Sharnita has enough motivation, environmental support, and specific strategies for her program to be successful? What do you think her biggest challenges will be?
- What can you learn from Sharnita's experience that will help you in your own behavior-change efforts? What strategies that she adopted will work for you?

Macronutrients, Micronutrients, and Energy

Q | We need more carbs than vitamins, right?

In an absolute sense, yes—but both are critical. In addition to the six classes listed in the previous section, nutrients can also be divided into macronutrients and micronutrients (Table 8-1). **Macronutrients** are nutrients that provide calories and that you need to consume in fairly large amounts: carbohydrates, proteins, and fats. Each class of macronutrient liberates en-

micronutrients Nutrients such as vitamins and minerals needed in small or trace amounts.

ergy with a different level of efficiency (carbohydrates being the most efficient), and the amount of calories each provides also differs (fats having the most). As you'll learn a little later in this chapter, macronutrients provide more than just calories, and each affects your health in different ways. A balance of macronutrients is best for health. Water doesn't provide energy, but it is also needed daily in large amounts.

Micronutrients (vitamins and minerals) are needed in smaller amounts but are just as critical. Micronutrients occur naturally in food, and many processed foods (such as

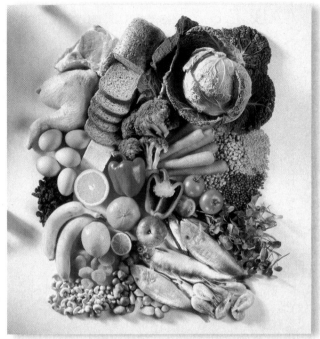

Choose a variety of foods daily to meet all your nutrient needs.

bread, cereal, orange juice, milk) are also fortified with micronutrients. Micronutrients do not provide calories; they provide necessary compounds for the liberation of energy from the macronutrients. Without the micronutrients, the macronutrients would not be able to effectively provide energy for everyday activities. They also help regulate many chemical reactions in the body that are critical for healthy functioning.

Q | Wouldn't I be healthier on an all-fruit diet?

An all-fruit diet would increase your intake of nutrients in four of the six essential nutrient categories—carbohydrates, water, vitamins, and minerals. However, you would be severely limiting your intake of the other two essential nutrients—protein and fat. Nutrients in all six categories are required for health. Carbohydrates, fats, and proteins all play specific roles in the human body, and none is more important than the others. Eating almost exclusively from only one or two nutrient categories will leave you with severe nutritional deficiencies that will harm your health in both the short and long terms. So, is an all-fruit diet healthy? Probably not. Is it necessary to eat fruit daily? Most definitely.

Q | What exactly is a calorie?

A **calorie** is a measure of the energy in a food as well as a measure of the energy burned through physical activity

calorie A measure of the energy in food; usually refers to a kilocalorie, or the amount of energy required to raise the temperature of 1 kg of water by 1°C.

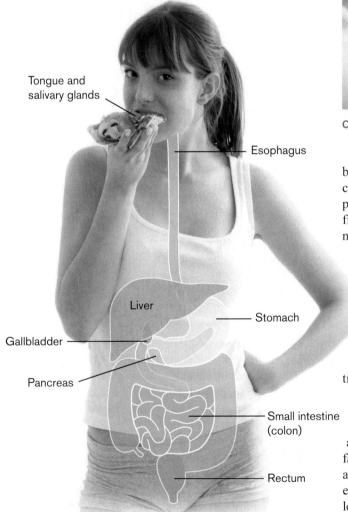

Figure 8-1 **The digestive system.** Food is partially broken down by chewing and is mixed with saliva and enzymes in the mouth. It passes through the esophagus to the stomach where it is dissolved by stomach acids. The liver, gallbladder, pancreas, and lining of the small intestine release enzymes and other chemicals that aid in digestion. Muscular contractions mix and move food through the digestive tract. Most digestion and absorption of nutrients take place in the small intestine. Undigested food is concentrated in the colon, collected in the rectum, and expelled via the anus.

Tongue and salivary glands

Esophagus

Liver

Stomach

Gallbladder

Pancreas

Small intestine (colon)

Rectum

TABLE 8-1 ESSENTIAL NUTRIENTS

	NUTRIENT CLASS	ENERGY	MAJOR FUNCTIONS	MAJOR SOURCES
MACRONUTRIENTS	**CARBOHYDRATE**	4 calories/gram	Energy for the body; nondigestible forms aid in elimination and help regulate glucose and cholesterol	Grains (breads, cereals), vegetables, fruits, milk products
	PROTEIN	4 calories/gram	Growth and repair of bone and muscle; components of cells, blood, enzymes, and certain hormones; energy for the body	Meat, poultry, fish, milk products, eggs, legumes, nuts
	FAT	9 calories/gram	Energy for the body; aid in absorption of certain vitamins; thermal insulation, cushioning of organs, and maintenance of cells	Meat, poultry, fish, milk products, eggs, nuts, seeds, some vegetables
MICRONUTRIENTS	**VITAMINS**	—	Regulation of body processes, including tissue growth and repair; liberation of energy; preservation of healthy cells, nerves, and immune function	Fruits, vegetables, grains
	MINERALS	—	Regulation of growth and development; liberation of energy	Many foods
	WATER	—	Digestion and absorption of food; lubrication, cushioning, and temperature control; medium for chemical reactions and transport of chemicals throughout the body	Water and other liquids,* fruits, vegetables

*Alcohol is a liquid that provides energy (7 calories/gram) but is not an essential nutrient.

(see the discussion of energy balance in Chapter 7). What we, and food labels, commonly call a "calorie" is technically a kilocalorie—the amount of energy required to raise the temperature of 1 kilogram of water by 1° Celsius.

As shown in Table 8-1, macronutrients provide different amounts of calories. Carbohydrates and protein provide 4 calories per gram, and fats provide 9 calories per gram (there are about 28 grams in an ounce). What this means is that per gram (or ounce), fat provides the most calories. A tablespoon of butter (which is mostly fat) and a tablespoon of sugar (all carbohydrate) weigh about the same, 11–12 grams, but the butter has more than twice the calories of the sugar.

Q If I go out drinking a couple nights a week, does that mean I consume more calories?

Yes, unless you eat less food on those days. Alcohol isn't an essential nutrient, but it does contain calories—7 calories per gram of alcohol. Some alcoholic beverages also contain carbohydrates, so their calorie total is higher. One standard 12-ounce beer has about 150 calories; 1.5 ounces of hard liquor, the amount in a shot or a typical mixed drink, has about 100 calories. Multiply your total number of drinks by these values to get the approximate calorie intake of one of your evenings out.

Alcohol has other effects on health beyond its calorie contribution; see Chapter 13 for more information.

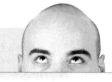

Mind Stretcher
Critical Thinking Exercise

Do you feel good after you eat or drink a healthy meal or snack? Do you feel bad after you consume foods and beverages you know are poor choices? Are your feelings physical or emotional, or both? Can you use your feelings to improve your eating habits?

Energy and Nutrient Recommendations

Q | How many calories should I eat every day?

Depending on your sex, age, weight, and activity level, you need between 1,600 and 3,600 calories per day to maintain your current weight (Table 8-2). Lab Activity 8-1 will help you more precisely determine the energy intake that is appropriate for you.

Where did these numbers come from? From the **Dietary Reference Intakes (DRIs),** one of the major tools for planning a healthy diet. The DRIs are established by the Food and Nutrition Board of the National Academies; they are based on the best available research and provide recommended intake levels of nutrients for Americans of all ages. For some nutrients, they also provide safe upper lim-

Dietary Reference Intakes (DRIs) A set of standards that includes recommended intakes of all essential nutrients, recommendations for balancing intakes of macronutrients, and upper safe limits for selected nutrients.

its, and intakes above those levels are likely to be harmful to health. Several different nutrient standards make up the DRIs, and you'll see those different standards discussed throughout the chapter. The goal of the DRIs is to provide guidance on nutrient intake levels that will prevent deficiencies and help reduce the risk of chronic disease.

Q | Do people have to count calories and add up all the nutrients in foods on a daily basis?

Not necessarily, although close tracking of your diet can be helpful from time to time, especially if you're trying to make changes. What is useful for everyone is a periodic check. Do you know how many calories you currently consume? How close are you to meeting the recommendations for individual nutrients? Lab Activity 8-2 will help you perform just such an analysis.

Keeping careful track of what you eat for several days can help give you a good picture of your current diet—and how you might improve it. Try to track your food intake on

TABLE 8-2 ESTIMATED CALORIE REQUIREMENTS FOR ADULTS, AGE 20 YEARS*

HEIGHT	ACTIVITY LEVEL**	CALORIES PER DAY	
		MEN	WOMEN
5 FEET (60 INCHES)	Sedentary	1,950–2,200	1,700–1,850
	Low active	2,150–2,400	1,900–2,100
	Active	2,400–2,700	2,150–2,300
	Very active	2,650–3,000	2,400–2,600
5 FEET 6 INCHES (66 INCHES)	Sedentary	2,200–2,500	1,900–2,100
	Low active	2,400–2,750	2,150–2,300
	Active	2,700–3,050	2,400–2,600
	Very active	3,000–3,410	2,700–2,950
6 FEET (72 INCHES)	Sedentary	2,450–2,800	2,150–2,350
	Low active	2,700–3,050	2,350–2,600
	Active	3,000–3,400	2,650–2,900
	Very active	3,350–3,850	3,000–3,300

*Values show the range for 20-year-olds with a body mass index (BMI) between 18.5 and 25.0. For each year above age 20, subtract 7 calories per day for women and 10 calories per day for men.

**Activity levels: *Sedentary* (activities of daily living); *low active* (activities of daily living plus the equivalent of 30 minutes per day of moderate activity); *active* (activities of daily living plus the equivalent of about 60–90 minutes per day of moderate activity); *very active* (activities of daily living plus the equivalent of about 150–240 minutes per day of moderate activity). Thirty minutes of vigorous activity is equivalent to about 60 minutes of moderate activity.

Source: National Academies, Institute of Medicine, Food and Nutrition Board. (2005). *Dietary reference intakes for energy, carbohydrate, fiber, fat, fatty acids, cholesterol, protein, and amino acids (macronutrients).* Washington, DC: National Academies Press.

Fast Facts

Invisible Calories?

Do the energy intake recommendations in Table 8-2 seem large to you? How many calories do you think you eat? Researchers have found that most people underestimate—by a significant amount—their energy intake, both in terms of individual meals and daily totals. Amounts vary, but underestimation by 15–25 percent is typical. The number is even higher for larger meals: One study of college students found that for large fast-food meals, calorie estimations were nearly 40 percent below the actual energy content of the meal! Are you an underestimator? Carefully track and measure all your food for a day or two for a reality check.

Source: Wansink, B., & Chandon, P. (2006). Meal size, not body size, explains errors in estimating the calorie content of meals. *Annals of Internal Medicine, 145*(5), 151.

both weekdays and weekends, especially if your schedule and eating patterns tend to vary. You don't have to meet the recommended intakes for each nutrient every day, but your average intakes should be in line with the Dietary Reference Intakes.

The most important thing on a daily basis is awareness. Are you paying attention to what—and how much—you are eating? Relatively small deviations from recommended intakes can add up over time. On average, Americans gain a pound a year between ages 20 and 60—a small change in one year but a big change over time!

Energy Density and Nutrient Density

Q | What are the most filling foods with the fewest calories?

Your question relates to the important concept of **energy density,** or the amount of energy in a food per unit of weight. Foods with high energy density have a large number of calories by weight—usually because they are high in fat, which has the most calories per gram, and low in water and fiber, which add weight

to foods without adding any calories. On the flip side, foods high in water and fiber have a low energy density, meaning they have a small number of calories by weight, so they can help fill you up without providing a lot of calories. For example, one small slice of cheese weighs about 1 ounce and has about 100 calories. For that same 100 calories, you could have any of these alternatives:

- five small (5-inch) carrots
- one large apple
- six apricots

Each of these servings of fruits and vegetables weighs about 8 ounces, so for the same 100 calories, you get to consume eight times the weight of food. If you want to fill up with fewer calories, try large portions of foods that are low in energy density. Many fruits, vegetables, and whole grains—if eaten without added sugars or fats—are low in energy density. It is OK to eat some foods with high energy density, but the energy density of your overall diet should be relatively low. And it's best if the high-energy-density foods you consume are also rich in nutrients.

Q | What are "super" foods— nutritionally rich, full of fiber, things like that?

"Super" foods is a good way to think about foods that rate high in **nutrient density,** Nutrient-dense foods are those that are naturally rich in vitamins, minerals, and other beneficial food compounds while providing relatively few calories. They are the best way to ensure adequate nutrients from a healthy level of energy intake. Good examples are vegetables, fruits, whole grains, fish, low-fat dairy products, and lean cuts of meat and poultry. To be considered nutrient dense, foods should remain as close to their natural state as possible—relatively unprocessed and without a lot of added sugars or fats. Don't confuse "nutrient-dense" foods with "energy-dense" foods. The former are packed with nutrients, the latter are packed with calories. Sometimes a food can be both (for example, nuts), and although it's good for you, you should not eat too much of it. You'll learn more about identifying nutrient-dense foods in the discussion of food labels on pp. 296–297 and in Chapter 9.

If you think of your daily calories in terms of a budget, you'll want to "spend" your calories wisely—get as much nutrient bang for your calorie buck as you can. Unfortunately, most adults choose many foods

energy density The amount of energy (calories) in a food per unit of weight.

nutrient density The amount of nutrients in a food per energy (calories) provided; a food high in nutrient density provides a substantial amount of vitamins, minerals, and other nutrients, and relatively few calories.

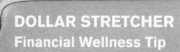

DOLLAR STRETCHER
Financial Wellness Tip

Substitute no-cost water for some of your more expensive beverages. Analysis of the nutrient density and energy costs of foods reveals that most popular sweetened beverages are not a low-cost source of any nutrients—bad for your financial budget and your calorie budget!

that are low in nutrient density. For example, top sources of calories in the diets of young adults ages 19 to 30 include sodas and sports drinks, grain-based desserts (cakes, cookies, doughnuts, and the like), alcoholic beverages, and pizza.[3] These choices are high in calories and low in nutrients, especially fiber, vitamins, and minerals.

The American Diet and the Recommended Diet

Q | I think my diet is about average—I eat what most people eat. Is that good or bad?

Like most Americans, you probably have room for improvement. As described at the beginning of the chapter, the typical American diet is too high in calories

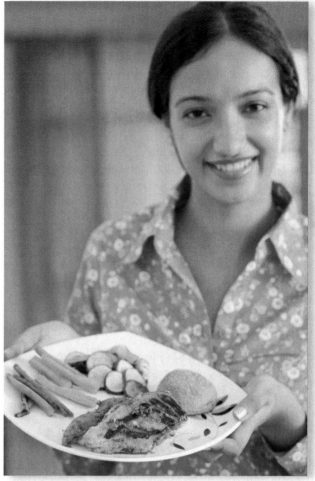

Pay attention to what you eat and how much you eat. Spend your calorie budget wisely by consuming nutrient-dense foods.

Intake as percent of goal or limit

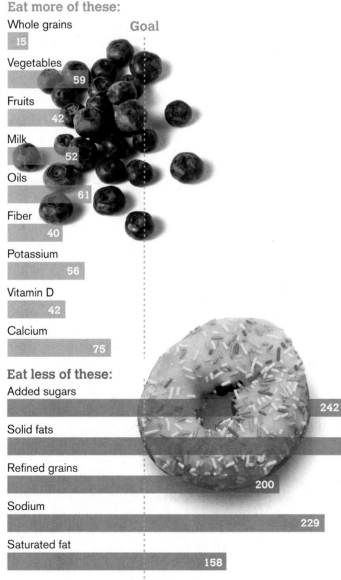

Eat more of these:

Whole grains — Goal — 15
Vegetables — 59
Fruits — 42
Milk — 52
Oils — 61
Fiber — 40
Potassium — 56
Vitamin D — 42
Calcium — 75

Eat less of these:
Added sugars — 242
Solid fats — 281
Refined grains — 200
Sodium — 229
Saturated fat — 158

Limit

and certain nutrients and too low in others (Figure 8-2). In the next sections, we'll review each class of nutrients and provide strategies for achieving a healthy intake—whether that means an increase or a decrease. The dietary recommendations in this chapter are based on the *Dietary Guidelines for Americans,* which are issued by the Departments of Agriculture and Health and Human Services every five years. The guidelines incorporate the Dietary Reference Intakes and are based on expert reviews of nutrition research. They provide authoritative advice about dietary habits that promote health and reduce risk for major chronic diseases. To learn more about the *Dietary Guidelines for Americans,* visit http://www .DietaryGuidelines.gov.

Figure 8-2 Dietary intakes of selected nutrients and foods in comparison to recommended intakes or limits. Americans consume too much added sugars, sodium, unhealthy fats, and refined grains and too little fiber and certain micronutrients.

Source: Dietary Guidelines Advisory Committee. (2010). *Report of the Dietary Guidelines Advisory Committee on the dietary guidelines for Americans, 2010* (http://www.cnpp.usda.gov/DGAs2010-DGACReport.htm).

Carbohydrates

Carbohydrates are one of the three classes of macronutrients; they are typically the source of the largest proportion of calories in the diet. Most people consume plenty of carbohydrates daily, because they are the main component of bread, pasta, cereal, grains, vegetables, fruit, and many other foods.

Carbohydrates are our primary energy source. When carbohydrates are digested, they are broken down into **glucose,** which circulates in the blood as a readily available energy source for cells. Glucose that is not used can be stored as **glycogen** in the liver and skeletal muscles. When energy is needed, glycogen can be converted back into glucose. However, there are limits to how much glucose can be stored as glycogen. Consumption of excess calories as carbohydrate can lead to weight gain and increased body fat.

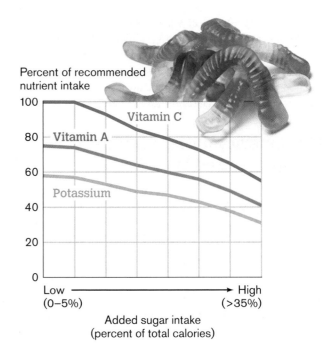

Figure 8-3 **Added sugars and intake of selected nutrients.** As added sugar intake goes up, intake of key vitamins and minerals goes down.

Source: Data from Marriott, B., Olsho, L., Hadden, L., & Connor, P. (2010). Intake of added sugars and selected nutrients in the United States, National Health and Nutrition Examination Survey (NHANES) 2003–2006. *Critical Reviews in Food Science and Nutrition, 50,* 228–258.

Simple and Complex Carbohydrates

Q | What is another name for simple carbohydrates?

carbohydrates A category of essential nutrients that includes sugars, starches, and dietary fiber.

glucose A simple carbohydrate derived from plant sources that circulates in the blood and is used to produce energy; also called blood sugar.

glycogen A form of stored glucose; primarily found in skeletal muscle and the liver.

simple carbohydrates Carbohydrates containing one or two units of sugar per molecule; occur naturally in fruits, milk, and other foods; commonly added to processed foods.

added sugars Simple carbohydrates added during processing and preparation of foods.

complex carbohydrates Carbohydrates such as starches and dietary fiber containing chains of many sugar units.

Simple carbohydrates are one of two general categories of carbohydrates—simple and complex—based on chemical structure. Simple carbohydrates contain one or two units of sugar per molecule, and many of them have a sweet taste. There are different types of simple carbohydrates, including glucose, sucrose, fructose, and lactose.

Simple carbohydrates occur naturally in fruits, honey, sweet potatoes, milk products, and some cereal products. Simple carbohydrates are also often added to foods during processing and preparation and at the table. These **added sugars** provide calories but few other essential nutrients, and high intake of added sugars is associated with unhealthy blood cholesterol levels, elevated blood pressure, poor vitamin and mineral intakes (Figure 8-3), and possibly weight gain.[4] Americans currently consume far above the recommended amount of added sugars. The top sources of added sugars are regular soft drinks, candy, cakes, cookies, pies, fruit drinks, and milk- and grain-based desserts (such as ice cream and sweet rolls). One typical 12-ounce regular soft drink has about 33 grams of added sugars, representing 130 calories.

Complex carbohydrates, which include starches and fiber, contain longer chains of many sugar units. Starches are found naturally in many foods, including grains, such as wheat, oats, rice, and barley; **legumes,** which are beans and peas (for example, pinto beans, kidney beans, lentils); and other vegetables. Most starches are broken down during digestion into simple sugars, which can then be used by the body. Some types of starches, such as those in legumes, are resistant to digestion and don't break down completely, so they can cause intestinal gas. Dietary fiber, discussed in more detail below, doesn't break down during digestion and passes relatively intact into the large intestine.

Grains are edible seeds of certain types of grasses (Figure 8-4). In foods, they can be in the form of **whole grains** or refined grains. In its natural state, a kernel of grain has three parts:

- *Bran:* An outer protective covering that is rich in fiber and contains several vitamins
- *Germ:* The inner part of the seed from which a new plant can sprout; a concentrated source of certain vitamins
- *Endosperm:* The large center of the seed, containing complex carbohydrates

When whole grains are refined, they are stripped of their germ and bran, leaving only the starchy endosperm. The

legumes Peas and beans, such as white, black, and pinto beans; soybeans; lentils; and chickpeas.

whole grain The entire grain kernel, including the bran, germ, and endosperm.

Wellness Strategies

Identifying Carbohydrates: Whole Grains and Added Sugars

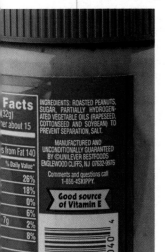

When you walk through a grocery store, you can easily find foods that contain added sugars and processed carbohydrates, especially in the aisles with packaged foods, baked goods, cookies, and candy. To find foods higher in complex carbohydrates, naturally occurring sugars, and whole grains, walk around the perimeter of the store and look for the fresh produce and other foods closer to their natural state. Many grain foods (bread, cereal, pasta) come in whole-grain forms—look for them!

To identify which packaged foods have whole grains and which have added sugars, you need to read ingredient lists. Look for the names listed below, and take note of their position on the ingredient list. If they are first, that means they are the primary ingredient (by weight) in a food product. For grains, you want the whole grain listed first. Don't be fooled by the name of the product—"wheat bread," "multigrain bread," and bread "made with whole wheat" are not necessarily whole-grain rich; check the ingredient list.

Total amounts of sugars are listed on food labels, but the amount on the label doesn't distinguish between naturally occurring sugars and added sugars. However, if a food

doesn't include any fruit or milk products, then all the sugar in the product likely comes from added sugars.

Choose foods with these whole grains high on the ingredient list:

Amaranth	Sorghum
Buckwheat	Triticale
Bulgur (cracked wheat)	Whole grain barley
Brown rice	Whole grain cornmeal
Millet	Whole rye
Oats and oatmeal	Whole wheat
Popcorn	Wild rice
Quinoa	

Limit foods with these added sugars on the ingredient list:

Brown sugar	Invert sugar
Corn sweetener	Lactose
Corn syrup	Maltose
Dextrose	Malt syrup
Fructose	Molasses
Fruit juice concentrate	Raw sugar
Glucose	Sucrose
High-fructose corn syrup	Sugar
Honey	Syrup

refining process converts whole grains to refined grains, producing products like white flour and white rice; it also removes most of the nutrients from the grain. For this reason, whole grains are a richer source of nutrients—

more nutrient dense—than refined grains and therefore recommended.

Some studies have found that whole-grain intake protects again cardiovascular disease, type 2 diabetes, certain types of cancer, and weight gain.[5] Most Americans do not consume adequate amounts of whole grains and thus miss out on the fiber, nutrients, and other beneficial compounds they contain. To improve the quality of your carbohydrate choices, choose whole grains over refined grains at least half the time. In addition, choose foods with naturally occurring sugars, and limit your consumption of added sugars. The box "Identifying Carbohydrates: Whole Grains and Added Sugars" will help you make good choices.

Q | What is the glycemic index?

Glycemic index (GI) is a measure of how quickly carbohydrates you consume increase the level of glucose in your blood. When you consume simple or complex carbohydrates, they are converted into sugar (glucose) in your body. Simple carbohydrates are more quickly and readily converted into glucose than many types of complex carbohydrates are. The higher a food's glycemic index, the faster and

glycemic index (GI)
A scale that quantifies the effect of a carbohydrate-containing food on the level of glucose in the blood.

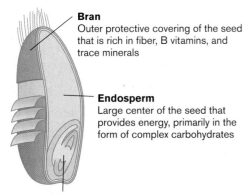

Bran
Outer protective covering of the seed that is rich in fiber, B vitamins, and trace minerals

Endosperm
Large center of the seed that provides energy, primarily in the form of complex carbohydrates

Germ
Part of the seed from which a new plant can sprout; provides fatty acids, vitamin E, B-vitamins, and antioxidants

Figure 8-4 Anatomy of a whole grain. Because whole grains include the bran, germ, and endosperm from the grain kernel, they are naturally higher in nutrients and dietary fiber than refined grains.

higher blood sugar levels increase —and the faster the subsequent drop when the glucose is used up. *Glycemic load* is a related measure, which takes into account the amount of carbohydrate in a food or a meal. For example, carrots have a high glycemic index but a small amount of carbohydrate, or a low glycemic load, so they don't cause as big a rise in blood sugar as a food with a high GI and a large amount of carbohydrate.[6] However, not every food with a low GI value is a good choice—for example, premium full-fat ice cream has a low GI but is very high in calories and fat—and GI isn't listed on food labels or easily calculated. For these reasons, using GI to choose foods can be difficult and complex. However, you can use the following general principles related to glycemic index to improve your food choices:

- Choose foods high in fiber, including whole grains, legumes, vegetables, and fruits.
- Choose fresh or raw foods rather than processed foods.
- Limit your intake of added sugars.

A food that causes a quick rise in blood sugar gives you a quick energy boost but then quickly leaves you feeling hungry again. A food with a lower GI value gives you more of a feeling of satiety (fullness) and keeps you satisfied longer, even if it has the same number of calories as the higher GI food. The dilemma is that when you're hungry, you're looking for something to give you a quick boost, and simple carbohydrates—like candy or a sweet beverage—can do that really well. But then you're hungry again before too long, which can be the start of a poor eating cycle. The better strategy is to avoid becoming overly hungry so you're not tempted to eat foods high in added sugars.

Recommended Carbohydrate Intake

Q How much carbohydrate should I eat daily? Is there an amount or percentage?

The Dietary Reference Intakes (DRIs) described earlier specify a minimum amount of carbohydrate that the body needs in order to function. It is a fairly small amount: 130 grams for adults, or about the amount in two baked potatoes. Most American should consume—and do consume—more. The DRIs also include recommendations for carbohydrate intake as a percentage of total daily calories, a value that depends on the amount of protein and fat consumed.

Acceptable Macronutrient Distribution Ranges (AMDRs) One of the standards that make up the Dietary Reference Intakes; recommended intake ranges for protein, fat, and carbohydrate as percentages of total daily calories.

The **Acceptable Macronutrient Distribution Ranges (AMDRs)** provide a range of healthy values for intake of all macronutrients. For carbohydrates, the range is 45–65 percent of total daily calories. If you're sedentary or have a low overall calorie in-

---

Fast Facts

I'll Take Some Sugar with My Sugar . . . and Fat and Alcohol

On average, Americans consume 83 grams (330 calories) of added sugars per day. Over the course of a year, that adds up to the equivalent of 65 pounds of granulated sugar! On a daily basis, those 330 calories of added sugars contribute to excess energy intake (too many calories) and poor intake of other nutrients (too few nutrients).

The other sources of "empty" calories in the American diet are alcohol and solid fats (such as butter and fats in fatty meats). Together, these three high-calorie, low-nutrient food sources contribute about 1,000 calories per day to the diet of the average American man and 700 calories per day to the diet of the average American woman, squeezing out healthier, more nutrient-dense foods.

The way to meet your nutrient needs without consuming too many calories is to focus on nutrient density and to limit intake of added sugars and other energy-dense, nutrient-poor foods and beverages.

Source: National Cancer Institute, Risk Factor Monitoring and Methods Branch. (2010). Usual energy intake from solid fats, alcoholic beverages & added sugars (SoFAAS). *Diet* (http://riskfactor.cancer.gov/diet/usualintakes/sofaas.html).

---

take, go with a value at the lower end of the range; if you're active, you should consume carbohydrates at the high end of the AMDR range.[7] For added sugars, a limit of no more than 25 percent of total daily calories is suggested—but most people should consume far less. In order to meet your nutrient needs at a healthy energy intake, you need to limit your consumption of empty calories from added sugars.

Lab Activity 8-2 will help you determine your current intake of carbohydrates, protein, and fats. If any are too high, you can then set goals for change.

Q Does eating a lot of carbs matter . . . can carbs make me fat?

Yes, they can, and so can fat, protein, alcohol, and ice cream—and iceberg lettuce and peas and pineapple! If you overeat, you can gain weight, regardless of which foods and beverages you consume. To change your body weight, you simply need to create a deficit or an excess of calories. If you eat more than you need, then you will eventually gain weight, and if you eat less than you need, you slowly lose weight. So, can carbohydrates make you fat? You bet. Can any food make you fat? Absolutely.

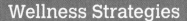

Wellness Strategies

Recommendations for Macronutrients

The Dietary Reference Intakes set several different types of standards for carbohydrates and the other macronutrients. Use these values to assess and plan your diet.

Minimum Adequate Intake

	Women	Men
Carbohydrate	130 grams	130 grams
Protein*	46 grams	56 grams
Fat**		
Omega-6 fatty acid (linoleic acid)	12 grams	17 grams
Omega-3 fatty acid (alpha-linolenic acid)	1.1 grams	1.6 grams

*Protein requirements can be calculated more precisely by multiplying body weight (in pounds) by 0.36 grams (see p. 279).
**See p. 280 for more on specific types of fats.

Acceptable Macronutrient Distribution Ranges

	Percent of Total Daily Calories
Carbohydrate	45%–65%
Fat (total)	20%–35%
Protein	10%–35%

Additional Recommendations

Added sugars	No more than 25% of total daily calories*
Dietary fiber	14 grams of dietary fiber per 1,000 calories consumed (about 25 grams per day for women and 38 grams per day for men)
Dietary cholesterol	As low as possible while consuming a nutritionally adequate diet
Saturated fats	As low as possible while consuming a nutritionally adequate diet
Trans fats	As low as possible while consuming a nutritionally adequate diet

*Added sugars should not displace other nutrients, and a much lower intake is appropriate for most people. The American Heart Association recommends limits of 150 calories (38 grams, equivalent to 9 teaspoons) per day for men and 100 calories (25 grams, equivalent to 6 teaspoons) per day for women.

Sources: National Academies, Institute of Medicine, Food and Nutrition Board. (2005). *Dietary Reference Intakes for energy, carbohydrate, fiber, fat, fatty acids, cholesterol, protein, and amino acids (macronutrients).* Washington, D C : National Academies Press. Johnson, R. K., and others. (2009). Dietary sugars intake and cardiovascular health: A scientific statement from the American Heart Association. *Circulation, 120,* 1011–1020.

A better question is, Can carbs make me healthy? And the answer is yes, they can. In fact, populations and cultures whose diets are high in complex carbohydrates tend to have lower rates of many of the chronic diseases that are common in the United States, including heart disease, diabetes, and certain cancers.[8] But the key to healthy carbohydrate intake is the types of carbohydrate you consume. Populations that favor diets high in simple or refined carbohydrates or both tend to have higher rates of many chronic diseases. As noted earlier, complex carbohydrates, especially whole grains, provide many health benefits—unlike added sugars.

Fiber

Q | What's the deal with fiber? Isn't that like prune juice for old people?

Fiber is for old people—and also for young people who want to grow old gracefully. **Dietary fiber** has tremendous health benefits, and populations that eat fiber-rich diets tend to have very low rates of many chronic diseases.[9] Fiber protects against cardiovascular disease, obesity, and type 2 diabetes, and it helps lower blood pressure and improve blood cholesterol and glucose levels. By adding bulk to your diet, fiber can make you feel full faster, reducing your appetite. It also helps promote digestive health.[10] Dietary fiber reduces constipation, and certain types of fiber may alleviate the symptoms of irritable bowel syndrome in some people.[11] (Irritable bowel syndrome is a common disorder of intestinal functioning characterized by abdominal pain, cramping, bloating, constipation, and diarrhea.) Although research findings are mixed, some studies have suggested that dietary fiber may reduce the risk of colon cancer.[12]

Dietary fiber is nondigestible carbohydrates, and there are two general types:

- **Soluble (viscous) fiber** soaks up water and turns into a gel during digestion. It slows the body's absorption of glucose, improves insulin sensitivity, and may delay the return of hunger after you eat. It also binds with cholesterol in the intestine for quick removal. Examples of foods that contain soluble fiber include peas, soybeans, oats, plums, bananas, the pulp (fleshy parts) of apples and pears, broccoli, carrots, and sweet potatoes.

dietary fiber Complex carbohydrates that cannot be broken down by the digestive system.

soluble (viscous) fiber Form of dietary fiber that soaks up water and turns into a gel during digestion; it may improve the body's insulin sensitivity and cholesterol levels.

■ **Insoluble fiber** binds water in the intestines, thereby making stool bulkier and softer, which speeds the transit of food through the digestive system and makes elimination easier and more complete. Examples of foods that contain insoluble fiber include whole grains, wheat bran, nuts and seeds, potatoes, the skin of apples and pears, flax, green beans, and cauliflower.

Consuming fiber, especially if you suddenly increase your intake, can temporarily increase intestinal gas and flatulence. However, given all the long-term benefits of dietary fiber, that's not a bad trade-off—and your body will adjust to increased fiber intake.

Q | What is the best way to get fiber into your diet?

insoluble fiber Form of dietary fiber that binds water but does not dissolve; it adds bulk to the diet and improves elimination.

Dietary fiber is found naturally only in plant foods. Virtually all plant foods have some amount of fiber, and some have particularly high levels (Figure 8-5). Recommended fiber consumption is based on calorie intake—14 grams per 1,000 calories—which works out to about 25 grams of fiber per day for women and 38 grams per day for men. On average, however, American adults consume only about 15 grams of fiber per day.

Grains, cereals, pasta, rice	Serving size	Fiber (grams)
Bran cereal	1/3 cup	9.1
Shredded wheat cereal	1 cup	5.6
Oat bran flakes cereal	1 cup	5.2
Rye (wafer) crackers	2	5.0
Whole wheat English muffin	1	4.4
Wheat bulgur, cooked	1/2 cup	4.1
Spaghetti, whole wheat	1/2 cup	3.1
Oat bran muffin, small	1	3.0
Barley, pearled, cooked	1/2 cup	3.0
Popcorn, air popped	1 1/2 cups	2.0
Oatmeal, plain, cooked	1/2 cup	2.0
Whole wheat bread	1 slice	1.9
Rye bread	1 slice	1.9
Brown rice	1/2 cup	1.8

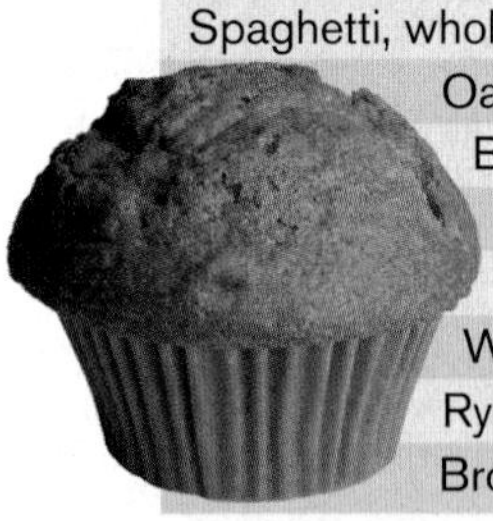

Fruits	Serving size	Fiber (grams)
Pear, medium	1	5.5
Avocado, cubed	1/2 cup	5.0
Apple, medium	1	4.4
Asian pear, small	1	4.4
Raspberries	1/2 cup	4.0
Blackberries	1/2 cup	3.8
Prunes, stewed	1/2 cup	3.8
Figs, dried	1/4 cup	3.7
Banana, medium	1	3.1
Orange, medium	1	3.1
Guava	1	3.0
Dates	1/4 cup	2.9
Apricots	3	2.1
Kiwifruit	1	2.1

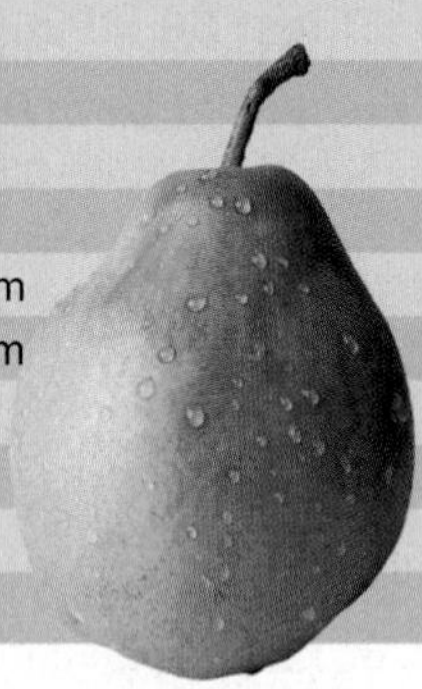

Legumes, nuts, seeds	Serving size	Fiber (grams)
Navy beans	1/2 cup	9.6
Split peas	1/2 cup	8.1
Lentils	1/2 cup	7.8
Pinto beans	1/2 cup	7.7
Black beans	1/2 cup	7.5
Kidney beans	1/2 cup	6.8
Lima beans	1/2 cup	6.6
White beans	1/2 cup	6.3
Chickpeas	1/2 cup	6.2
Soybeans (mature)	1/2 cup	5.2
Almonds	1 oz	3.5
Sunflower seed kernels, dry roasted	1 oz	3.1
Pistachio nuts	1 oz	2.9
Pecans	1 oz	2.7

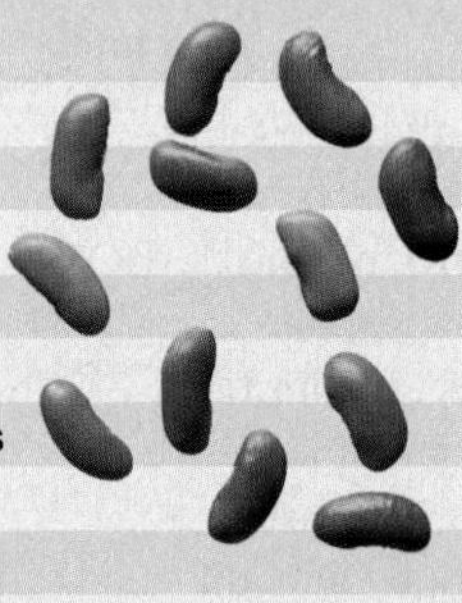

Vegetables	Serving size	Fiber (grams)
Artichoke hearts	1/2 cup	7.2
Green peas	1/2 cup	4.4
Sweet potato, medium, baked with skin	1	3.8
Potato, medium, baked with skin	1	3.8
Soybeans, green	1/2 cup	3.8
Pumpkin, canned	1/2 cup	3.6
Spinach, frozen, cooked	1/2 cup	3.5
Sauerkraut, canned	1/2 cup	3.4
Winter squash, cooked	1/2 cup	2.9
Tomato paste	1/4 cup	2.7
Collards, cooked	1/2 cup	2.7
Broccoli, cooked	1/2 cup	2.6
Okra, cooked	1/2 cup	2.6
Turnip greens, cooked	1/2 cup	2.5

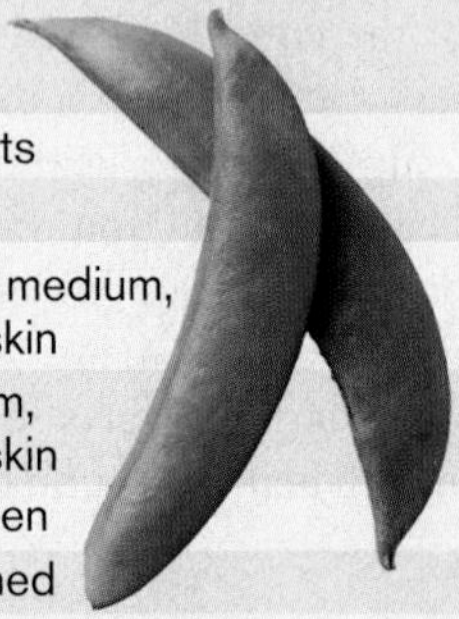

Note: All the food servings listed in this table have fewer than 200 calories.

Figure 8-5 Fiber content of selected high-fiber foods

Source: Data from U.S. Department of Agriculture, Agricultural Research Service, Nutrient Data Laboratory. (2009). *USDA national nutrient database for standard reference,* Release 22 (http://www.ars.usda.gov/ba/bhnrc/ndl).

You can increase your fiber intake by regularly consuming whole-grain products (ones with a whole grain first on the food ingredient list), whole fruits with the skin, legumes, and high-fiber breakfast cereals, which also make nutritious and delicious snacks. Many foods that are high in fiber are also rich in other nutrients and—if they're not prepared with lots of added fats—low in calories, meaning they're nutrient dense.

If you feel overwhelmed or confused about how to get enough fiber, just remember to favor complex carbohydrates and whole foods, fruits, and veggies, and you'll likely meet the daily requirements for healthy carbohydrate intake.

Protein

Q | I don't eat meat. Protein is just for athletes anyway, isn't it?

Protein is for everyone. It's an essential macronutrient that is the major structural component of all the cells in your body. You need protein for the repair and growth of muscle and bone. Proteins and their components also function as enzymes and hormones, in cell membranes and blood, and as carriers of important molecules throughout the body. Like carbohydrates, proteins provide about 4 calories per gram; however, the energy in protein is not liberated quite as easily, so protein is not considered a primary source of energy or fuel for the body.

Complete and Incomplete Proteins

Q | Is red meat the best kind of protein?

Red meat is an excellent source of protein, but there is more to the story. Protein is made up of molecules called **amino acids**—that is, amino acids are the building blocks of the body's protein molecules. There are twenty amino acids, eleven of which can be made by the body and nine of which cannot. *Essential amino acids* are the nine that cannot be made by the body and must be supplied in the diet. Your body can make the eleven *nonessential amino acids* if you consume enough essential amino acids and calories. You can easily obtain essential amino acids if you eat a variety of protein-containing foods, including but not limited to red meat.

Complete proteins contain all the essential amino acids and are found in animal foods and soy: meat, fish, poultry, soybeans and soy products, eggs, and dairy products. (Some of the less widely available grains such as quinoa and amaranth are also complete proteins.) Foods that lack one or more of the essential amino acids are referred to as **incomplete proteins.** Except for soy, plant sources of protein—beans and other vegetables, nuts, seeds, and grains—are incomplete proteins. Meeting protein needs is easy when you include a variety of both types of proteins in your diet, but vegetarians can obtain adequate protein by combining different types of plant proteins (see below).

When selecting animal proteins, consider the type and amount of fat and the total number of calories. Some food sources of animal protein are high in both unhealthy saturated fats and calories; you can choose healthier, more nutrient-dense alternatives. Table 8-3 shows the protein and saturated fat content of some popular protein sources, along with some lower fat alternatives. Fish and shellfish tend to be low in saturated fat, and the fat in many types of fish is a type that has been shown to improve heart health.

Plant sources of protein naturally contain little or no saturated fat, although fats may be added during processing. For plant proteins, your concern should be consuming a variety of sources. Different types of plant proteins are deficient in different amino acids, so combinations of these incomplete proteins create complete proteins. So-called complementary protein pairs include legumes and grains, legumes and nuts, and legumes and seeds. You don't have to consume complementary proteins in the same meal; a variety of plant foods consumed over the course of a day can provide all essential amino acids.[13] It is, however, easy to combine proteins in one meal: pinto beans and a tortilla, hummus with pita bread, vegetable chili with cornbread, salad with chickpeas and sunflower seeds, or split pea soup with rye crackers. Plant foods can be a source of protein for both vegetarians and nonvegetarians. In addition, they contain fiber and are lower in fat and calories than many animal protein sources—in many cases, they are also less expensive.

To sum up the answer to your question, red meat is a valuable source of complete protein, but eating a variety of proteins is healthier than sticking to any single protein source. If you don't eat red meat—and many people do

protein A category of essential macronutrient; a compound made of amino acids.

amino acids Molecules that are the building blocks of proteins; the 9 essential amino acids cannot be made by the body and must be obtained from food; the 11 nonessential amino acids can be made by the body.

complete proteins Dietary sources of protein that provide all the essential amino acids; found in animal foods and soy.

incomplete proteins Dietary sources of protein that are missing one or more essential amino acids; found in plant sources of protein.

DOLLAR STRETCHER
Financial Wellness Tip

Economize on protein by buying small portions of lean meat, poultry, and fish on sale. Fattier cuts may be cheaper, but more goes to waste. Choose less expensive protein sources often; these include plant proteins and nonfat dairy products.

TABLE 8-3 PROTEIN, SATURATED FAT, AND ENERGY CONTENT OF SELECTED PROTEIN SOURCES

FOOD	PROTEIN (GRAMS)	SATURATED FAT (GRAMS)	CALORIES
Regular ground beef patty (30% fat)	21.6	6.2	232
Extra lean ground beef patty (5% fat)	22.4	2.5	145
Veggie burger or soyburger patty	11.0	1.0	124
Fried chicken breast (½) with skin	31.2	2.4	218
Roasted chicken breast (½) without skin	26.7	0.9	142
Salami, sliced (3 oz.)	19.5	8.9	323
Roast beef, fat trimmed (3 oz.)	21.9	3.4	177
Turkey breast, sliced (3 oz.)	11.3	0.1	94
Regular cheddar cheese (1 oz.)	7.1	6.0	114
Low-fat cheddar cheese (1 oz.)	6.9	1.2	49
Whole milk (1 cup)	7.7	4.6	149
Low-fat (1%) milk (1 cup)	9.7	1.8	118
Nonfat milk (1 cup)	8.3	0.1	83
Yogurt, fruit, low-fat (8 oz.)	9.9	1.6	232
Yogurt, plain, nonfat (8 oz.)	14.0	0.3	137
Egg (1 large)	6.3	1.6	78
Salmon (3 oz.)	18.8	2.1	175
Tuna, canned in water (3 oz.)	20.1	0.7	109
Shrimp (3 oz.)	17.8	0.2	84
Tofu (½ cup)	10.0	0.9	94
Soybeans (½ cup)	14.3	1.1	149
Lentils (½ cup)	8.9	0.1	113
Pinto beans (½ cup)	5.8	0.2	103
Kidney beans (½ cup)	6.7	0.1	108
Spaghetti (½ cup)	4.1	0.1	110
Whole-wheat bread (1 small slice)	3.6	0.2	69
Flour tortilla (8-inch)	3.8	0.9	144
Peanut butter (2 tablespoons)	7.7	2.6	188
Sunflower seed kernels, roasted (1 oz.)	5.5	1.5	165
Pumpkin seeds, roasted (1 oz.)	5.3	1.0	126

Source: Data from U.S. Department of Agriculture, Agricultural Research Service, Nutrient Data Laboratory. (2009). *USDA national nutrient database for standard reference,* Release 22 (http://www.ars.usda.gov/ba/bhnrc/ndl).

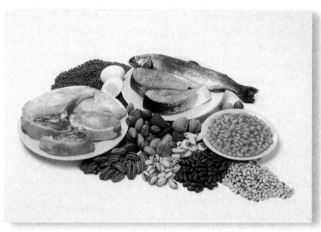

When selecting animal proteins, choose those that are low in unhealthy fats. For plant proteins, consume a variety of protein sources over the course of the day to obtain all essential amino acids.

avoid meat for cultural, religious, ethical, or health reasons—you can meet your daily protein requirement with other lean complete proteins such as chicken, fish, or soy or with a combination of incomplete proteins such as beans, nuts, grains, and vegetables.

Recommended Protein Intake

Q | I hear a lot about protein—how much am I supposed to eat?

Healthy adults need to consume about 0.36 grams of protein per pound (0.8 grams per kilogram) of body weight. Here are some examples:

- 36 grams of protein per day for a 100-pound adult
- 54 grams of protein per day for a 150-pound adult
- 72 grams of protein per day for a 200-pound adult

Lab Activity 8-1 will help you set a personal protein goal based on the Dietary Reference Intakes.

The Acceptable Macronutrient Distribution Range (AMDR) for protein is 10–35 percent of total daily calories. If your diet is relatively low in calories, then the percent of total daily calories from protein may need to be at the higher end of the range in order to meet your daily requirement. For example, for a 200-pound person with a diet of 1,700 calories per day, 72 grams of protein would be 17 percent of total daily calories; with a diet of 3,000 calories per day, 10 percent.

Some people need more protein: Infants, children, adolescents, and women who are pregnant or breastfeeding have different requirements, up to 0.59 grams per pound of body weight for a woman who is breastfeeding. The Dietary Reference Intakes state that athletes do not need additional protein, but the American College of Sports Medicine recommends a somewhat higher protein intake for both endurance athletes (0.54–0.64 grams per pound)

and resistance athletes (0.54–0.77 grams per pound) who are engaged in serious training.[14] Athletes typically consume high-calorie diets, so this higher protein intake can be achieved with food (supplements are not recommended) and remain within the AMDR for protein.

Diets very high in protein—above the AMDR—are not recommended. Some studies have found that very-high-protein diets can have a negative effect on kidney function and bone density in some people.[15] There is no evidence that consuming high levels of protein from foods or supplements, or taking supplements of specific amino acids, will improve athletic performance. For weight loss, high-protein diets are no better than other types of diets. In the long term, it is the total energy content of the diet that matters for weight management, not the macronutrient distribution (see Chapter 9).

On average, Americans consume about 15 percent of total daily calories as protein, so most Americans consume adequate amounts.[16] Of more concern than a shortfall in protein intake is the nutrient profile of the most common sources of protein in the U.S. diet—high in calories and solid fats.

Q | Do I need to eat extra protein from supplements to build muscle?

READ ONLINE

Fats

Q | I know, I know—fats are bad and should always be avoided, right?

No. Not all fats are bad—and some are essential. **Fats** are needed in sufficient quantities for cellular integrity, healthy reproduction, absorption of fat-soluble vitamins, support and cushioning of organs, and thermal insulation. As described earlier, fats also provide energy (9 calories per gram). Consuming healthy fats in limited amounts can boost your health. Choosing the wrong fats can increase your risk of cardiovascular disease and type 2 diabetes, and consuming too much fat can lead to weight gain, just as consuming excess calories from any other source does.

Types of Fats

Fats in food are made up of different types of fatty acids. These fatty acids are found in the form of **triglycerides,** which contain three fatty-acid molecules and a glycerol molecule. Fatty acids are chains of carbon atoms with hydrogen atoms attached to some or all of the carbon atoms. Chemical differences—in the length of carbon

fats A category of essential macronutrient; an organic compound made up of fatty acids; lipid.

triglycerides Major form of fat found in foods and stored in the body, consists of three fatty-acid molecules and a glycerol molecule.

chains, the types of bonds between the carbon atoms, and the number of hydrogen atoms attached to the carbon chains—give rise to the differing effects of various types of fats on health. Most food fats contain a mix of different types of fatty acids. Let's review the types of fats and their effects on health.

Q | What's the difference between saturated and unsaturated fats?

The difference is in their chemical structure and behavior in the body (Figure 8-6).

- **Saturated fatty acids:** All the bonds between carbon atoms on the chain are single bonds, and every available bond from each carbon atom is attached to a hydrogen atom. In other words, the fatty acid chain is "saturated" with hydrogen atoms. Saturated fats are generally solid at room temperature.
- **Unsaturated fatty acids:** One or more of the available bonds on the carbon chain is not attached to a hydrogen atom, and neighboring carbon atoms form a double bond. Fatty acids with one double bond are called *monounsaturated* and those with two or more double bonds are called *polyunsaturated.* Unsaturated fats are usually liquid at room temperature and are called oils.

Food fats typically contain multiple types of fatty acids, and the predominant types determine the fat's characteristics. Butter is about two-thirds saturated fat and one-third unsaturated fat, so it is fairly solid at room temperature. Corn oil is about 85 percent unsaturated fatty acids, so it is liquid at room temperature. Generally speaking, saturated fats are found primarily in animal products, whereas unsaturated fats come from plant sources. There are exceptions: Fish contains polyunsaturated fatty acids, and certain plant oils (coconut and palm) are highly saturated.

saturated fatty acid A fatty acid with a carbon chain full of hydrogen atoms; usually from animal sources and solid at room temperature.

unsaturated fatty acid A fatty acid with a carbon chain that includes one or more carbon-carbon double bonds; usually from plant sources and liquid at room temperature. Monounsaturated fatty acids have one carbon-carbon double bond, and polyunsaturated fatty acids have two or more double bonds.

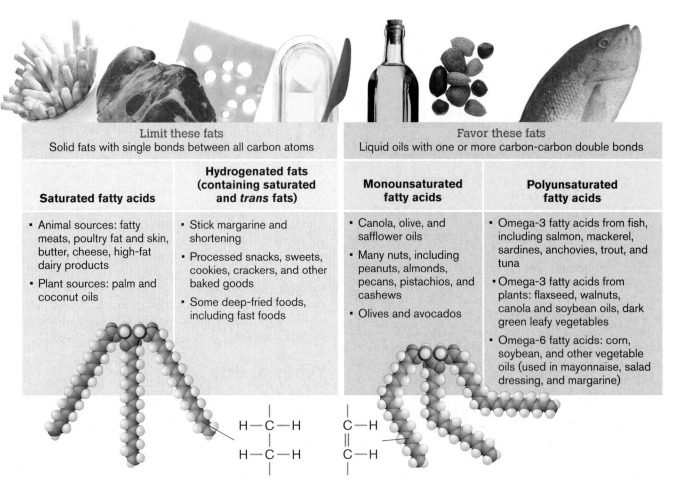

Limit these fats
Solid fats with single bonds between all carbon atoms

Favor these fats
Liquid oils with one or more carbon-carbon double bonds

Saturated fatty acids

- Animal sources: fatty meats, poultry fat and skin, butter, cheese, high-fat dairy products
- Plant sources: palm and coconut oils

Hydrogenated fats (containing saturated and *trans* fats)

- Stick margarine and shortening
- Processed snacks, sweets, cookies, crackers, and other baked goods
- Some deep-fried foods, including fast foods

Monounsaturated fatty acids

- Canola, olive, and safflower oils
- Many nuts, including peanuts, almonds, pecans, pistachios, and cashews
- Olives and avocados

Polyunsaturated fatty acids

- Omega-3 fatty acids from fish, including salmon, mackerel, sardines, anchovies, trout, and tuna
- Omega-3 fatty acids from plants: flaxseed, walnuts, canola and soybean oils, dark green leafy vegetables
- Omega-6 fatty acids: corn, soybean, and other vegetable oils (used in mayonnaise, salad dressing, and margarine)

Figure 8-6 Types of fats. Although all food fats are in the form of triglycerides, fatty acids differ in their chemical properties and structure, which affects their behavior in the body and their long-term impact on health.

Q | Why is saturated fat so unhealthy for you?

When you consume saturated fats, they act on your liver to increase the amount of low-density lipoproteins (LDL), or "bad" cholesterol, in your blood. High levels of LDL increase your risk for heart attack and stroke. Saturated fat is also associated with insulin resistance in cells, which increases your risk for type 2 diabetes. Our bodies can make all the saturated fats we require, so saturated fatty acids are not an essential nutrient—we don't actually need to eat any! Replacing some of the saturated fats in your diet with unsaturated fats can reduce your risk for a variety of serious health problems.

Saturated fats occur naturally in many foods from animal sources, including fatty cuts of beef and pork; poultry with skin; and cream, butter, cheese, and other dairy products made from whole milk or reduced-fat (2 percent) milk. Many processed foods—fried and baked desserts and snack foods, for example—also contain high levels of saturated fat. Top sources of saturated fat in the U.S. diet include cheese, pizza, grain- and dairy-based desserts, sausage and other fatty meats, whole and reduced-fat milk, and mixed dishes containing beef and chicken.[17]

Q | What are *trans* fats, and why are they so bad?

Trans fats are produced during the process of **hydrogenation,** in which hydrogen atoms are added to polyunsaturated fatty acids, turning some of them into saturated fatty acids. Food manufacturers use this process because hydrogenated fats have a longer shelf life and can be reused for frying; they also improve the texture of some baked goods. Because they are solid or semisolid at room temperature, hydrogenated vegetable oils are used to create shortening, margarine, and spreadable fats.

Typically, only some of the carbon-carbon double bonds are converted to single bonds during hydrogenation, resulting in a "partially hydrogenated" oil. The partial hydrogenation of oils affects the remaining double bonds on the carbon chains, changing their shape to a configuration referred to as *trans.* Like saturated fats, **_trans_ fatty acids** raise bad LDL, but they also lower HDL (high-density lipoproteins, or "good" cholesterol)—a double blow to heart health. Hydrogenated fats contain both saturated fats and *trans* fats and so should be limited in your diet.

Trans fats are found in foods fried in hydrogenated oils or shortening, such as french fries and doughnuts, as well as many types of baked goods, including cookies, cakes, pastries, pie crust, and biscuits. Stick margarines can be another source. Small amounts of *trans* fats also occur naturally in some meat and dairy products, but it's unclear if these naturally occurring *trans* fats are as bad for health as those that have been manufactured.

In response to the significant negative health effects of *trans* fats, the U.S. Department of Agriculture in 2006 mandated that *trans* fat content be listed on food labels, and some cities began banning it in restaurant foods. Food manufacturers have started reducing or eliminating *trans* fat from their products, and it's possible that artificially produced *trans* fats will cease to be a part of our national diet. In the meantime, read food labels and use caution when you see the word *hydrogenated* in the ingredient list or *trans* fat listed on the food label. When it comes to *trans* fat, the less you consume, the better. Ideally, the only *trans* fats in your diet should be those that occur naturally.

Q | What are omega fatty acids?

When you see *omega* in reference to a fat, it is an indication of the chemical structure of a polyunsaturated fat. In omega-3 fatty acids, the first carbon-carbon double bond starts with the third carbon from the end of the carbon chain; similarly, in omega-6 fatty acids, the first double bond is at the sixth carbon from the end.

The two essential fatty acids in the human diet are both polyunsaturated:

- Alpha-linolenic acid (ALA) is an omega-3 fatty acid found in fairly high concentrations in flaxseeds and flaxseed oil, walnuts and walnut oil, soybeans and soybean oil, and canola oil. The body converts ALA into other types of fats. The top food source of ALA in the American diet is salad dressing.
- Linoleic acid is an omega-6 fatty acid widespread in commonly used food oils, including safflower, sunflower, and corn oils. Lack of linoleic acid in the diet can cause hair loss and poor wound healing.

hydrogenation A process that adds hydrogen atoms to polyunsaturated fats to produce a more solid and stable fat; hydrogenated fats include saturated fatty acids and standard and *trans* forms of unsaturated fatty acids.

trans fatty acid An unsaturated fatty acid with an atypical chemical shape that affects its functioning in the body; found naturally in small amounts in certain foods and produced during the process of hydrogenation.

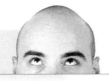

Mind Stretcher
Critical Thinking Exercise

When you make your daily food choices, do you ever consider basic dietary guidelines and nutritional recommendations? Do you look at food labels and the other nutritional information provided in stores and restaurants? What criteria do you use in selecting foods? If you were a public health official, what strategies would you use to get people like yourself and your peers to put more emphasis on nutrition recommendations in making food choices?

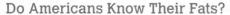

Research Brief

Do Americans Know Their Fats?

The first step to making healthy choices about fats is being able to identify the different types of fats and how they affect health. How do Americans stack up? Although knowledge has improved in the past few years, there are still information gaps. A 2008 survey found the following among a representative sample of American adults.

Knowledge of the relationship between different fats and heart disease

Who knows that consumption of . . .	Percent
Saturated fat increases risk of heart disease	77%
Trans fat increases risk of heart disease	73%
Hydrogenated oils increase risk of heart disease	56%
Polyunsaturated fat decreases the risk of heart disease	44%
Monounsaturated fat decreases the risk of heart disease	41%
Vegetable oils decrease the risk of heart disease	24%

Knowledge of sources of fats

Who can name one food source of . . .	Percent
Saturated fats	79%
Trans fats	72%
Polyunsaturated fats	59%
Monounsaturated fats	53%

Who can name three food sources of . . .	Percent
Saturated fats	30%
Trans fats	17%

How would you have done on the survey? If you're still confused about the different types of fats, review Figure 8-6 and the other information in this section of the chapter. If you've got it straight, then put your knowledge into action. Check foods labels and other sources of nutrition information to make healthy choices.

Source: Eckel, R. H., and others. (2009). Americans' awareness, knowledge, and behaviors regarding fats. *Journal of the American Dietetic Association, 109*(2), 288–296.

Don't get bogged down in the chemistry of fats! Because you will often see news stories about omega-3 and omega-6 fats, you just need a little background to put the information in context.

Q I hate tuna, but heard it has fats that are good for you. Is this true?

Yes. Some fish are rich in particular types of omega-3 fatty acids with long names—eicosapentaenoic acid (EPA) and docosahexaenoic acid (DHA). These fats are considered heart-healthy because they reduce blood clots, decrease inflammation, normalize heart rhythms, and lower the risk of developing or dying from high blood pressure, coronary heart disease, and stroke for some people. These omega-3 fatty acids are found in many fish, including salmon, herring, sardines, trout, tuna, mackerel, and anchovies. The body can also synthesize these compounds from plant sources of alpha-linolenic acid (ALA, described above), but the process is very inefficient and doesn't produce much EPA and DHA.

Because of the health benefits of these omega-3 fats, health authorities recommend that we eat several servings of fish per week. There are cautions about eating certain types of fish, which may be contaminated by mercury and other heavy metals (see Chapter 9 for more on food safety).

If you don't like tuna, then try other types of fish and seafood—and try them prepared in different ways. If you don't like any type of fish or seafood, you can obtain some healthy omega-3 fats from plant sources such as flaxseed and walnut oils, although as described above, they yield very small amounts of EPA and DHA.

Cholesterol

Q Is there good and bad cholesterol in foods?

Not exactly, no. **Dietary cholesterol** is a waxy substance in the cell walls of animal tissues—so it is found only in animal products. The top sources of dietary cholesterol in the American diet are egg yolks, dairy products, and meat (beef, chicken, sausage, bacon, and so on). There is no dietary requirement for cholesterol because your body can manufacture all the cholesterol it needs.

How does dietary cholesterol relate to blood cholesterol? The two are different types of cholesterol. Most blood cholesterol is produced by your liver, with only about a quarter or less coming from the foods you eat. Blood cholesterol circulates through your body, carried in protein packages called lipoproteins.

dietary cholesterol A waxy substance in the cell walls of animal tissues; in humans, produced by the liver and consumed in animal products.

- *Low-density lipoprotein (LDL)* carries cholesterol from the liver to the rest of the body. High levels of LDL can cause dangerous accumulation of cholesterol on the walls of blood vessels.
- *High-density lipoprotein (HDL)* carries cholesterol from the body back to the liver, where it can be eliminated.

You can see why LDL and HDL are referred to as "bad" and "good" forms of blood cholesterol.

High intake of dietary cholesterol can raise levels of blood cholesterol, including bad LDL, but it is not considered as much of a culprit as dietary saturated and *trans* fats. These two dietary fats promote cholesterol production by the liver, which is where most of blood cholesterol comes from. So, consuming dietary cholesterol in moderation is OK.

Plant foods contain related cellular compounds called **phytosterols.** These compounds are similar in structure to cholesterol and they compete with dietary cholesterol for absorption during digestion. What this means is that phytosterols reduce the amount of dietary cholesterol absorbed by the body—a health benefit![18] Phytosterols are found naturally in plant foods and are sometimes added as supplements in margarine spreads, salad dressings, and other foods. Phytosterol supplements may be recommended for some people with high blood cholesterol or heart disease.

phytosterol A plant-based compound that competes with dietary cholesterol for absorption by the body, resulting in lower blood cholesterol levels.

Recommended Fat Intake

Q | How much fat should I consume in one day to have a healthy amount?

As you've seen, there are many recommendations related to your fat intake—for both type and amount. Most Americans get plenty of fat in their diet and meet the requirement for essential fatty acids, which is equivalent to about 4 teaspoons of vegetable oil (see p. 275). The Acceptable Macronutrient Distribution Range for fat is 20–35 percent of total daily calories. Most of that should come from unsaturated fats from plant and fish sources instead of saturated and *trans* fats from animal fats and hydrogenated oils. Replacing some of the saturated and *trans* fats in your diet with unsaturated fats is a great change to make for reducing your risk of chronic disease.

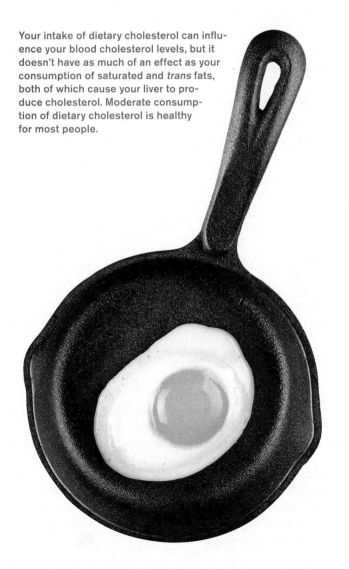

Your intake of dietary cholesterol can influence your blood cholesterol levels, but it doesn't have as much of an effect as your consumption of saturated and *trans* fats, both of which cause your liver to produce cholesterol. Moderate consumption of dietary cholesterol is healthy for most people.

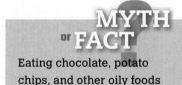

Eating chocolate, potato chips, and other oily foods makes acne worse.

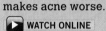 WATCH ONLINE

Water

Q | Why is drinking water important?

Water is a vital nutrient. It is needed for the digestion and absorption of food; it is the main ingredient in blood; and it provides lubrication, cushioning, and temperature control throughout the body. Adult males are about 60 percent water by weight, and adult females about 55 percent water by weight. To maintain a healthy water balance and sustain life, you must consume enough fluids to balance what you lose through urine, sweat, evaporation in the lungs, and bowel movements.

Sources of Water

Liquids, fruits, and vegetables are good food sources of water, though almost all foods contain some water.

Q | Can I drink juice instead of water?

Juice, like all types of fluids you consume, can help you meet your daily water requirement. On average, fluids are the source of about

Wellness Strategies

Tips for Meeting Dietary Fat and Cholesterol Recommendations

When you complete Lab Activity 8-2, you'll find out where you stand in relation to most of the guidelines for fat and cholesterol intake. Then develop strategies for change that are right for you.

Targets

- Overall fat intake: 20%–35% of total daily calories
- Saturated fat: 10% or less of total daily calories (initial goal), working toward 7% or less of total daily calories
- *Trans* fat: Avoid artificially produced *trans* fats; the small amount of *trans* fats in the diet should be from natural sources
- Dietary cholesterol: 300 mg or less per day for healthy adults, 200 mg or less per day for people with or at high risk for cardiovascular disease or type 2 diabetes

General Strategies

- Read food labels and nutrition information available at restaurants to identify the type and amount of fat in the foods you commonly eat; use the information to make good choices
- Trim obvious fat from cuts of meats
- Monitor and limit portion sizes of foods high in unhealthy fats and cholesterol

Substitutions to Try

Instead of:	Try:
Regular cheese	Low-fat or fat-free cheese, or select a favorite cheese and cut your portion size in half
Full-fat ice cream and other desserts	Low-fat or fat-free ice cream, frozen yogurt, and dessert toppings
Pizza with cheese and meat toppings	Pizza with vegetable toppings; ask for half the usual amount of cheese
Sausage, bacon, salami, high-fat lunch meats	Canadian bacon, sliced turkey, other lower-fat lunch meats
Butter, stick margarine	Tub or squeeze margarine spreads, vegetable oils
Cream- or cheese-based salad dressings, sour cream	Vegetable-based salad dressings, low-fat or nonfat sour cream or plain yogurt
Pasta with cream sauce or alfredo sauce	Pasta with tomato or other vegetable-based sauce
Fried chicken or fish	Baked chicken (without skin) or fish
Ground beef, ribs, pork chops, prime grades of beef	Ground turkey, veggie burgers, extra-lean ground beef, sirloin steak, choice grades of beef
Biscuits, muffins, coffee cake, pastries	Fruit, yogurt, or small serving of a sweet treat
Fruit pie with crust	Baked fruit crisp (no pastry crust)

---

80 percent of daily water intake, and the water in foods the remaining 20 percent. Many fruits and vegetables are very high in water content.

Water is usually the best source for meeting the body's hydration needs. That said, many people consume other types of beverages daily, some healthier than others. Milk is an important source of calcium, especially for children. However, some people have trouble digesting milk; see the box "Living with . . . Lactose Intolerance." Orange juice is a favorite breakfast drink and contains lots of vitamin C and potassium, but orange juice fortified with calcium is also available and usually has as much calcium as milk. Fruit juice can be a good source of water if it fits in your overall nutrient and calorie needs. Although whole fruits are more nutrient dense than fruit juice, 100-percent fruit juices are healthier beverage choices than fruit drinks or punches (which often have little fruit and much added sugar) or other types of beverages high in calories and sugar.

Q Does soda count? Can I have soda instead of water?

As a source of water, yes, soda counts. Plain water, juice, soda, coffee, tea, and alcoholic beverages all count. But although soda is a favorite beverage of many, it often isn't the best choice. Regular soda is loaded with added sugars, has no vitamins or minerals, and contains phosphoric acid, which can speed the body's excretion of calcium.[19] Unfortunately, soda consumption in children, adolescents, and some other population groups has replaced milk consumption.[20] Although the short-term effects of this may be negligible, there is concern that over the long term, drinking soda instead of milk may result in lower bone mineral density.[21] Lower bone density in young people can place them at greater risk for osteoporosis later in life. Drinking empty calories as sodas may also be linked with increased rates of overweight and obesity in children.

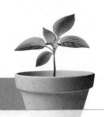

Living with . . .

Lactose Intolerance

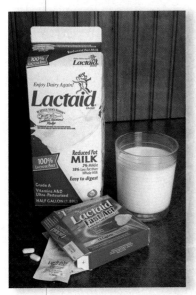

Lactose intolerance is the inability to digest significant amounts of lactose, the predominant sugar in milk. This condition may affect more than 30 million Americans. Its occurrence is lowest among European Americans and higher among African Americans, Latinos, Asian Americans, and Native Americans.

The problem stems from a shortage of the enzyme lactase, which is normally produced by cells lining the small intestine. Lactase breaks down milk sugar into simpler forms that can then be absorbed into the bloodstream. When there is not enough lactase to digest the amount of lactose consumed, the results, although not usually dangerous, may be distressing. Common symptoms include nausea, cramps, bloating, gas, and diarrhea, which can begin shortly after eating or drinking foods containing lactose.

The best treatment for lactose intolerance is prevention, which usually occurs through trial and error. Many people who are lactose intolerant can consume some lactose—the equivalent of 1 cup of milk—without developing symptoms and so can consume small servings of dairy products throughout the day. For those who react to very small amounts of lactose or have trouble limiting their intake of foods that contain it, nonprescription lactase enzymes can convert the lactose in milk to a more digestible form. Lactose-reduced milk and other dairy products are available at most supermarkets. These products contain all the nutrients found in regular dairy products.

If you are lactose intolerant, make sure your diet includes the recommended amount of calcium even if you don't consume dairy products. Nondairy foods high in calcium are green vegetables such as broccoli and kale and fish with soft, edible bones such as salmon and sardines. Recent research indicates that yogurt with active cultures may be a good source of calcium for many people with lactose intolerance, even though it is fairly high in lactose. Evidence shows that the bacterial cultures used to make yogurt produce some of the lactase enzyme required for proper digestion of lactose.

Sources: NIH Consensus Development Conference: Lactose Intolerance and Health. (2010, February). *Final panel statement* (http://consensus .nih.gov/2010/lactosestatement.htm). National Digestive Diseases Information Clearinghouse. (2009). *Lactose intolerance* (http://digestive.niddk .nih.gov/ddiseases/pubs/lactoseintolerance).

Fast Facts

Water of Life

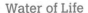

A person can survive much longer without food than without water. How long a person can survive without water depends on the person and the conditions. A baby or a child left in a hot car, an athlete exercising in hot weather, or a senior left alone without air conditioning during a heat wave might become dehydrated and overheated and die within just a few hours. In less extreme conditions, an adult might live for 7–10 days without water—but he or she would be very ill. A person can live for more than a month without food.

Source: Environmental Protection Agency. (2007). *Water trivia facts* (http://www.epa.gov/safewater/kids/water_trivia_facts.html).

Can you drink sodas instead of water? Absolutely. Should they be your primary beverage? Definitely not. When you have a choice, choose water—it is calorie-free and cost-free.

Recommended Intake of Water

Q Do I really need eight glasses of water a day?

Drinking eight glasses of water a day was considered the norm for a long time. However, the latest U.S. dietary guidelines concluded that the combination of thirst and usual drinking patterns (especially consumption of fluids with meals) is sufficient to maintain a normal level of hydration in most cases. Individual needs are variable and depend on factors such as daily physical activity level and heat exposure. The average water intake of people between 19 and 30 is about 3.7 liters (13 cups) for men and 2.7 liters (9 cups) for women—the totals are from drinking water and other beverages as well as the water contained in foods.[22]

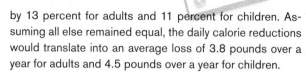

Research Brief

A Tax on Sweetness?

The rise in obesity among Americans has been associated with eating more meals away from home and drinking more caloric sweetened beverages. Together, sodas, energy drinks, and sports drinks are now the leading source of calories for Americans ages 14–30. These beverages contain added sugars but few if any other nutrients.

Some organizations and state and local governments have suggested a tax on caloric sweetened beverages. A recent study analyzed the effects of a hypothetical tax that would increase the price of caloric sweetened beverages by 20 percent. Researchers estimated that the tax would reduce the total calorie intake from the taxed beverages by 13 percent for adults and 11 percent for children. Assuming all else remained equal, the daily calorie reductions would translate into an average loss of 3.8 pounds over a year for adults and 4.5 pounds over a year for children.

What do you think? If you consume these types of beverages, would such a tax reduce your intake? What do you think of the general strategy of taxing "empty" calories?

Source: Smith, T. A., Lin, B.-H., & Lee, J.-Y. (2010). *Taxing caloric sweetened beverages: Potential effects on beverage consumption, calorie intake, and obesity.* USDA Economic Research Service report no. ERR-100 (http://www.ers.usda.gov/Publications/err100/).

How can you tell if you are drinking enough water? Do you rarely feel thirsty? Do you produce at least 1.5 liters (6–7 cups) of slightly yellow urine per day? If so, then your fluid intake is probably sufficient. Healthy people who regularly participate in physical activity or are exposed to excess heat may need more purposeful drinking to maintain adequate hydration levels. See Chapter 3 for more specific recommendations for fluid intake during exercise.

Vitamins and Minerals

Q | Are minerals different from vitamins?

Both vitamins and minerals are micronutrients, but vitamins are organic and minerals are inorganic. What that means is that vitamins contain carbon and minerals don't. Humans need about fourteen different vitamins and seventeen different minerals.

Vitamins are divided into two groups: *water-soluble* (vitamin C and the B vitamins) and *fat-soluble* (vitamins A, D, E, and K). Water-soluble vitamins travel throughout the body in the bloodstream, and excess amounts are excreted in the urine, so these vitamins need to be regularly replaced in the body. Fat-soluble vitamins are absorbed differently and can be stored by the body in the liver and fatty tissues.

Minerals, also called elements, are divided into two groups: *major minerals* and *trace minerals.* The major minerals (at least 100 milligrams needed daily) include sodium, calcium, phosphorus, magnesium, potassium, and chloride. The trace minerals, or those needed in much smaller amounts, include copper, fluoride, iodine, iron, selenium, and zinc. Although the daily requirement for the trace minerals is much lower than the major minerals, they are no less important.

vitamins Organic (carbon-containing) compounds needed in small quantities by the body for normal functioning.

minerals Inorganic compounds essential for normal metabolism, growth and development, and regulation of cell activity.

Q | What do vitamins and minerals do?

Vitamins are necessary to regulate certain body functions and processes, including tissue growth and repair, the release of energy from nutrients, preservation of healthy cells, and the maintenance of nerves, skeletal tissue, red blood cells, and immune function. Without adequate vitamin intake, these processes will not work optimally. In addition, some vitamins are believed to help reduce the risk of chronic diseases; see the discussion of antioxidants on p. 290 for more information. Minerals perform functions similar to those of vitamins, including the liberation of energy and the regulation of growth and development. To learn more about what specific vitamins and minerals do for you, see Tables 8-4 and 8-5.

If you consume significantly less than the recommended amount of a particular vitamin or mineral, symptoms of a deficiency disease can develop. For example, people who consume little or no vitamin C for a month or longer will develop scurvy, whose symptoms include weakness, bleeding gums, and tooth loss. Full-blown deficiency diseases are rare among Americans. However, many people do not consume recommended amounts of certain vitamins and minerals, and although the shortfalls may not be sufficient to cause a deficiency disease in the short term, there can be long-term effects. For example, below-recommended intakes of calcium and vitamin D can limit peak bone-mass development; in later life, this increases the risk of osteoporosis, fractures, and related disabilities.

Sources and Recommended Intakes of Vitamins and Minerals

Q | How much calcium and iron do I need to be healthy?

Dietary Reference Intakes (DRIs) have been established for the essential vitamins and minerals—

TABLE 8-4 VITAMINS: SOURCES, FUNCTIONS, AND RECOMMENDED INTAKES

VITAMIN	MAJOR FUNCTIONS	KEY FOOD SOURCES	RECOMMENDED DAILY INTAKE*
FAT-SOLUBLE VITAMINS			
VITAMIN A	Maintenance of normal vision, immune system functioning, reproduction and fetal development, skin and the surface linings of the nose, mouth, and digestive tract	Liver and other organ meats, oily fish, eggs, milk and other fortified dairy products, dark-colored fruits and leafy vegetables (e.g., tomatoes, red peppers, sweet potatoes, kale, carrots)	Males: 900 µg Females: 700 µg
VITAMIN D	Absorption of calcium and phosphorus for maintenance of healthy bones and teeth; support for healthy cellular metabolism	Fortified dairy products, orange juice, cereals; eggs, liver, oily fish (skin also produces vitamin D in response to exposure to sunlight)	Males: 15 µg (600 IU) Females: 15 µg (600 IU)
VITAMIN E	An antioxidant that protects cells from damage by free radicals; may help prevent chronic disease	Vegetable oils, whole grains, nuts, seeds, leafy green vegetables	Males: 15 mg Females: 15 mg
VITAMIN K	Blood clotting, bone metabolism	Leafy green vegetables, Brussels sprouts, cabbage, soy, asparagus, green beans, dried plums	Males: 120 µg Females: 90 µg
WATER-SOLUBLE VITAMINS			
BIOTIN	Synthesis of fats, glycogen, and amino acids	Egg yolk, legumes, nuts, cereals, yeast, liver; smaller amounts in fruits and meat; also synthesized by intestinal bacteria	Males: 30 µg Females: 30 µg
CHOLINE	Maintenance of cell membranes; precursor for acetylcholine, a neurotransmitter involved in muscle control, memory, and other functions	Milk, eggs, liver, pork, fish, soy milk, peanuts	Males: 550 mg Females: 425 mg
FOLATE	Metabolism of DNA, RNA, and amino acids; synthesis of new cells; prevents one form of anemia	Enriched grain products, green vegetables (spinach, broccoli, asparagus), orange juice, legumes, beets, whole grains, liver	Males: 400 µg Females: 400 µg
NIACIN	Energy metabolism	Meat, fish, poultry, enriched and whole-grain breads and cereals, leafy green vegetables, potatoes, peanuts	Males: 16 mg Females: 14 mg
PANTOTHENIC ACID	Energy metabolism, synthesis of fats, neurotransmitters, hormones, and hemoglobin	Chicken, beef, fish and shellfish, whole grains, legumes, egg yolk, oats, potatoes, tomatoes, broccoli	Males: 5 mg Females: 5 mg
RIBOFLAVIN (VITAMIN B-2)	Energy metabolism, many cellular processes	Wide variety of foods, including milk, meats, grains, and fortified cereals	Males: 1.3 mg Females: 1.1 mg
THIAMINE (VITAMIN B-1)	Required for metabolism of carbohydrates and protein	Enriched, fortified, and whole-grain foods; organ meats, leafy green vegetables, nuts, legumes	Males: 1.2 mg Females: 1.1 mg
VITAMIN B-6	Metabolism of amino acids and glycogen; support for cellular functioning and immune response	Meat, chicken, fish, liver and other organ meats, whole grains, nuts, legumes, fortified products	Males: 1.3 mg Females: 1.3 mg
VITAMIN B-12	Synthesis of amino acids, DNA, red blood cells; support for nervous system functioning	Fish and seafood, meat, poultry, fortified grain products, milk and yogurt	Males: 2.4 µg Females: 2.4 µg
VITAMIN C	Aids in iron absorption, promotion of healing, immune function, and protein metabolism; an antioxidant that protects cells from damage by free radicals	Most vegetables and fruit, especially citrus fruits, tomatoes, berries, potatoes, green vegetables	Males: 90 mg Females: 75 mg

*Recommended daily intakes for adults ages 19–30; for information on other age groups and life stages, including pregnancy, visit http://iom.edu/Activities/Nutrition/SummaryDRIs/DRI-Tables.aspx; to calculate your personal DRIs, go to the Interactive DRI website (http://fnic.nal.usda.gov/interactiveDRI).

Sources: Adapted from Food and Nutrition Board, National Academies. (2010). *Dietary Reference Intakes: Vitamins* (http://fnic.nal.usda.gov/nal_display/index.php?info_center=4&tax_level=3&tax_subject=256&topic_id=1342&level3_id=5140). Dietary Guidelines Advisory Committee. (2010). *Report of the Dietary Guidelines Advisory Committee on the dietary guidelines for Americans, 2010* (http://www.cnpp.usda.gov/DGAs2010-DGACReport.htm).

TABLE 8-5 SELECTED MINERALS: SOURCES, FUNCTIONS, AND RECOMMENDED INTAKES

MINERAL	MAJOR FUNCTIONS	KEY FOOD SOURCES	RECOMMENDED DAILY INTAKE*
CALCIUM	Formation of bones and teeth, control of blood clotting, muscle and nerve functioning	Milk and other dairy products, calcium-set tofu, fortified orange juice and bread, green leafy vegetables, broccoli, bones in fish	Males: 1,000 mg Females: 1,000 mg
FLUORIDE	Maintenance of tooth and bone structure; prevention of dental caries	Fluoridated water, tea, certain fish eaten with bones	Males: 4 mg Females: 3 mg
IODINE	Essential part of thyroid hormones, regulation of body metabolism	Iodized salt, seafood, processed foods	Males: 150 µg Females: 150 µg
IRON	Component of hemoglobin, myoglobin, and enzymes; regulation of cell growth and differentiation; prevention of anemia	Meat and poultry, fish and seafood, fortified grain products, legumes, dark-green vegetables, dried fruit, pumpkin seeds	Males: 8 mg Females: 18 mg
MAGNESIUM	Maintenance of normal muscle and nerve function, energy transfer, activation of many enzymes	Widespread in foods, especially nuts, seeds, whole grains, legumes, leafy green vegetables, soymilk, yogurt	Males: 400 mg Females: 310 mg
PHOSPHORUS	Maintenance of acid-base balance, bone growth and maintenance, energy storage and transfer in cells, synthesis of DNA and RNA	Widespread in foods, especially milk and other dairy products, fish, seeds, whole grains, meat, poultry	Males: 700 mg Females: 700 mg
POTASSIUM	Maintenance of body water balance and cellular function; assists in muscle contraction; blunts rise in blood pressure from excess sodium; decreases bone turnover and recurrence of kidney stones	Fruits and vegetables, especially leafy greens, cantaloupe, bananas, orange juice, mushrooms, potatoes, tomato sauce, legumes, diary products, nuts, fish, pork	Males: 4,700 mg Females: 4,700 mg
SELENIUM	Defense against oxidative stress from free radicals; regulation of thyroid hormone action	Seafood, meat, eggs, whole grains, nuts	Males: 55 µg Females: 55 µg
SODIUM	Maintenance of body water balance, acid-base balance, cellular function	Salt, soy sauce, and processed foods with added salt, especially lunch meats, canned soups and vegetables, salty snacks, processed cheese	Males: 1,500 mg Females: 1,500 mg
ZINC	Synthesis of amino acids, RNA, DNA; aids in wound healing and immune response; important for proper senses of taste and smell	Whole grains, meat, eggs, liver, seafood (especially oysters)	Males: 11 mg Females: 8 mg

Sources: Adapted from Food and Nutrition Board, National Academies. (2001). *Dietary reference intakes: Electrolytes and water* (http://fnic.nal.usda.gov/nal_display/index.php?info_center=4&tax_level=3&tax_subject=256&topic_id=1342&level3_id=5140). Dietary Guidelines Advisory Committee. (2010). *Report of the Dietary Guidelines Advisory Committee on the dietary guidelines for Americans, 2010* (http://www.cnpp.usda.gov/DGAs2010-DGACReport.htm).

that is, they include standards for the amounts individuals should consume to prevent nutrient deficiencies and reduce the risk of chronic diseases. There are two sets of standards: **Recommended Dietary Allowances (RDAs)** and *Adequate Intakes (AIs).* RDAs are set at intakes established to meet the needs of almost all individuals; if there is insufficient data to set an RDA, then an AI value is set. The DRIs are reviewed and updated as new research is completed. Regardless of the type of standard (RDA or AI), the DRIs represent the best available information on healthy vitamin and mineral intakes. The recommendations shown in Tables 8-4 and 8-5 are for young adults (ages 19–30); for information on other age groups and life stages, including pregnancy, visit the Web site for the Food and Nutrition Board (http://www.iom.edu/fnb). To calculate your personal DRIs, go to the Interactive DRI Web site (http://fnic.nal.usda.gov/interactiveDRI).

Q | Is it truly possible, without eating thousands of extra calories per day, for someone to get all the recommended daily vitamins?

Yes, most healthy adults can meet all their vitamin and mineral needs by eating nutrient rich foods—without taking supplements and without exceeding moderate calorie intake. There are a few situations for which supplements or extra care might be required; these are described in more detail on pp. 294–295.

Vitamins and minerals are abundant in food, especially in unprocessed whole grains, vegetables, fruits, legumes, lean meats, and nonfat dairy products. They are also added to some processed foods, including breakfast cereals. However, a diet high in empty calories from added sugars, solid fats, and alcohol and low in nutrient-dense foods *can* leave you short on some vitamins and minerals—another reason to choose nutrient-dense foods. If the dietary analysis you complete in Lab Activity 8-2 indicates you need to increase your intake of a particular vitamin or mineral, refer to Tables 8-4 and 8-5 for particularly good food sources.

A few vitamins are also produced by the body. Biotin (vitamin B₇) is produced by bacteria found naturally in your intestines. Vitamin D is produced by the skin in response to exposure to sunlight. See p. 292 for more on vitamin D.

Q | Can you overdose on vitamins?

Yes, more is not necessarily better, and too high an intake of certain vitamins and minerals can harm your health—but this usually occurs only from taking high doses in supplement form. Because the fat-soluble vitamins can be stored in the body, they pose a higher risk for overload toxicity than water-soluble vitamins do. Thus, taking megadoses of vitamins A, D, E, and K can be toxic.[23]

You can also overdose on minerals. For example, megadoses of calcium can cause digestion problems and possibly kidney damage; taking too much phosphorus can deplete your body's stored calcium; and overdoses of iron can be dangerous, especially in children. Excess intake of a vitamin or mineral may cause illness immediately, or a problem may develop over time.

In part because of these risks, the Dietary Reference Intakes include a limit for certain micronutrients, called the **Tolerable Upper Intake Level (UL).** The UL is the highest level of daily intake of a nutrient that is likely to pose no risk of adverse health effects for most people (Table 8-6). The UL for vitamin A for healthy adults, for example, is 3,000 micrograms a day; for vitamin E, 1,000 milligrams a day; for calcium, 2,500 milligrams a day; and for iron, 45 milligrams a day. ULs have been set only for nutrients for which there is adequate evidence. If a vitamin or mineral does not have a UL, that doesn't mean a high intake is safe.

Vitamin A is a special case: High doses of vitamin A (retinol, from animal sources) can be harmful; among other concerns, high-dose retinol has been linked to birth defects in infants if consumed during pregnancy. The body can also make vitamin A from other compounds, including the carotenoids found in colorful fruits and vegetables like carrots and red peppers. These plant sources of vitamin A are not toxic in the same way as animal sources, so the UL for vitamin A applies only to retinol.

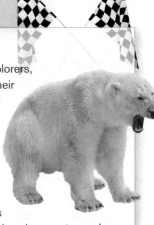

Fast Facts

Lethal Liver?

In 1912, two Antarctic explorers, stranded with no food, ate their six sled dogs, including the dogs' vitamin A–rich livers. Both explorers became ill, and one died from what was the first documented case of lethal vitamin A poisoning. The highest levels of vitamin A in nature are found in the livers of animals adapted to very cold environments, such as seals, sea lions, and walrus. An ounce of moose liver has seven times the amount of vitamin A as an ounce of chicken liver. The highest levels are thought to be in polar bears: If eaten in one meal, the liver of a polar bear has enough vitamin A to kill a human. So, if offered roasted polar bear liver, politely decline.

Source: Nataraja, A. (2002). Man's best friend? *Student BMJ Archive* (http://archive.student.bmj.com/issues/02/05/life/158.php).

TABLE 8-6 TOLERABLE UPPER INTAKE LIMITS (ULS) FOR ADULTS FOR SELECTED VITAMINS AND MINERALS

	DAILY INTAKE LIMIT
CALCIUM	2,500 mg
CHLORIDE	3,600 mg
CHOLINE	3,500 mg
COPPER	10,000 µg
FLUORIDE	10 mg
FOLATE	1,000 µg *
IODINE	1,100 µg
IRON	45 mg
MAGNESIUM	350 mg *
MANGANESE	11 mg
NIACIN	35 mg *
PHOSPHORUS	4,000 mg**
SELENIUM	400 µg
SODIUM	2,300 mg ***
VITAMIN A	3,000 µg ****
VITAMIN B6	100 mg
VITAMIN C	2,000 mg
VITAMIN D	100 µg
VITAMIN E	1,000 mg *
ZINC	40 mg

*From supplements or fortified foods only; there is no evidence of adverse effects of consumption from naturally occurring sources.
**Athletes and others with high energy intakes appear to be able to consume higher levels of phosphorus from food without ill effect.
***For adults with or at risk for hypertension, the UL for sodium is 1,500 mg/day.
****From preformed vitamin A (retinol) only.

Source: Food and Nutrition Board, National Academies. (2010). *Dietary Reference Intakes: UL for Vitamins and Elements* (http://fnic.nal.usda.gov/nal_display/index.php?info_center=4&tax_level=3&tax_subject=256&topic_id=1342&level3_id=5140).

Again, it is unlikely that you could consume a toxic dose of a vitamin or mineral unless you were taking high doses in supplement form. However, it is important to note that there aren't any known benefits of consuming vitamins and minerals in amounts above recommended levels.

Q | Can I take vitamin pills instead of eating vegetables?

That's a bad idea. Although supplements can supply needed vitamins, whole foods contain hundreds of substances that may promote health and prevent disease in as-yet-unknown ways. Compounds known as **antioxidants** may protect cells from unstable molecules known as **free radicals**; damage caused by free radicals may lead to cancer, heart attacks, and stroke. (Free radicals are produced through normal metabolism, but environmental factors such as smoking or exposure to sunlight or pollution can boost free radical production and activity.) Antioxidants such as beta-carotene, lycopene, and vitamins C and E interact with and stabilize free radicals. Antioxidants are one member of a broader class of compounds known as **phytochemicals**—chemicals found in plants that may affect health but have not been classified as essential nutrients.

Good sources of antioxidants and other phytochemicals include many of the nutrient-dense foods that have been mentioned throughout the chapter:[24]

- Yellow, orange, and red fruits and vegetables, including carrots, tomatoes, cantaloupe, winter squash, sweet potatoes, apricots, mangos, watermelon, papaya, pink grapefruit, raspberries, plums, and red and purple grapes
- Leafy deep-green vegetables such as spinach, collards, and chard
- Other deeply colored foods, including blueberries, blackberries, and saffron
- Cruciferous vegetables, including broccoli, cauliflower, cabbage, kale, bok choy, and Brussels sprouts
- Members of the allium family, including onions, garlic, and leeks
- Legumes, almonds and other nuts, wheat germ, and safflower, corn, and soybean oils
- Tea, red wine, dark chocolate
- Whole grains

Current evidence supports consuming a diet high in food sources of antioxidants and other disease-protecting nutrients instead of taking antioxidant or other types of supplements. There is no evidence that multivitamin/mineral supplements prevent chronic diseases in healthy people.[25] And little is confirmed about the effects of supplements of individual nutrients—vitamins, minerals, or antioxidants. In some cases, researchers have found that high intakes from foods reduce the risk of chronic disease but intake from supplements actually increases risk. Your best bets are healthy, whole foods—a variety of whole grains and colorful fruits and vegetables. And don't overdo the wine and dark chocolate! Although

antioxidant A compound that protects cells from damage by free radicals by reacting with them or counteracting their effects.

free radicals Unstable, highly reactive molecules created during normal metabolism and in response to environmental factors; may aid the development of cancer, cardiovascular disease, and other diseases of aging by reacting with and damaging DNA and other parts of cells.

phytochemical A naturally occurring chemical in plant-based foods that may help prevent or treat chronic disease.

Research Brief

Beta-carotene and Smokers

Beta-carotene is one of the carotenoids that the body can convert into vitamin A; it can also act as an antioxidant. After a number of studies found a lower lung cancer risk among people with higher blood levels of beta-carotene, several research trials tested whether high doses of beta-carotene supplements over an extended time would lower smokers' risk of lung cancer. The findings were surprising: The risk of developing and dying from lung cancer actually went up among the smokers taking beta-carotene compared with smokers not taking the supplement. The excess risk disappeared after the participants in the studies stopped using the supplements. Further review of the findings found that consumption of fruits and vegetables reduced the risk of lung cancer.

What are possible explanations for the findings? One may be the interaction of the effects of smoking on beta-carotene; it appears that cellular changes caused by smoking alter the actions of beta-carotene to produce more free radicals rather than reducing the number of these cell-damaging compounds. Beta-carotene supplements have not been found to be harmful (or beneficial) in non-smokers. In addition, there may be different effects from consuming supplements compared with beta-carotene in whole foods. Carrots and red peppers, for example, are rich in beta-carotene, but they also contain many other substances—and their benefits may be the result of a variety of phytochemicals working in combination. Two points you should take away from the research:

■ Don't smoke—smokers, regardless of whether they take beta-carotene supplements, have much higher rates of lung cancer and premature death than nonsmokers do.
■ Base your diet on nutrient-dense whole foods rather than relying on supplements.

Source: Druesne-Pecollo, N., and others. (2010). Beta-carotene supplementation and cancer risk: A systematic review and meta-analysis of randomized controlled trials. *International Journal of Cancer, 127*(1), 172–184.

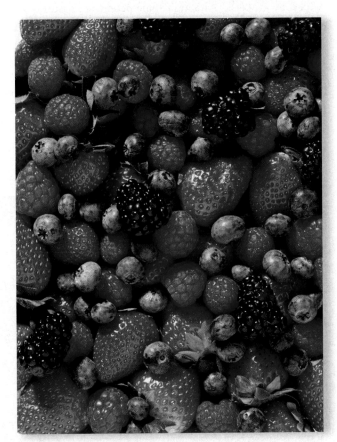

Consume foods rich in antioxidants and other phytochemicals—including whole grains and colorful fruits and vegetables—to help reduce your risk of many chronic diseases. Don't rely on supplements, which don't have all the benefits of whole foods.

both wine and chocolate contain antioxidants, you also need to consider whether the alcohol in wine and the calories in both have a place in your diet—and your life.[26]

Don't use vitamin supplements or fortified foods as an excuse to base your diet on highly processed foods. Such foods are typically devoid of vitamins and minerals, and some may even speed the loss of vitamins and minerals from your body. They also have none of the antioxidants and other phytochemicals just described. Choose nutrient-dense whole foods—processed foods should make up only a small part of your daily diet.

Q Does preparing foods in certain ways alter the vitamin and mineral content of the foods? [ ] READ ONLINE

Vitamins and Minerals of Special Concern

Based on recent studies, public health officials have identified one vitamin and three minerals of special concern: Americans currently consume too little calcium, vitamin D, and potassium and too much sodium.[27]

Q I put milk on my cereal but that's about it for dairy. Am I short on calcium?

CALCIUM AND VITAMIN D—CRITICAL FOR STRONG BONES. You could be—the majority of American are short on

osteoporosis Loss of bone mass and density, causing bones to become fragile.

both calcium and vitamin D. The only group whose average calcium intake meets recommended levels is males ages 19–50, and except for children and adolescent males, no group meets the recommended vitamin D intake.[28] Completing Lab Activity 8-2 will help you check your current intakes.

Calcium and vitamin D are both critical in the formation of healthy bones and teeth. Calcium is the main component of your bones, and vitamin D is necessary for your body to absorb and use calcium from your diet. Calcium deficiency can lead to reduced bone mass and **osteoporosis,** a weakening of the bones that can cause fractures and disability later in life (see the box "Got Calcium . . . and Exercise?"). In addition to its importance in bone health, vitamin D is also being investigated for its role in preventing a number of chronic diseases, including cardiovascular disease and certain forms of cancer.

Everyone should pay attention to calcium and vitamin D intakes. The richest source of both is fluid milk, which naturally contains calcium and is fortified with vitamin D. Other dairy products such as yogurt and cheese also provide calcium, but check labels to see the amount per serving. Nondairy sources of calcium include fortified soy milk or orange juice, tofu prepared with calcium sulfate, canned sardines or salmon with bones, green vegetables (broccoli, collards, spinach, and the like), almonds, edamame (green soybeans), and white beans.

Few foods naturally contain vitamin D. Oily fish such as salmon and tuna are the best sources, with smaller amounts found in liver, cheese, and egg yolks. In addition to milk, some other dairy products, breakfast cereals, and certain brands of orange juice and yogurt may also be fortified with vitamin D.

Your skin naturally produces vitamin D in response to sun (ultraviolet radiation) exposure, but many health authorities are hesitant to suggest that people spend more time in the sun due to the risk of skin cancer. Factors that reduce the skin's synthesis of vitamin D include cloud or smog cover, dark skin color, use of sunscreen, early or late time of day, winter season, and higher geographic latitudes.

In the United States, there is sufficient ultraviolet radiation for year-round vitamin D production only at latitudes below a line extending between Los Angeles, California, to Columbia, South Carolina. If you live north of this line, then for at least part of the winter, the intensity of the sun's radiation is insufficient to support the synthesis of vitamin D by your skin; dietary intake is required.[29]

To reach the intake goals for both calcium and vitamin D, start by consuming more foods naturally rich in or fortified with these nutrients. If increasing your intake of food sources isn't enough, you can also consider calcium and vitamin D supplements. See pp. 294–296 for general advice and cautions on choosing supplements.

Q | I really like pretzels and other salty snacks. Is that a problem?

SODIUM AND POTASSIUM—A BETTER BALANCE FOR BETTER BLOOD PRESSURE. It can be. Salt is sodium chloride, and although sodium is an essential mineral, excess consumption is unhealthy. High intake of sodium raises blood pressure and can contribute to full-blown hypertension, an established risk factor for heart attack, stroke, and kidney disease. Blood pressure also rises with age, and more than 90 percent of U.S. adults develop high blood pressure in their lifetime—meaning virtually everyone is at risk. Although some people are more sensitive to the effects of sodium than others, reducing sodium intake is an important goal for everyone.

Potassium intake is also key, because potassium can lower blood pressure and also reduce sodium's effects on blood pressure. Reducing sodium intake while increasing potassium intake has been shown to reduce deaths from cardiovascular disease as well as cut medical costs. Other benefits of potassium include decreased bone loss and reduced risk of kidney stones.

Americans are currently out of balance with sodium and potassium:[30]

- *Sodium:* The suggested upper limit for sodium intake is 2,300 mg/day, but the average intake is nearly 3,500 mg/day. For much of the population—middle-aged and older adults, people with hypertension, and African Americans—an even lower intake of 1,500 mg/day is recommended, and many health experts recommend this lower number for everyone.
- *Potassium:* The recommended intake is 4,700 mg/day, but the average intake is only about 3,200 mg/day for men and 2,400 mg/day for women.

What can you do? Learn to like less salty foods! Luckily, the preference for super-salty foods is an acquired taste, and your taste buds will adjust within a few weeks or months. You

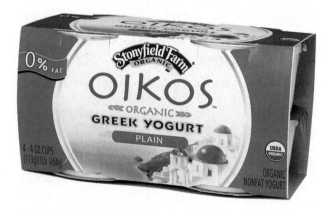

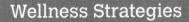

Wellness Strategies

Got Calcium . . . and Exercise? Tips for Reducing Your Risk for Osteoporosis

Calcium is critical in the development of optimal bone density and the prevention of osteoporosis. *Osteoporosis* by definition means "porous bone" and is a sign that bone has lost calcium for strength and matrix for support. Once this occurs, the bone becomes fragile and can easily fracture, especially from a fall but in severe cases even after something as simple as a sneeze. Among seniors, fractures are a major cause of disability and often lead to the loss of the ability to live independently. About 25 percent of hip-fracture patients over age 50 die in the year following their fracture.

Bone is living, growing tissue that is constantly "remodeling"—old bone tissue is removed (resorbed) and new bone tissue is formed. The process happens rapidly as you grow, with bone formation exceeding bone resorption, and you reach peak bone density by about your mid-20s. Among adults, about 10 percent of the bone tissue in the skeleton is remodeled each year. After about age 30, bone resorption slowly begins to exceed bone formation, leading to slow loss of bone density.

Bone loss accelerates during aging, especially in post-menopausal women (the drop in estrogen levels that occurs during menopause accelerates the rate of bone loss). Because women start out with less bone mass than men and then lose it more rapidly, women are more likely than men to develop osteoporosis. However, the condition occurs in both sexes, and about 20 percent of the 10 million Americans with osteoporosis are men.

To reduce your risk of developing osteoporosis, build maximum bone mass in your young adult years and then work to maintain it with these strategies:

- Get your recommended intakes of calcium and vitamin D.
- Engage in regular weight-bearing exercise, activities in which you are supporting your own weight, like walking, jogging, dancing, and resistance training.
- Avoid smoking and excessive alcohol intake.

Sources: National Institute of Arthritis and Musculoskeletal and Skin Diseases. (2009). *Osteoporosis overview* (http://www.niams.nih.gov/Health_Info/Bone/Osteoporosis/default.asp). National Osteoporosis Foundation. (2010). (http://www.nof.org).

can still enjoy salty foods from time to time, but make them special treats and limit your portion sizes. The vast majority of sodium in the American diet—80–85 percent—comes from salt added by food manufacturers during processing. (Naturally occurring sodium accounts for about 10 percent, and salt added at the table or during cooking accounts for the remaining 5–10 percent.) What this means is that you have to check food labels for sodium content and make choices accordingly. Reducing the sodium in the American diet to recommended levels will likely also require a broad public health effort—perhaps with mandatory reductions in the sodium content of certain types of foods.

Increasing your potassium intake is more straightforward—there are many rich food sources! Americans are low in potassium because they don't eat enough fruits and vegetables. Try some of the following good sources of potassium:

- white and sweet potatoes
- legumes
- tomatoes, tomato sauce, and tomato juice
- bananas
- oranges and orange juice
- papaya, apricots, and peaches
- cantaloupe, honeydew, and watermelon
- many vegetables, including beet greens, spinach, brussels sprouts, artichokes, broccoli, collards, cucumber, celery, kale, snap beans, turnip greens, carrots, corn, red peppers
- yogurt
- many types of fish, including halibut, rockfish, haddock, salmon, tuna, and cod

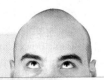

Mind Stretcher
Critical Thinking Exercise

Should reduced-sodium foods continue to be "niche" foods—a small proportion of processed foods sold in our stores and quick service restaurants? What do you think of the idea of regulations requiring food manufacturers to slowly but significantly reduce the salt in all processed foods? What about a system of taxes that would make lower-sodium foods less expensive for consumers? How would you balance consumer preferences for salty foods with the costs of consumption of those foods in terms of chronic disease prevalence and medical care costs?

Special Recommendations for Specific Groups

Q | My girlfriend is a vegetarian. Does she get all her vitamins that way?

Is she a vegan? If not, it is unlikely she will experience any real vitamin deficiencies. The popularity of vegetarian diets has risen in recent years, along with an interest in avoiding meat and meat products for environmental, philosophical, or health reasons. However, there has not been a parallel increase in vitamin deficiencies.

Vegans are vegetarians who eat no animal products whatsoever, in contrast to other types of vegetarians who may eat dairy products, eggs, or fish and just avoid meat and poultry (see Chapter 9 for more on vegetarian diets). Vitamin B_{12} is a concern because only animal foods naturally contain vitamin B_{12}; although it takes a long time for vitamin B_{12} deficiency to develop, the symptoms are serious and include permanent neurological damage. Many cereals are fortified with vitamin B_{12}, so many vegetarians get their intake that way. Vegans who do not consume any foods fortified with vitamin B_{12} should consider taking a dietary supplement.

Iron can also be a concern for vegetarians, because the iron found in plant foods is more difficult for the body to absorb than the iron found in meat and poultry. Vegetarians need to consume extra iron to make up for the lower absorption. Vitamin C helps the body absorb iron, so consuming vitamin C–rich foods along with iron-rich foods is beneficial. Problems with low iron are seen mostly in women of reproductive age, especially women with a heavy menstrual flow. Iron deficiency can lead to **anemia,** or low levels of hemoglobin, the component of blood that transports oxy-

gen. This is particularly problematic during pregnancy, when the blood needs to deliver oxygen to the fetus as well as the mother. Iron deficiency may also hinder athletic performance in endurance events, which require oxygen delivery over a sustained period.

If your girlfriend's age makes pregnancy a possibility, then a special recommendation for folic acid also applies to her. See Table 8-7 for more information about this and other recommendations for specific groups or circumstances.

anemia Below-normal number of red blood cells or lack of sufficient hemoglobin, resulting in reduced oxygen-carrying capacity of the blood; most often caused by insufficient iron, which is needed to produce hemoglobin.

Choosing and Using Supplements

Q | How do I know which nutrient supplements to take?

As described in this chapter, the best approach is to obtain your essential nutrients from food rather than relying on supplements. Whole foods have the benefits of antioxidants and other phytochemicals as well as dietary fiber. Most people can achieve recommended intakes of all micronutrients by consuming nutrient-dense foods.

There is no evidence that supplements prevent chronic diseases in the general, healthy population. For some special population groups, particular supplements may be beneficial, but in other cases, nutrient supplements can be harmful (recall the box "Beta-carotene and Smokers" on p. 291).

Review the results of the dietary assessment you complete in Lab Activity 8-2. If you are short on any nutrients according to the Dietary Reference Intakes (DRI) recommendations for you, make changes in your diet first and then reassess your status before going ahead with a supplement.

If you cannot obtain enough of a particular nutrient through dietary sources, or if medical tests indicate a problem such as iron-deficiency anemia, then a supplement of a particular nutrient may be appropriate for you. But take care: Some supplements can interact with drugs or other supplements. For example, calcium reduces the effectiveness of certain antibiotics and medications used to treat seizure disorders. Follow the directions for use carefully, and check with your health care provider if you are taking any prescription or over-the-counter drugs.

Avoid high-dose supplements unless prescribed by your physician to treat a specific deficiency. There is no need to exceed the DRI, and high-dose supplements may be ineffective or even harmful. For example, your body absorbs calcium best in doses of 500 mg or less, so higher-dose supplements can be a waste of money. Also be sure to consider your combined intake from all supplements plus fortified foods; if you don't pay attention, you might consume a particular nutrient above the tolerable upper intake limit (UL) set by the Dietary Reference Intakes (see Table 8-6).

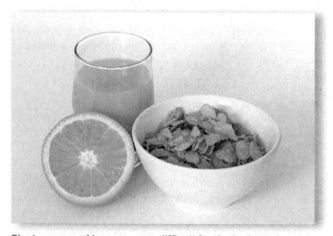

Plant sources of iron are more difficult for the body to absorb, and strict vegetarians need to consume about twice as much iron as people with nonvegetarian diets. Eating vitamin C–rich foods along with iron-rich foods is helpful because vitamin C helps the body absorb iron.

TABLE 8-7 DIETARY REFERENCE INTAKE ADJUSTMENTS FOR SPECIAL CIRCUMSTANCES

GROUP	RECOMMENDATION
WOMEN OF CHILDBEARING AGE	**Folic acid:** All women capable of becoming pregnant should consume 400 µg of folic acid from fortified foods or supplements in addition to naturally occurring food folate from a varied diet. Folate reduces the risk of neural tube defects, including spina bifida, in a developing fetus. Because the neural tube develops very early in pregnancy, before a woman may know she is pregnant, the recommendation applies to all women of reproductive age.
SMOKERS	**Vitamin C:** People who smoke should consume an additional 35 mg/day of vitamin C over that needed by nonsmokers.
PEOPLE OVER AGE 50	**Vitamin B$_{12}$:** Many older adults cannot absorb vitamin B$_{12}$ from foods, so people over 50 should meet their recommended intake by consuming fortified foods or supplements.
VEGETARIANS	**Iron, zinc, and vitamin B$_{12}$:** If plant foods are the only source of iron and zinc, then the iron and zinc requirements are approximately twice those of nonvegetarians. Vegans also need to consume vitamin B$_{12}$ (found naturally only in animal foods) from fortified foods or supplements.
ATHLETES ENGAGING IN REGULAR INTENSE EXERCISE	**Iron:** Average iron requirements are 30–70 percent higher for athletes than for people engaging in typical levels of physical activity.

Source: Adapted from Food and Nutrition Board, National Academies. (2006). *DRI: Dietary Reference Intakes: The essential guide to nutrient requirements.* Washington, DC: National Academies Press.

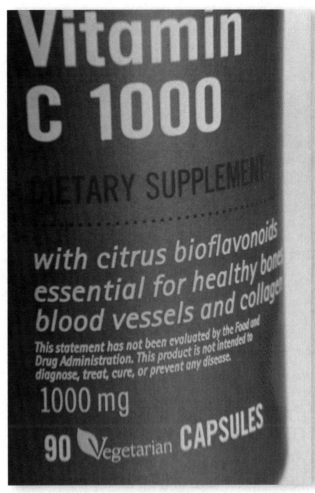

Dietary supplements are not regulated in the same ways as drugs and foods. Although they may carry claims about the product's effects on health, they must also print a warning that these claims have not been evaluated by the FDA.

Q How do I know if my vitamin supplements are any good?

It is actually quite difficult to determine the quality of supplements, because they are not regulated by the Food and Drug Administration (FDA) the way drugs are. Unlike over-the-counter and prescription drugs, supplements do not have to be proven to be safe or effective before they can be sold. If a supplement is found to be unsafe, then the FDA can take action to remove it from the market.

Supplements are not intended to diagnose, treat, or prevent disease, so they cannot claim they are effective for any of those functions. Don't take vitamins because you think they can do things like increase muscle mass, fend off sleep, reduce stress, or prevent the common cold; effects such as these have not been proven.

In terms of quality, the FDA doesn't analyze the content of supplements. However, it does set manufacturing standards designed to ensure that supplements contain the ingredients listed on the label, are not contaminated, and are appropriately packaged and labeled. If you take vitamin supplements, buy them from well-known companies, which usually have the highest quality control. You can also look for "seals of approval" from independent organizations that test supplements for proper manufacturing and accurate labeling. These seals do not guarantee that a supplement is safe or effective, but they do offer some assurance that they contain what is listed on the label. Organizations that offer product certifications include ConsumerLab .com (http://www.consumerlab.com/seal.asp), U.S. Pharmacopeia (http://www.usp.org/USPVerified/ dietarySupplements), and NSF (http://www.nsf.org/ business/dietary_supplements).

Food Labels: An Important Tool for Consumers

Q | What do the percentages on food labels mean?

The percentages refer to **Daily Values (DVs),** a set of standards used on food labels to help you place the food in the context of your overall daily diet. The Daily Values are based on a diet of 2,000 calories per day, and although you may need more or less, the DV is a good benchmark. For some nutrients, including fiber, calcium, and iron, the DV is a goal. For others, including sodium and saturated fat, the DV is a limit, and the less you eat of these substances, the better.

Only certain nutrients are required to be listed on food labels—those that are considered most important for consumers when they evaluate foods. See Figure 8-7 for tips to help you use food labels to make healthier choices.

Q | Are the listings on food labels actually facts? How accurate are they?

Food labels should be accurate. Manufacturers are responsible for ensuring the accuracy of food labels on their products, but the FDA conducts random tests and can take action if a company is in violation of the regulations.

Consumers should keep three points in mind about food labels. First, numbers can be rounded off on food

DOLLAR STRETCHER
Financial Wellness Tip

Don't buy unnecessary supplements, especially those in expensive specialty beverages, bars, and powders. Use only supplements you truly need, and start by checking cereal boxes. Many fortified ready-to-eat cereals offer high nutrient density and value.[31]

labels. A product that contains fewer than 5 calories per serving can be called "calorie-free," and perhaps most importantly, a product that has less than 0.5 mg of *trans* fat per serving can be said to contain zero *trans* fat. If you consume a lot of these products with small amounts of *trans* fat, your total intake can add up. To be sure that a product really has no *trans* fat, check the ingredient list for hydrogenated fats; if you see them on the list, then the product contains some *trans* fats.

Second, use caution when reading the claims and other information on the front of food packages. Some aspects of packaging and some types of claims are more closely regulated than others. For example, a food package can have a picture of fruit on the front but not actually contain fruit. The label "low fat" is regulated and specifically means 3 grams of fat or less per typical serving, whereas the labels "low carb" and "low glycemic index" are not regulated and don't have consistent meanings. For more on the complex world of food-label regulations, visit the FDA Web site (http://www.fda.gov/Food/ LabelingNutrition/LabelClaims).

Finally, consider the full profile of a food. A breakfast cereal that prominently labels itself as low in fat and sodium isn't necessarily a healthy choice if it includes a huge amount of added sugar. Potato chips that have no *trans* fat are still high in overall fat, salt, and calories. Fat-free isn't calorie-free. Your best bet is to limit your consumption of highly processed foods and eat more fruits, vegetables, and whole grains.

Assessing Your Diet for Energy and Nutrient Intakes

Q | How do I know if I'm eating the right amounts of the right things? Is my diet good, bad, or OK?

There are different ways to assess your diet. The lab activities for this chapter will help you estimate how many calories you need to maintain your weight as well as how your current diet stacks up against the nutrient recommendations. In Chapter 9, you'll

Daily Values (DVs)
Nutrient-intake standards used on food labels that quantify the nutrients as percentages in a 2,000-calorie-per-day diet.

Nutrition Facts

Serving Size 1/2 package (285g)
Servings per Container 2

Amount per Serving

Calories 300   Calories from Fat 60

	% Daily Value*
Total Fat 6g	9%
Saturated Fat 2.5g	13%
Trans Fat 0g	
Cholesterol 30mg	10%
Sodium 600mg	25%
Potassium 420mg	12%
Total Carbohydrate 45g	15%
Dietary Fiber 5g	20%
Sugars 12g	
Protein 15g	

Vitamin A 40%	•	Vitamin C 15%
Calcium 10%	•	Iron 8%

*Percent Daily Values are based on a 2,000 calorie diet. Your daily values may be higher or lower depending on your calorie needs.

	Calories	2,000	2,500
Total Fat	Less than	65g	80
Sat Fat	Less than	20g	25g
Cholesterol	Less than	300mg	300mg
Sodium	Less than	2,400mg	2,400mg
Total Carbohydrate		300g	375g
Dietary Fiber		25g	30g

Calories per gram:
Fat 9 • Carbohydrate 4 • Protein 4

Check serving size, number of servings, and calories

- The label information is based on ONE serving, but many packages contain more. Look at the serving size and how many servings you are actually consuming. If you consume double the serving size, then you must double everything listed on the label, including calories.
- Fat-free doesn't mean calorie-free. Lower-fat items may have as many calories as full-fat versions.

Limit saturated fat, *trans* fat, cholesterol, sodium, and added sugars

- For heart health, limit unhealthy fats and sodium. Check ingredient list for hydrogenated fats, which are the source of artificial *trans* fats.
- Limit foods with added sugars, which add calories but not other nutrients.

Look for foods rich in potassium, dietary fiber, vitamins A and C, calcium, and iron

- Get the most nutrients for your calories. Look for foods that are high in healthy nutrients and low in calories, unhealthy fats, and sodium.
- Potassium isn't required to be listed on all food labels, but it should appear on foods that have significant amounts. Look for it.
- A food that has 20% or more of the Daily Value is high in a nutrient.

Choose lean protein sources

- When evaluating a food for its protein content, make choices that are lean, low-fat, or fat-free. Compare how much protein a serving of the food provides with the total fat and calories. Get the most protein for your calories and fat.

Remember the Daily Values

- The % DV is a general guide to help you link nutrients in a serving of food to their contributions to your total daily diet. Foods may be high (20% DV or more) or low (5% DV or less) in particular nutrients.
- The % DV is based on a 2,000-calorie diet; you may need more or less.

Don't forget to check the ingredients list

- For whole-grain foods, a whole grain should appear first on the list.
- To limit added sugars, make sure that sugars are not among the first few items in the list.
- If hydrogenated fats appear on the list, the food contains at least some *trans* fats.

Figure 8-7 Nutrition Facts label. The information on food labels can help you make healthier choices. Use labels to evaluate individual foods and to compare different brands or types of similar foods.

Source: Adapted from U.S. Department of Agriculture. (2006). *Nutrition facts label* (http://www.fda.gov/Food/LabelingNutrition/ConsumerInformation/ucm121642.htm).

learn more about different eating plans—another way to look at your diet. As you complete the tracking needed to assess your diet, take time to be accurate in your listing of what you eat and how much. As mentioned earlier in the chapter, many people underestimate their portion sizes and energy intakes, which can affect nutrient analysis. A few days of careful data collection will give you a realistic picture of your typical diet. Then you can determine if you need to make changes to bring your diet in line with the recommendations for lifelong health and wellness.

Summary

A healthy diet will help you feel good, maintain a healthy body weight, and minimize your risk for many chronic diseases. A healthy diet also allows you to be physically active and reach all of your fitness goals. Make good choices, and enjoy your food.

Choose a healthy balance of protein, carbohydrate, and fat to meet your energy needs. Favor nutrient-dense foods, and avoid high-calorie (energy-dense) foods that provide little besides calories. Give special priority to foods rich in nutrients for which you fall short of recommended intakes. For many Americans, these nutrients include dietary fiber, vitamin D, calcium, and potassium.

To meet your nutrient needs within appropriate energy intakes, focus on the advice from the *Dietary Guidelines for Americans*:

- Know your personal calorie needs, and stay within those limits.
- Reduce excessive calorie intake from added sugars, solid fats, and highly processed foods (especially those low in fiber and high in sodium and sugar). Avoid or limit sugar-sweetened beverages.
- Eat more vegetables, legumes, fat-free and low-fat dairy products, seafood, fruits, and fiber-rich whole grains.
- Consume smaller portions, especially of high-calorie foods.
- Check food labels to monitor calories, portion sizes, and nutrients.

Assess your diet periodically to help yourself stay on track. Eat well, and be well!

More to Explore

Dietary Guidelines for Americans
http://www.DietaryGuidelines.gov
Interactive Dietary Reference Intakes
http://fnic.nal.usda.gov/interactiveDRI
National Institutes of Health, Office of Dietary Supplements
http://ods.od.nih.gov
Nutrient-Rich Foods Coalition
http://www.nutrientrichfoods.org
Nutrition.gov
http://www.nutrition.gov
U.S. Food and Drug Administration: Food Labeling
http://www.fda.gov/Food/LabelingNutrition/ConsumerInformation
U.S. Food and Drug Administration: National Nutrient Database
http://www.nal.usda.gov/fnic/foodcomp/search

Determining Energy and Macronutrient Intake Goals

☑ **SUBMIT ONLINE**

NAME	DATE	SECTION

This lab includes instructions for making several calculations:

- Daily calorie requirement
- Daily protein requirement
- Estimated target macronutrient intake (percentages and grams)

You can use the information from this lab to help you set important nutrition goals.

Daily Calorie Requirement

If your weight is stable, your current daily energy intake is the number of calories you need to maintain your weight at your current activity level. However, people often underestimate the size of their food portions, and so energy goals based on estimates of current calorie intake from food records can be inaccurate. You can also estimate your daily energy needs using formulas developed as part of the Dietary Reference Intakes.

Equipment

- Weight scale
- Tape measure or other means of measuring height
- Calculator (optional)

Preparation: None

Instructions

Measure your height (in inches) and weight (in pounds), and then identify the appropriate physical activity coefficient (PA) from the table below. Plug these values, along with your age, into the appropriate formula for your sex.

Height: [   ] inches   Weight: [   ] lbs.

PHYSICAL ACTIVITY COEFFICIENTS FOR ENERGY NEEDS CALCULATION

		PHYSICAL ACTIVITY COEFFICIENT (PA)	
PHYSICAL ACTIVITY LEVEL	DESCRIPTION*	MEN	WOMEN
Sedentary	Activities of daily living	1.00	1.00
Low active	Activities of daily living plus the equivalent of about 30 minutes per day of moderate activity	1.12	1.14
Active	Activities of daily living plus the equivalent of about 60–90 minutes per day of moderate activity	1.27	1.27
Very active	Activities of daily living plus the equivalent of about 150–240 minutes per day of moderate activity	1.54	1.45

*30 minutes of vigorous activity is equivalent to about 60 minutes of moderate activity.

Formula for Men

$$[864 - (9.72 \times age)] + \{PA \times [(6.44 \times weight) + (12.78 \times height)]\}$$

Step 1. $9.72 \times$ age ☐ years = ☐

Step 2. $864 -$ result from step 1 ☐ = ☐ *(Result may be a negative number)*

Step 3. $6.44 \times$ weight ☐ lbs. = ☐

Step 4. $12.78 \times$ height ☐ inches = ☐

Step 5. Result from step 3 ☐ + result from step 4 ☐ = ☐

Step 6. PA (from table) ☐ × result from step 5 ☐ = ☐

Step 7. Result from step 2 ☐ + result from step 6 ☐ = ☐ **calories per day**

Formula for Women

$$[387 - (7.31 \times age)] + \{PA \times [(4.94 \times weight) + (16.78 \times height)]\}$$

Step 1. $7.31 \times$ age ☐ years = ☐

Step 2. $387 -$ result from step 1 ☐ = ☐ *(Result may be a negative number)*

Step 3. $4.94 \times$ weight ☐ lbs. = ☐

Step 4. $16.78 \times$ height ☐ inches = ☐

Step 5. Result from step 3 ☐ + result from step 4 ☐ = ☐

Step 6. PA (from table) ☐ × result from step 5 ☐ = ☐

Step 7. Result from step 2 ☐ + result from step 6 ☐ = ☐ **calories per day**

Results

Daily calorie requirement for weight maintenance: ☐ **calories per day**

Daily Protein Requirement

The Dietary Reference Intakes also provide a formula you can use to calculate the amount of protein you should average daily to meet your body's needs.

Equipment

- Weight scale
- Calculator (optional)

Preparation: None

Instructions

Measure your weight (in pounds) and plug in the appropriate value from the table below.

Weight: ☐ lbs.

DIETARY PROTEIN REQUIREMENTS BY AGE AND LIFE STAGE

AGE/LIFE STAGE	GRAMS OF PROTEIN PER POUND OF BODY WEIGHT
Ages 14–18	0.39 g/lb.
Ages 19 and older	0.36 g/lb.
Pregnant	0.50 g/lb.
Breast-feeding	0.59 g/lb.

For athletes engaged in heavy training: The *Dietary Reference Intakes* states that athletes need no additional protein, but the American College of Sports Medicine recommends a somewhat higher protein intake for both endurance athletes (0.54–0.64 gram per pound) and resistance athletes (0.54–0.77 gram per pound). Use a value in one of these ranges if you feel it is appropriate for you.

Protein requirement = weight: ☐ lbs. × value from table ☐ g/lb. = ☐ g

Results

Daily protein requirement: ☐ **grams per day**

Estimated Target Macronutrient Intakes

After calculating your daily calorie and protein requirements, your next step is to set intake goals for all three classes of macronutrients—protein, fat, and carbohydrate.

Equipment

Calculator (optional)

Preparation: None

Instructions

You can allocate your total daily calories among the three classes of macronutrients to suit your preferences. Just make sure that your values fall within the Acceptable Macronutrient Distribution Ranges (AMDRs) set by the Food and Nutrition Board of the National Academies, that the three percentages you select total 100 percent, and that the percentage you set for protein is sufficient to meet the protein need you calculated in the previous section of the lab.

NUTRIENT	AMDR (% OF TOTAL DAILY CALORIES)	YOUR GOALS (% OF TOTAL DAILY CALORIES)
Protein	10%–35%	☐ %
Fat	20%–35%	☐ %
Carbohydrate	45%–65%	☐ %
TOTAL		100%

To translate your percentage goals into daily intake goals expressed in calories and grams, multiply the percentages you've chosen by your total calorie intake and then divide the result by the corresponding calories per gram. Use the total daily calorie goal you calculated in the first part of this lab activity and the percentage goals you set in the chart above.

Nutrient	Total calories per day	×	Macronutrient percentage goal (expressed as a decimal)	=	Calories per day of macronutrient	÷	Calories per gram of macronutrient	=	Grams per day of macronutrient
Protein*		×	0.	=	cal/day	÷	4 cal/g	=	g/day
Fat		×	0.	=	cal/day	÷	9 cal/g	=	g/day
Carbohydrate		×	0.	=	cal/day	÷	4 cal/g	=	g/day
Sample for carbohydrate	*2,000*	×	*0.50*	=	*1,000 cal/day*	÷	*4 cal/g*	=	*250 g/day*

*Check the value calculated for protein to ensure it is at or above the protein requirement you calculated in the previous section of the lab. If it is below that number, adjust your target macronutrient percentages (raise protein, lower fat or carbohydrate or both) until your protein consumption meets the DRI.

Summary of Results

Total Daily Energy Intake: [ ] calories per day

MACRONUTRIENT	PERCENT OF TOTAL DAILY CALORIES	GRAMS PER DAY
Protein	%	g/day
Fat	%	g/day
Carbohydrate	%	g/day

Reflecting on Your Results

Are you surprised with your results? Was the value calculated for your total daily calorie requirement what you expected? If not, is it higher or lower? Do your results match what you thought about your energy intake and nutrient requirements?

Planning Your Next Steps

To determine how close you are to meeting your personal intake goals, keep a running tally over the course of the day. For packaged foods, food labels list the calories and the number of grams of fat, protein, and carbohydrate. Nutrition information is also available in many quick-service restaurants, in grocery stores, in nutrition analysis software, and online. By checking these resources, you can track your total intake of calories, fat, protein, and carbohydrate and assess your current diet. (Lab Activity 8-2 will take you through a detailed analysis of your diet, including energy, macronutrients, and key vitamins and minerals.) As a first step here, describe the strategies you'll use to track your current diet to determine how it compares to the goals and requirements you calculated in this lab activity.

Source: Formulas, calorie, and protein requirements, and AMDRs from Food and Nutrition Board, Institute of Medicine, National Academies. (2002). *Dietary Reference Intakes: Energy, carbohydrate, fiber, fat, fatty acids, cholesterol, protein, and amino acids.* Washington, DC: National Academy Press.

SUBMIT ONLINE

NAME   DATE   SECTION

In this lab you'll analyze one day's diet. For a more complete and accurate assessment of your diet, average and then analyze the results from several different days, including a weekday and a weekend day.

Equipment

Access to the energy and nutrient content of your foods and beverages. Information is available from food labels, restaurant nutrition guides, and the free online USDA food composition database (http://www.nal.usda.gov/fnic/foodcomp/search).

Preparation: None

Instructions

Record the foods you consume over the course of the day; be as accurate as possible in determining your portion sizes for the "Amount" column. Use the chart printed below, a nutrition analysis software program, or the free online nutrition analysis at MyPyramid Tracker (http://www.mypyramidtracker.gov). If you are performing the analysis by hand using the chart in this lab, do the best you can to include complete information on everything you eat.

DAY OF THE WEEK (CIRCLE):   M   T   W   TH   F   SA   SU

Food	Amount	Calories	Protein (g)	Carbohydrate (g)	Fiber (g)	Added sugars (g)*	Fat (g)	Saturated fat (g)	Cholesterol (mg)	Sodium (mg)	Potassium (mg)**	Vitamin A (µg RE)	Vitamin C (mg)	Calcium (mg)	Iron (mg)
Sample: Wheat bread	1 slice	70	4	12	2	2	1	0.2	0	135	70	0	0	30	1

* Added sugars: Don't include naturally occurring sugars from fruit and milk in this column. Sugar content information for a food usually doesn't distinguish between naturally occurring sugars and added sugars. However, if a food doesn't include any fruit or milk products, then the sugar in the product likely all comes from added sugars. Track the major sources of added sugars in your diet.

** Potassium: Not listed on every food label, but potassium content is given if the food contains a significant amount.

Results

Calculate your totals: Complete the chart below by totaling the values in each column. (If you used MyPyramid Tracker or another online or software tool, copy your day's totals into the chart.) In addition, calculate the percentage of total daily calories for protein, carbohydrate, fat, and saturated fat using the following formula:

$$\frac{(\text{number of grams of energy source}) \times (\text{number of calories per gram of energy source})}{\text{total daily calories}}$$

Note: Fat and saturated fat provide 9 calories per gram; protein and carbohydrate provide 4 calories per gram. For example, if you consume 60 total grams of fat and 2,000 calories, the percentage of total calories from fat is:

$$\frac{(60 \text{ grams of fat}) \times (9 \text{ calories per gram of fat})}{2,000 \text{ calories}} = 27\% \text{ total daily calories as fat}$$

Fill in the recommended totals or limits: Use the calorie and macronutrient values from Lab Activity 8-1 or choose values from Table 8-2 and the boxes "Recommendations for Macronutrients" and "Tips for Meeting Dietary Fat and Cholesterol Recommendations" on pp. 275 and 284. For vitamins and minerals, select the appropriate recommendations from Tables 8-4 and 8-5. The "reference recommendations" in the chart are basic DRI and AMDR guidelines for young adults; your individual recommendations may differ. For personalized recommendations, you can also visit the Interactive DRI website (http://fnic.nal.usda.gov/interactiveDRI).

	Calories	Protein (g)	Protein (% of total calories)	Carbohydrate (g)	Carbohydrate (% of total calories)	Fiber (g)	Added sugars (g)	Fat (g)	Fat (% of total calories)	Sat. fat (g)	Saturated fat (% of total calories)	Cholesterol (mg)	Sodium (mg)	Potassium (mg)	Vitamin A (µg RAE)	Vitamin C (mg)	Calcium (mg)	Iron (mg)
Your totals																		
Recommended totals or limits																		
Reference recommendations			10–35%		45–65%	14 g per 1,000 cal			20–35%		<10%	<300 mg	<2,300 mg	4,700 mg	900 or 700 µg	90 or 75 mg	1,000 mg	8 or 18 mg

Reflecting on Your Results

How did your diet stack up against the recommendations? Were there any areas of concern—nutrients for which you consumed more or less than the recommended amounts? The recommendations are averages, so you don't have to meet every guideline every day, but your analysis does provide a benchmark. Were you at all surprised by the results?

Planning Your Next Steps

Choose one nutrient for which you could improve your intake—either increase or decrease—in order to bring it in line with the guidelines. Develop at least three strategies for improving your intake of that nutrient. Looking at the daily food record you used for your analysis, what foods might you add, subtract, or substitute?

If your typical daily diet meets all the recommendations, congratulations—and keep it up!

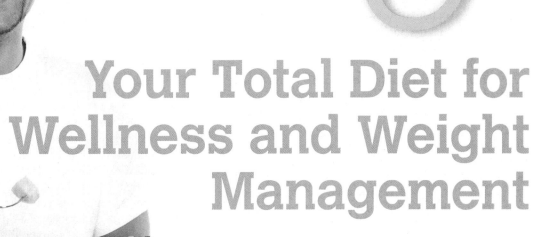

9

Your Total Diet for Wellness and Weight Management

>> **COMING UP IN THIS CHAPTER**

Learn how to combine foods into a healthy eating plan ›
Improve your food selection, preparation, and safety
skills › Evaluate strategies and products for weight loss
and maintenance › Learn recommended techniques for
healthy weight gain › Identify symptoms of eating
disorders › Assess your eating habits and create a realistic
plan for improvement

Wellness Connections

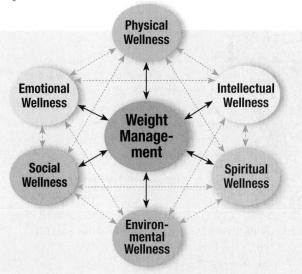

How does weight management relate to wellness? A healthy body weight is important for
physical wellness in both the short and long term,
affecting your physical functioning today and your
risk for chronic diseases in the future. Your weight
and your control (or lack of control) over your eating
habits affects self-esteem, self-efficacy, and emotional and spiritual wellness. Social wellness is also
closely linked to what you eat, where you eat, and
your weight status. How do others affect your food
choices, and how does your weight affect your interactions with others?

Successful weight management depends on intellectual wellness, especially your ability to evaluate
food choices, plan ahead for challenging situations,
and be a critical consumer of the many products and
services advertised for weight loss. It also depends

on your environment. The weight-management environment in our country is challenging—with too
many opportunities to eat too much and too few opportunities for physical activity. What can you do to
meet this challenge—and help change the environment for the better?

Maintaining a healthy body weight is a challenge for many Americans. The food supply doesn't match the recommended diet—it contains too many calories overall and too high a proportion of calories from less-than-ideal sources. The fast pace of our lives doesn't help our efforts to eat healthfully, and there are many powerful environmental influences supporting unhealthy choices and behaviors. With more than two-thirds of American adults overweight or obese, successful weight management is a public health problem that needs to be addressed to reduce the rates of heart disease, type 2 diabetes, and certain cancers.

As an individual, you can take charge of your own food choices as you do your best to navigate an unhelpful environment. You need to keep in mind that a diet for weight management isn't a temporary thing, separate from your usual way of eating. Your weight management diet is the foods you eat every day and the total dietary pattern you follow over time. Your overall goals are to be a mindful eater, paying attention to what you eat and how much you eat, and to choose foods you enjoy that meet your nutrient needs without exceeding your energy needs.[1] Eating is fun—enjoy it!

This chapter introduces several different dietary patterns associated with good health and long-term weight management, and it presents guidelines for making sound choices at home and when you eat out. It also provides the tools you need to evaluate weight-loss products and services. Finally, it introduces symptoms and treatments of eating disorders.

Planning a Healthy Diet

Q | How can I know what to eat and what to avoid with all the contradictory information out there?

Knowing what to eat can be a challenge these days; there are many sources of information, and it can be difficult to identify which ones are reliable. A couple of well-researched tools from the federal government provide information for everyday use—the Dietary Guidelines for Americans and the Dietary Reference Intakes (DRIs)—both of which were discussed in Chapter 8. In this chapter, we'll introduce MyPyramid, the food plan from the U.S. Department of Agriculture (USDA) that translates recommended nutrient intakes into a dietary pattern that allows you to get all the nutrients you need without consuming too many calories. Additional food plans have also been linked to reduced risk of chronic diseases; these include the Dietary Approaches to Stop Hypertension (DASH) and certain Mediterranean-style dietary patterns. We'll also briefly describe these eating patterns.

Although specific details are the subject of ongoing research, most of the basics of dietary advice have remained constant over time. For example, the first time the Dietary Guidelines for Americans were issued—more than thirty years ago—they recommended increased consumption of fruits, vegetables, and whole grains and reduced intake of saturated fats, salt, and processed carbohydrates. The recommendations are the same today, with even more long-term research studies to support them. Don't let fads and controversies obscure the consistent dietary advice to eat moderate portions of nutrient-dense foods.

USDA's MyPyramid

Q | Is there still such a thing as food groups? If so, how many fruits and vegetables should I eat?

Yes, dietary recommendations are still based on food groups. The USDA's **MyPyramid** food guide includes five basic food groups—grains, vegetables, fruits, milk, and meat and beans—as well as specific recommendations for intake of oils (Figure 9-1). The different widths of the food group bands in Figure 9-1 indicate how much food you should eat from each group. The MyPyramid graphic also includes a reminder for daily physical activity, which is important for both weight management and prevention of chronic diseases. *(The information in the chapter about MyPyramid is cur-*

MyPyramid The USDA-recommended eating plan based on five food groups plus oils; designed to ensure a balanced intake of essential nutrients within energy intake limits.

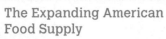

Fast Facts

The Expanding American Food Supply

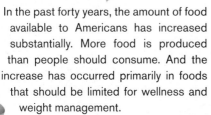

In the past forty years, the amount of food available to Americans has increased substantially. More food is produced than people should consume. And the increase has occurred primarily in foods that should be limited for wellness and weight management.

	Approximate per capita daily calories	
	1970	**2010**
Food supply (total)	3,200	3,900
Food supply (adjusted total)*	2,175	2,700
Added fats and oils and dairy fats	400	650
Flour and cereal products	425	625
Caloric sweeteners	400	450
Everything else (meat, eggs, nuts, dairy, fruits, vegetables)	925	950

*Adjusted for spoilage and waste

Source: USDA Economic Research Service. (2010). *Food availability (per capita) data system* (http://www.ers.usda.gov/Data/FoodConsumption).

Figure 9-1 **USDA's MyPyramid.** MyPyramid includes five main food groups plus oils (yellow band). Its key messages are these:

- Make half your grains whole.
- Vary your veggies.
- Focus on fruits.
- Know your fats.
- Get your calcium-rich foods.
- Go lean with protein.

Source: U.S. Department of Agriculture. (2005). *MyPyramid* (http://www.mypyramid.gov).

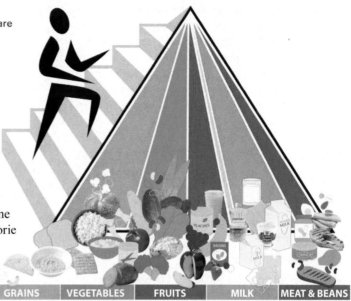

rent as of November 2010, but updates are likely; check for them at http://www.mypyramid.gov.)

To determine the amount of food you should consume from each group, you first need to know your overall calorie intake. Refer to your results from Lab 8-1 (or look at Table 8-2) for an approximation of your daily calorie needs. Next, find the appropriate column in Figure 9-2 for your recommended food intake pattern.

Daily Amounts of Food from Each Group

Calorie level	1,600	2,000	2,400	2,800	3,200
Grains	5 oz eq	6 oz eq	8 oz eq	10 oz eq	10 oz eq
Whole grains	3 oz eq	3 oz eq	4 oz eq	5 oz eq	5 oz eq
Other grains	2 oz eq	3 oz eq	4 oz eq	5 oz eq	5 oz eq
Vegetables	2 c	2½ c	3 c	3½ c	4 c
Dark green vegetables	1½ c/wk	1½ c/wk	2 c/wk	2½ c/wk	2½ c/wk
Orange/red vegetables	4 c/wk	5½ c/wk	6 c/wk	7 c/wk	7½ c/wk
Legumes	1 c/wk	1½ c/wk	2 c/wk	2½ c/wk	3 c/wk
Starchy vegetables	4 c/wk	5 c/wk	6 c/wk	7 c/wk	8 c/wk
Other vegetables	3½ c/wk	4 c/wk	5 c/wk	5½ c/wk	7 c/wk
Fruits	1½ c	2 c	2 c	2½ c	2½ c
Milk	3 c	3 c	3 c	3 c	3 c
Meat and beans	5 oz eq	5½ oz eq	6½ oz eq	7 oz eq	7 oz eq
Oils	22 g (5 tsp)	27 g (6 tsp)	31 g (7 tsp)	36 g (8 tsp)	51 g (11 tsp)
Remaining (discretionary) calories*	22 g (5 tsp)	27 g (6 tsp)	31 g (7 tsp)	36 g (8 tsp)	51 g (11 tsp)

Food group amounts shown in cup (c) or ounce equivalents (oz eq). Oils are shown in grams (g) and approximate teaspoons (tsp). Vegetable subgroup amounts are per week. Quantity equivalents for each food are:

- Grains, 1 ounce equivalent: ½ cup cooked rice, pasta, or cooked cereal; 1 ounce dry pasta or rice; 1 slice bread; 1 small muffin (1 oz); 1 ounce ready-to-eat cereal.
- Fruits and vegetables, 1 cup equivalent: 1 cup raw or cooked fruit or vegetable, 1 cup fruit or vegetable juice, 2 cups leafy salad greens. Legumes can count toward the daily meat and beans total OR as vegetables.
- Meat and beans, 1 ounce equivalent: 1 ounce lean meat, poultry, fish; 1 egg; ¼ cup cooked dry beans; 1 Tbsp peanut butter; ½ ounce nuts/seeds.
- Milk, 1 cup equivalent: 1 cup milk or yogurt, 1½ ounces natural cheese, or 2 ounces of processed cheese.

* The discretionary calorie allowance represents the additional calories remaining after choosing nutrient-dense, low-fat, no-sugar-added foods in each food group.

Figure 9-2 **MyPyramid food intake patterns based on daily calorie intake**

Source: Adapted from Dietary Guidelines Advisory Committee. (2010). *Report of the Dietary Guidelines Advisory Committee on the dietary guidelines for Americans, 2010* (http://www.cnpp.usda.gov/DGAs2010-DGACReport.htm; p. B2-20).

(You can also visit http://www.MyPyramid.gov to download a personalized plan and to see intakes for calorie levels not shown in Figure 9-2.) The chart shows the amount of food—in cups, ounces, teaspoons—that you should consume each day from each food group. Note that the vegetable group is divided into subgroups to help you get an appropriate variety of nutrients; these subgroups will be described in more detail a little later in the chapter.

Q How can I possibly eat the amount of food recommended by MyPyramid and not get fat?

You can—but you must choose wisely. To consume the recommended amounts of food within your calorie limit, follow these three guidelines:

- Choose nutrient-dense foods from each group.
- Stay within the limit for discretionary "extra" calories.
- Watch your portion sizes.

MyPyramid food patterns are based on nutrient-dense foods. If you select low-fat or nonfat foods without added sugars within each food group, you'll meet your nutrient needs with some calories left over. Remember the idea of a calorie budget we introduced in Chapter 8? You spend a certain number of calories on the essential foods, and then you may have some calories left over for extras such as these:

- Fats or sweeteners added to foods (for example, butter or syrup)
- Foods or beverages that are mostly fat, added sugars, or alcohol (for example, candy, soda or energy drinks, or beer)
- Higher-calorie forms of foods—those with solid fats or added sugars—for some of your servings from the basic food groups (for example, a sweetened cereal, a slice of full-fat cheese, or a piece of chicken with skin)
- Additional servings from any food group

The bottom row on the chart in Figure 9-2 shows the approximate number of discretionary calories available at each calorie level. You'll notice it's a fairly small number! This is where many Americans get into trouble—they consume too many calories as solid fats, added sugars, and alcohol, exceeding a healthy calorie intake and squeezing out the essentials (Table 9-1). If you do that, you'll gain weight and be short on nutrients. Remember, the number for discretionary calories in Figure 9-2 is a *limit,* and it assumes that all your other food choices are nutrient-dense, low-fat or nonfat, and have no added sugars. Suggestions for good choices within each food group are provided a little later in the chapter.

As you consider your food choices, don't focus just on what you need to limit—that can make you feel deprived. Instead, think about all the great-tasting foods you can enjoy every day.

TABLE 9-1 TYPICAL AMERICAN DIET VERSUS MYPYRAMID, ADJUSTED TO A 2,000-CALORIE/DAY DIET FOR COMPARISON

	MYPYRAMID RECOMMENDATION	TYPICAL DIET
GRAINS	6.0 cups	6.4 cups
WHOLE GRAINS	3.0 cups	0.6 cup
VEGETABLES	2.5 cups	1.6 cups
FRUIT	2.0 cups	1.0 cups
MILK	3.0 cups	1.5 cups
MEAT AND BEANS	5.5 ounce-equivalents	5.1 ounce-equivalents
OILS	27 g (6 tsp.)	18 g (4 tsp.)
SOLID FATS	16 g (~ 1 Tbsp.)	43 g (~ 3 Tbsp.)
ADDED SUGARS	32 g (~ 2½ Tbsp.)	79 g (~ 6 Tbsp.)
ALCOHOL	—	10 g (~ ¾ of a beer or glass of wine)

Source: Dietary Guidelines Advisory Committee. (2010). *Report of the Dietary Guidelines Advisory Committee on the dietary guidelines for Americans, 2010* (http://www.cnpp.usda.gov/DGAs2010-DGACReport.htm).

Another way to stay within your calorie limits is to monitor your portion sizes. Many people significantly underestimate the amount of food they eat. Do you put a teaspoon of margarine or butter on your baked potato—or more like a quarter cup? Is your serving of pasta half a cup—or two cups? And just how big was that bagel? To help retrain your eye to be more accurate at estimating portion sizes, take some time to check food labels, measure foods with a measuring cup or spoon, and just pay attention what you have in your hand or on your plate (Figure 9-3). Practice monitoring your portions for a few days or a week, and you'll get much more accurate. Using visual cues can help you eat less, especially when faced with the very large portion sizes in restaurants.

Finally, don't forget about alcohol—those calories count! In addition, drinking alcoholic beverages has other effects on health, and intake limits are suggested because of those effects: no more than an average of one drink per day for women and two drinks per day for men. See Chapter 13 for much more on alcohol.

Q | Can all foods fit into a healthy diet?

Yes, they can, but remember frequency and portion size—not too often and not too much. For example, you can have your favorite dessert, but if it's high in fat, sugar, and calories, you need to consume a small portion, and probably not every day. It's the overall quality of your diet that matters, and a good dietary plan is one that is sustainable, enjoyable, and provides a variety of healthy foods. The majority of your diet should be healthy, nutrient-dense foods—but there's room for "fun foods" as well. Thinking that you will never again eat a favorite food makes eating a chore and sets you up for failure. Chocolate chip cookies, grandma's apple pie, and chips and salsa have a place in a healthy diet, but the wise eater limits the amount of these foods within the course of a day or week. Even Sesame Street's Cookie Monster knows that "a cookie is a sometime food."

Next, we'll take a look at each of the food groups in MyPyramid, with suggestions for good choices and portion sizes.

Q | Do big, warm cinnamon rolls count as grains?

GRAINS: MAKE HALF YOUR GRAINS WHOLE. Yes, but they also probably use up all your daily discretionary calories—and more—without providing many nutrients. Although amounts vary, a commercially prepared cinnamon roll can have up to 800 calories and 30 grams (2½ tablespoons) of fat, along with refined flour and about 50 grams (¼ cup) of added sugars. You will have spent a lot of your daily calorie budget without getting many nutrients in return. A cinnamon roll can be an occasional "fun food" in your diet. What about "low-fat" cinnamon rolls? Well, they may have slightly less fat but probably provide almost as many calories—and just as few nutrients—as their full-fat counterpart.

When you choose foods, don't think just about what you're avoiding (such as some fat grams); think about what you are gaining in terms of fiber, vitamins, minerals, and phytochemicals. Instead of that cinnamon roll for breakfast, try some healthy hot or cold cereal or whole-grain toast. Many breakfast foods have whole-grain versions, so breakfast is a great opportunity for incorporating whole grains into your diet. Add some fruit and nonfat milk or yogurt, and you're off to a great start.

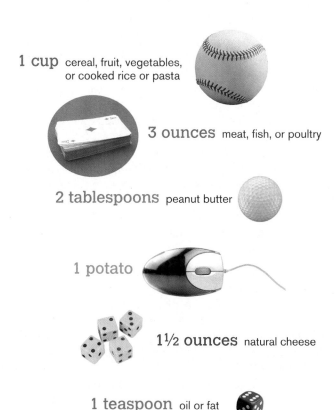

1 cup cereal, fruit, vegetables, or cooked rice or pasta

3 ounces meat, fish, or poultry

2 tablespoons peanut butter

1 potato

1½ ounces natural cheese

1 teaspoon oil or fat

Figure 9-3 Visual guide to portion sizes. Train your eye to accurately estimate portion sizes by comparing them to everyday objects such as a baseball, golf ball, deck of cards, computer mouse, and dice.

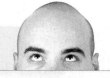

Mind Stretcher
Critical Thinking Exercise

Do you sometimes overeat? If so, are you more likely to overeat in certain situations, at certain times of day, or with particular people? Do you overeat when you're in a certain frame of mind—stressed, angry, or tired, for example? How can you use this information to improve your ability to manage your food choices and weight?

Q If I order sandwiches on wheat bread, is that whole grain?

Probably not. As described in Chapter 8, you need to check ingredient lists or ask to determine if "wheat bread" is actually a whole-grain choice. If it is, a whole grain will be the first ingredient on the list. Whole grains are recommended because they have more fiber, vitamins, minerals, and phytochemicals than refined grains. At least half your daily grain intake should be in the form of whole grains—whole-wheat bread or pasta, whole-grain cereal, brown rice, and so on.

MyPyramid eating patterns give recommendations for grain intake in terms of ounce-equivalents. For example, for a 2,000-calorie diet, six ounce-equivalents of grains are recommended, with three of those coming from whole grains. Each of the following represents one ounce-equivalent:

- 1 slice of bread or half an English muffin
- 1 small muffin, roll, or biscuit (2- to 2½-inch diameter)
- 1 cup cereal flakes
- 1/2 cup cooked pasta, rice, or cereal
- 1 small tortilla (6-inch diameter)

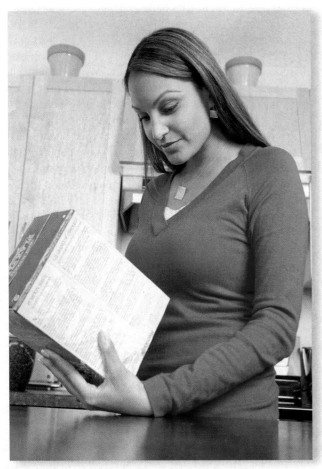

To get all your nutrients within your calorie budget, choose nutrient-dense foods from every food group.

Q Aren't french fries veggies?

VEGETABLES: VARY YOUR VEGGIES. Technically speaking, they are—in fact, they're one of the most consumed vegetables in America.[2] Although french fries are potatoes, and potatoes are vegetables, most of the calories in fries come from added fats. French fries are not a nutrient-dense choice from the vegetables group, and a single serving of fast-food fries will likely use up your day's discretionary calorie budget (and a good deal of the day's sodium limit). They're a once-in-a-while food choice.

If you're like most Americans, you need to eat more vegetables overall and choose ones with little added fat. For a 2,000-calorie diet, MyPyramid recommends a total of 2½ cups of vegetables per day. The following count as 1 cup of vegetables:

- 1 cup of raw or cooked vegetables—sliced, chopped, or mashed
- 2 cups raw leafy greens
- 1 large ear of corn (8–9 inches)
- 1 medium sweet or white potato (2½- to 3-inch diameter)

For vegetables, MyPyramid also includes specific recommendations for variety. To get all the vitamins, minerals, fiber, protein, and phytochemicals that the vegetable food group has to offer, you need to choose vegetables from five subgroups:

- Dark green vegetables: Broccoli, spinach, collards, mustard greens, turnip greens, kale, raw leafy greens that are dark in color (romaine, escarole, watercress)
- Orange and red vegetables: Carrots, pumpkin, sweet potato, winter squash, tomatoes
- Legumes (dry beans and peas): Black-eyed and split peas, chickpeas; black, kidney, pinto, white, and soy beans (for MyPyramid, a serving of legumes can be counted either as a vegetable or as a meat alternative)
- Starchy vegetables: White potatoes, green peas, yellow or white corn
- Other vegetables: Cabbage, cauliflower, celery, cucumbers, green beans, head lettuce, mushrooms, onions, summer squash

You don't have to include every subgroup every day, but choose vegetables from several of them each day, and you'll meet the weekly recommendations shown in Figure 9-2. Americans currently consume a fair amount of starchy vegetables, iceberg (head) lettuce, and tomatoes, but they need to add more legumes and dark green and orange vegetables to their diets.

Add some color to your vegetable choices! Visit the *Fruits and Veggies Matter* Web site (http://www.fruitsandveggiesmatter.gov) for ideas and recipes. Most canned and frozen vegetables are as good a choice as fresh vegetables, especially if little or no salt or fat has been added. For regular canned vegetables, draining and rinsing can reduce the amount of sodium.

Fast Facts

Top Five Ways to Gain Weight in College

1. **Avoid fruit and vegetables.** These not only provide lots of vitamins and minerals, but their high fiber and water content leaves you feeling fuller—and less tempted to overeat. They're high in nutrient density and low in energy density.

2. **Skip breakfast.** This is a surefire way to overeat later in the day—and often with poor food choices.

3. **Drink regular soda, energy drinks, and sports drinks.** One can or bottle provides 150–300 calories, all coming from added sugars, and no nutrients.

4. **Eat from snack machines.** The choices are usually loaded with calories, salt, and fat. Instead, bring your own healthier snacks to school or work, and eat regularly throughout the day to avoid hunger attacks.

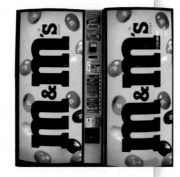

5. **Linger at the buffet.** Residence dining-hall buffets are a great way to increase your calorie intake while enjoying the social atmosphere. When given a choice of foods, such as at a buffet, people are likely to sample the variety and eat more than when their options are limited. So eat like you would at home, picking your favorite entrée and side dishes—and don't go back for more.

Q Is a fruit "drink" the same thing as juice?

FRUITS: FOCUS ON FRUIT. Probably not. Only beverages that are 100-percent fruit juice can be labeled *juice* without some type of qualifier. So beverages called *fruit juice drink, fruit punch, fruit cocktail,* or *fruit-ade* have something in them besides fruit juice—typically, added sugars. Any beverage that contains juice should be labeled with the percentage: for example, "50% juice."

You can count juice toward your daily MyPyramid fruit servings if it is 100-percent juice; such juices are nutritionally similar to whole fruits.[3] However, it's best to consume whole fruits, too, because they have fiber and are often lower in calories than juice. For example, a medium orange is the caloric equivalent of 4 ounces (1/2 cup of juice)—and most people typically drink larger servings of juice. Over time, those extra calories from juice can add up, so it is wise to choose whole fruits for a good proportion of your

intake from this group. And limit fruit drinks and punches, with their large amounts of added sugars.

For a 2,000-calorie diet, MyPyramid recommends a total of 2 cups of fruit per day. The following count as 1 cup of fruit:

- 1 cup of fresh, canned (in juice or water), or frozen fruit
- 1 cup of 100% fruit juice
- ½ cup dried fruit
- ½ grapefruit; 1 small apple; 1 medium pear; 1 large peach, banana, or orange

Q Eating fruit is expensive and inconvenient. Any suggestions?

Fresh fruit can be expensive and inconvenient—both issues for college students—because it doesn't have a long shelf life. Here are some strategies for minimizing cost and waste:

- Purchase prepackaged bags of fresh fruits with a long shelf life, such as apples and oranges.
- Freeze fresh fruit that you can't eat before it's too ripe, or buy fruit already frozen; fruit lasts a long time in the freezer and is a great addition to cereal, yogurt, and smoothies or eaten alone as snacks.
- Buy canned fruit on sale—but make sure you choose fruit that is packed in juice or water rather than in syrup.
- Watch for sales and check around your campus or community for the most inexpensive places to buy fruits and vegetables, including farmer's markets.
- Pool your fruit buying and eating with several students or neighbors to save time and money.

Q How can hamburger and pinto beans count as the same thing?

MEAT AND BEANS: GO LEAN WITH PROTEIN. The meat-and-beans group is MyPyramid's protein group; all the foods in the group are good sources of protein. Both hamburger and pinto beans provide protein, so they are both in this group, along with poultry, fish, pork, eggs, tofu, nuts, and seeds. Pinto beans and other legumes can count either toward your daily vegetable intake or toward your intake from the meat-and-beans group. As described in Chapter 8, plant protein sources other than soy are incomplete proteins; if you eat only plant proteins, you need to consume a variety over the course of the day to meet your protein requirements. If you don't add fats to plant proteins, they are excellent choices—high in protein, fiber, and other nutrients—and are strongly recommended by the *Dietary Guidelines for Americans.* Animal sources of protein do provide complete proteins; to stay within your calorie budget, choose those that are low in saturated fat. For example, very lean ground beef is a wiser choice than high-fat sausage.

Because so many types of foods are included in this group, MyPyramid provides recommendations in terms of ounce-equivalents. For a 2,000-calorie diet, 5½ ounce-equivalents are recommended from the group. Each of the following counts as 1 ounce-equivalent:

- 1 ounce cooked lean meat, poultry, or fish
- 1 egg
- 1 tablespoon peanut or almond butter
- 2 tablespoons hummus
- ¼ cup legumes or tofu
- ½ ounce (1 tablespoon) nuts or seeds

Vegetarian or meat-eater, you can find affordable healthy foods to meet your goals for this food group. See Chapter 8 for more information on complete and incomplete protein sources.

Q I don't like milk. Do I have to drink it?

MILK: GET YOUR CALCIUM-RICH FOODS. No. MyPyramid recommends 3 cups of milk or the equivalent per day. Other types of foods besides liquid milk count for this food group. The following are equivalents:

- 1 cup of milk or yogurt
- 1½ ounces of natural cheese (cheddar, swiss, parmesan)
- ¹⁄₃ cup shredded cheese
- 2 ounces of processed cheese (American)
- ½ cup ricotta cheese

Cottage cheese and ice cream count, but because they are lower in calcium, larger portion sizes are required to equal 1 cup of milk: 2 cups of cottage cheese and 1½ cups of ice cream. For ice cream, the fat and added sugars count toward your discretionary calorie total. The same goes for other dairy foods: If you choose sweetened products (flavored milk or yogurt, for example), the added sugars count toward your discretionary calorie allowance, as do any fat calories from milk, yogurt, or cheese that isn't low-fat or nonfat.

For people who are lactose intolerant, lactose-free products are available, as are enzyme preparations that make milk more digestible (see Chapter 8). If you avoid all dairy products, other foods—including calcium-fortified beverages like orange juice and soy milk—can provide calcium, although you may miss out on some of the other nutrients in dairy products.

Q Is it a good idea to eliminate oil since it's just pure fat?

OILS: RECOGNIZE AND CHOOSE HEALTHY FATS. No, absolutely not. As described in Chapter 8, fats are necessary for life. However, there are good fats and not-so-good fats.

DOLLAR STRETCHER
Financial Wellness Tip

When food shopping, compare the unit cost and not just the price of the package (for example, 4 pounds for $8 is better than 2 pounds for $5). In addition, look at the top and bottom shelves and the ends of aisles for the best values. The most expensive items are usually at or just below eye level midway down the aisle.

The oils recommended in MyPyramid are the good fats—those that provide the essential fats for your diet without a lot of the unhealthy saturated and *trans* fats that cause health problems. You need at least the equivalent of a few teaspoons of liquid oils each day to meet your need for fats in the diet. These can come from vegetable oils used in cooking, from salad dressings or mayonnaise, or from the oils in foods like fish, nuts, and avocados. Monounsaturated and polyunsaturated fats have a place in your daily diet; for a 2,000-calorie diet, 27 grams or about 6 teaspoons of oils per day are recommended. Table 9-2 provides a guide to the amount of oils in some common foods. Check food labels to identify the types and amounts of fats in processed foods.

It's easy to meet your daily requirement for oils, although many Americans currently do not, because too many of their fats are the less healthy types. As a reminder, the not-so-good fats are those that are solid at room temperature, like butter and shortening and the fats in animal products like beef, chicken, and pork. All these solid fats

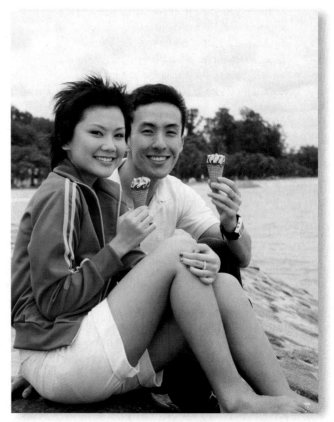

All foods can fit in a healthy diet, even sweet treats—just not too much and not too often. Make a healthy overall dietary pattern a priority, and stay committed to being a mindful eater.

TABLE 9-2 OIL CONTENT OF COMMON FOODS

FOOD	AMOUNT OF FOOD	AMOUNT OF OIL
VEGETABLE OIL	1 Tbsp.	1 Tbsp. (14 g)
SOFT (*TRANS*-FREE) MARGARINE	1 Tbsp.	2½ tsp. (11 g)
MAYONNAISE	1 Tbsp.	2½ tsp. (11 g)
MAYONNAISE-TYPE SALAD DRESSING	1 Tbsp.	1 tsp. (4 g)
ITALIAN DRESSING	2 Tbsp.	2 tsp. (8 g)
THOUSAND ISLAND DRESSING	2 Tbsp.	2½ tsp. (11 g)
OLIVES, RIPE, CANNED	8 large	1 tsp. (4 g)
AVOCADO	½ medium	3 tsp. (15 g)
PEANUT BUTTER	2 Tbsp.	4 tsp. (16 g)
PEANUTS, DRY ROASTED	1 oz.	3 tsp. (14 g)
ALMONDS, DRY ROASTED	1 oz.	3 tsp. (15 g)
SUNFLOWER SEEDS	1 oz.	3 tsp. (14 g)
SALMON STEAK	3 oz.	2 tsp. (8 g)
TUNA, CANNED IN OIL	3 oz.	1 tsp. (5 g)

Sources: USDA. (2008). How do I count the oils I eat? *Inside the Pyramid* (http://www.mypyramid.gov/pyramid/oils_count_print.html). USDA, Agricultural Research Service. (2009). USDA national nutrient database for standard reference, Release 22. *Nutrient Data Laboratory Home Page* (http://www.ars.usda.gov/ba/bhnrc/ndl).

count toward your discretionary calorie total. Unhealthy *trans* fats are from hydrogenated vegetable oils; try to avoid all non-natural sources of *trans* fats in your diet.

Q | What's the easiest way to know if I'm eating well?

MAKING MYPYRAMID WORK FOR YOU. The best way to assess your eating pattern is to do an analysis. Although tracking your food intake might not sound like a lot of fun, eating well is important, so some effort is warranted. MyPyramid is designed to help you meet all nutrition goals—appropriate energy and nutrient intakes and chronic disease prevention—so assessing your diet against the food-intake pattern for your calorie level is a good place to start. You can use the tracking form in Lab Activity 9-1 or an online tool such as the free one at http://www.mypyramid.gov. This and other online tools typically ask you to enter all the foods eat, with as much precision as possible (for example, ½ cup oatmeal, 1 tablespoon maple syrup, 1 cup milk). Although you can get some information by analyzing one day's intake, the more days you do, the more accurate the information. It's usually best to include at least one weekday and one weekend day, be-

cause eating patterns often differ. It's also important to put in *everything* you eat and drink, not just the items you think will make your diet look good.

Q | Where do I get information? How do I figure out what I'm really supposed to eat?

The message is the same for each food group: Choose moderate portions of nutrient-dense foods. Food labels, the MyPyramid Web site (http://www.mypyramid.gov), and the USDA food composition database (http://www.nal.usda.gov/fnic/foodcomp/search) are all good sources of information. With some practice, however, you won't have to look up every food every time; you'll know the nutritional quality of the foods you eat most often, and you can check labels of any new processed foods you're considering buying. See the box "Making Nutrient-Dense Food Choices" for some guidelines on getting the most from your calories. The MyPyramid Web site also includes sample menus and recipes to help get you started.

In the future you may find additional tools in your local grocery stores. The FDA plans to have tight regulations

Wellness Strategies

Making Nutrient-Dense Food Choices

Grains

- Choose whole grains at least half the time. Look for whole-grain cereals, bread, and pasta.
- Watch your portion sizes for foods like bagels and muffins. Commercially prepared baked goods are often supersized and can represent 4 or more ounce-equivalents for the grains food group.
- Instead of sweetened breakfast cereals or regular granola, try an unsweetened cereal topped with cut-up fruit or a small portion of reduced-fat granola.
- Instead of pasta with cheese or white sauce (alfredo), choose pasta with vegetables or red sauce (marinara) most often.
- Limit the number and portion size of grain foods high in fat and sugar such as pastries and croissants. Choose whole-grain toast or bread most of the time.

Vegetables

- Unless prepared with added fat, nearly all vegetables are nutrient-dense choices. Choose a colorful variety of vegetables and load up your plate.
- Add extra vegetables to breakfast scrambles, sandwiches, soups, and salads.
- Instead of fried vegetables, try steamed, roasted, or oven-baked vegetables.
- Instead of cheese or white-sauce toppings for potatoes, broccoli, and other vegetables, try herbs, lemon juice, or salsa.

Fruits

- Unless prepared with added sugar or fat, nearly all fruits are nutrient-dense choices. Choose fresh fruit and 100-percent fruit juice most of the time.
- Instead of sweetened applesauce and canned fruit packed in syrup, try unsweetened applesauce and canned fruit packed in juice.
- Limit the number and portion size of fruit desserts like pies and pastries. Choose whole fruits most of the time.

Meat and Beans

- Unless prepared with added fat, legumes and other plant protein sources are nutrient-dense choices.
- Nutrient-dense animal proteins include beef (loin, round) with the fat trimmed off, chicken without skin, fish, low-fat lunch meats, and canadian bacon.
- See Chapter 8 for more suggestions of protein sources that are low in unhealthy fats.

Milk

- Instead of sweetened fruit yogurt, try plain fat-free yogurt with fresh or frozen fruit.
- Instead of whole milk and full-fat cheeses, try low-fat or fat-free types.

Solid Fats

- All solid fats count toward your discretionary calorie total.
- Choose low-fat or fat-free versions of cream cheese and sour cream.
- Instead of regular margarine or butter, try lower-fat spreads.

Added sugars

- All added sugars count toward your discretionary calorie total.
- Instead of regular soda, sports and energy drinks, or sweetened teas, try water, unsweetened tea, or seltzer mixed with 100-percent fruit juice.
- Limit the number and portion sizes of candy, cookies, cakes, and other desserts. Choose fresh or dried fruit or frozen 100-percent-fruit-juice bars most of the time.

Sources: Adapted from USDA. (2009). Choose "nutrient-dense" forms of food. *Steps to a Healthier Weight* (http://www.mypyramid.gov/STEPS/nutrientdensefoods.html). Nutrient Rich Foods Coalition. (2007). *Nutrient Rich Foods Teaching Tools* (http://www.nutrientrichfoods.org/for_health_professionals/teaching_tools.html).

on "front-of-package" labels, so that manufacturers can't make false or misleading claims. For now, though, consumers should use information on both sides of the label, especially the Nutrition Facts panel, which provides almost everything you need to know to make healthy food choices.

Q | I never eat breakfast and always end up at the vending machine. What do you recommend?

Finding time to eat a good breakfast can be difficult, especially if you have early classes. Skipping breakfast, however, is a sure-fire way to be really hungry later in the morning, and for some people, this makes it harder to concentrate during class. Research has shown that skipping breakfast makes you much more likely to gain weight and more likely to make poor nutritional choices when you do eat get around to eating.[4] Vending machines definitely provide a quick source of calories but not a good choice of calories—or even a good use of your money.

Whether you live at home or in a dorm, try to make a little time for breakfast in the morning. Healthy and quick choices include unsweetened cereal with fruit and low-fat milk, low-fat granola with nonfat yogurt, and whole-grain toast or bagels topped with a *trans*-free margarine spread or 1–2 tablespoons of peanut butter. Peanut butter provides

Research Brief

Moderate, Regular Eating Decreases the Risk of Obesity

People who think they can lose weight by skipping meals need to think again. A recent study showed that people who eat more frequently during the day have almost half the incidence of obesity than people who eat less often. About five hundred people were asked to report their diets five times over one year. Those who ate four or more times a day (generally three meals and a snack) were *45 percent less likely to be obese* than those who ate three or fewer meals daily.

People who regularly skipped breakfast were *450 percent more likely to be obese* compared to regular breakfast eaters. There was no indication that eating at night contrib-uted to greater weight, after taking into account total calories. Eating breakfast or dinner away from home, however, was associated with higher weight, potentially due to larger portions and more fat in restaurant food.

What does this mean for you? Eat regularly, and eat breakfast. If you don't have time for a sit-down breakfast, get up a little earlier or plan ahead and pack a breakfast to go.

Source: Ma, Y., Bertone, E. R., Stanek III, E. J., Reed, G. W., Hebert, J. R., Cohen, N. L., Merriam, P. A., & Ockene, I. S. (2003). Association between eating patterns and obesity in a free-living U.S. adult population. *American Journal of Epidemiology, 158*(1), 85–92.

---

both oils and protein and can help keep you feeling full. A small glass of 100-percent juice is also a good choice.

Bacon, sausage, pancakes, waffles, sugary cereals, and other foods with a lot of fat or sugar should be saved for special occasions—and then in modest portions. And don't overdo the caffeinated coffee and tea—too much caffeine can leave you jittery and unable to focus—or the typical add-ons of cream and sugar.

If you don't have time to sit down and eat, pack something ahead of time to get you through the morning. Ideally, you should eat 300–500 calories within two or three hours of waking; otherwise, you'll be dragging through those early classes and ravenously hungry by midday. Perishable foods should be eaten within two hours of being taken out of the refrigerator (or longer if they're in an insulated pack), which should give you enough time to eat your breakfast on the go. Good foods to pack are bagels or bread with peanut butter, whole fruit, yogurt, and dry packaged cereals. Most residence dining halls will pack a meal for you if you have a meal plan, so you can just stop by the cafeteria on your way to class and pick up your morning meal. If you live off campus, plan ahead and pack your own breakfast.

Q | **What are some easy snacks that are healthy?**

Healthy snacks should be part of your eating plan, and there are many options that can help you meet your recommended MyPyramid food group intakes. Just take care not to stock your refrigerator with energy-dense, nutrient-poor packaged baked goods, chips, sweetened beverages, and candy. Good snack options include moderate portions of the following foods:

- Whole-grain crackers, plain or with peanut butter, salsa, or hummus or another bean dip
- Low-fat microwave popcorn
- Fruit (fresh, canned, or dried)
- Carrot and celery sticks, bell pepper strips, broccoli florets
- Nonfat yogurt with fruit (if you have a blender, make a smoothie from nonfat yogurt and frozen fruit chunks)
- Single-serving containers of unsweetened applesauce or fruit juice—or pack your own in reusable containers for a less expensive option that also helps reduce trash
- Nuts and seeds
- Cereals, especially those with little or no added sugar
- Homemade trail mix, made from cereal, nuts and seeds, and dried fruit
- Hard-cooked egg
- 100% fruit juice
- Cup of vegetable soup

Energy, protein, and granola bars are easy to carry, but read the labels carefully before you buy them because some are very high in calories, saturated fat, and added sugars.

Pay attention when you snack so that you don't eat more than you intend to. Take out exactly how much you plan to eat before you call a friend, start your homework, turn on the television, or engage in another activity that will take your focus away from how much you're eating. Don't forget to include your snacks in your dietary analysis. Snacks count!

Vegetarian Diets

Q | **I'm a vegetarian. Can I still use MyPyramid?**

Yes. MyPyramid has information for all types of eaters, including vegetarians, children, and pregnant and lactating mothers. There are

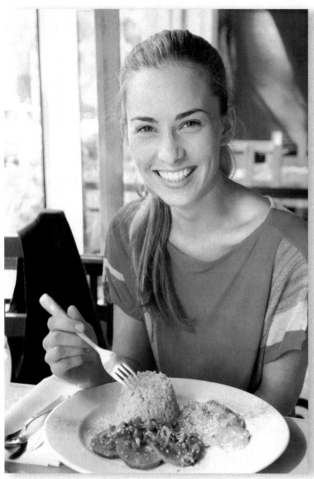

Vegetarian diets can meet all nutrient needs. But just as for a nonvegetarian diet, nutrient-dense choices from each food group is key.

vegetarian options in each food group, depending on what type of vegetarian diet you follow. **Vegans** eat only plant foods and avoid all animal products. Other vegetarians avoid flesh foods but include dairy (lacto) or egg (ovo) products, or both. Thus, **lacto-vegetarians** eat plant foods and dairy products, and **lacto-ovo-vegetarians** eat plant foods, dairy products, and eggs.

About 5 million Americans consistently follow a vegetarian diet, and many more consume vegetarian meals at least some of the time; this latter group is sometimes referred to as *partial vegetarians*.[5] Common reasons for choosing a vegetarian diet include health concerns, economic and ethical considerations, religious beliefs, and concern for the environment and animal welfare. Vegetarian diets tend to be lower in saturated fat and cholesterol and higher in fiber, potassium, folate, and other micronutrients and phytochemicals; these differences may help explain lower rates of heart disease, hypertension, and type 2 diabetes among vegetarians.

vegan A dietary pattern composed exclusively of plant foods, with no animal products.

lacto-vegetarian A dietary pattern composed of plant foods and dairy products.

lacto-ovo-vegetarian A dietary pattern composed of plant foods, eggs, and dairy products.

If you're a vegetarian, visit the special section on the MyPyramid Web site with advice for you. The general guidelines are the same—select nutrient-dense choices from each food group.

Healthy vegetarian protein sources from the meat and beans group include eggs (for ovo-vegetarians), legumes, nuts and nut butters, and various soy products, including tofu, tempeh, and veggie burgers. By selecting a variety of plant proteins over the course of the day, vegetarians can obtain all the essential amino acids (see Chapter 8).[6]

Lacto- and lacto-ovo-vegetarians can follow the general guidelines for selecting foods from the milk group—choosing low-fat and nonfat options most of the time. Vegans can choose non-dairy sources of calcium. As described in Chapter 8, vegetarians need to take special care to consume adequate amounts of iron, zinc, and vitamin B_{12}. Recall that consuming vitamin C–rich foods along with iron-rich foods can help the body absorb iron. Vitamin B_{12} is found only in animal foods and so must be obtained from fortified foods or supplements.

If you are or are thinking about adopting a vegetarian diet, or if you just want to learn more, consult the following Web sites: MyPyramid: Vegetarian Diet (http://www.mypyramid.gov/tips_resources/vegetarian_diets.html); MedlinePlus: Vegetarian Diet (http://www.nlm.nih.gov/medlineplus/vegetariandiet.html); and the Vegetarian Resource Group (http://www.vrg.org).

DASH and Other Dietary Plans

Q | What other eating plans are there?

There are many eating plans available—in books, online, from weight-loss programs—and some are better options than others. Two eating patterns that the *2010 Dietary Guidelines for Americans* links to reduced risk of chronic disease are the **DASH (Dietary Approaches to Stop Hypertension) diet** and some Mediterranean-style diets.[7]

The DASH diet, as its name indicates, was originally developed to help people reduce blood pressure. It emphasizes whole grains, vegetables, fruits, and low-fat dairy products and includes poultry, seafood, and nuts; it limits red meat, sweets, sodium, and sugar-containing beverages.[8] The DASH diet comes in several versions, including one with sodium intake reduced to the level recommended for people with or at risk for high blood pressure—this group includes anyone with hypertension, African Americans, and middle-aged and older adults.

Research has found that the DASH diet, especially its low-sodium version, significantly reduces blood pressure and improves heart function. Blood pressure goes down within just a few weeks of starting on the DASH plan.

DASH diet Dietary Approaches to Stop Hypertension, a dietary pattern designed to reduce blood pressure that emphasizes potassium-rich vegetables and fruits and low-fat dairy products; includes whole grains, poultry, fish, and nuts and limits sodium, red meat, and added sugars.

Mediterranean diet A dietary pattern associated with cultures bordering the Mediterranean Sea; the pattern emphasizes whole grains, fruits, vegetables, legumes, nuts, seeds, fish, and olive oil and limits meat, saturated fat, and full-fat dairy products.

When combined with exercise and weight loss, the DASH diet has even more benefits, including greater reductions in blood pressure, improved cognition, reduced insulin sensitivity, and improved cholesterol levels.[9] Like MyPyramid, the DASH diet can be the basis for a weight-reducing diet and is a good choice for everyone. For more about DASH, including meal plans and recipe ideas, visit the Web site for the National Heart, Lung, and Blood Institute (http://www .nhlbi.nih.gov/hbp/prevent/h_eating/h_eating.htm).

Q | What's the Mediterranean diet? It sounds exotic.

The Mediterranean diet is a pattern associated with the traditional diets of the cultures that border the Mediterranean Sea. Although the diets vary among and within these countries, they have some common features, which are referred to as the **Mediterranean diet** (Figure 9-4):[10]

- Staples include unrefined grains, vegetables, legumes, fruits, and nuts and seeds, with high overall fiber intake.
- Fish and (in non-Islamic countries) wine are often served at meals.
- Olive oil is the primary source of added fats.
- Consumption of saturated fat, meat, and full-fat dairy products is limited.

As you can see, many aspects of this dietary pattern are consistent with the recommendations in MyPyramid and DASH. The Mediterranean diet has a total fat consumption near or over the limit suggested by the Dietary Reference Intakes, but most of that fat is from healthy, unsaturated oils. It is primarily a plant-based diet and is linked to lower rates of several chronic diseases—another healthy choice for you!

Developing Practical Skills

Now that you know the basics of eating patterns associated with good health, it's time to put that knowledge to work in your everyday life. To do that, you need to develop your skills at planning meals, shopping, cooking, and selecting foods when eating out. You also need the basics on food safety so that you can prepare meals and eat leftovers without worrying about foodborne illness, toxins, or allergens.

Meal Planning and Preparation

Q | What am I supposed to do if I don't know how to cook? Help!

Not having any cooking experience can be a roadblock. Most everyone can put together simple breakfasts and meals—cereal with fruit, basic sandwiches—that don't require much, if any, cooking. But for more complex meals, you may feel stuck. If you don't have access to a campus dining hall or a friendly roommate who cooks, you may have to rely more on prepared foods while you learn some basic cooking skills.

In terms of planning meals, think about your goals according to MyPyramid. Most Americans don't eat enough whole grains, low-fat dairy, fruits, and vegetables, so start there. For breakfast, have whole-grain cereal or toast, fruit, and milk or yogurt. Have at least two servings of vegetables at lunch and dinner, and snack on fruit. Frozen and canned vegetables are easy to fix, and many have directions and even recipe ideas on their labels. Go for lean protein sources, such as sliced turkey in a sandwich or legumes in your salad. The sites listed in the box "Resources for Meal Planning and Cooking" have lots more ideas; see especially the sample menus created for MyPyramid and DASH.

Wine In moderation

Meats and sweets Less often

Poultry, eggs, cheese and yogurt Moderate portions daily to weekly

Drink water

Fish and seafood Often, at least two times per week

Fruits, vegetables, grains (mostly whole), olive oil, beans, nuts, legumes, seeds, herbs and spices Base every meal on these foods

Illustration by George Middleton © 2009 Oldways Preservation and Exchange Trust www.oldwayspt.org

Be physically active; enjoy meals with others

Figure 9-4 **Mediterranean Diet Pyramid** The Mediterranean diet is based on minimally processed foods from plant sources, with olive oil as the principal type of fat. For more information on the Mediterranean diet and tips for incorporating it into your daily diet, visit the Oldways Web site (http://www .oldwayspt.org).

Source: © 2009 Oldways Preservation and Exchange Trust. *2009 Mediterranean Diet Pyramid* (http://www.oldwayspt.org/mediterranean-diet-pyramid).

A growing number of prepared foods provide good nutritional options. Most grocery stores carry a vast line of breakfasts, lunches, and dinners that just need to be heated. Of course, many of these foods have a lot more sodium and fat than if you cooked them yourself—and they are more expensive—but they can be helpful in a pinch, especially if you buy them on sale. Be sure, before you buy, to read the nutrition labels and comparison shop in terms of both price and nutrition. Even options that call themselves "healthy" are likely to be relatively high in sodium, so if you do consume a packaged entrée, watch your sodium intake the rest of the day. To reduce the high levels of sodium in rice mixes, frozen stir-fry meals, and similar foods, use only half the seasoning packet; add your own spices to boost the flavor with less sodium. For convenience foods that call for the addition of butter or margarine, use only half the amount to reduce added fats.

Another good move is to load up on fresh fruit and vegetables, many of which can be eaten raw or with minimal cooking, such as steaming or heating in a microwave. You'll get plenty of vitamins, minerals, and fiber with little cooking time and effort. Many prepared entrées have less than a full serving of vegetables, so supplementing them with additional vegetables can help you meet your MyPyramid goals. You can add vegetables to many types of convenience foods—rice and pasta mixes, tomato-based pasta sauces, frozen pizza, creamed soups, and casserole mixes.

Next, start to develop food preparation and cooking skills. Start with a few simple things. You don't need to learn to cook fancy dishes; a few basic pots, pans, and utensils are all you need. Everyone can follow basic directions in a recipe. You could also take a cooking class—a great investment of time for learning an important life skill. Although you might not be able to include this course in your academic curriculum, there is a good chance your school offers non-credit cooking classes or you can find them at the local YMCA, recreation department, or community center. Also, a number of Web sites can teach you how to cook even if you've never opened an oven. Don't let the fear of cooking keep you from eating well: Take a cooking class, use more fruits and vegetables, purchase healthier prepared foods.

Eating Away from Home

Q | I live on campus. What kind of food should I eat in the dining hall?

You might be tired of reading it, but the advice remains the same: Your best choices are moderate portions of nutrient-rich foods. Your dining hall likely offers plenty of these—along with some not-so-healthy options that should be once-in-a-while foods. For example, it's up to you to choose whole-grain cereals or egg-white omelets often, and to save the chocolate-chip waffles, bacon, and danish pastries for occasional treats.

How much do you know about the foods that are available? Many campus dining halls have ingredient lists and nutrition data available—in print or online. They may also identify the dishes by category, such as vegetarian, vegan, low-calorie, or heart healthy. Check out the information that's available, and use it to make good choices. Also take note of the portion sizes the information is based on—and make appropriate adjustments. If you aren't sure what something is or what's in it, ask.

Good options include the following:

- Whole-grain cereals, breads, and pasta; read the ingredient list or ask if you're not sure—just because a bread looks brown doesn't mean it's a whole-grain
- Oatmeal (without a lot of added sweeteners) and egg-white omelets for hot breakfasts
- Fresh fruit—always a good choice
- Salads topped with fresh vegetables, legumes, and seeds; limit high-fat toppings like croutons and cheese, and select a low-fat or oil-based salad dressing served on the side
- Vegetable or broth-based soups; having a cup of soup or a glass of water before you eat can help fill you up
- Sandwiches and wraps containing some combination of lean meat, low-fat cheese, and lots of veggies; use salsa, vinegar, or mustard for flavor
- Lean chicken and beef dishes; grilled, broiled, or baked fish
- Vegetarian pasta and bean dishes with tomato-based sauces and little added fat
- Just about any vegetable fixed without added fat—load up your plate
- Nonfat yogurt

Q | What are the best fast-food choices? What about other types of restaurants?

Fast-food restaurants are tempting because they are fast, relatively inexpensive, and consistent—you know what you'll get. However, many classic fast-food choices are problematic due to both what they provide and what they don't provide: Many are high in calories, total fat and saturated fat, and sodium, and they're low in fiber and many micronutrients. A fast-food meal can use up a large chunk of your daily calorie budget without giving you an equal helping of nutrients in return.

There are better options at many fast-food restaurants—salad with dressing on the side, for example, or a grilled chicken sandwich. Size also matters: A small burger and fries might contain 500 calories and 5 grams of saturated fat, whereas a double cheeseburger, large fries, and a large shake has closer to 2,500 calories and 40 grams of saturated fat (and an entire day's supply of sodium). For additional tips for fast-food restaurants and traditional sit-down restaurants, see the box "Tips for Eating Out" on page 320. Many of the strategies suggested for dining-hall eating also apply to restaurants.

Wellness Strategies

Resources for Meal Planning and Cooking

The Web sites listed below are a good place to start looking for ideas. Not every recipe at every site is a healthy choice, but you can use your knowledge of nutrition to make wise choices.

MyPyramid Menu Planner: Helps you plan menus for a day or a week using the MyPyramid recommendations for you or your family.

http://www.mypyramidtracker.gov/planner

National Heart, Lung, and Blood Institute's Deliciously Healthy Eating Recipes: Includes recipes as well as an illustrated food-preparation glossary.

http://hp2010.nhlbihin.net/healthyeating

National Heart, Lung, and Blood Institute's recipe booklets: Includes heart-healthy recipes, the DASH eating plan, and Latino and African American dishes.

http://www.nhlbi.nih.gov/health/public/heart/obesity/lose_wt/recipes.htm

University of New Hampshire Health Services: *Good Eats: Quick & Easy Food for Busy College Students:* Includes recipes like "Breakfast Bulgur While You Shower," "Five-Minute Quesadillas," and "Starving Student's Simple Supper."

http://www.unh.edu/health-services/good_eats

Iowa State University Extension: Spend Smart, Eat Smart: Provides suggestions for saving money along with easy and quick recipes.

http://www.extension.iastate.edu/foodsavings/

Try the "Sandwich Building" activity to learn more about creating healthy sandwiches:

http://www.extension.iastate.edu/nutrition/sandwich

Centers for Disease Control: Fruits and Veggies Matter: Go to the recipes section to find ways to use just about any fruit or vegetable.

http://www.fruitsandveggiesmatter.gov

Nutrient Rich Foods Coalition Recipes: A database of recipes that meet the Coalition's criteria for nutrient richness; you can search the database by ingredient, meal, total time, or difficulty level.

http://www.nutrientrichfoods.org/recipes

USDA Recipe Finder: A database of recipes organized not only by ingredient, meal, and cost but also by specific nutrition goals (e.g., less saturated fat) and preparation time.

http://recipefinder.nal.usda.gov

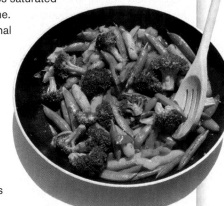

Eat Better America: This commercial site recommends specific brands in some recipes, but you can use whatever brands you find locally; the recipes follow recognized dietary guidelines and include nutritional information.

http://www.eatbetteramerica.com

YumYum Student Recipes and **Cookin' for College:** Not every recipe on these sites is a healthy choice, but the sites also include student-oriented tips and how-to information. The Cookin' for College site includes video clips showing how to make some of the recipes.

http://www.yumyum.com/student
http://www.cookinforcollege.com

Here are additional time- and money-saving tips:

- Shop sales, use coupons, and buy nonperishables in bulk.
- Share shopping and cooking responsibilities with roommates and friends; start a "dinner club" with other students to take turns cooking and share costs.
- Cook a big batch of a dish that freezes well (for example, soups, stews, and pasta dishes); save the leftovers to reheat later in the week.
- Cook from scratch when you can, to avoid expensive convenience foods and to give you more control over the amount of added fat, salt, and sugar. For example, plain rice or pasta is less expensive and lower in sodium than a flavored packaged mix, and the same goes for oatmeal (plain oats in a large container versus flavored packets).

---

foodborne illness An illness caused by consuming foods or beverages contaminated with disease-causing organisms.

Food Safety and Technology

Food safety is often in the news, with recalls of contaminated foods or outbreaks of **foodborne illness.** Food safety is a concern for both large-scale commercial food producers and people cooking at home. Technological developments also affect our food supply, and consumers must make decisions about whether to purchase particular types of foods, including those certified organic. Food allergies are also an important issue for some people.

Wellness Strategies

Tips for Eating Out

Fast-Food Restaurants

- Order small burgers or grilled chicken sandwiches without cheese, mayonnaise, or "special" sauces.
- For sandwiches, choose whole-grain bread, rolls, or pita with lean meats and lots of vegetables; pickles, onions, hot peppers, lettuce, tomatoes, mustard, and fat-free dressings add flavor without fat.
- Skip the chips in favor of fruit (if available), or have pretzels instead.
- Skip the fries, order the kid's portion, or share them with a friend.
- For pizza, get the thin crust and ask for half the amount of cheese and twice the vegetables instead of meat toppings.
- Order salads with lots of vegetable toppings and a low-fat dressing on the side; avoid or limit creamy full-fat dressings, cheese toppings, and croutons.
- Drink water, 100-percent juice (small size), unsweetened tea, or low-fat milk instead of a milk shake or regular soda.
- Have frozen yogurt or a fruit salad for dessert rather than pie, cookies, or a milk shake

Sit-Down Restaurants

- If you know where you're going, look for the menu online and plan what you'll order.
- Don't skip lunch if you're going out to dinner, because you'll be more likely to make poor dinner choices if you're super hungry; have a small lunch or snack.
- Feel free to ask the server questions about how a dish is prepared and to request changes or substitutions.
- If you want to avoid overeating, it's usually best to order a menu item rather than heading for the buffet.
- Skip the appetizers, unless you want to order one instead of an entrée.
- If portions are large, share with a friend or take half home; ask for the to-go box when you order and place half the food in it as soon as you're served.
- Ask for salad dressing, gravy, and sauces to be served on the side.
- Foods that are fried, stuffed, or covered with cheese (e.g., au gratin, scalloped) or a cream sauce (e.g., alfredo, hollandaise) are high in calories and unhealthy fats; choose grilled, broiled, roasted, baked, flame-cooked, or steamed dishes.
- Try fresh fruit or sherbet for dessert.

Q | Isn't food safety a worry only for people with jobs preparing or serving food?

FOODBORNE ILLNESS. No. Food safety is for everyone. Although many people worry about pesticides and other chemicals in their food, the biggest threats come from **pathogens,** viruses and bacteria and other disease-causing microorganisms that contaminate food and cause foodborne illness. Each year, foodborne illness affects more than 75 million Americans, causing 325,000 hospitalizations and about 5,200 deaths.[11] Most cases of foodborne illness, also called food poisoning or stomach flu, last only a few days and are characterized by nausea, vomiting, diarrhea, and fever. For otherwise healthy people, these symptoms are unpleasant but not serious. Higher-risk populations (older adults, pregnant women, infants and children, and people with compromised immune function) can suffer much more serious outcomes. If you become ill with symptoms of foodborne illness, drink plenty of fluids and wash your hands frequently to avoid spreading the infection; consult a health care provider if you have a high fever or your symptoms are very severe and don't improve within three days.

The most common causes of foodborne illness are the bacteria *Salmonella, Campylobacter,* and *E. coli* O157:H7 and the group of viruses called norovirus. These pathogens are present on many foods when you purchase them, especially animal products and fresh produce. However, cross-contamination can taint most any other food; your hands, cutting boards, kitchen counters, knives, and refrigerator shelves are all places where a pathogen can travel from one food to another. You cannot see or smell these pathogens on food.

There is no way to ensure that all the food coming into your home is free of pathogens, so you need to practice safe food handling and storage to prevent illness. Figure 9-5 summarizes the basic four steps for food safety: clean, separate, cook, and chill. Here are some additional tips:

- Wash fruits and vegetables under running water just before eating, cutting, or cooking. Wash them even if you plan to peel them. Scrub firm produce, such as melons and cucumbers, with a clean produce brush.
- Remove and discard the outermost leaves of a head of cabbage or lettuce.

pathogen A microorganism that causes disease, such as a virus or bacterium.

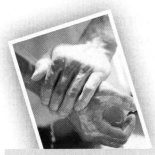 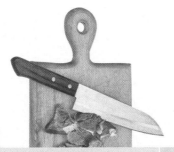 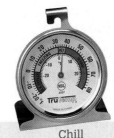

Clean	Separate	Cook	Chill
• Wash hands with soap and warm water for 20 seconds before and after handling food. If soap isn't available, use an alcohol-based gel. • Run cutting boards and utensils through the dishwasher or wash them in hot soapy water after each use. • Keep countertops clean by washing with hot soapy water after preparing food.	• Use one cutting board for raw meat, poultry, and seafood and another for salads and ready-to-eat food. • Keep raw meat, poultry, and seafood and their juices apart from other food items in your grocery cart. • Store raw meat, poultry, and seafood in a container or on a plate so juices can't drip on other foods.	• Use a food thermometer; you can't tell food is cooked safely by how it looks. • Stir, rotate the dish, and cover food when microwaving to prevent cold spots where bacteria can survive. • Bring sauces, soups, and gravies to a rolling boil when reheating.	• Cool the fridge to 40°F or below, and use an appliance thermometer to check the temperature. • Chill leftovers and takeout foods within 2 hours, and divide food into shallow containers for rapid cooling. • Thaw meat, poultry, and seafood in the fridge, not on the counter; don't over-stuff the fridge.

USDA Recommended Safe Minimum Internal Temperatures

Beef, veal, lamb, steaks, and roast	Fish	Pork	Beef, veal, lamb, ground	Egg dishes	Turkey, chicken, and duck, whole, pieces, and ground
145°F	**145°F**	**160°F**	**160°F**	**160°F**	**165°F**

Figure 9-5 **Four basic steps for food safety.** For additional information, visit http://www.foodsafety.gov and http://BeFoodSafe.gov

Sources: Adapted from U.S. Department of Agriculture. (2007, June). *Four easy lessons in safe food handling* (http://www.fsis.usda.gov/be_foodsafe/BFS_Brochure_Text/index.asp). U.S. Department of Agriculture. (2006, April). *"Is it done yet?"* (http://www.fsis.usda.gov/is_it_done_yet).

■ Keep foods at a safe temperature until served. Cold foods should be held at 40°F or below. Hot foods should be kept at 140°F or above.

■ Don't eat unsafe foods, including unpasteurized milk or juice, cookie dough containing raw eggs, or raw or undercooked eggs, fish, oysters, hamburgers, and other meats.

■ Clean your refrigerator regularly.

Researchers who have studied college students' food-handling practices have found that the majority don't follow the recommendations.[12] Take a few extra minutes to follow the basic steps for food safety to reduce the risk of foodborne illness for yourself and the people around you.

Q | Can I still eat the pizza leftover from Friday night?

Assuming it's been refrigerated and it isn't yet Tuesday, you're probably OK, because leftover pizza can safely last for three or four days. Refrigeration is key for leftovers, because pathogens can multiply rapidly at temperatures between 40°F and 140°F. Foods should be eaten within two hours of being taken out of the refrigerator. Table 9-3 provides guidelines for how long it's safe to store food in the refrigerator and freezer. These guidelines assume that your refrigerator is cold enough. Researchers studying food safety practices among college students found that the average refrigerator was above the maximum recommended temperature of 40°F, increasing the risk for foodborne illness.[13] Have you checked your refrigerator's temperature? Use an inexpensive appliance thermometer to ensure the refrigerator is kept at an appropriate temperature. It's also a great tool after a power outage to determine if the food in the fridge is still safe to eat.

Q | My mom checks a roast with a meat thermometer, but I don't have one. Is it really necessary?

Yes, the best way to determine if meat is cooked to a safe temperature is to use a meat thermometer to measure its internal temperature. "Done" according to color or time

TABLE 9-3 SAFE REFRIGERATOR AND FREEZER STORAGE FOR FOODS

CATEGORY	FOOD	REFRIGERATOR (≤40°F)	FREEZER (≤0°F)
LEFTOVERS	Cooked meat or poultry	3–4 days	2–6 months
	Chicken nuggets or patties	3–4 days	1–3 months
	Pizza	3–4 days	1–2 months
	Quiche with filling	3–4 days	1–2 months
SALADS	Egg, chicken, ham, tuna, macaroni salads	3–5 days	Don't freeze
HOT DOGS	Opened package	1 week	1–2 months
	Unopened package	2 weeks	1–2 months
LUNCHEON MEAT	Opened package or deli sliced	3–5 days	1–2 months
	Unopened package	2 weeks	1–2 months
BACON, SAUSAGE	Bacon	7 days	1 month
	Sausage, raw (chicken, turkey, pork, beef)	1–2 days	1–2 months
HAMBURGER, OTHER GROUND MEATS	Hamburger, ground beef, turkey, veal, pork, lamb, mixtures	1–2 days	3–4 months
FRESH BEEF, VEAL, LAMB, PORK	Steaks	3–5 days	6–12 months
	Chops	3–5 days	4–6 months
	Roasts	3–5 days	4–12 months
FRESH POULTRY	Chicken or turkey, whole	1–2 days	1 year
	Chicken or turkey, pieces	1–2 days	9 months
FISH	Lean fish	1–2 days	6 months
	Fatty fish	1–2 days	2–3 months
	Cooked fish	3–4 days	4–6 months
SOUPS, STEWS	Vegetable or meat added	3–4 days	2–3 months
EGGS	Raw in shell	3–5 weeks	Don't freeze
	Hard-cooked	1 week	Don't freeze
MAYONNAISE	Opened jar	2 months	Don't freeze
DAIRY	Milk	1 week	3 months
	Yogurt	1–2 weeks	1–2 months
	Cheese, hard, opened	3–4 weeks	6 months

Sources: Adapted from FoodSafety.gov. (2010). Storage times for the refrigerator and freezer. *Keep Food Safe* (http://www.foodsafety.gov/keep/charts/storagetimes.html). U.S. Food and Drug Administration. (2006). *To Your Health! Food Safety for Seniors* (http://www.fda.gov/Food/ResourcesForYou/Consumers/Seniors/ucm182679.htm).

in the oven isn't necessarily the same thing as "safe." Research has shown that neither color nor time adequately indicates that meat is completely cooked. The color of roast or ground beef, for example, is no longer considered a safe indicator. Similarly, for whole poultry, checking whether the juices from the bird are clear, the meat is no longer pink, or the legs easily pull away from the body are common but inaccurate techniques. The only safe way is to use a meat thermometer. Reusable ones cost a few dollars, and checking the temperature takes only 10–30 seconds. See Figure 9-5 for recommended safe internal temperatures.

Q What's mad cow disease?

🖥 **READ ONLINE**

Q So, is everyone allergic to peanuts?

FOOD ALLERGIES. Not everyone, but peanuts are one of the most common food **allergens** and cause severe reactions in some people. About 6–8 percent of children under age 4 and 3.7 percent of adults have some form of food allergy, and exposure to the allergen can have serious consequences. Food allergies are different from food intolerances such as lactose intolerance, which you learned about in Chapter 8. In a food *allergy,* the body's immune system mistakenly identifies the food as a harmful substance and releases histamine and other chemicals into the bloodstream. A food *intolerance* has a different underlying cause—such as the absence of an enzyme needed to fully digest a food (as in lactose intolerance) or a sensitivity to a substance (such as MSG)—and is usually less severe than an allergy.

Symptoms of food allergies include coughing or wheezing, flushed skin, rash or hives, tingling or itchy sensations in the mouth, swelling of the lips or tongue, nausea, abdominal cramps, and diarrhea. In some cases, a severe reaction known as *anaphylaxis* occurs, characterized by constriction of the airways in the lungs, swelling of the throat causing suffocation, and severe lowering of blood pressure and shock. Anaphylaxis is a medical emergency. Prompt treatment with epinephrine during the early stages of anaphylaxis can help slow and reduce the severity of the allergic reaction. People with severe allergies may carry an auto-injector with epinephrine (for example, an EpiPen) for this purpose.

To help reduce accidental exposure to allergens, people with food allergies should read food labels and ask questions when eating food from a restaurant or a dining hall. By law, any food that may contain one or more of eight major food allergens—milk, eggs, fish, shellfish, tree nuts (such as walnuts and almonds), peanuts, wheat, or soybeans—must list the allergens on the label. If you have a reaction to a food and are unsure if it's due to intolerance, allergy, or foodborne illness, talk with your physician.

allergen A substance that is capable of producing an allergic reaction in the body's immune system; most food allergens are proteins.

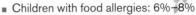

Fast Facts

Food Allergies

- Children with food allergies: 6%–8%
- The most common food allergens among children: Eggs, cow's milk, peanuts, tree nuts
- Adults with food allergies: 3.7%
- The most common food allergens among adults: shellfish, peanuts, tree nuts, fish, eggs
- Annual episodes of food-induced anaphylaxis: 30,000
- Annual deaths from food-induced anaphylaxis: 100–200
- Leading causes of fatal and near-fatal food-allergic reactions: peanuts and tree nuts
- Percentage of people with food allergies experiencing an unintended exposure during a two-year period: 50%

Source: National Institute of Allergy and Infectious Diseases. (2010). Quick facts. *Food Allergy* (http://www.niaid.nih.gov/topics/foodallergy/understanding/pages/quickfacts.aspx).

Q Fish is supposed to be healthy, but doesn't it contain mercury?

FISH AND MERCURY. Some fish does contain mercury, which is a concern for human health. Mercury gets into the water from human activities (burning of gas and other fossil fuels) and from natural sources such as volcanic eruptions. It is picked up by microorganisms, which are eaten by larger organisms, and then even larger ones, and so on. Through this process of *bioaccumulation,* large predatory fish such as sharks and swordfish contain the highest levels of mercury.

In terms of your health, you have to balance the risks from mercury in fish with the benefits of consuming fish. Fish and shellfish contain high-quality protein; they are low in saturated fat; and many types contain heart-healthy omega-3 fatty acids (see Chapter 8). Nearly all fish and shellfish contain traces of mercury, which for most people poses little health risk because the body can eliminate it. Some varieties contain higher levels of mercury, which can be harmful to an unborn baby or a young child's developing nervous system. Because of this, the Food and Drug Administration (FDA) and the Environmental Protection Agency (EPA) make these recommendations for women who are or may become pregnant, nursing mothers, and young children:[14]

- Do not consume shark, swordfish, king mackerel, or tilefish; these fish contain the highest levels of mercury.

- Limit consumption of albacore ("white") tuna to no more than 6 ounces per week; it has more mercury than canned light tuna.
- Do eat up to 12 ounces per week of a variety of fish and shellfish that are lower in mercury, including salmon, pollock, catfish, canned light tuna, and shrimp.
- For local, recreationally caught fish, pay attention to fish-consumption advisories issued by federal, state, and local governments (http://www.epa.gov/mercury/advisories.htm).

Q | Are organic foods better than regular foods?

ORGANIC FOODS. This question has been and will be debated for a long time—and the answer also depends on your definition of *better.* Organic farming began in the late 1940s and has more recently become quite popular. After every outbreak of foodborne illness, there tends to be a spike in interest in organic food. But is organic safer or more nutritious?

Organic refers to how the food is produced—without use of genetic engineering, ionizing radiation, chemical fertilizers, hormones, pesticides, and sewage sludge, and only by using tillage and cultivation practices such as crop rotation, cover crops, and fertilization with properly treated crop and animal wastes.[15] Advantages of organic compared to typical commercial farming include conservation of water and soil resources, recycling of animal waste, fewer chemicals released, improved soil fertility, promotion of crop diversity, and protection of farm workers, livestock, and wildlife from potentially harmful pesticides. Organic foods can, however, be contaminated by pesticides from nearby conventional farms and by viruses and bacteria, especially if farms do not follow USDA rules about use of animal manures.[16]

Other differences between organic and conventional foods include these:[17]

- *Nutrition:* Research findings have been mixed, with some studies finding higher levels of nutrients in organic foods and some finding no differences between organic and conventional crops. Weather, soil, and growing conditions also affect the nutritional content of foods.
- *Chemical residues:* Organic foods contain fewer pesticide residues in terms of both the number and the overall amount of chemicals. However, both organic and nonorganic foods must not exceed government-set safety thresholds for pesticide residues, and the benefits of levels of chemicals below these thresholds are unclear. In general, domestically grown fruits and vegetables have lower chemical residues than imported crops.
- *Foodborne illness:* Research findings have been mixed. On the one hand, organic meat products reduce the risk of exposure to prion diseases (such as "mad cow") and certain chemical residues. On the other hand, some organic production requirements may inherently increase the risk of certain types of bacterial or fungal contamination.
- *Cost:* Organic foods usually cost more—sometimes slightly more, sometimes substantially more—due to increased production costs and in some cases lower crop yields. In addition, because they have no preservatives, some organic foods may have a shorter shelf life.
- *Taste:* Again, research findings have been mixed, with some people stating they can tell the difference and prefer the taste of organic foods and other people noticing no taste differences.

It's up to you to weigh the pros and cons of organic foods and decide what's right for you. *Consumer Reports* and the Organic Center (http://www.organic-center.org) make specific recommendations about the foods with the highest pesticide residues based on government test data. If you want to purchase organic foods, note that they are labeled in three different categories:

- "100% Organic" foods contain all organic ingredients.
- "Organic" foods must contain at least 95 percent organic ingredients.
- "Made with Organic" foods must contain at least 70 percent organic ingredients.

Foods in the first two categories can display the USDA Organic seal.

Q | Do irradiated foods give off radiation?

FOOD IRRADIATION. No. Food irradiation is the process of exposing food to ionizing radiation in order to kill bacteria, viruses, and other disease-causing and spoilage-causing organisms. The food does not become radioactive, and although there may be small chemical changes, the nutritional value of the food is essentially unchanged and the shelf life may increase.[18] Medical devices are frequently sterilized with similar technology to eliminate infection risk. Even NASA uses irradiation to help prevent astronauts from getting foodborne illness in space—which would be really unpleasant! The effects of irradiation on food and on animals and people eating irradiated food have been studied extensively, with many benefits and few if any risks identified.

The Centers for Disease Control and Prevention (CDC) states that food irradiation is a safe and effective means of preventing many serious foodborne diseases that are transmitted through meat, poultry, fresh produce, and other foods. In the past, American consumers responded negatively to the idea of food irradiation, but attitudes may be changing as foodborne illness becomes a greater concern. Foods treated with irradiation can be identified by the radura symbol.

One caution: The fact that a food has been irradiated doesn't mean you can relax your home food-safety measures! If it's exposed to pathogens, food can still become contaminated after it's been irradiated.

Making Changes for the Better

Q | What are the best ways to break bad eating habits?

Apply basic techniques of behavior change along with sound nutrition principles. Start by assessing your diet and your commitment to change. Is improving your diet a priority for you? It needs to be in order to make changes in long-standing eating habits. Do you already have a good idea what eating patterns you'd like to change? Even if you do, it's best to do a reality check by monitoring your current eating habits—keep track not just of what you eat but also what else is going on. Where were you, who were you with, and how did you feel?

Assess your dietary pattern against MyPyramid (see Lab Activity 9-1), and then set an appropriate SMART goal. For example, if your analysis shows that your fruit intake is very low, you might tackle that first. Turn your general goal—"eat more fruit"—into a specific one: "In the next two months, I will increase my consumption of fruit from 3 cups per week to 2 cups per day. Because I do not want to increase my overall calorie intake, at the same time I will decrease my intake of sweetened beverages from three per day to two per day."

Next, start on the path to change with strategies and interim goals such as these:

- Make a list of the fruits you like that are available at the local market, campus cafeteria, and snack truck, along with their prices. Then develop a plan of fruits to buy or select at the start of your program.
- Set specific behavioral goals. For example, "I will eat fruit for breakfast at least three days this week and five days next week." Or "I will carry an apple or an orange for an afternoon snack three days this week." Or "Instead of a regular soft drink, I will have water or diet soda during my afternoon work break."
- Change your environment to make success more likely. For example, you may need to not only buy fruit but also put it in the front of the refrigerator or on the counter to remind you of the change you're trying to make. If you usually buy a sweetened drink from a particular vending machine or mini-market, don't go near those places for a little while to help avoid the temptation.

Small measurable changes are quite achievable. Once you get started with a plan like this, you are more likely to experience early successes, which will encourage you to keep moving forward. After a while, eating fruit will become a habit that you don't have to think much about. Additional suggestions and examples for improving eating habits are found throughout this chapter.

Healthy Weight Loss and Maintenance

If you're like most Americans, maintaining a healthy weight will be a challenge at some point in your life. Although the basics of weight change are simple—the energy balance equation—the complex set of factors affecting your eating and exercise patterns are not all under your control. For successful weight management, you need a strong commitment, clear goals, and as many strategies and supports as you can make use of. And you need to stick with it. A diet for weight management isn't a temporary thing—it's a lifelong eating pattern!

Focus on Energy Balance

Think back to the energy balance concept introduced in Chapter 7, with its "Energy In" and "Energy Out" sides. Here we'll look more closely at neutral, positive, and negative energy balance:

- *Neutral energy balance* means you're taking in the same number of calories that you're using and your weight will remain stable.
- *Positive energy balance* means you're consuming more calories than your body is using and you will gain weight.
- *Negative energy balance* means you're consuming fewer calories than your body is using and you will lose weight.

On a very basic level, changes in weight are due to changes in one or both sides of the energy balance. Remember, when your body gains weight from a positive energy balance, that's what it was designed to do. For most of human

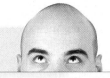

Mind Stretcher
Critical Thinking Exercise

Have you ever tried to lose weight? What strategies did you use? Were they successful? Did you stick with your program and maintain your weight loss over time? Why or why not? What did you learn about yourself and your environment? Based on your experiences, what might you try differently in the future, and what advice can you offer others?

existence, food was scarce and physical activity was required for survival; body-fat stores protected people from starvation if the food supply decreased and provided the extra energy needed for physical exertion, growth, and reproduction. So, storing excess energy as fat is a basic physiological response that improved survival—a positive thing, at least before the food supply became constant (and excessive) and the need for physical activity in daily life nearly vanished!

Q | My weight's fine right now, but should I eat a little less each year since we burn fewer calories as we get older?

Yes. If your weight is currently stable and healthy, you should strive to maintain it. It's much easier to prevent weight gain than to lose weight after you've put it on. Over time, weight maintenance will mean slightly decreasing your calorie intake to adjust for age-related decreases in metabolism. The Dietary Reference Intakes decrease recommended calorie intakes by 7–10 calories per year. That's not much, but it adds up over time—and most Americans gain weight as they age. If your level of physical activity changes, you also need to account for that. Even if your weight is stable and healthy, if the results from the lab activities for Chapter 8 and this chapter indicate that your dietary pattern could stand some improvement—more whole grains or fruits, for example, or less sodium—then make that the focus of your behavior-change efforts.

Q | With all the weight loss info out there, what's the best way to lose weight?

Weight gain results from a positive energy balance, and weight loss comes from tipping the balance in the other direction. Sounds simple—and in theory it is. But to do so, you must overcome powerful internal and external forces that shape your eating and activity habits.

Here's the basic strategy: To lose weight, you must tip the balance in the negative direction. A pound of weight is equivalent to 3,500 calories, so to lose a pound, you need to create a negative energy balance of 3,500 calories. Experts recommend weight loss at a pace of 1–2 pounds per week, which would be the equivalent of a daily negative energy balance of 500–1,000 calories. You can create this negative energy balance through changes in both the "Energy In" and "Energy Out" sides of the balance: by taking in fewer calories, doing more physical activity—or both, which is usually best. It's easier to make big shifts in energy balance by cutting intake calories—a regular soda is the calorie equivalent of about 30 minutes of brisk walking—but physical activity is beneficial for both weight loss and maintenance and your overall wellness.

Fast Facts

Is the "Freshman 15" for Real?

It's often said that college freshman gain weight during their first year in college, a phenomenon known as the "freshman 15." But is it for real? Do students really gain 15 pounds during their first year in college? Studies have indeed consistently found weight gain—but the average gain is only 2–5 pounds. However, if the trend of weight gain continues, it could turn into a problem. So, while you're studying and negotiating all the changes that come with the first year of college, don't forget to choose nutrient-rich foods and moderate portion sizes.

Source: Vella-Zarb, R. A., & Elgar, F. J. (2009). The "freshman 5": A meta-analysis of weight gain in the freshman year of college. *Journal of American College Health, 58*(2), 161–166.

Consider the example of someone who currently takes in about 2,400 calories per day and isn't very active. To create a negative calorie balance of 500 calories per day, he might cut 400 calories per day from his food intake and burn an additional 100 calories through 20–30 minutes of brisk walking. Simple, yes? But in practice, quite challenging. Let's take a closer look at strategies for tackling both sides of the energy balance.

Q | Can I use My-Pyramid as a weight-loss plan?

REDUCING ENERGY IN. Yes, absolutely. MyPyramid can help you create an eating pattern that reduces calorie intake and ensures you still get all your essential nutrients. Once you know your target energy intake, you can select the appropriate MyPyramid plan. So, if you currently consume 2,400 calories and want to cut that by 400 calories per day, follow MyPyramid's 2,000-calorie-per-day plan. Consume the recommended amount of food from each food group *and* keep your discretionary calories below the limit. Visit http://www.MyPyramid.gov to get the specifics for your target energy intake as well as other helpful resources; you can also use the site to track both your daily diet and physical activity. Bringing your diet in line with MyPyramid will likely involve the basic changes emphasized throughout this chapter: Choose moderate portions of nutrient-dense foods and limit your consumption of empty calories from solid fats, added sugars, and alcohol. Refer to p. 314 for the discussion of making good choices within the food groups.

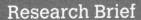

Research Brief

Comparing Diets: Does Macronutrient Composition Matter?

A recent study compared the effects of weight-loss diets with different percentages of energy from fat, protein, and carbohydrate. The study followed a group of overweight adults for two years, which is a relatively long period for a weight-loss study—but important because many dieters are successful for six months or a year but then regain weight. In terms of fat, protein, and carbohydrate percentages, the four diets were 20/15/65, 20/25/55, 40/15/45, and 40/25/35. Key findings from the study included the following:

- After six months, average weight loss across the four diets was about 13 pounds; people on all the diets began to regain weight after twelve months.
- After two years, weight loss was similar across all four diets and about 9 pounds among the 80 percent of participants who completed the trial.
- Everyone who lost weight showed improvements in chronic-disease risk factors such as waist circumference, blood pressure, LDL cholesterol, and blood insulin levels.
- Satisfaction with the diet and reported levels of hunger, cravings, and satiety (fullness) were similar for all the dietary patterns.
- Participants whose target diet was significantly different from their baseline diet (much higher in protein or lower

in carbohydrate, for example) shifted their diet in the direction of the target but did not achieve or maintain the target.
- Commitment and adherence to the diet, indicated by greater frequency of attendance at group instructional sessions, was similar across the diets and associated on an individual level with greater weight loss.

The researchers concluded that reduced-calorie diets result in weight loss regardless of which macronutrients they emphasize. They found that the amount of weight loss depended on the size and consistency of the reductions in calorie intake. Large changes in the composition of the diet were difficult for people to maintain over time, and they tended to return to their starting macronutrient pattern. A very positive finding was that relatively modest amounts of weight lost translated into clear improvements in chronic disease risk factors.

So, if you're considering different eating patterns for weight loss—pick one that is reasonable and that you think you can stick to. Adherence is much more important than any particular combination of macronutrients.

Source: Sacks, F. M., and others. (2009). Comparison of weight-loss diets with different compositions of fat, protein, and carbohydrates. *New England Journal of Medicine, 360*(9), 859--873.

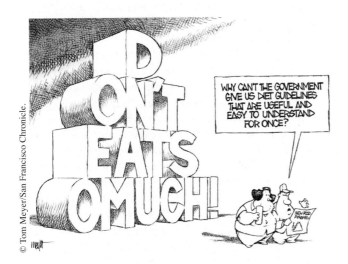

Q | Which causes more weight loss—cutting carbs or fat?

Cutting calories causes weight loss, regardless of the source of the calories. So far, research into macronutrient composition—whether some

specific combination of fat, protein, and carbohydrate is best for weight loss—indicates that no one pattern is best.[19] As long as it's reasonable, the best macronutrient pattern is one with a lower calorie intake that the dieter can stick with over time.[20] The biggest problem with the effectiveness of "diets" is that people don't stick with them: Weight goes down and then goes back up, often further up than before the diet. Even successful dieters tend to stray from the initial dietary plan, especially if it's far removed from their typical eating habits. For example, people often start "low-carb" diets by cutting carbs, but slowly over time their carbohydrate intake moves back toward where it started. What matters for success in weight loss and maintenance is what happens to overall calorie intake.

What does that mean for you? If you're considering different eating patterns—say relatively low-fat or high-protein—as long as the options are all reasonable, choose the pattern that appeals most to you. Does it fit your budget, schedule, and food preferences? Does it accommodate any special health concerns you have? If you have a chronic condition, talk to your physician before making any significant changes to your diet. Because of your particular health concerns, one pattern might be better than another for you. And don't stray from the basic guidelines for healthy nutrient intakes. Remember, a successful dietary pattern for weight management needs to be maintained for the long haul.

Q | Isn't temporarily cutting way back on calories the best way to lose weight?

No. Cutting back significantly on calories may be the most intuitive method of weight loss, and it does usually work—but only for a short time. This approach generally leads to uncomfortable feelings of extreme hunger along with quick weight regain. Whenever you restrict your food intake, there is a good chance that you will eventually compensate by overeating and putting back all the weight you lost—and possibly more. To maintain weight loss, you'll need to permanently reduce your calorie intake, so you need to find an energy-intake level that you can maintain over time. The lowest daily calorie intake recommended is 1,200 calories for women and 1,500 calories for men.

Complete fasting is even worse, because it leads to dehydration and feelings of lethargy, difficulty concentrating, sleeplessness, irritability, and more—none of which are recommended for academic success. Most of the weight you lose during a fast is water weight, which quickly returns (and is important to replenish). Coming off the fast may prompt you to go on something of an eating binge—again, not leading to long-term weight loss.

Extreme calorie restriction should be reserved only for situations where it's medically indicated and should be

DOLLAR STRETCHER
Financial Wellness Tip

Create your own 100-calorie snack options—save money, boost nutrients, and reduce packaging. Pack small servings of fruit, raw vegetables, yogurt, whole-grain crackers, and low-fat granola. Make your own trail mix from whole-grain cereal, nuts, seeds, and dried fruit.

closely supervised by a physician. Anyone severely restricting calories for unsupervised weight loss may be at risk of or already suffering from an eating disorder (see the section later in the chapter for more on eating disorders).

As previously stated, the best approach to safe and effective long-term weight loss is to combine a modest decrease in calorie intake with a moderate boost in physical activity—and to maintain it. Although this common-sense approach doesn't make the cover of most magazines, it usually works. Plus, as little as 1 pound per week of weight loss can add up to a lot over time—especially if you are likely to maintain the weight loss. You can opt for trying to lose "30 pounds in 30 days" or a similarly unrealistic diet plan. However, you're likely to be back where you started and trying again just a few months later.

Q | OK, cut calories. How do I find out how many calories are in the foods I eat?

If you eat in a residence dining hall, you may have to ask an employee for information, although more and more colleges are making this information available online. Fast-food chains regularly make calorie and nutrition information available, but sit-down restaurants rarely have nutrition information available.[21] Refer to the tips on eating out (p. 320) to help reduce calories.

If you prepare your own meals and snacks, then use food labels to quickly determine your calorie intake. Pay attention to the serving size on the label, because your portion size might be considerably larger than one serving as defined by the label. For example, the label on the microwave popcorn box might say 180 calories per serving but also say that there are three servings per bag; if you eat the entire bag, that's 540 calories. Reading food labels may slow down your shopping and meal preparation for a bit, but it won't be long before you have a good sense of the calorie content of your typical foods. Calorie content information is also available through the MyPyramid Web site (http://www.mypyramid.gov) and the USDA nutrient database (http://www.nal.usda.gov/fnic/foodcomp/search).

Checking the calorie content of food—and keeping track of it—is a great weight management strategy.[22] Studies of people who've lost weight and successfully kept it off show that self-monitoring works: One recent study found that those who tracked what they ate lost twice as much weight as those who did not; the record-keeping was most effective when done frequently, in detail, and close to meal and snack times.[23]

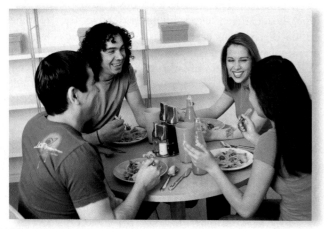

Successful weight management strategies include knowing your calorie needs, monitoring portion sizes, reducing intake of empty calories, and eating more fruits, vegetables, and whole grains. And don't forget to enjoy your food!

Research Brief

Choice versus Obligation: "Healthy" Foods, "Tasty" Foods, and Hunger

A common scenario is to make a healthy choice at one meal and then compensate or overcompensate for it later. For example, you might go out for lunch and order a chicken salad with light dressing instead of a burger with fries, but when you get home you eat half a bag of cookies as a "reward" for achieving a health goal or because you feel in some way deprived. How much of this behavior is based on actual hunger and how much on patterns of thinking? Researchers have recently conducted several experiments with college students to explore how the perception of a food affects subsequent hunger levels.

In one study, the researchers asked a group of students to eat a chocolate-raspberry protein bar. Half the students were told it was a "new health bar" full of protein, vitamins, and fiber and with no artificial sweeteners; the other half were told it was a "tasty and yummy" chocolate bar with a chocolate-raspberry core. When later asked about their hunger levels, students who ate the "health" bar rated themselves as hungrier than students who ate the identical "tasty" bar. In a similar study, students were given a piece of bread described either as "nutritious, low-fat, and full of vitamins" or as 'tasty, with a thick crust and soft center." When offered pretzels after the slice of bread, the students who ate the "low-fat" bread ate more pretzels—about 60 percent more—than those who ate the identical bread described as "tasty."

What these studies show is that characterizing a food as healthy seemingly tricks people into feeling hungrier—they perceive a "healthy" food as less satisfying, regard-less of its ingredients, and act accordingly. In the study with bread and pretzels, researchers also asked participants if they were concerned about their weight. Students who responded yes ate fewer pretzels than those not concerned about weight. This finding shows the effects of commitment to a weight-management goal—reduced likelihood for rebound eating after the consumption of a healthy food.

What if people are given a choice rather than having a "healthy" food imposed on them? In a third study, the researchers offered students a choice of protein bars (chocolate-raspberry or honey-peanut), with one randomly described as "healthy" and the other as "tasty." Students were allowed to choose which bar they wanted. In these circumstances, there were no differences in hunger ratings between the students who chose the "healthy" bar and those who chose the "tasty" bar. When allowed to make a healthy choice themselves, rather than having it imposed on them, students did not respond by feeling hungrier. Choosing healthy foods out of a personal commitment eliminated the hunger boost—again showing the power of perception.

What does this mean for you? If you commit yourself to the goal of choosing healthy foods and managing your weight, you may be less likely to feel deprived and hungry. But be aware of your cognitive and emotional responses to food choices, and try not to react to healthy food choices by "rewarding" yourself with more food.

Source: Finkelstein, S. R., & Fishbach, A. (2010). When healthy food makes you hungry. *Journal of Consumer Research, 37*(3), 357–367.

Q How can I not eat junk when I'm stressed out?

It may be tough, but you can develop food-free strategies to deal with stress or choose healthier snacks for stressful times. You've brought up a very important issue related to weight management—that we all eat for reasons other than hunger, including stress, boredom, or fatigue or the desire to socialize. Tracking your eating habits and your reasons for eating can make you a more mindful eater and more aware of how your thoughts and emotions affect your eating habits. With this awareness comes the opportunity to develop strategies for positive change. If you arrive home from work or class every afternoon feeling stressed and immediately turn to an unhealthy snack, try some strategies to break the pattern. Drop your book bag or purse just inside your door and then go walk for ten minutes to blow off steam. Grab the phone and call a friend, but don't eat mindlessly while you talk on the phone.

You can also stock your room or kitchen with healthier snacks and place them in front of all the other foods. Engage in some positive thinking about your healthy snack—praise yourself for making a good choice and focus on how good it tastes. How you think about foods can affect your levels of hunger and satisfaction; see the box "Choice versus Obligation."

MYTH or FACT

As a general rule, avoid eating after 9 p.m., because those calories are usually stored as body fat.

▶ WATCH ONLINE

Q I'm trying to watch my weight, but there's food everywhere. How can I win?

Americans have both the luxury and burden of living in a society where food choices are abundant, relatively inexpensive, and quite tasty! The temptations are everywhere. Growing up, how often did you have access to an unlimited amount of your favorite foods with ice cream after every meal? It's no wonder so many college students find themselves at risk for putting on weight. Dining halls and food courts provide environments where friends gather, linger, and eat, focusing on socializing and not calorie awareness. At other times—if you feel overwhelmed by school, job, or family responsibilities—you may feel so pressed for time that both healthy eating and physical activity move to the bottom of your priority list. Our environments and schedules are not always conducive to weight management.

What can you do? You can take control of part of your environment—your residence—and make changes to aid in your weight management program. Swap out the empty-calorie foods and beverages and stock up on lower-calorie, nutrient-rich options you enjoy. Put the healthier choices in plain view and make them easy to choose—cut vegetables, whole fruit, whole-grain crackers, and low-fat yogurt make grab-and-go snacks or meals. For parts of your environment you can't change, temporary avoidance might help until you are more comfortable with your new eating pattern. For example, if the food court is your downfall, pack your lunch and eat elsewhere; invite a few friends along. To tackle the dining hall, try some of the strategies suggested on p. 318.

Be aware of environmental influences on your eating habits—from television ads to the arrangement of foods in the grocery store and dining hall—to lessen their impact on you. Support efforts on your campus or in your community to create a more weight-management-friendly environment, such as smaller-portion options at the food court, easier-to-find nutrition information about dining-hall foods, and new walking trails. And make weight management a priority in your life; try some of the behavior change strategies suggested in Chapter 2 for boosting commitment, including completing an analysis of the pros versus cons of change.

Q | Why does weight loss seem to plateau?

It's not uncommon for the rate of weight loss to slow down. At the start of a weight-loss program, you may quickly lose some fluid weight, after which you will lose weight more slowly. Weight lost after the first few weeks is likely to be body fat—so although the losses may be smaller, they're the type of losses you want! If you plateau after a number of weeks or months, you may not realize that you've started eating more—or losing part or all of your negative energy balance. Try monitoring of your food intake more closely to see what's going on.

Sometimes, a plateau is OK. You may have reached a new state of energy balance based on your new eating and exercise pattern. You've lost fat and pounds and should now focus on weight maintenance. Many people lose weight and then regain it, so maintaining a small-to-moderate weight

Fast Facts

Dorm Food: 22,000 Calories Per Room and Counting

A recent study inventoried food and beverages in the dorm rooms of college students. The researchers found an average of about fifty food items per room, representing more than 22,000 calories. The most common items were salty snacks, cereal or granola bars, main dishes, desserts or candy, and sugar-sweetened beverages. Few students had low-calorie beverages, 100-percent fruit or vegetable juices, dairy products, fruits, or vegetables. Items purchased by parents were higher in calories and fat than items purchased by students.

If this sounds like an inventory of the food your room, then do some environmental control in order to meet your dietary goals. Stock up on foods you should eat more of, and don't keep foods you're trying to limit. And have a little chat with your parents before their next visit or care package.

Source: Nelson, M. C., & Story, M. (2009). Food environments in university dorms: 20,000 calories per dorm room and counting. *American Journal of Preventive Medicine, 36*(6), 523–526.

loss is an important accomplishment. Weight management requires a lifelong commitment and keeping up with all the strategies that allowed you to lose the weight in the first place. Keep monitoring your food intake to make sure your calorie intake doesn't start creeping up, along with your weight. Close monitoring will keep you on track.

There's a physiological explanation for why weight loss tends to slow—even if you are maintaining your negative calorie balance. A pound is still a pound, and 3,500 calories is still 3,500 calories, but something is going on in your body. The largest component of the "Energy Out" part of the energy balance is your resting metabolic rate. When you cut your caloric intake, your body compensates by reducing your metabolic rate. You might say, "But doesn't my body know I *want* to lose the weight?" Unfortunately for us in the twenty-first century, the human body is designed to preserve fat for future emergencies requiring energy. The drop in metabolic rate is about 8 calories per pound lost per day, which translates into about 80 fewer calories burned by the body per day if you've lost 10 pounds.[24] That's one of the reasons why it's easier to prevent weight gain than to maintain weight loss.

Exercise is critical for maintaining weight loss and preventing weight regain. The calories you burn during exercise ("Energy Out") help you maintain your energy balance without severely restricting your food intake. Let's look next at the "Energy Out" part of the energy balance.

Q | What's the best exercise for weight loss?

INCREASING ENERGY OUT. The best exercise program for weight loss is the one you'll keep doing—and preferably it will include both aerobic exercise and strength training. Aerobic exercise helps you use energy ("Energy Out") and can be an important part of your negative energy balance for weight loss. The more energy you use during exercise, the more you can eat and still create a negative energy balance—or a neutral energy balance once you're in the maintenance phase. For long-term maintenance of weight loss, you need an energy intake you can stick with along with burning energy through exercise.

The amount of exercise needed to lose weight and maintain weight loss varies from person to person, but many people need more than 300 minutes per week of moderate-intensity aerobic exercise (or 150 minutes of vigorous exercise) in order to lose weight and maintain the loss. Participants in the National Weight Control Registry—an ongoing study of people who've lost a substantial amount of weight and kept it off—engage in an average of one hour of exercise per day, which amounts to about 2,600 calories (energy) used per week through moderate-intensity exercise.[25] You can try different amounts and intensities of exercise to determine what works best for you. Any amount of exercise is better than none, so develop a program that fits your life.

Strength training is also critical. It helps maintain your muscle mass, which will otherwise decrease as you lose weight: It takes muscular work to move your body around, so when your body weighs less, your muscles don't have to work as hard. Remember the fitness principle of reversibility! If you want to avoid a drop in muscle mass as you lose weight, work your muscles with strength training.

In addition to helping with weight loss, exercise has many other direct health and wellness benefits. A program that combines a reduction in calories with an increase in exercise will have the best results for your health.[26] Make time for exercise and be as active as you can. Refer to Chapters 3–6 for more on creating a complete fitness program.

Q | What are realistic, practical techniques for weight loss?

GETTING STARTED. First, make sure you are motivated and committed to losing weight. Weight-loss programs are challenging, so do a careful analysis of pros versus cons. If you haven't already analyzed your diet (Lab Activities 8-1 and 9-1), that should be your next step. You have to learn about your current eating patterns and habits in order to identify barriers and strategies for change.

As for any other type of behavior change, set a SMART goal. If you set a body weight goal in Lab Activity 7-2

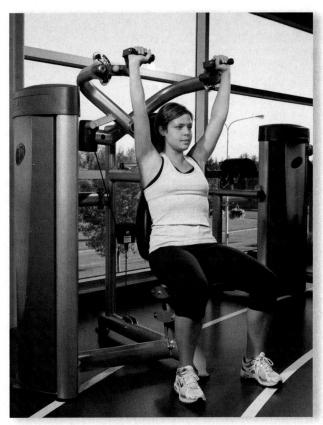

Exercise is a key part of a healthy lifestyle for weight management. Endurance activities burn calories, and strength training maintains muscle mass and helps reduce the drop in metabolic rate that comes with weight loss.

based on body composition assessment, you can use that as your long-term goal. (Alternatively, you could set a lifestyle or behavior goal, such as reducing servings of desserts or calories from sweetened beverages.) For someone who is overweight, a weight loss of 10 percent will reduce the health risks associated with excess body fat. If you're significantly overweight and need help setting a goal, talk with your health-care provider.

Make sure your goal is SMART—pay special attention to developing a goal that is both achievable and realistic. It's more realistic to set a modest goal—and then achieve and maintain it—than to set an extremely challenging goal that you are unlikely to reach. Break up your goal into small steps. Each small success will increase your self-efficacy and provide an opportunity to reward yourself.

Next, develop strategies and techniques for your program. You'll need specific ways to create a negative calorie balance, by reducing food intake or increasing physical activity, or both. You'll also need strategies for dealing with your key challenges, from the food court on campus to stress from late-night studying; see the box "Tips and Techniques for Successful Weight Management" for ideas. Be sure to identify resources that can support your efforts and people who can help you succeed.

Wellness Strategies

Tips and Techniques for Successful Weight Management

Create Realistic Goals and Plans

- Set a realistic SMART goal; good goals for wellness include preventing or stopping weight gain or achieving a small, maintainable weight loss.
- Break your long-term goal into small steps.
- Create a dietary plan whose energy intake is no lower than 1,200 calories per day for women or 1,500 calories per day for men. Choose a level of energy intake that you can maintain over time.

Monitor Your Behavior and Progress

- Track your food intake and your physical activity.
- Weigh yourself regularly (the practice is associated with better outcomes, but if you find it particularly stressful, skip it).

Manage Portion Sizes and Hunger

- Check food labels for both the calories per serving and the total number of servings in the package.
- Measure and weigh your food portions using a measuring cup and spoon and a food scale until your "eye" is accurate.
- Serve food on small plates and in small bowls to make small servings seem more generous.
- Serve yourself reasonable portions; when you eat at home, don't keep the serving dishes on the table.
- Start meals with a glass of water, a cup of vegetable soup, or a high-fiber food to help fill you up.
- Eat slowly to give the hunger center of your brain the 15–20 minutes it needs to catch up with what you've eaten. Take small bites, chew your food, and pay attention to the flavors in your foods.
- When you finish, clear the table and put the leftovers away.
- Don't eat foods like chips, crackers, or cookies out of the bag or box. Take a moderate portion and serve it in a bowl or on a plate.
- Every day, eat four or five regular snacks and meals, including breakfast, spreading your food intake across the day. Eat small snacks between meals to avoid getting overly hungry.
- Refer to the tips on pp. 318–320 about eating in campus dining halls and in restaurants.

Make Healthy Dietary and Activity Changes

- Choose foods that are high in nutrient density and low in energy density. See the tips on p. 314 for making nutrient-dense food choices.
- Focus your calorie cuts on added sugars, solid fats, alcohol, and some refined grains. Maintain or increase your intake of fruits, vegetables, whole grains, and lean protein and dairy foods.
- Watch your beverage intake; limit sweetened drinks and alcoholic beverages.
- Eat at home when you can. Prepare healthy, flavorful foods you enjoy.
- Engage in aerobic and strength-training exercises regularly. Even small increases in physical activity help with weight management.
- Visit http://www.smallstep.gov for additional ideas.

Change Your Environment

- Remove energy-dense foods from your residence; stock up on healthy foods and snacks.
- Place nutrient-rich choices in visible, easy-to-reach places, in front of less healthy options.
- Keep food away from the TV and computer; having it in easy reach leads to mindless overeating.
- Avoid, at least temporarily, settings where you typically overeat. Identify cues for overeating, such as the break room at your job, and change or avoid them.

Take Care of Yourself

- Get adequate sleep.
- Manage your stress in healthy ways, such as exercise, relaxation techniques, and talking with friends.
- Develop strategies for dealing with other emotional triggers for eating, including anger or boredom.
- Maintain a positive body image; see Chapter 7 for tips.
- Engage in positive self-talk about your weight-management efforts; enjoy your food and imagine the beneficial effects of healthy food choices on wellness.
- Get support from friends and family; tell people what you are doing and ask for their help.

Lab Activity 9-2 will help you develop your weight management program. Once you've got your plan in place, you're ready to get started!

Weight-Loss Plans, Products, and Procedures

Stores are full of plans and products promising easy weight loss. But just because a diet book has been advertised or a

supplement has made it to store shelves doesn't mean it's safe and effective for weight loss. Use your critical thinking skills to evaluate any product related to weight loss.

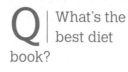

Q | What's the best diet book?

Any diet that sounds too good to be true probably is. Evaluate any diet plan critically. Avoid diets that promise rapid, easy weight loss or

Behavior Change Challenge

Video Case Study

▶ WATCH ONLINE Meet Edgar

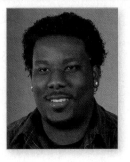

Edgar is a college student who wants to improve his diet by eating less junk and fast food and by choosing smaller portions. He'd like to change because he plans to do personal training and wants to be in better shape than his prospective clients; he's also thinking about how he'll look at the beach during the summer. Edgar's challenges include his motivation level and the fact that he loves the convenience of fast food and dislikes new foods and most vegetables. Watch the video to learn more about Edgar and his plan. As you watch the video, think about the following questions:

- What strategies and techniques would you suggest to help Edgar overcome the challenges and road-blocks he faces? Think about the stages of change and techniques described in Chapter 2.
- What can you learn from Edgar's experience that will help you in your own behavior change efforts?

say that there's no need to cut calories or to exercise. Also steer clear of diets that involve extreme or gimmicky eating patterns, such as special food combinations, very rigid or complex eating rules or menus, or very limited food selections. Any healthy dietary approach should advocate variety and moderation. Visit the American Dietetic Association's Web site for consumers (http://www.eatright.org/public) and look for the section on "Diet Reviews" to read reviews of over one hundred diet books. If you need help in developing a personalized weight-loss plan, talk with your physician or a registered dietitian.

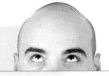

Mind Stretcher
Critical Thinking Exercise

Analyze a weight-loss plan from a book or commercial program. What are the plan's major guidelines and parameters? How does the plan stack up against what you learned from your text about healthy diet, exercise, and weight-loss strategies? What are the plan's major strengths and weaknesses?

Q Do I need to join an expensive program, with foods, meetings, and all that? 📖 READ ONLINE

Q Weight-loss supplements are advertised everywhere. Which are best?

There are more supplements available than any reasonable person would know what to do with, and they all make fairly astounding claims about weight loss. However, no supplement has been proven safe and effective for weight loss. A recent study of a variety of weight-loss supplements found that none appeared to work any better than a placebo for weight loss.[27]

Most advertised weight-loss supplements contain products, natural or synthetic, which attempt to increase your metabolism or suppress your appetite. On the surface, this seems rather logical and effective. In reality, it is not. Inundating your body with unregulated chemicals is potentially harmful. Marketers, however, like to note that these products are "natural," implying that they must be good for you. The truth is that natural isn't always good, that some supplements are contaminated with other compounds, and that in some cases and combinations, supplements can be dangerous or even fatal. In 2004, the FDA banned the sale of dietary supplements containing ephedra, stating the products carried unacceptable health risks, including high blood pressure, insomnia, irregular heart rate, heart attack, stroke, and death. While on the market, ephedra products made up less than 1 percent of all dietary supplement sales but accounted for 64 percent of adverse events associated with supplements.[28] This despite the fact that ephedra is a "natural" product derived from a plant.

As described in Chapter 8, supplements are not regulated the same way as prescription or over-the-counter drugs are, and they do not have to be proven safe or effective before being sold. Some supplements are believed to carry risks, and the long-term effects of many are unknown (Table 9-4).[29] Although ingredients are listed on the label, there is no guarantee that the supplement contains those ingredients in those proportions. In addition, there have been high-profile cases of supplement contamination. The FDA has found that supplements promoted for weight loss, bodybuilding, and sexual enhancement are more likely than those in other categories to be contaminated with prescriptions drugs, steroids, and other chemicals.[30]

Q Can I take a pill, eat whatever I want, and still lose weight?

No. A number of prescription drugs are available for weight loss, but none allow for unlimited eating! Prescription drugs are usually recommended only for people with a BMI over 30, although they may be recommended for people with lower BMIs if they have significant obesity-related health problems.[31]

TABLE 9-4 SELECTED SUPPLEMENTS MARKETED FOR WEIGHT LOSS

PRODUCT	CLAIM	FACT
BITTER ORANGE	Increases calories burned	■ Contains synephrine, similar to banned ephedra and possibly with similar effects and risks ■ Long-term effects unknown
CHITOSAN	Blocks fat absorption	■ Relatively safe but won't cause significant weight loss ■ May cause constipation, bloating, and gastrointestinal distress ■ Long-term effects unknown
CHROMIUM	Reduces body fat and builds muscle	■ Relatively safe but won't cause weight loss ■ Long-term effects unknown
CONJUGATED LINOLEIC ACID (CLA)	Reduces body fat, builds muscle, decreases appetite	■ May increase muscle and reduce body fat, but won't reduce total body weight ■ Causes diarrhea, indigestion, and gastrointestinal distress
COUNTRY MALLOW	Decreases appetite, increases calories burned	■ Contains ephedra; likely unsafe ■ Banned by the FDA
EPHEDRA	Decreases appetite	■ Increases heart rate and constricts blood vessels; linked to high blood pressure, heart-rate irregularities, sleeplessness, seizures, strokes, and death ■ Although banned by the FDA, still available, especially as tea
GREEN TEA EXTRACT	Increases calories burned and fat metabolism while decreasing appetite	■ Limited evidence to claims about weight loss ■ Causes vomiting, bloating, indigestion, and diarrhea ■ May contain large amounts of caffeine
GUAR GUM	Blocks absorption of fat, increases feeling of fullness	■ Relatively safe but won't cause weight loss ■ Causes diarrhea, flatulence, and gastrointestinal distress ■ Can cause intestinal obstruction
HOODIA	Decreases appetite	■ No reliable evidence to support weight loss claim; safety unknown

As of 2010, one prescription medication was approved for long-term use for weight loss: orlistat (brand name Xenical). Other drugs may be prescribed for shorter periods of time, but because people usually regain weight when they stop taking drugs, long-term use is typically needed for success. Orlistat inhibits the absorption of up to 30 percent of the fat you consume, meaning those calories aren't absorbed; however, if you eat more than about 15 grams of fat with a meal, you may experience side effects including loose stools or diarrhea, gas with an oily anal discharge, oily spotting of undergarments, and more frequent or hard-to-control bowel movements. Studies have found modest weight loss among users of the drug: after twelve months, about 6 pounds on average for those taking orlistat.[32]

A lower-dose version of orlistat, known under the brand name Alli, is approved for over-the-counter use for adults. It works the same way as the prescription version, blocking about 25 percent of the fat you eat from being absorbed;

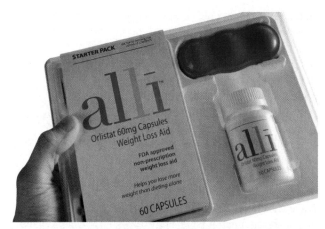

In order for success, all medical treatments for obesity—prescription and over-the-counter drugs and surgery—also require lifestyle changes, including a reduced-calorie diet and exercise.

it has the same potential side effects. Like all weight-loss drugs, Alli is intended for use along with a reduced-calorie diet and exercise. To avoid weight gain after stopping the medication, you must continue with your diet and exercise program.

All drugs have potential risks and side effects. In 1997 and again in 2010, prescription weight-loss drugs were removed from the market because they were found to have serious potential cardiovascular risks. Also in 2010, the FDA warned users of orlistat and Alli of a rare but serious side effect (liver failure) in a small number of people using the drugs.[33] For anyone considering use of a weight-loss medication, the health risks from the drug must be balanced against the risks from overweight or obesity. For some people, use of prescription medications can help jump-start their weight-loss efforts and reduce the health risks associated with obesity. But as with any other weight-loss method, the key is to stick with the lifestyle changes—reduced calorie diet, increased physical activity—over the long term.

Q | Gastric bypass or liposuction: Which is a better choice for losing a lot of weight?

Gastric bypass is a surgical procedure for the morbidly obese, undertaken only in cases where other approaches to weight loss have failed and after a thorough medical and psychological evaluation. It involves creating a small pouch by stapling or removing portions of the stomach, reducing the amount of food that can be eaten and also bypassing part of the small intestine, thereby also preventing the absorption of some calories and nutrients. (In a related procedure, an adjustable band is placed around the top of the stomach to allow only a small amount of food to enter.) *Liposuction* is quite different: it's an elective cosmetic procedure that

is not intended to produce any significant weight loss but instead to "reshape" certain areas of the body by removing primarily subcutaneous fat.

Neither type of surgery is something you should consider just to lose some weight. Both have risks, including complications such as bleeding, infection, and blood clots. Gastric bypass is an option only after a careful evaluation that concludes that excess body fat (usually a BMI of at least 35 or 40) is creating serious health problems such as diabetes, hypertension, and heart disease. Additionally, neither procedure teaches long-term skills for managing body weight. Although gastric bypass surgery makes the stomach smaller, it's still possible to regain a considerable amount of weight if dietary changes are not maintained. Liposuction has no significant weight-loss benefits, and the aesthetic gains will quickly disappear if there isn't a change toward healthier eating and increased physical activity.

Just as for any weight-loss approach, surgery needs to be accompanied by a lifelong commitment to behavior change, healthy eating and physical activity habits, and appropriate medical follow-up. For more on surgery and other approaches to weight loss, visit the Web site of the Weight-control Information Network (http://win.niddk.nih.gov).

Healthy Weight Gain

Q | I need to gain some weight but I don't want flab. Do I just eat more?

You do need to eat more, but you need to be careful about the foods you choose—and you need to exercise. Although the primary problem related to weight in the United States today is excess body weight, some people are underweight. Although being underweight can result from an eating disorder or a chronic disease, it can also be a concern for athletes and naturally thin people who wish to be bigger, stronger, and more muscular. Elderly people may become underweight due to a gradual loss of taste and smell or the inability to prepare healthy meals. Although being underweight isn't usually thought of as a health risk, people who are significantly underweight (BMI <18.5) have much higher rates of premature death. Older people who are underweight are at higher risk for falls and broken bones, often the result of osteoporosis. Also, at any age, men who are chronically underweight are at greater risk for erectile dysfunction.

Even though you need to increase your calorie intake to gain weight, those calories should come from healthy foods. Eating more empty calories will cause you to gain weight but also increase your risk for a number of chronic diseases. Remember the positive energy balance: You need to eat about 3500 extra calories to gain a pound. Aim for foods that are both nutrient rich and energy dense; you don't need expensive supplements. Here are some weight-gain strategies:

- Eat five or six times a day—regular meals and snacks. Don't drink a big glass of water or other beverage right before or while you're eating; leave room in your stomach for more healthy food!
- Add concentrated sources of calories, such as nut butters and nonfat milk powder, to some of your typical foods.
- For breakfast, have an extra slice of whole-grain toast or a muffin topped with peanut butter. Make hot cereals with milk instead of water, and add dried fruits and nuts.
- Top salads with legumes, sunflower seeds, avocados, and dressings made with unsaturated vegetable oils.
- For dinner, try larger portions of baked chicken or fish and whole-grain pasta or rice.
- Good snack choices include whole-grain crackers with peanut butter, nuts and seeds, dried fruit, yogurt, and low-fat granola.

One other important note: Be realistic about your goal. Body size and muscularity are partly determined by your genes. If everyone in your family has a thin body type, then you can add muscle but you won't be able to radically change your build.

Q | What kind of workout should I do to gain weight? Avoid cardio?

Not exactly. Exercise is critical for healthy weight gain—you want to gain weight in the form of increased muscle size and not increased fat stores. Although you shouldn't completely avoid endurance exercise, resistance training is more important to increase muscle size. Keep up with your cardio training, but don't overdo it; too many calories burned during aerobic exercise can make it more difficult to add weight.

To increase muscle size, you need to strength train and apply the overload principle: Do more than you're currently doing. For hypertrophy, the American College of Sports Medicine recommends a program with moderate resistance (70%–85% of 1-RM), 8–12 repetitions per set, 1–3 sets per exercise, and a rest interval of 1–2 minutes between sets.[34] People new to weight training should work out two or three days per week, and people at an intermediate level can train four days per week using upper- and lower-body split routines. Include a variety of upper- and lower-body exercises in your program, and be patient—adding muscle and gaining weight takes time to do right. And recall that men have a greater capacity for hypertrophy than women. Refer to Chapter 5 for much more on creating an effective muscle-fitness program.

Eating Disorders

This chapter has emphasized choosing a moderate, nutrient-rich diet for wellness and weight management. Although you need to be concerned about your body composition and weight in terms of your health, your weight management goals need to be realistic and take into account your genes,

lifestyle, and personal circumstances. For someone who is overweight, a small amount of weight loss has significant health benefits. Focus on good health and don't be overconcerned with body weight and shape.

Many body sizes and shapes are associated with good health, and a positive body image is also important for wellness. Our cultural ideals for body type and weight have been moving away from the size and shape of the average American for decades, and media emphasis on unattainable body types can hurt body image. A negative body image detracts from emotional wellness and can contribute to the development of an eating disorder. Don't compare yourself to perceived cultural and media ideals; set body-weight goals according to what is healthy and realistic for you. See the suggestions in Chapter 7 for maintaining a positive body image.

Q | My roommate eats twice as much as I do. Are some people just immune to gaining weight?

Although some people are blessed with a set of genes that prevents them from gaining weight, most of us are not so lucky! Your roommate may have these genes but more likely is suffering from an **eating disorder.** There are three primary types of eating disorders:

- **Anorexia nervosa,** characterized by extreme thinness and intense fear of gaining weight
- **Bulimia nervosa,** characterized by frequent bouts of binge eating following by purging or excessive exercise to compensate for the extra calories consumed
- **Binge-eating disorder,** characterized by binge eating without compensatory purging

Each type of eating disorder is distinguished by specific behaviors and risks (Table 9-5). All are dangerous, especially anorexia, which has one of the highest death rates of any psychological disorder.[35]

According to the National Institute of Mental Health, women and girls are most likely to develop eating disorders, but about 5–15 percent of people with anorexia or bulimia and 35 percent of those with binge-eating disorder are male.[36] Many people with eating disorders have other psychological problems, including depression, anxiety, or substance abuse. Eating disorders most often develop during adolescence or young adulthood, but they can also develop in childhood or later in adulthood.

For some people, eating disorders develop after a period of dieting, but the underlying causes are complex.

eating disorder A severe disturbance in eating patterns and behavior involving insufficient or excessive food intake.

anorexia nervosa An eating disorder characterized by extreme thinness, intense fear of gaining weight, distorted body image, and disturbed eating behaviors.

bulimia nervosa An eating disorder characterized by frequent binge-purge cycles, or rapid consumption of an unusually large amount of food followed by compensatory purging through vomiting, fasting, excessive exercise, or use of laxatives or diuretics.

binge-eating disorder An eating disorder characterized by binge eating, in which an individual rapidly consumes an unusually large amount of food; binges are not followed by purges, and most people with the disorder are overweight.

TABLE 9-5 EATING DISORDERS: CHARACTERISTICS AND RISKS

	CHARACTERISTICS	SYMPTOMS AND RISKS
ANOREXIA NERVOSA	■ Emaciation, relentless pursuit of thinness, and unwillingness to maintain a normal, healthy weight ■ Distorted body image (seeing oneself as overweight even when dangerously thin) ■ Intense fear of gaining weight ■ Extremely disturbed eating behavior ■ Weight loss through excessive diet and exercise, use of self-induced vomiting, or misuse of laxatives, diuretics, or enemas ■ Lack of menstruation	■ Thinning of bones ■ Brittle hair and nails ■ Dry and yellowish skin, growth of fine hair over body ■ Anemia, muscle weakness and loss ■ Severe constipation ■ Low blood pressure, slowed breathing and pulse, lethargy ■ Drop in internal body temperature ■ Depression, anxiety, obsessive behavior ■ Death from complications (cardiac arrest, electrolyte and fluid imbalances, suicide)
BULIMIA NERVOSA	■ Recurrent, frequent binge-purge cycles: eating an unusually large amount of food followed by compensatory purging (vomiting or use of laxatives or diuretics), fasting, or excessive exercise ■ Feeling a lack of control over eating ■ Fear of gaining weight ■ Unhappiness with body size and shape ■ Disgust or shame about eating behavior ■ Normal weight or slightly underweight	■ Electrolyte imbalance ■ Gastrointestinal problems (reflux disorder, irritation from laxative abuse) ■ Worn tooth enamel and decaying teeth from exposure to stomach acids ■ Chronically inflamed and sore throat ■ Kidney problems from diuretic abuse ■ Dehydration from purging fluids ■ Depression, social withdrawal ■ Death from complications (cardiac arrest from irregular heartbeat)
BINGE-EATING DISORDER	■ Recurrent, frequent episodes of binge eating; no compensatory purging ■ Feeling a lack of control over eating ■ Disgust or shame about eating behavior ■ Overweight or obesity	■ Risks from excess body weight, including high blood pressure and type 2 diabetes ■ Depression

Source: Adapted from National Institute of Mental Health. (2009). *Eating Disorders* (http://www.nimh.nih.gov/health/publications/eating-disorders/complete-index.shtml).

People with low self-esteem, feelings of inadequacy or lack of control, and extremely negative body image may be more likely to develop an eating disorder. People with bulimia are often impulsive, whereas those with anorexia tend to be controlling or perfectionist. Additional risk factors for eating disorders include a history of being teased about body shape or weight, a history of physical or sexual abuse, past failed attempts at dieting, relationship problems, or involvement in a sport that emphasizes thinness. Cultural ideals and social influences on eating patterns can also play a role. For a person with an eating disorder, behaviors such as extreme dieting, bingeing, and purging may provide a sense of control or a way to deal with stress and other painful emotions.

Q | How can I tell if a friend has an eating disorder?

Someone with anorexia will be extremely thin or rapidly losing weight. Other behaviors associated with anorexia include repeated weighing, skipping meals or avoiding eating in front of others, taking tiny portions, and eating in a ritualistic way such as counting out food items or bites. People with anorexia may also shop and cook for friends but not eat themselves. Although it may be hard to understand, people with anorexia may be unaware they have an eating disorder and may vehemently deny that they are too thin.

People with bulimia or binge-eating disorder are usually of normal weight or overweight, so they are more difficult to identify. People who binge are usually aware and ashamed of their behavior and try to hide it, concealing food and eating in secret. When someone has bulimia, others may notice large stashes of food that seem to disappear quickly, frequent trips to the bathroom after meals, excessive and rigid exercise regimens, discolored teeth (from vomiting), and withdrawal from usual activities and friends.

Eating disorders are serious, sometimes life-threatening conditions that require medical and psychiatric treatment. If you suspect someone has an eating disorder, talk to her or him. Communicate your concerns in a caring way, and offer specific examples of your friend's eating or exercise behaviors that you've noticed and that you're worried about. Express your support and offer to help find a counselor, nutritionist, or other health care professional.

Q | Are eating
disorders
permanent?

No, but this doesn't mean they are easy to treat. The first step in treating an eating disorder is acknowledging its presence, which can be particularly difficult for someone with anorexia. A troubling recent development has been the spread of pro-eating-disorder Web sites that describe, endorse, and support anorexia and bulimia. These sites provide tips for things like purging techniques and hiding rapid weight loss from others. By providing advice and support, these sites may normalize the extreme behaviors, making them appear safe and also making it more difficult for people to confront the severity of their condition.[37]

Once a problem is recognized, the person needs to seek help from a health care professional with training and experience treating eating disorders. Referrals are available from the National Eating Disorders Association (800-931-2237; http://www.nationaleatingdisorders.org). The treatment plan depends on the nature of the symptoms and any physical problems. For example, someone with anorexia who is extremely thin and experiencing an irregular heart rhythm will likely need to be treated in the hospital, at least to start. In other cases, outpatient therapy can be appropriate. Treatment may involve medication, psychotherapy, and nutritional counseling.

If you suspect someone has an eating disorder, including yourself, it's best to address the issue, not avoid it. Eating disorders can be life threatening, but when they are acknowledged, they can be successfully treated. You don't have to struggle with an eating disorder for the rest of your life—help is available.

Summary

A healthy diet is one that allows you to meet your nutrient needs without exceeding your energy needs for weight management. It contains moderate amounts of enjoyable, nutrient-rich foods, with occasional servings of favorite once-in-a-while foods. Several dietary patterns meet the goals of a healthy diet, including the USDA's MyPyramid, the DASH diet, the Mediterranean diet, and a variety of vegetarian eating patterns. For most Americans, bringing their current diet in line with a healthy dietary pattern requires eating more fruits, vegetables, whole grains, lean meats, fish, and low-fat dairy, while limiting intake and portion sizes of foods and beverages high in calories from solid fats, added sugars, and alcohol.

Skills that can help you maintain a healthy eating pattern include preparing foods at home, making wise choices when eating out, and using good food-safety practices. For successful weight loss and maintenance, permanent changes to eating and exercise habits are needed to produce a healthy energy balance. Most weight-loss products do not promote safe and effective long-term results. Prescription drugs and surgery should be considered only when other weight-control measures have been unsuccessful and body weight is causing serious health problems. Like severe obesity, eating disorders are serious medical conditions that require treatment.

Put weight management in the proper perspective—it is important but it should not be all that you think about. Eating should be a pleasurable activity. Be adventurous and try different foods; just make sure to do everything in moderation, including regular exercise. Enjoy your food, eat well, and be happy!

More to Explore

American Dietetic Association
  http://www.eatright.org/Public
DASH Eating Plan
  http://www.nhlbi.nih.gov/hbp/prevent/h_eating/h_eating.htm
FoodSafety.gov
  http://www.foodsafety.gov
Health Canada: Food and Nutrition
  http://www.hc-sc.gc.ca/fn-an/index-eng.php
MedlinePlus: Weight Control
  http://www.nlm.nih.gov/medlineplus/weightcontrol.html
MyPyramid
  http://www.MyPyramid.gov
National Eating Disorders Association
  http://www.NationalEatingDisorders.org
Nutrition.gov
  http://www.nutrition.gov
Weight-control Information Network
  http://win.niddk.nih.gov

🔲 **SUBMIT ONLINE**

NAME　　　　　　　　　　　　　　　　**DATE**　　　　**SECTION**

This lab asks you to compare your diet to the pattern recommended by MyPyramid. You can complete the analysis for one day, but for a more complete and accurate assessment of your diet, average and then analyze the results from three days, including a weekday and a weekend day.

Equipment: None

Preparation: None

Instructions

Fill in the target total intake goals for each food group for your energy level from Figure 9-2. Make as many copies of the log as you need, depending on the number of days you're assessing. Track the amount of foods from each food group you consume over the course of the day in terms of ounce-equivalent, cups, and so on. Complete the analysis using the log below or the free online nutrition analysis available at MyPyramid Tracker (http://www.mypyramidtracker .gov). If you complete the analysis online, you can repeat it periodically to see how your diet changes.

Day of the week (circle): M T W Th F Sa Su

☐ **= 1 cup or ounce-equivalent** ▷ **= ½ cup or ounce-equivalent**

GROUP / AMOUNTS		CHECK NUMBER CONSUMED	MY TOTAL	TARGET TOTAL*
Grains (1 oz.-eq. = 1 slice bread, 1 cup dry cereal, ½ cup cooked rice or pasta)	Whole-grain	☐ ☐ ☐ ☐ ☐ ☐ ☐ ☐ ▷	oz.-eq.	oz.-eq.
	Other	☐ ☐ ☐ ☐ ☐ ☐ ☐ ☐ ▷	oz.-eq.	oz.-eq.
Vegetables (1 cup raw or cooked vegetables, 2 cups leafy greens)		☐ ☐ ☐ ☐ ☐ ☐ ☐ ☐ ▷	cups	cups
Fruits (1 cup fruit or juice, ½ cup dried fruit)		☐ ☐ ☐ ☐ ☐ ▷	cups	cups
Milk (1 cup milk/yogurt, 1½ oz. natural cheese, 2 oz. processed cheese)		☐ ☐ ☐ ☐ ☐ ▷	cups	cups
Meat & beans (1 oz.-eq. = 1 oz. meat, 1 egg, ¼ cup legumes, 1 Tbsp. peanut butter, ½ oz. nuts/seeds)	Low-sat-fat	☐ ☐ ☐ ☐ ☐ ☐ ☐ ☐ ▷	oz.-eq.	oz.-eq.
	High-sat-fat	☐ ☐ ☐ ☐ ☐ ☐ ☐ ☐ ▷	oz.-eq.	oz.-eq.
Oils (tsp.)		☐ ☐ ☐ ☐ ☐ ☐ ☐ ▷ ☐ ☐ ☐ ☐ ☐ ☐ ☐	tsp.	tsp.

*Target total from Figure 9-2 or http://www.MyPyramid.gov.

Additional information

Number of vegetable subgroups consumed (dark green, orange/red, starchy, legume, other): ☐
Other foods eaten that don't fit into the groups:

Comments (including environmental cues—locations, people, day/times—that triggered overeating or poor choices):

Results

Complete the chart below by averaging your totals for the number of days you tracked and then comparing them to the recommended MyPyramid totals for each group. (If you used MyPyramid Tracker or another online or software tool, copy your results into the chart.)

GROUP / AMOUNTS		MY AVERAGE TOTAL	TARGET TOTAL*
Grains	Whole-grain	oz.-eq.	oz.-eq.
	Other	oz.-eq.	oz.-eq.
Vegetables		cups	cups
Fruits		cups	cups
Milk		cups	cups
Meat & beans	Low-sat-fat	oz.-eq.	oz.-eq.
	High-sat-fat	oz.-eq.	oz.-eq.
Oils		tsp.	tsp.

Average number of vegetable subgroups consumed (dark green, orange/red, starchy, legume, other): [ ]

Other foods eaten that don't fit into the groups:

Reflecting on Your Results

How did your diet stack up against the recommendations? Were there any areas of concern—food groups for which you consumed more or less than the amounts recommended for you? The recommendations are averages, so you don't have to meet every guideline, every day, but your analysis does provide a benchmark. Were you at all surprised by the results?

Planning Your Next Steps

Choose one food group for which you could improve your intake—either increase or decrease your overall intake or improve the quality of your choices—in order to bring it in line with the guidelines. Develop at least three strategies for improving your intake from that food group. Consider the foods you ate during your analysis: Where could you make changes? What foods might you add, subtract, or substitute?

If your typical daily diet follows the MyPyramid pattern, congratulations—and keep it up!

🖱 SUBMIT ONLINE

NAME	**DATE**	**SECTION**

Equipment: None

Preparation: None

Instructions

Identify the Pros and Cons of Weight Loss for You

PROS	CONS

Set a SMART Goal: If you set a body-weight goal in Lab Activity 7-2 based on body-composition assessment, you can use that as your long-term goal. You can also set a lifestyle or behavior goal. Make sure your goal meets all the SMART criteria.

Calculate a Negative Calorie Balance: If you've set a body-weight goal, complete the following calculations to determine your weekly and daily negative-calorie-balance goals and the number of weeks to achieve your target weight.

1. Current weight ☐ lb. − target weight (from Lab 7-2) ☐ lb. = total weight to lose ☐ lb.

2. Total weight to lose ☐ lb. ÷ weekly weight loss* ☐ lb. = time to achieve target ☐ weeks

3. Weekly weight loss target ☐ lb. × 3,500 cal./lb. = weekly negative calorie balance ☐ cal./week

4. Weekly negative calorie balance ☐ cal./week ÷ 7 days per week = daily negative calorie balance ☐ cal./day

*A loss of no more than 1–2 pounds per week is recommended for most people.

To achieve your weight-loss goal on schedule, you must achieve the daily negative calorie balance by decreasing your calorie consumption (eating less) or increasing your calorie expenditure (being more active), or both. A combination of the two strategies will probably be most successful.

Strategies for Reducing Energy In: Identify at least three strategies for reducing calorie intake. You might eliminate certain items from your typical daily diet (sweetened beverages, high-calorie snacks) or substitute lower-calorie choices (low-fat milk instead of whole milk). Be realistic. Calculate the total calories saved by your strategies.

1.	
2.	
3.	
Others:	Total calories cut: _____

Strategies for Increasing Energy Out: Identify at least three realistic strategies for increasing calorie expenditure, and calculate the total extra calories burned by your strategies. Use the activity calorie costs in Table 7-6.

1.	
2.	
3.	
Others:	Total calories expended: _____

Strategy check: Add up your calories cut and calories expended [   ]
Have you met your negative calorie balance goal? If not, go back and make additional adjustments.

Changes to Habits or Environment: Develop strategies to help make your targeted change; look for ideas in the Wellness Strategies boxes throughout the chapter. For example, if reducing portion sizes is part of your plan, you might measure your portions for a week or use a smaller plate. Identify at least three strategies to make changes to your habits or environment to support your behavior change efforts.

1.
2.
3.
Others:

Monitoring: Tracking some part of your effort—what you're eating and/or your physical activity—boosts your changes of success. Develop a plan for self-monitoring and briefly describe what you'll do.

Confidence Check: Your plan is in place, and you're ready to start. How confident do you feel that you can engage in the strategies you've selected and stay on track? Rate your confidence level from 1 (least confident) to 10 (most confident). If your confidence is shaky, why is that? Identify a key roadblock or possible derailment, and identify a way to address it. Review the behavior change techniques in Chapter 2 if needed.

Confidence level (1–10): _____   Key challenge and method for addressing it:

Results, Reflection, and Planning for the Future

Follow your plan for a week, and see how it goes; then review your progress. Did you meet your goals? Did you try all the strategies you planned? Which ones, if any, did you skip? Why? After you review your progress, identify at least one change to your plan that will help you be more successful going forward.

Progress to date: Change to plan to boost success:

Keep trying and stick with it! Your efforts over the long term are what matters.

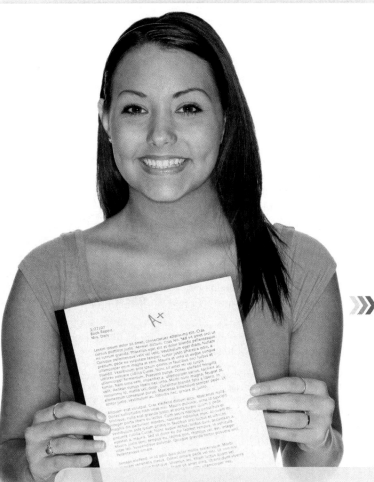

>>> **COMING UP IN THIS CHAPTER**

Discover the physiology of stress and relaxation > Become aware of the factors that affect your experience of stress > Recognize the effect stress has on your health and performance > Identify the sources of stress in your life > Develop personalized strategies for managing stress

Wellness Connections

How does stress relate to overall wellness? Your physical wellness status can be a cause of stress if you are ill, fatigued, or unfit. Similarly, taking action to improve your physical wellness—through exercise, healthy eating, and adequate sleep—greatly reduce the effects of stress. Emotional wellness is also connected, with positive and negative emotions both causing and being caused by stress in your life. Optimism, enthusiasm, and the ability to express feelings all help in stress management. And dealing successfully with stress brings feelings of accomplishment, boosting self-esteem. Positive spiritual wellness can also help you cope by helping you to focus on what is truly important to you.

How's your social network? Negative relationships or lack of supportive people in your life increase stress, whereas strong social support is a great stress buffer. Intellectual wellness is also critical for stress management, especially in terms of your ability to manage your time, make wise financial decisions, and address life's challenges. Cognitive

abilities are impaired by high levels of stress and by negative behaviors, such as drinking alcohol, that some people use to cope with anxiety. Finally, don't forget the role of your environments—are they loud, demanding, and stressful, or do you spend time in comforting environments that are pleasing to the senses? Any steps you take to improve your environment can affect all wellness dimensions in positive ways and reduce your stress.

S tress is the focus of this chapter. You can experience stress from both positive events (getting married, graduating) and negative events (losing a job, death of a family member). You can never eliminate stress: You need it in your life to be challenged and to grow. But too much negative stress is unpleasant in the short term and increases your risk of getting sick or injured; over the long term, excess stress can contribute to health problems such as high blood pressure and heart disease. Stress can also affect relationships, job performance, and schoolwork.

This chapter will help you identify the sources of stress in your life, and more importantly, it will help you cope positively with stress. Successful stress management is essential for optimal wellness. You'll learn effective stress-management strategies as well as techniques to help you relax and recoup when you feel the weight of the world is on your shoulders.

Stress and the Stress Response

One of the first steps for successful stress management is recognizing the physical and emotional changes that occur when you are stressed. Sometimes, they can be dramatic.

> ### Fast Facts
>
> **What Percent Are You?**
>
> - 30 percent of Americans feel that stress affects their ability to get things done at least once a week.
> - 47 percent of Americans say they have lain awake at night due to stress.
> - 52 percent of Americans are concerned about the level of stress in their lives.
> - 64 percent of young adults say relationships are a significant source of stress.
> - 69 percent of Americans say work has a significant impact on stress levels.
> - 71 percent of Americans name money as the number-one factor that affects their stress level.
>
> **Sources:** American Psychological Association. (2009). *Stress in America 2009* (http://www.apa.org/news/press/releases/2009/11/stress.aspx). American Psychological Association. (2008). *Stress in America 2008* (http://www.apa.org/news/press/releases/2008/10/stress-women.aspx).

What Is Stress?

Q I don't get it. Everyone tells me they're stressed out about finals, but I feel fine. Is stress overrated?

stressor A specific physical or psychological event, condition, or demand that triggers stress.

stress The collective physical and emotional changes we experience in response to a stressor.

homeostasis A stable state of physiological functioning (metabolic equilibrium) actively maintained by complex biological mechanisms that operate via the autonomic nervous system.

acute stress A state of stress experienced in response to an immediate perceived threat, real or imagined.

stress (fight-or-flight) response Physiological changes in reaction to a stressor that prepare an individual for a physical response (to fight or to flee).

No. Stress affects nearly everyone. Although your friends are stressed about finals, something else might trigger stress for you—money, job, family, friends, relationships, time management. Specific events that trigger stress are called **stressors**—physical or emotional demands from your external or internal environment. The list of potential stressors is nearly endless, and stressors vary from individual to individual.

Although most of us know when we are feeling stress and probably wish we had less of it in our lives, it's not simple to define. **Stress** is the collection of physical and emotional changes we experience in response to the demands of stressors. Your friends may perceive final exams as a source of potential harm (bad grades!), so they experience stress and all its related physical and emotional symptoms.

The Stress Response: Fight or Flight

Q When I'm feeling especially stressed, my cheeks feel hot and my palms get sweaty. Is this normal?

Yes. The human body undergoes a series of automatic physiologic reactions when exposed to a potential stressor—including changes that can make your cheeks hot and your palms sweaty.

Under normal circumstances, your body is in a fairly relaxed and stable state of functioning called **homeostasis.** Your breathing and heart rates are relatively low and steady, and other body processes function at a "normal" level—maintaining body temperature, digesting food, producing energy, and so on.

Everything changes when you are exposed to a stressor that you perceive as a threat—a state of **acute stress.** Through a series of rapid physiologic reactions that occur outside conscious control, your body prepares itself to meet the challenge posed by the stressor. These physiological changes are collectively known as the **stress response** or the **fight-or-flight response,** which emphasizes the body's preparation for a physical response to the stress, getting you ready to fight or to flee. For example, your cardiovascular system increases blood flow to muscles to get them ready to work; the specific changes that occur during the stress response are shown in Figure 10-1. Many systems increase their functioning, and some nonessential systems slow or stop so that resources can be used elsewhere.

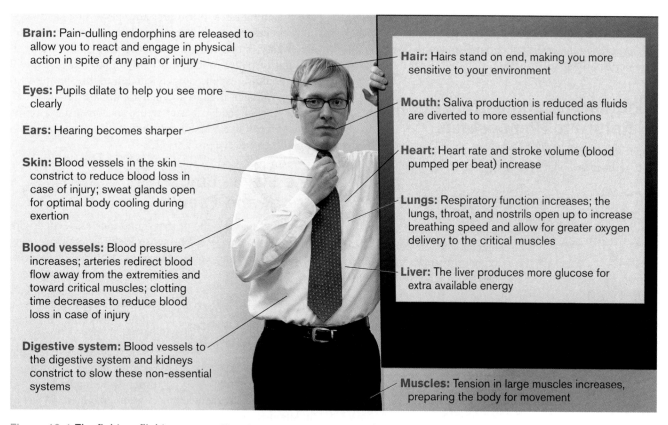

Brain: Pain-dulling endorphins are released to allow you to react and engage in physical action in spite of any pain or injury

Eyes: Pupils dilate to help you see more clearly

Ears: Hearing becomes sharper

Skin: Blood vessels in the skin constrict to reduce blood loss in case of injury; sweat glands open for optimal body cooling during exertion

Blood vessels: Blood pressure increases; arteries redirect blood flow away from the extremities and toward critical muscles; clotting time decreases to reduce blood loss in case of injury

Digestive system: Blood vessels to the digestive system and kidneys constrict to slow these non-essential systems

Hair: Hairs stand on end, making you more sensitive to your environment

Mouth: Saliva production is reduced as fluids are diverted to more essential functions

Heart: Heart rate and stroke volume (blood pumped per beat) increase

Lungs: Respiratory function increases; the lungs, throat, and nostrils open up to increase breathing speed and allow for greater oxygen delivery to the critical muscles

Liver: The liver produces more glucose for extra available energy

Muscles: Tension in large muscles increases, preparing the body for movement

Figure 10-1 The fight-or-flight response. The stress response prepares the body for a physical response to a stressor.

autonomic nervous system (ANS) Branch of the nervous system that provides unconscious control of basic body processes; consists of two divisions, sympathetic and parasympathetic.

sympathetic nervous system A division of the autonomic nervous system that quickly generates the fight-or-flight response in reaction to a perceived threat; it accelerates key body processes to prepare the body for physical action.

parasympathetic nervous system A division of the autonomic nervous system that balances the actions of the sympathetic nervous system by slowing body processes, returning the body to homeostasis once a stressor has passed.

The stress response prepares the body for a physical reaction to a threat regardless of whether a physical reaction is required or whether the perceived threat is real or imagined, external or internal. The stress response is quite necessary in times of real emergency. But if you're only imagining something stressful or if the stressor doesn't require a physical response—an upcoming exam or social situation, for example—then the fight-or-flight response isn't very appropriate. Moreover, chronic exposure to the stress response can harm your health, which will be described in more detail later in the chapter.

Q | Which hormone is responsible for helping the body cope with stress?

The stress response involves many body systems, and several hormones play key roles. When the brain senses a stressor, it activates the **autonomic nervous system (ANS),** which pro-

vides unconscious controls of critical internal body processes, such as the heart and breathing rates and digestion. The two branches of the ANS play different roles in the body's response to stress: The **sympathetic nervous system** generates the fight-or-flight response, and the **parasympathetic nervous system** helps return the body to homeostasis once the threat has passed.

When a stressor activates the sympathetic nervous system, it releases **adrenaline** (epinephrine) and **cortisol.** These hormones are chemical messengers that bind to cells in the body and trigger the fight-or-flight response. Although beneficial for that brief period of need, sustained high levels of these hormones can have negative health effects, including a dampening of the immune system.[1]

Another stress hormone is **oxytocin,** which acts as a neurotransmitter in the brain. Women release oxytocin during labor to assist in cervical dilation and also during breast-feeding to

adrenaline A hormone secreted by the adrenal glands, which sit on top of the kidneys; it binds to cells in the body and helps trigger the immediate changes of the fight-or-flight response, including increases in heart rate, blood pressure, and energy supplies.

cortisol A hormone secreted by the adrenal glands, which sit on top of the kidneys; it is secreted in response to stress and helps trigger the changes of the fight-or-flight response, including increased blood glucose, altered immune function, and reduction in nonessential body functions.

oxytocin A hormone that acts as a neurotransmitter in the brain; in women, it facilitates dilation of the cervix during labor and the letdown reflex during breast-feeding; it also facilitates trust, empathy, and social bonding.

"let down" their milk.[2] However, oxytocin also suppresses the stress response, more so in women than men. Gender differences in the effects of chronic stress are discussed in greater detail below.

Counterbalancing Fight or Flight: A Return to Homeostasis

Once the crisis triggered by a stressor is over, the body usually returns to a relatively unstressed state, or homeostasis.

Q | How do I know when I'm finally relaxed again?

From a physiological perspective, your body will experience a decrease in metabolism, heart rate, and blood pressure. Your muscles relax and your breathing slows. However, this ultra-calm state isn't likely to last long because we usually operate in a state of readiness to respond to perceived threats. In this state, our heart and breathing rates, blood pressure, blood flow, and other body processes are all "normal." Although our palms are not sweaty in this state, it doesn't take much for the fight-or-flight response to kick in. If we are too relaxed, it will be difficult to respond quickly enough to threatening situations, whether a saber-toothed roommate or an errant driver. If your body doesn't return to homeostasis on its own, you can use relaxation techniques to elicit the *relaxation response*; see pp. 370–372.

The Stress Emotions: Anger and Fear

Anger and fear are the primary emotions associated with stress. When the stress response kicks in, you may feel yourself becoming angry (the urge to "fight") or fearful (the urge to run, or "flight").

Q | What's wrong with getting angry? Everybody does it.

ANGER. Anger may be a helpful response in some situations, but in others, it can be inappropriate or even harmful. Anger is a natural response to something we perceive as a threat, whether real or imagined. Types of threats that produce the feeling of anger include betrayal, injustice, and other wrongs. Anger can be caused by an external event, such as a traffic jam, or an internal event, such as a personal financial problem.

Anger, which is a primitive survival emotion, produces both emotional and physiological changes. Anger can be useful in certain situations. For example, in the face of imminent danger, it can provide the courage to defend ourselves and our loved ones or motivate us to improve. But anger can also be problematic, especially if your emotions rage out of control and lead to physical harm to you or others. Harmful manifestations of anger include the following:

- Shouting at people or using violent words
- Being unable to deal with difficult situations without anger
- Using or being tempted to use aggression or violence
- Using anger to make yourself feel better
- Being recognized as an angry person and feared or avoided by others
- Avoiding situations because you fear your own temper

People who are frequently and inappropriately angry are also at increased risk for anger-linked health problems, including hypertension, heart disease, and a decrease in immune functioning.[3]

Q | Should I just vent when I'm feeling angry?

No. Common wisdom tells us to blow off steam or vent when we're angry, but this is rarely a good approach. Releasing anger in an uncontrolled way reinforces and escalates the feeling rather

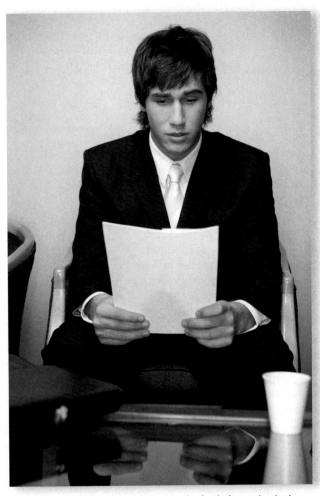

The fight-or-flight reaction prepares the body for a physical response to a stressor, whether such a response is needed or not. You will experience physical and emotional changes until the crisis or challenge is over, and then your body will return to homeostasis.

Wellness Strategies

Dealing with Anger

If you feel yourself becoming angry in a situation in which expressing your feelings is inappropriate or unhelpful, then you need to find a positive way to deal with your anger. Try the following strategies:

- Reason with yourself. Engage in self-talk to calm yourself, especially if the situation isn't really worth getting angry about.
- Convert your anger into a more constructive behavior. If getting angry isn't going to improve the situation, what will? If the problem can't be solved, what else could you do right now that would be useful?
- Step back or remove yourself from the situation, giving yourself a time-out.

- Practice a relaxation technique to diffuse your anger, such as deep breathing (p. 370), or another strategy to decrease your feelings of anger.

If you find your anger often leading to the need to practice one of these strategies, it may be helpful to keep a journal of the circumstances that produce these feelings. You should quickly begin to see patterns, which can help you better handle your anger. By becoming aware of your triggers and responses, you can better learn to minimize and manage feelings of anger—and the accompanying stress.

than addressing the situation or helping you regain your emotional composure.

What about suppressing anger? That can also have a negative impact if anger remains uncontrolled. People who hold in their angry feelings may develop a hostile, cynical attitude and try to get back at others indirectly—this is known as passive-aggressive behavior. These patterns of thinking and behavior can damage health and relationships.

Because anger is a normal emotion, it's important to learn to manage it in positive ways. If you feel your anger building, ask yourself these three questions:[4]

1. Is this situation important enough to get angry about?
2. Am I justified in getting angry?
3. Will expressing my anger make a positive difference?

If the answer to all three questions is yes, then a calm expression of your anger may be appropriate. This means stating your feelings or needs in an assertive but not aggressive or demanding manner. Assertive communication

involves respecting the feelings and views of everyone—leading to a calming of tempers rather than an escalation of anger.

If you answer no to any of the three questions, then you need to find a way to calm yourself; see the box "Dealing with Anger."

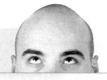

Mind Stretcher
Critical Thinking Exercise

Think about the last time you got terribly angry. What did you do? How did you express your anger? How did you feel afterward? Do you think your anger was justified and your response appropriate? Would you say that you successfully handled the stressful moment? Make a list of other ways you could have responded to the situation. Do you think any of these alternative reactions would have resulted in a more positive or productive outcome?

Q I don't really fear anything. Does stress always cause fear?

FEAR AND ANXIETY. Often, but not always. **Fear** is the other primary stress emotion—the "flight" in the fight-or-flight response. The word *fear* is often used interchangeably with the word **anxiety.** Fears may be categorized as rational (useful) or irrational (useless). Useful fears are reactions to real events that are life threatening and require a response to avoid or survive the danger. Being trapped inside a burning building elicits a rational, useful fear, because it will help you try to get out quickly. This feeling of fear will usually disappear when the stressor is eliminated.

Irrational fears are unreasonable or excessive. An irrational fear can be a **phobia,** which is a persistent, irrational, intense fear of a specific object, activity, or situation. Irrational fears can be so powerful that they interfere with daily functioning and cause a variety of mental, emotional, and physical problems. Social phobia, or fear of embarrassment or humiliation in social situations, may eventually lead to avoidance of all social interaction, creating complete social isolation.

The fear reaction is also altered in people who have post-traumatic stress

fear Anxiety or apprehensiveness about a possible or probable situation or event.

anxiety A persistent state of worry, unease, and nervousness not directed at any particular threat; can be a normal reaction to stress or, if excessive, may indicate a psychological disorder.

phobia A persistent, intense, irrational fear of a specific object, activity, or situation; a form of anxiety disorder.

disorder (PTSD). Anyone can develop PTSD after a frightening event, but it is most common among veterans of war and survivors of abuse, disasters, and other serious crises. People with PTSD feel fearful or stressed even when there is no danger; they may be constantly on edge and experience nightmares and flashbacks of the trauma. PTSD is usually treated with psychotherapy or medication, or both.

Q | What's the difference between normal anxiety and too much anxiety?

Anxiety, worries, doubts, and fears are a normal part of life. It's perfectly normal to worry about midterms, finals, and financial aid. The difference between normal and disordered anxiety is the frequency of the anxiety and whether it disrupts daily functioning. For example, after hearing about a shooting at a university on the other side of the country, the average person might feel a temporary sense of unease and worry. A person with disordered anxiety, however, might be unable to sleep for days, worrying about a worst-case scenario in which his or her university is attacked—and maybe even taking excessive preventive measures.

If your anxiety is so constant that it interferes with your ability to function and relax, you may have what's known as *generalized anxiety disorder.* Maybe you worry excessively about things that are unlikely to happen, or you feel tense and anxious all day long for no real reason. Maybe you worry about the same things that other people do—money, relationships, family problems, difficulties at work or school—but you take these worries to a higher level: "The economy is in the tank; I'm sure I will get fired" or "She hasn't handed our tests back yet; I must have done terribly." A constant, excessively high level of anxiety can cause physical problems, such as body aches, insomnia, and exhaustion, and eventually lead to difficulty maintaining a normal lifestyle and make relaxation almost impossible.

Q | So what do I do to not worry so much?

"If you can solve your problem, then what is the need of worrying?" asked an 8th-century Buddhist scholar named Shantideva. "If you cannot solve it," he continued, "then what is the use of worrying?" So the easy answer is to stop worrying. But doing that can be hard. Different strategies are appropriate for different people. For some, substituting planning and problem-solving for worrying can help; for others, a relaxation technique is most beneficial. Self-help doesn't work for everyone, but here are some relatively effective psychosocial techniques any worrier can try:

- *Self-monitoring* involves noticing when you begin to feel anxious and recording when and where the feelings began, their intensity, and the symptoms. The goal is to become familiar with your patterns of worry, which will eventually enable you to better prepare for worrisome situations and to begin to adjust your thinking.
- *Cognitive therapy* attempts to make thought patterns more positive—to reappraise worry. Creating more positive and realistic thoughts ("I can help the situation get better") reduces worrisome thoughts.
- *Worry exposure* may be the most challenging technique. It involves exposure to situations and ideas that create worry in order to become used to the worry and to see that worrying and anxiety do not cause negative events.

If you find that your worries are interfering with your daily life, talk to a counselor or other health professional.

Factors Affecting Your Experience of Stress

Q | Why do we all respond so differently to stress?

Personality, life experience, social setting, typical patterns of thinking, and even gender all have an effect on how each of us responds to life's ups and downs. Stress is an individualized experience. Don't feel bad—or make someone else feel bad—if you aren't stressed out by the same things as your friends or family members.

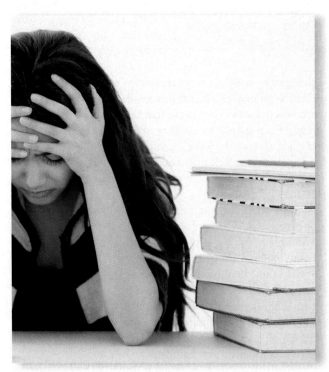

Worry—about grades, money, relationships—is perfectly normal. But if anxiety is so severe or constant that it disrupts your daily functioning and prevents you from ever relaxing, you may have an anxiety disorder.

Research Brief

Forgive and . . . Improve Your Health?

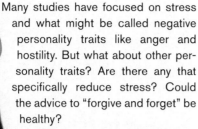

Many studies have focused on stress and what might be called negative personality traits like anger and hostility. But what about other personality traits? Are there any that specifically reduce stress? Could the advice to "forgive and forget" be healthy?

A group of researchers recently looked at how forgiveness affects responses to stress. They studied a group of students, first giving them an assessment measuring "trait forgiveness"; those who rate high in this trait consistently reconcile with people who have wronged them and don't hold grudges, seek revenge, or focus on harm caused by others. Study participants were then exposed to a social stressor (an interview about a recent incident that angered them) and a stressful task (a series of math problems done out loud without the aid of paper and pencil). Before, during, and after the tasks, participants' blood pressure, heart rate, and heart function were monitored.

What did the researchers find? Students who rated high in trait forgiveness had lower blood pressure throughout the test. This means their blood pressure was lower for the baseline measurement, didn't rise as high in response to the stressors, and returned to baseline levels more quickly once the stressors had passed. The results of the study suggest that forgiveness is associated with lower blood pressure and can protect the heart from the long-term effects of stress. More research is needed, but "forgive and forget" may be good advice to follow.

Source: Friedberg, J. P., Suchday, S., & Shelov, D. V. (2007). The impact of forgiveness on cardiovascular reactivity and recovery. *International Journal of Psychophysiology, 65:* 87–94.

Personality

Q | Personality-wise, who are the most stressed people?

It's not entirely clear. **Personality** is a collection of qualities or traits that characterize an individual, including emotional, intellectual, and social factors. Personality may be expressed in patterns of thinking, feeling, and behavior; in approaches to different situations; and in interactions with others. There are many models or theories of personality. Some researchers have looked at collections of characteristics, called personality "types," and others have looked at particular traits, such as those you might use to describe a friend or family member (for example, honest, intelligent, shy, assertive, hard-working, low-key).

Researchers in the 1950s developed a model of personality based on two patterns of behavior:

- **Type A:** Being rushed, ambitious, impatient, time conscious, goal driven, competitive, aggressive, and quick to anger; having difficulty relaxing
- **Type B:** Being patient, easygoing, and adaptable to changing circumstances

Although widely used in the popular media, the type A/B model of personality has been criticized as an over-simplification. Certain aspects of the type A behavior pattern—anger and hostility—have been associated with an increased risk of cardiovascular disease and possibly other health problems.[5] People who are type A may also be more likely to feel stressed and to have more difficulty dealing with their stress.

Q | Can I change my personality?

Not really, but you can change patterns of thinking and behavior that cause problems for you. Your personality is the result of heredity as well as social, psychological, and behavioral factors. The prenatal environment may also play a role in the development of personality and responses to stress: If a mother has a high level of cortisol during pregnancy, the fetus has a similarly high level.[6] This exposure to excess cortisol in the womb can affect the receptors for stress-related substances in the brain, which may make the baby more susceptible to stressors later in life.

Experience also plays a significant role in individual personality development. Every situation you are exposed to from birth on helps to form your personality, and how you respond to different events provides you with experience handling stressful situations.

personality A collection of emotional, intellectual, and social qualities or traits that characterize an individual.

type A personality A personality type characterized by traits of urgency, impatience, hostility, excessive competitiveness, and drive for success.

type B personality A personality type characterized by traits of relaxation, patience, and adaptability.

Think about the personality traits of your parents and siblings and how they react to stress. Not everyone in a family has a similar personality or deals with stressors in the same way. But by observing others and being aware of your own thoughts and behaviors, you can learn about why you react the way you do. With strategies such as self-talk and relaxation techniques, you can reshape problematic responses to stressors even if you can't change your basic personality traits.

Gender

Do men and women handle stress differently? Consider the following example:

Together, Jaymes and Maisha have been trying to start a custom furniture business while still in school. Jaymes has worked with furniture his whole life, and Maisha is majoring in business, so this seems like a logical extension for them and a plan for their future. Their days are long and pressured, and both feel the constant strain of balancing school, work, and their 18-month-old daughter, Bailey. Yet despite equally tension-filled lives, Maisha and Jaymes handle the stress in totally different ways. "When I have a bad day, I'll come home and play with Bailey, then call some friends and tell them what happened," says Maisha. "When Jaymes has a bad day, it's so obvious, because he won't talk about anything. He internalizes everything." Maisha worries that keeping everything to himself isn't good for Jaymes.

Q | My guy friends really can't seem to deal with stress. Why do girls just seem to get it?

Subtle hormonal and evolutionary differences may help explain the differences you've noticed. Researchers looking at both biological and behavioral responses to stress have found that women are more likely to deal with stress by "tending and befriending"—nurturing those around them and reaching out to others. And they've found that men are more prone to initiate a confrontation or to withdraw, similar to the fight-or-flight response.[7]

Women's and men's differing responses may be due to cultural differences in what is considered gender-appropriate behavior, but there is also a biological component. In the initial response to stress, men and women release the same stress hormones, cortisol and adrenaline. Women, however, also secrete oxytocin, which mitigates the production of cortisol and adrenaline. Men also produce oxytocin during stressful times, but its effects are diminished by testosterone, which men produce in significantly greater quantities than women. Therefore, oxytocin may enhance relaxation in women and provide some protection from the damaging effects of stress hormones.

Gender differences in response to stress may have a profound effect on wellness and may be one of the reasons women typically enjoy a longer life expectancy than men.

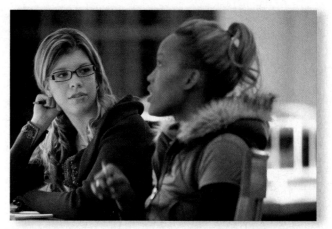

Women are more likely than men to respond to stressors with a tend-and-befriend pattern of behavior, which reduces anxiety, increases feelings of attachment, and helps women build and maintain social support networks.

Higher levels of oxytocin facilitate social interaction and feelings of attachment.[8] The increased oxytocin level and associated "tend-and-befriend" behavior pattern increase relaxation and reduce hostility, thereby reducing the health risks from anger. They also help women build and maintain strong social networks, another factor linked to improved health and greater life expectancy. Although women are three times more likely to suffer from depression related to stress, they seem to have stronger coping mechanisms for stress than do men.

These gender differences may have their roots in evolution. Females traditionally tended to their offspring in the face of danger rather than fighting, which was left to the males. Additionally, socializing might have been a protective measure, because the bigger the social circle, the greater the protection from physical harm. These differences are still seen today. Reports show that on days women report high stress at work, their children report that their mothers are especially loving and nurturing; men, however, tend to withdraw from their family on high-stress days. Further, on the days men face particularly stressful days at work, they also report having more stress at home.[9]

In terms of stress, men might be well advised to act more like women. To seek social support, or tend and befriend, is health protective.

Ways of Thinking: Cognitive Patterns

Cognitive factors have an important role in determining your responses to a stressor and how you cope with it.

Q | Why does it seem my friends handle stress so differently than I do?

On the surface, it can seem that everyone handles stress differently. However, when you look closely, you'll notice

Wellness Strategies

How to Think Constructively and Reduce Your Stress

"Constructive thinking" is an idea that has been around for some time. According to this idea, the way people think largely dictates how successful they will be in life. Therefore, how "super-achievers" think is quite different from how average achievers think. For instance, super-achievers don't worry about things they can't control, and they are less sensitive to disapproval and rejection. To think like a super-achiever, try some of these strategies:

- Don't linger on rejection; instead, let it drive you to succeed.
- Think in ways that facilitate effective action: "I can make the dean's list."
- Stay focused on the present; don't get distracted by irrelevant issues.

- Use failure as a learning tool, not as a sign of your self-worth. For example, basketball great Michael Jordan missed many more shots than he made!
- Accept people for who they are; don't judge them compared to you or some arbitrary standard.
- Think like an optimist and be realistic.
- Finally, know that "you are what you think," so think in a way that makes you feel good and moves you toward greater success in life.

Source: Epstein, S. (1998). *Constructive thinking: The key to emotional intelligence.* Westport, CT: Praeger.

that people often follow the same series of steps when they are confronted with a stressor. This cognitive process, known as the **transactional model of stress,**[10] outlines how we all assess and approach a stressful situation:

Step 1: *Primary appraisal* is the initial reaction to a stressor, when you determine whether the stressor presents harm ("am I OK, or am I in trouble?"). If you think you're OK, then you are likely to move on. If you think you're in trouble, then you intuitively go to the next step.

Step 2: *Secondary appraisal* allows you to determine how much control you feel you have over the threat ("what can I do now?"). If you feel lots of control, then you will have minimal stress. No perceived control means lots of stress and going to step 3.

Step 3: *Coping* is deciding what to do about the threat. You base this decision on the situation and everything around you—people, material resources, thoughts, emotions, cost vs. benefit of different actions, and so on.

Step 4: *Reappraisal* occurs after you have addressed the stressor. At this point, you decide if the threat still exists. If so, you begin the appraisal process again; if not, you move on.

transactional model of stress A four-step framework for evaluating our ability to cope with a stressor before deciding how to respond and then assessing whether the response was successful.

attribution theory A theory of about how we explain success or failure after a stressful event—whether the outcome is due to external or internal factors.

According to transactional theory, we all follow a similar pattern of thinking when we deal with stress, even if it doesn't seem so from the outside.

Attribution theory provides another window into our responses to stress; it focuses on how we assess our success or failure after a stressful event.[11] This theory asserts that

the more successful we are in coping with stress, the more likely we are to take full responsibility for our actions ("I aced the test because I worked hard at it"). Conversely, if we can't effectively deal with a stressor, it is easier to attribute our lack of success to some external force ("I failed the test because I have a terrible teacher"). Interestingly, when we fail at something, we are likely to attribute our failure to an external force. However, when rivals fail, we typically attribute their failure to a cause within them! The box "How to Think Constructively and Reduce Your Stress" suggests strategies for modifying your thinking style in positive ways.

Q | Why do I get so down on myself when I'm stressed?

Certain thought patterns and ways of thinking—including ideas, beliefs, expectations, and perceptions—can contribute to your stress level and have a negative impact on your health. We often create distress with illogical thinking, unrealistic expectations, and negative beliefs that reinforce painful emotions. Feeling certain that you will never be able to pass math or that you'll never get a job are typical negative thinking patterns of college students. This type of thinking can make things seem worse than they really are. In this way, much of our stress and emotional suffering comes from our own minds.

Two types of coping strategies for dealing with negative self-talk and stressors are *problem-focused coping* and *emotion-focused coping.*[12] Problem-focused coping involves attempting to do something practical and constructive about the stressor—to change the stressful circumstance for the better. Examples are finding a tutor to help prepare for a math test and participating in mock job interviews at the career center.

Emotion-focused coping involves attempting to regulate emotions elicited by a stressful event—to feel less anxious and upset about the stressful circumstance. Emotion-focused coping can have different outcomes, depending on the exact nature of the coping strategies. For example, attempting to deal with emotions through avoidance or denial is often unsuccessful because it does nothing to deal with the impact of a stressor. However, other emotion-focused coping techniques can help. *Emotional-approach coping* involves working through the emotions associated with a stressor with techniques such as self-talk, talking with others, and journal writing. This approach should be used cautiously, however, because it can have negative health effects for people who tend to dwell on negative thought patterns and emotions.

Which coping technique works best? The most effective technique varies from person to person and depends on the situation. However, we often choose coping methods that are familiar, regardless of their effectiveness—change is uncomfortable, so we stick with what we know. For example, a student may habitually avoid job interviews and social situations because they make her uncomfortable, and she may believe that she is effectively coping with these stressors by avoiding them, but she creates other problems for herself by doing so. Or someone who smokes to relieve stress may be trying to quit smoking, but when things get stressful she goes to her comfort zone—smoking.

The best advice may be to recognize your stress and to try different coping strategies. Give each coping strategy a chance to work—it may take time to build your problem-solving skills or to obtain the benefits from emotional-approach coping.

Stress and Wellness

Stress comes in all shapes and sizes, and if they are not effectively addressed, so do the associated problems. Stress affects your physical and mental performance, your risk for cardiovascular and other chronic diseases, and the functioning of your immune system.

Stress and Performance

The link between stress and performance is often highlighted during sporting events, especially big events like the Super Bowl, Wimbledon, and the Olympics. Some athletes do quite well under this pressure (such as Peyton Manning, Serena Williams, Michael Phelps), but others don't perform as expected. Stress affects performance at all levels of sport—college, high school, and even peewee. Why some athletes rise to the occasion while others never seem quite "on" on the big day is often related to how they handle stress. They are all physically well conditioned, but as coaches are fond of saying, "Winning is 10 percent physical and 90 percent mental."

Performance isn't just about sports. Your ability to "perform" under stress is also about taking tests, speaking in public, having a job interview, dating, and much more.

Q I'd rather drop a class than give a presentation in it. Why does stress make public speaking so much worse for me?

As stress and anxiety increase, so do performance and efficiency—but only up to a point. Some degree of stress can be beneficial, especially for physical performance. The fight-or-flight response is quite possibly the ultimate performance enhancer—it enabled our ancestors to survive! The heightened senses, increased heart rate and blood flow, increased energy production, and other physiological changes of the stress response can be essential to success in an athletic event.

Stress-related performance improvements happen in nonsporting events as well. Public speaking tends to be very stressful for most adults, college students included. An optimal level of stress helps speakers excel—they become energized, are more aware of their surroundings, and feel confident about delivering a great speech.

However, as most of us have experienced, this relationship between stress and improved performance is not entirely linear. Instead, once the stress level crosses a certain threshold, the effect on performance is negative. In sports this can happen due to excess nervous energy—an example is a novice runner who is so excited that he goes out too fast, only to falter badly towards the end. During a speech, an intense stress response can impair memory, focus, and concentration—so that the speaker forgets lines and can't focus on questions from the audience.

The relationship between stress and performance, in which some stress is good but too much is not, is known as the **Yerkes-Dodson law,** or the inverted U hypothesis (Figure 10-2). Developed in the early 1900s by psychologists Robert Yerkes and John Dodson, the peak of the inverted U represents the point at which the amount of stress (physical and mental arousal) helps maximize performance. If there is too little or too much stress, performance is likely to suffer. The amount of stress needed for peak performance differs from person to person and event to event.

At times it may be impossible to avoid high-stress situations in which you have to perform at a high level, such as a class speech or some type of lab-skills test. According to the Yerkes-Dodson law, if you *overlearn* the task, or practice it enough so that it becomes second nature, you should be able to perform to your potential regardless of the situation.

Yerkes-Dodson law The principle that some stress (arousal) is beneficial to performance, but too much is detrimental; also called the inverted U hypothesis.

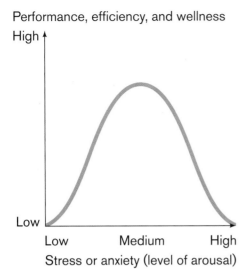

Performance, efficiency, and wellness

Figure 10-2 Yerkes-Dodson law: Stress and performance.
Performance and efficiency are enhanced by a certain amount of stress or anxiety. A moderate amount of stress challenges people to perform at their highest level. Too little stress means too little challenge and little or no motivation or improvement. Too much stress causes both wellness and performance to decline.

Stress and Overall Health

Q | Can stress really make me sick?

Yes it can. People with unresolved chronic stress and people who handle stress poorly are at increased risk for a wide range of stress-related health problems. Conditions that can be caused or worsened by stress include cardiovascular disease, impairment of the immune system, digestive and metabolic disorders, and depression and other mental health problems.[13]

How much stress is too much? It depends on the individual and his or her coping resources. Warning signs of excess stress in each of the dimensions of wellness are listed in Figure 10-3.

Acute versus Chronic Stress

Q | What does stress do to the body over time?

Short-term, acute stress typically results in the fight-or-flight response and its associated changes. Acute stress can have health effects—muscle tension, headache, heartburn, and so on—but these problems are usually temporary and diminish when the stress response ends and the body returns to homeostasis. In contrast, the effects of **chronic stress** can be more serious and long-lasting.

chronic stress Stress that lasts a long time or occurs frequently.

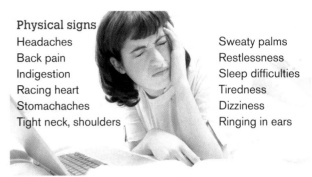

Physical signs
Headaches
Back pain
Indigestion
Racing heart
Stomachaches
Tight neck, shoulders
Sweaty palms
Restlessness
Sleep difficulties
Tiredness
Dizziness
Ringing in ears

Emotional signs
Crying
Anxiety
Anger
Overwhelming sense of nervousness
Boredom—no meaning to things
Edginess—ready to explode
Loneliness
Feeling powerless to change things
Unhappiness for no reason
Easily upset

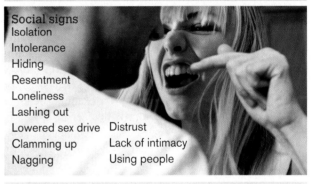

Social signs
Isolation
Intolerance
Hiding
Resentment
Loneliness
Lashing out
Lowered sex drive
Clamming up
Nagging
Distrust
Lack of intimacy
Using people

Behavioral signs
Excess smoking
Grinding teeth
Bossiness
Substance abuse
Compulsive gum chewing
Compulsive eating
Critical of others
Inability to get things done

Intellectual signs
Trouble thinking clearly
Inability to make decisions
Lack of creativity
Thoughts of running away
Memory loss
Constant worry
Forgetfulness
Loss of sense of humor

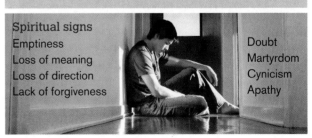

Spiritual signs
Emptiness
Loss of meaning
Loss of direction
Lack of forgiveness
Doubt
Martyrdom
Cynicism
Apathy

Figure 10-3 Stress warning signals

An early model of how chronic stress affects health is the **general adaptation syndrome (GAS),** proposed by researcher Hans Selye. This model has three stages:

- *Alarm reaction:* The acute reaction to a stressor (fight or flight)
- *Resistance:* The body's attempt to adapt to the demands of a persistent stressor (such as negative work environment, chronic physical pain, care-giving, unhappy relationship)
  - *Exhaustion:* The state of impaired functioning that occurs if a persistent stressor exhausts the body's resources for coping

Selye's model also distinguishes between positive and negative stress. A positive stressor, or **eustress,** enhances physical or mental functioning (for example, strength training or a challenging school project). Negative stressors, or **distress** (for example, death of a family member or job loss), can cause emotional pain, anxiety, or injury, especially if the stress isn't resolved in an effective manner. Chronic exhaustion and distress are associated with increased risk for health problems.

Recent research has focused on **allostatic load,** which is the cumulative physical damage of chronic exposure to stress hormones. A high allostatic load may result from frequent or chronic stressors, poor coping with stressors, inability to shut down the stress response, or an uneven stress response in different body systems. When people's allostatic load exceeds their ability to adapt and cope, they are at increased risk for a variety of health problems.[14]

Underlying Factors in Stress-Related Health Problems

Q How does stress tear you down physically?

The links between stress and illness can be difficult to pinpoint because there is no standard measure of stress and there are significant individual differences in how people react to stressors and cope with stress. Two pathways of causality can be examined: behavioral and biological.

While under stress, people may engage in behaviors that either enhance or hurt their health. Negative health behaviors associated with stress include poor sleep, little or no physical activity, poor eating habits, smoking or drinking more, and avoiding regular or symptom-specific medical care. People who are stressed and engage in unhealthy behaviors are at elevated risk for developing health problems, having worse outcomes from disease, and even experiencing higher rates of premature mortality.

As described earlier, the physiological response to a stressor involves the release of cortisol, adrenaline, and other hormones that control the fight-or-flight response. The actions of these hormones are beneficial for acute stress but can cause problems if a person is exposed to frequent or chronic stressors. Concentrations of the hormones may build up if the body doesn't have the time or resources to recover. These hormones raise blood pressure and cholesterol levels, alter glucose metabolism, and suppress the immune system. They also cause an inflammatory response in the body, and chronic inflammation has been linked to many health problems, including cardiovascular disease, allergies, and certain forms of cancer.

Stress and Specific Conditions

Q Can stress be a factor for serious physical conditions?

Yes. Stress is a risk factor for both serious chronic diseases and minor health problems. Stress can contribute to the development of cardiovascular disease; increase the risk for infections like colds; and cause headaches, skin changes, and digestive problems (Table 10-1). As described in the last section, negative health behaviors that may increase when a person is under stress—including smoking, drinking, and poor eating habits—also raise the risk for many serious health outcomes.

Remember, however, that some level of stress is beneficial and can even improve performance. Also, it's impos-

---

MYTH or **FACT?**

Ulcers are caused by stress.

▶ WATCH ONLINE

general adaptation syndrome (GAS) A model of the body's response to chronic stress; the three phases are alarm (fight-or-flight response), resistance, and exhaustion.

eustress A positive stressor that enhances physical or mental functioning; it is typically short-term and may feel exciting or motivating.

distress A negative stressor that causes emotional pain, anxiety, or injury; it may be short- or long-term and cause anxiety and other unpleasant feelings.

allostatic load Cumulative physical damage of chronic exposure to the stress response, especially the effects of stress hormones.

Mind Stretcher
Critical Thinking Exercise

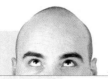

What types of stressors are of greatest concern to you? Do the major stressors in your life include both positive and negative experiences (eustress and distress)? Are these stressors new to your life as part of your college experience, or are they the same types of stressors that have given you trouble in the past?

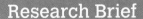

Research Brief

Hostility and Hypertension Risk in Young Adults

Researchers followed a group of more than three thousand young adults (ages 18–30) for fifteen years, assessing psychosocial factors and the rate of hypertension. Hostility was one of the psychosocial factors measured during the study, with each participant assessed for hostility with established criteria. After fifteen years, they found that the people who rated high for hostility had nearly twice the risk of hypertension compared to people who rated low for hostility. The precise mechanism for this increased risk is un-clear, but it may relate to the effects of the stress response on hormone levels and the cardiorespiratory system.

Hostility is a trait that is linked to elevated stress and increased risk of health problems, so if you are frequently very angry and hostile, take steps to change. Learn and practice calmer responses to life's frustrations.

Source: Lijing, L., and others. (2003). Psychosocial factors and risk of hypertension. *JAMA, 290*(16), 2138–2148.

sible to avoid stress no matter where you live or what you do. You shouldn't fear stress or feel that any one stressful event will cause you to get sick or contract a terrible disease. In fact, the majority of people confronted with traumatic life events remain disease-free. As you'll see later in the chapter, there are many positive steps you can take to manage the stress in your life and reduce your risk of developing a stress-related health problem.

Sources of Stress

Stressors can come at you from all sides. Your friends and family, your job, your schoolwork, and even your patterns of thought and behavior can be stressors. Major underlying causes of stress are change and fear of the unknown: "Can I handle college?" "Will I make new friends right away?" "Will I still have enough time to keep up with my job

TABLE 10-1 STRESS-RELATED HEALTH PROBLEMS

CONDITION	POTENTIAL EFFECTS OF ACUTE AND CHRONIC STRESS
CARDIOVASCULAR DISEASE	Damage to arteries from increased blood pressure, heart rate, blood-fat and glucose levels, and inflammation
INFECTIONS AND OTHER PROBLEMS RELATED TO IMMUNE FUNCTIONING	Increased risk of an acute infection or a flare-up of a chronic infection (for example, genital herpes) due to suppression and dysregulation of immunity; changes in immunity may reduce the body's ability to fight cancer
BODY COMPOSITION AND FAT DISTRIBUTION	Increased glucose and insulin in the blood from the stress responses encourage the body to store fat; long-term exposure to cortisol is linked to weight gain and abdominal obesity
DIABETES	Excess glucose contributes to glucose intolerance, insulin resistance, and type 2 diabetes; acute stressors may destabilize blood glucose levels in people with diabetes
MENTAL HEALTH DISORDERS	Increased risk for development or worsening of certain psychological disorders, including depression
HEADACHES	Muscle tension in the head, neck, and shoulders is linked to tension and migraine headaches
DIGESTIVE PROBLEMS	Worsening of heartburn; changes in how quickly food moves through the digestive tract, leading to diarrhea or constipation
SKIN CHANGES	Increases sensitivity and worsening of acne, psoriasis, and hives
SLEEP	Disruption of sleep patterns

responsibilities?" When thinking about stressors, *change* is the operative word. You might think something can't be stressful if it produces a good outcome, but that is not how stress works. Starting college is a joyous occasion but quite stressful. Graduating from college is even more exciting—and even more stressful. One problem with creating lists of stressors is that, as you've learned, stress is perceived differently by everyone. And it isn't necessarily the outcome that defines an event as stressful, but the type and amount of change that occur.

Life Experiences Large and Small

Q | I understand that things like marriage, divorce, and losing a job are stressful, but why do little things seem to cause so much stress?

Major life events—including marriage, a serious illness, getting or losing a job, and the death of a friend or family member—are obviously big changes, and they cause stress. We all experience big changes in our lives that we need to cope with. What major changes have occurred in your life in the past few years? Think about events such as starting or returning to college, moving to a new residence, changing jobs, the birth or adoption of a child, and so on. These major changes are significant potential stressors. The most serious challenges are big changes that are both negative and not under our control.

However, the more routine aspects of your day can also create stress. Daily hassles include things like struggling to keep up with homework and job responsibilities, doing too many things at once, feeling a lack of privacy, having problems with transportation, and being stuck in a noisy environment. Small stressors can add up and overwhelm your ability to cope. The busier and more successful you become, the more daily hassles you may have to face.

Mind Stretcher
Critical Thinking Exercise

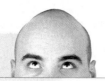

Make a list of the daily hassles you commonly encounter, such as being awakened too early by loud neighbors, standing in a long line for lunch, or repeatedly misplacing your keys. Divide your list into two groups: avoidable and unavoidable. For each stressor that is potentially avoidable, describe a strategy for eliminating it from your life. For stressors that are unavoidable, make a list of effective coping mechanisms.

Time Pressures

Q | Time is my problem. How do I make more of it!?

Typical reasons for a time crunch include classes, work, social relationships, family, studying, sleeping, eating, parenting, and caregiving for family members. Managing your time is made even more difficult by an ever-changing schedule. Within each school term, each day varies, and your schedule changes again with each new term or break. No wonder college students struggle so much with managing time! Effective time management strategies that can help you get more done each day, minimize stress, and improve your quality of life are described in the next section of the chapter.

Job and Financial Pressures

Q | What is rated the most stressful thing?

As we've discussed, the assessment of stressors varies from person to person. However, in surveys of Americans, money and work consistently top the list of stressors (Table 10-2). Chronic workplace stress has been linked to cardiovascular disease and premature mortality: Studies following thousands of

TABLE 10-2 TOP STRESSORS REPORTED BY AMERICAN ADULTS

STRESSOR	PERCENT REPORTING STRESSOR AS SIGNIFICANT
Money	71%
Work	69%
The economy	63%
Family responsibilities	55%
Relationships	51%
Family health problems	47%
Housing costs	47%
Personal health concerns	47%
Job stability	44%
Personal safety	27%

Source: American Psychological Association. (2009). *Stress in America: Executive summary.* Washington, DC: APA (http://www.apa.org/news/press/releases/stress-exec-summary.pdf).

Wellness Strategies

Getting Through Tough Economic Times

If you are stressed about job insecurity, job loss, or financial problems, try some of the following strategies:

- *Keep things in perspective.* Recognize the good aspects of life and retain hope for the future. Appreciate the positive things that happen every day.
- *Strengthen connections with your family and friends.* They can provide important emotional support.
- *Engage in activities* such as physical exercise, sports, and hobbies that can relieve stress and anxiety.
- *Develop new employment skills*—a practical and effective problem-focused method of coping as well as a way

of directly addressing financial difficulties. Returning to school is one such strategy.

- *Volunteer in your community.* It reduces stress, gets your mind off your problems, and broadens your network.
- *Focus on making things better, not on what has gone wrong.* Don't compare your current situation with the past. If you've had a major setback, give yourself time to heal and then move on.

Source: Substance Abuse and Mental Health Services Administration. (2009). *Getting Through Tough Economic Times* (http://www.samhsa.gov/economy). Visit the Web site for additional information and advice.

---

workers over time found that in men, the risks for chest pain, heart attack, and death rose along with the reported incompetence of their bosses, and the risks increased the longer the study participants worked in the same stressful environment. On the positive side, the more competent the participants thought their bosses were, the lower their risk of developing heart disease.[15] Although most studies on stress, work, and disease haven't proven cause-and-effect relationships, it's not unreasonable to assume that dissatisfaction at work can translate into great risk for ill health or premature death. How we interact with others in the workplace is important to our health and quality of life; and because we spend so much time at work, these relationships clearly count.

Although there is no consensus about the top stressor for college students, concerns relating to money (work, loans, and so on), academics, roommates, and relationships are often near the top of the list. Job-related stressors vary: The job needs and expectations of a full-time freshman living in a residence hall differ from those of a commuting parent attending night classes part-time while holding down a full-time job. Whereas the part-time student already has an income, the new freshman may feel a desperate need to get one. However, the part-time student likely has many financial obligations, and going back to school simply adds to that burden.

Typically, students who work more than twenty hours per week have worse health profiles than those working fewer hours. Sleeping less, eating less-healthy foods, smoking and drinking more,

and having a higher BMI have all been noted more frequently in students with heavy work schedules, and more students tend to work, and for more hours, as they progress through college.[16]

Some of the stress management strategies discussed later in the chapter are especially helpful for job and financial stress, including time management, goal setting, and problem solving. Here, see the suggestions in the box "Getting Through Tough Economic Times."

Q | I have to work to help pay for college. What is the best job so I can still get good grades?

If there is an ideal job to pay college bills without cutting into study time, it has yet to be discovered! However, jobs that are related to your major area of study are a good choice, if available. These jobs can provide on-the-job-training, may help prepare you for classes, and can serve as a springboard to future internships and jobs. Although you will have the burden of time commitment no matter what job you choose, if it is one that helps the academic cause, you are likely to enjoy it more, plan better, and use it to be more successful. On the other hand, if you are working a job you dislike, with terrible hours and unfriendly co-workers, then you may be adding stressors to your already stressed life! Some find that working on campus has the advantage of minimizing commuting time. Campus jobs may not pay as well as some off-campus jobs and may be difficult to come by (at least the really good ones), but persistence usually pays off. Also,

DOLLAR STRETCHER
Financial Wellness Tip

Having a budget and sticking to it can greatly reduce stress from your finances. Start by tracking all your income and expenses for two to four weeks. You can use this data to help set a long-term budget. Try a free or low-cost computer program or smart phone app to more easily track and sort expenses by category.

some college faculty have grant money available to pay students a small salary to assist with research. This can be a great way to make some money, learn more about your field, and build a relationship with your instructors.

Relationships and Families

Q | I really miss my friends from back home. Is this normal with so many new friends around?

It's both normal and common—so much so that we might even refer to it as being "friendsick" instead of homesick. Starting college disrupts your network of friends, with the disruption being greater the farther away from home you go—and it's a lot of work to build a new group of friends. Having a support group at the start of college helps: for example, meeting your new roommates in advance, being part of a sport or academic team, or just knowing others headed to the same college. College and university administrators are well aware of the benefits of built-in friends, and this may be a large reason behind freshman live-in policies and residence hall learning communities. Surveys consistently show higher rates of retention for students who live on campus and get involved in learning communities[17]—not to mention the better opportunity to establish friendships that can last a lifetime. So stick with it, don't get caught up worrying what your old friends are up to, and focus on developing new friendships at college.

Q | What advice can you give about stress and college success for those of us who aren't 19 and have kids and jobs and don't have time to be full-time students?

You're not alone. Each fall brings more nontraditional students (age 25 or older) to college campuses. More than one-third of all students enrolled in U.S. colleges and uni-

versities, or about 7 million, are nontraditional. Although this percentage has remained relatively constant since the 1980s, recently there has been a slight increase, particularly from military veterans. Women constitute a majority of both traditional (55 percent) and nontraditional (58 percent) college students. Only about one-third of U.S. college students live in residence halls, but two-thirds work, and most of them have more than one job.[18]

Although nontraditional students are much more likely to attend college part-time, they usually have the added burdens of a full-time job, parenting, caretaking, and many other family responsibilities. Many four-year colleges treat all students as if they were the traditional 18- to 21-year-olds, which can be frustrating for older students. Two-year colleges have a much higher percentage of older and non-traditional students and tend to also provide programs and services matched to the needs of that population.

Nontraditional students have a myriad of life responsibilities, and adding school can be a challenge. You will need to do some creative time management and select a manageable course load, and you'll need the support of your family and coworkers to succeed. Unlike students on the "four-year plan," you need to focus on each course individually, making sure to succeed in small steps while keeping a firm focus on your long-term goal.

Social and Environmental Stressors

Your social and physical environments can also contain stressors. Social stressors include interacting with new people, facing tough competition or discrimination, and using English if it isn't your first language. Stressors in the physical environments include crowded or loud residences, poor public transit, and extreme weather. New college students face numerous social and environmental challenges as they learn to navigate their new school. Many schools don't officially count enrollment until the third week of classes, because so many students find these stressors too much to handle and drop out. However, most are able to adjust and adapt, although sometimes with difficulty. Adjusting to college can be one the most difficult social and environmental challenges you will ever face. The rewards for persevering, however, are large and lifelong, as anyone who made it through will tell you.

Q | I've never shared a bedroom before. How am I supposed to live with someone I've never met?

Having a roommate, a first-time experience for many first-year students in four-year colleges, may be the most stressful initial experience in college life. Even worse is when a housing crunch forces you to have multiple roommates in a room designed for only two. This is a social and environmental stressor rolled into one! Just

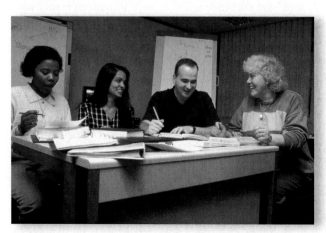

Traditional and nontraditional students may have different stressors, but both groups face challenges and changes that they must work through in order to adapt to college life and succeed in meeting their goals.

Research Brief

Parenting and College: Just One More Stressor

Parenting is wonderful, and you've heard your friends say, "I can't believe I was ever happy before my child was born." They seem so blissful, full of pride and joy. However, researchers have found that parents have significantly higher levels of depression than childless adults do, and although men and women handle parenting stress differently, it still comes down to worry about their kids. The worries are even worse for single parents.

Parents enjoy their children, but parenting, especially in the United States, is challenging. Parents in the United States tend to be isolated. We don't have the luxury of grandparents and other family members nearby to help out. In addition, parents are typically reluctant to talk about the difficult parts of raising children, of which there are many!

The reality, however, is that parenting is joyful but it takes a lot of work and can be quite challenging. And your worries for your "little angel" last a lifetime.

Source: Evenson, R. J., & Simon, R. W. (2005). Clarifying the relationship between parenthood and depression. *Journal of Health and Social Behavior, 46*(4), 341–358.

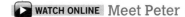

remember that meeting and interacting with new people can be one of the best rewards of college.

Communication and respect are keys to living with someone new. Start by learning about each other: What are your study and sleep habits (morning person or night owl)? Your tolerance for noise and clutter? How do you want to handle visitors, shared expenses, and borrowing or using each other's clothes, food, hair dryers, and so on? Setting "house rules" will help things run more smoothly; some schools even suggest roommate contracts to reduce misunderstandings. If you have a disagreement, try discussing it calmly and coming to some sort of compromise. If needed, talk with the resident assistant or advisor. Respecting your roommate includes common courtesy, such as not talking with others about things that happen in private space and not posting photos or unkind comments on Facebook.

What is your top stressor? Is it one of the categories of stressors already described or something related to academic work, such as evaluation of your tests, papers, and projects or the pressure to meet academic requirements and earn high grades? Is it adjusting to a roommate, developing new relationships, competing for grades, choosing a major,

Behavior Change Challenge

Video Case Study

▶ **WATCH ONLINE** Meet Peter

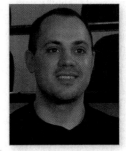

Peter is married and works full time as a corrections officer. Both he and his wife also attend school. Peter recognizes that he is stressed about his job and his many commitments, and he wants to develop strategies so that he can deal more effectively with stress. Watch the video to learn more about Peter, his behavior-change goals and strategies, and how successful he is over the course of his program. As you watch the video, think about the following questions:

- Do you think Peter has enough motivation and specific strategies for his program to be successful?
- What can you learn from Peter's experience that will help you in your own behavior change efforts? What strategies that he adopted will work for you?

Mind Stretcher

Critical Thinking Exercise

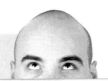

Think about all the environments where you spend time, including your classrooms, the student union, your workplace, and your residence. Are some more stressful than others? List the environments in order from the most stressful to the least stressful. Indicate next to each one the reason you think it is stressful or nonstressful. Then start at the top of your list and record three or more ways to reduce the stressful impact each of these environments has on you.

or one of the many other challenges related to college life? It's impossible to list all the stressors faced by college students, and something that was quite stressful during your first or second year may seem insignificant later on.

Managing Stress

Now that you've identified your major stressors, it's time to think about coping strategies. What are you doing now to manage stress? What else could you do? In surveys, more

Wellness Strategies

Stress Management: What Not to Do

Don't use tobacco, drugs, or alcohol: These substances provide temporary relief from stress, but they are highly addictive and lead to a host of health problems. Also, use of these substances doesn't do anything to address the underlying causes of your elevated stress level.

Don't binge eat: Eating causes the brain to release chemicals that dull pain and contribute to feelings of well-being. Although eating your favorite foods may seem comforting, using food to reduce stress is bound to lead to more problems, including weight gain and possibly even eating disorders.

Don't give up emotionally: Sometimes we can feel so overwhelmed we want to just give up. However, feeling completely helpless can be both psychologically and physically damaging. Find small, practical things you can do to improve a negative situation, or try a relaxation technique.

Don't be inflexible: Holding tightly to your patterns of thinking and behavior in the face of change is not the best way to handle stress. We all feel comforted by doing what we normally do, but remaining stuck in familiar but unsuccessful patterns usually creates even more stress.

Don't avoid the situation: Behavioral or cognitive avoidance will only make the situation worse the next time.

than 90 percent of Americans report trying some form of stress-management strategy (Table 10-3). However, not all of these methods of coping are recommended! Too much food or too much TV or Internet can become stressors themselves.

TABLE 10-3 AMERICAN ADULTS' TOP 10 STRESS-MANAGEMENT TECHNIQUES

TECHNIQUE	PERCENT REPORTING USE OF TECHNIQUE
Listen to music	49%
Exercise or walk	44%
Read	41%
Watch TV or movies for more than 2 hours/day	36%
Spend time with family or friends	36%
Play video games or surf the Internet	33%
Nap	32%
Pray	32%
Eat	28%
Spend time doing a hobby	27%

Source: American Psychological Association. (2009.) *Stress in America: Executive summary* (http://www.apa.org/news/press/releases/stress-exec-summary.pdf).

No one stress-management technique is best for everyone, but there are enough good techniques that everyone can find something helpful. What won't work is doing nothing or continuing to do what you've always done—unsuccessfully (see the box "Stress Management: What Not to Do").

Time Management

By managing your time wisely, you can minimize stress and improve your quality of life. Time-management techniques help you identify, prioritize, schedule, and execute tasks, projects, and goals in a successful and satisfying way. They can help you avoid time traps, including procrastination, lack of focus, and poor multitasking. Effective time management is challenging but well worth the effort.

Q I thought computers were supposed to make me use my time better, but every time I log on, I waste tons of time! What can I do?

Going online is a journey, and many people wander in unproductive ways. Strategies to minimize wasted computer time include setting online time limits, planning your Web destinations before logging on, and sticking to your original task (researching a term paper, for example). For social-networking sites like MySpace and Facebook, set aside a certain time each day to visit them, and don't let it compete with time designated for other work. When doing schoolwork, log out of your social sites, and turn off your cell phone when working on important projects. If you eliminate the temptations, you are more likely to get your work done.

Wellness Strategies

Time-Management Tips

Keep a time diary: If you can't seem to get a handle on your time, try keeping a time diary for a few weekdays and a few weekend days. Using fifteen-minute blocks, write down everything you do on those days. Take a close look and see where you can use your time. Live in an urban area? Maybe you can take a bus or train to work or school to catch up on reading. Live in suburbia? Maybe you can car pool. Watch a lot of TV? Cut back or record the shows and skip the commercials during playback. Consider whether you can incorporate exercise into daily tasks, such as using satellite parking and taking a vigorous walk to the main campus. A diary or log will make it easier to see how to manage your time better and accomplish more.

Divide your time into small blocks: Use the ten-minute rule for overwhelming or difficult assignments. Work on the task for a minimum of ten minutes, and if it is still difficult, put it down and move on to something else on your list. More often than not, you will find that after ten minutes of work, the task doesn't seem so bad and the end is in sight. Even if the task is pleasant but will take a lot of time, breaking it down into small blocks makes it much easier to complete.

Avoid distractions. Little distractions can add up to lots of wasted time. Keeping your instant-messaging program open while you are working on a paper is a time waster, as is watching TV while trying to work. Keep your focus on the task at hand, and you will be more productive. If you have roommates, go to the library or computer lab, but don't sit next to friends and try to socialize while working (and close Facebook!).

Do things right the first time: Taking the time to understand the professor's instructions or the boss's intentions will allow you to do the job right and not have to go back repeatedly for clarification. If the instructions aren't clear from the outset, ask before starting. This strategy should free up more time to spend on other important tasks.

Don't try to save time by skipping healthy habits: Get enough sleep, eat well, and get plenty of exercise. These all take time, time that you feel pressed for, but in the long run you will do better. If you don't remain physical healthy, you are not likely to perform well in class, at work, or anywhere else. Cutting back on sleep may give you more hours to work, but you'll be much less efficient; in fact, you're likely to accomplish more if you sleep longer and do your work while well rested. Taking the time to be healthy should be one of your top priorities in life, because shortchanging yourself on healthy habits has both short- and long-term negative health consequences.

Q | Do I really need a planner?

Most people who effectively manage their time will tell you the secret is to have some type of planner—and to use it. Making a daily schedule is one of the most effective time-management strategies. People who use planners don't forget or miss deadlines, and they plan ahead. Some use paper-and-pencil-planners; others use a cell phone, a PDA, or a computer program. The time you spend using a planner will pay off!

Use your planner to prioritize. Enter your deadlines and projects, and create a to-do list to schedule and chunk your work. Divide your list into two columns or categories: Group A for the highest priority, must-do tasks, and Group B for less-important items that can wait for your attention. Make sure to set aside enough time to complete the Group A items. For large projects, break the work up into chunks and schedule plenty of time; don't wait until the last minute to get started. Review and update your lists at either the start or the end of each day.

Creating and following a to-do list allows you to focus on what is currently most important and frees you from worrying that you should be working on something else. This focus alone will reduce your stress and make you more productive. A to-do list also allows you to see how much time you have available, helping you to say no to things that are either unimportant or not possible with your current schedule. Saying no is hard for many of us, but it is a big part of managing time and reducing stress. Realize that it is better to say no and competently complete what you are working on, rather than take on too many new tasks and do them poorly, if at all. See the box "Time-Management Tips" for additional strategies.

Cognitive Strategies

What and how you think determines the level of stress in your life. Yes, certain events may be out of your control, but regardless of the source of the potential stressor, how you think about it ultimately determines its impact on you.

Q | Does positive thinking really work to stop me from worrying?

ENGAGE IN REALISTIC SELF-TALK. A main goal of stress management is to clear up the distorted way we often perceive situations, stressful or not. By examining your patterns of thinking, you can better recognize

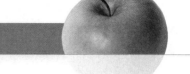

Wellness Strategies

ABCDE Model for Effective Thought Remodeling

Psychologist Albert Ellis believed that people cause themselves stress and emotional pain with their belief systems. He developed the ABCDE model to help people do cognitive restructuring and engage in more positive and realistic self-talk.

A: Identify your *adversity* (for example, "I lost my part-time job").

B: Identify your instinctive *beliefs* about the adversity ("I can't pay my bills").

C: Identify the *consequences* of those beliefs ("I'll have to quit college").

D: Begin to *dispute* those beliefs ("I can certainly find another job").

E: Become *re-energized* when you successfully dispute a belief ("I can stay in school!").

Source: Ellis, A. (1985). Expanding the ABC's of rational-emotive therapy. In M. J. Mahoney & A. Freeman (Eds.), *Cognition and psychotherapy* (pp. 313–323). New York: Plenum.

---

self-defeating thoughts, negative statements, and irrational beliefs that undermine your mood, behavior, and health. We all engage in these thoughts at least occasionally ("I can't possibly get this paper done on time"), but knowing how to deal with this negative thinking is the way out. Once you can recognize your negative self-talk, you can begin to restructure your thoughts, making them more positive, affirming, and realistic ("It won't be easy, but I can get this paper done"). Review the discussion of self-talk in Chapter 2; also see the box "ABCDE Model for Effective Thought Remodeling" for suggestions. Many people use the ABCDE model informally, because it's a logical approach to managing stress. Try applying this model to a current stressor in your life.

Q | I just can't seem to get over my bad quiz grade. What's the best way to move on?

Some of us get hung up on a bad grade, while others may be worried about paying for next semester. Moving on isn't always easy, but it's critical to reducing unhealthy stress. In addition to the ABCDE model, cognitive strategies for managing stressors of all types include focusing on the present, setting realistic goals, and developing problem-solving techniques.

FOCUS ON THE PRESENT. One of the great stressors is worrying about yesterday or tomorrow and not focusing on what is happening right now. You may have done poorly on your last quiz, but where do you stand overall in the course? Have your other assignments been OK? Was it just the first quiz of the semester? Does the instructor drop your lowest quiz score? Once you begin to focus on where you are today, you can relax and have a more positive outlook ("She does drop the lowest quiz score, so I should be OK").

SET REALISTIC GOALS. As described in Chapter 2, realistic goals are key for successful behavior change—and

they are just as important for stress management. To have the goal of an A for every assignment this semester is likely to set you up for stress. Instead, make your goal to get an A in the class (assuming you have a history of A-type success), and if a few assignments are less than perfect, you still have a chance at an A for the course—with much less stress. Often, the goals we set for ourselves are not realistic. Although you need to shoot for the stars in order to progress, it is important that you are in a position to reach them. If you have never exercised before, you shouldn't plan on a marathon this spring. Instead, attempt a local 5K. If you've never received an A in college, it may be too much to shoot for straight As this coming semester. Instead focus on one class for an A, and do your best in all the others.

Use an appropriate frame of reference: Recognize your strengths and weaknesses, and then set realistic goals based on them. If writing isn't your strength, your goal could be to improve on that during the upcoming semester. If you haven't been too good at getting assignments done on time, then that could be a realistic goal. If you set small, achievable goals, you can put the pieces in place to make them happen.

DEVELOP PROBLEM-SOLVING SKILLS. Developing effective problem-solving skills is another way to reduce stress. To do this, it is best to have realistic goals, focus on the present (you can't solve what has already happened), and keep a positive outlook ("I can do this!"). Here are four basic steps in problem-solving:

1. Identify the problem and describe it as accurately as you can. If it's large, break it down into manageable parts.
2. Brainstorm as many solutions to the problem as you can. Can you change the stressful circumstance? If not, can you change how you think about it?
3. Consider the positive and negative aspects of each potential solution, and then select the approach you think is most promising.
4. Evaluate the effectiveness of the solution you tried. If you don't think it worked, try one of your other possible solutions.

Wellness Strategies

Cognitive Stress-Management Techniques

Accept things you cannot change, and find a way to work within any limitations. This is a much better approach then being forever mad about something. If math isn't your strength, don't try to tough it out. Find a math tutor (available for free on most campuses) or online help resources. Make it as pleasant an experience as possible.

Laugh a little—or a lot. Laughter makes you feel good. It may lower blood pressure, reduce stress hormones, increase muscle flexion, boost immunity, and trigger the release of the body's natural painkillers. Don't be afraid to laugh out loud at a joke, a funny movie or cartoon, or some other humorous experience. Laugh when you are alone or in a crowd. It will brighten your mood and the mood of those around you.

Slow down: Try to pace instead of race. Plan ahead and allow enough time to get the most important things done. College students often think they work best under deadlines. All this really shows is that they are bad planners. Ask any professor and she will tell you that students who plan ahead and pace themselves usually do the best. Waiting until the last minute often results in many mistakes.

Let it go. The world won't end because you got a bad grade on a quiz or didn't have time to clean the kitchen. Don't beat yourself up for little things.

Problem-solving skills can often be developed by watching others who are successful (for example, "She always works on the assignment the same day it is given") and asking for advice ("How do you manage your time so well?"). Once you've observed other people's strategies, a little trial and error will show you which ones work best for you.

See the box "Cognitive Stress-Management Techniques" for additional tips.

Healthy Relationships and Social Support

We all need a sense of connectedness and belonging. Healthy and supportive relationships have consistently been shown to reduce stress and improve overall health and well-being. However, all relationships are not equally supportive. A network of supportive friends, or even just one supportive friend, can be vital to your well-being. Some key skills for relationship building are described in this section; see also the box "How to Win Friends—and Keep Them."

Q I can't seem to make any new friends. What can I do differently?

The first step is to meet new people. The more people you have in your life, the more likely you are to have a truly supportive relationship with at least one of them. For full-time students starting college, the pool of potential friends is one of the great benefits of living in a residence hall. Getting a job, volunteering, joining an intramural club, and participating in academic group projects are all ways to meet new people. Of course, by doing the things that you find interesting, you are more likely to find people who share your interests!

The second step is to make time for your friends. You can't maintain good relationships if you contact your friends only when it's convenient for you. Instead, you need to occasionally go out of your way for others and show them you truly care. Making time also includes showing up on time for events and remembering birthdays

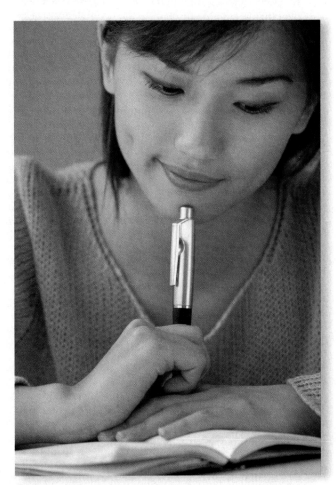

Effective problem-solving involves identifying and describing a problem, coming up with and evaluating possible solutions, and then giving one a try.

Wellness Strategies

How to Win Friends—and Keep Them

More than seventy-five years ago, Dale Carnegie wrote *How to Win Friends and Influence People,* one of the first self-help books. It is still in circulation today and has sold more than 15 million copies worldwide. He postulates that selling is all about making friends, and his key points include these:

- Become genuinely interested in other people.
- Smile.
- Remember that a person's name is to that person the sweetest and most important sound in any language.

- Be a good listener; encourage others to talk about themselves.
- Talk in terms of the other person's interests.
- Make the other person feel important—and do it sincerely.

Source: Carnegie, D. (1981). *How to Win Friends and Influence People* (rev. ed.). New York, NY: Simon & Schuster. (Original work published 1936)

---

and special occasions. These actions go a long way toward cultivating long-lasting relationships.

Another step in beginning and maintaining relationships is being a good listener. When people have encountered a stressful event, what they need most is someone to listen to them. Being truly listened to can have profound effects on us. It increases feelings of self-worth and creates a greater sense of personal connection. Listening is not easy for everyone, yet we can all benefit greatly from its healing power. Here are some tips for active listening:

- Ask people about their feelings and really pay attention to what they say. One of the easiest mistakes to make while listening is to think about what you want to say next instead of focusing on what the person is saying to you. Listen carefully and don't constantly interrupt.
- Reflect back what you hear, so the other person knows you really understand. You might repeat key points to show you are listening and to make sure you have understood them correctly.
- Focus your questions, comments, and attention on the other person. Put your feelings and needs aside for the time being. You want your friends to do the same for you when you are the one who needs to be listened to.

Q | Some of my friends have told me I'm rude, but I don't know why they say that. How can I know?

Have you ever thought you were saying something kind, but it turned out you offended someone? We may have good intentions with what we want to say, but it doesn't always work out that way. By taking a closer look at your patterns of communication, you might find that you can make changes that will help you maintain good relationships with others.

There are three general patterns of communication:

- **Passive communication** involves failing to honestly express feelings, thoughts, and beliefs, usually in order

to avoid conflict. This allows others to violate our rights, and the outcome is usually feelings of resentment and victimization.

- **Aggressive communication** involves directly standing up for personal rights and expressing thoughts, feelings, and beliefs in a way that is emotionally honest but in a way that may make others feel humiliated, degraded, belittled, or intimidated.
- **Assertive communication** involves standing up for personal rights and expressing thoughts, ideas, feelings, needs, and beliefs in direct, honest, and appropriate ways that are sensitive to others.

Although assertive people may sometimes be seen as aggressive, there is quite a difference. Imagine a situation in which a friend is twenty minutes late. An aggressive response would be a you-message: "You're late, and you've ruined my day by making me late." An assertive response would be an I-message: "I will have to adjust my schedule now that our meeting is starting late." The difference between assertive and aggressive communication is clear. Although each lets it be known that the friend's lateness has caused a problem, the assertive expression is kinder, indicating some level of sympathy, acknowledging that everyone occasionally runs late. Assertive communication will help you maintain relationships while still expressing your thoughts and feelings. Here are some tips for communicating assertively:

- **Use confident body language:** Stand up straight, look people in the eye (but don't stare them down), and relax.

passive communication A communication style in which the goal is to avoid confrontation; by failing to express honest feelings, beliefs, or thoughts, we allow our rights to be violated.

aggressive communication A communication style in which the primary goal is to get what we want, even if it requires manipulation and belittling others; needs and desires are clearly expressed but with a lack of consideration for the feelings or welfare of others.

assertive communication A communication style in which the primary goal is to solve a problem, finding a balance between our own needs and the needs of others; needs and wants are clearly expressed and in a way that is respectful and sensitive to others.

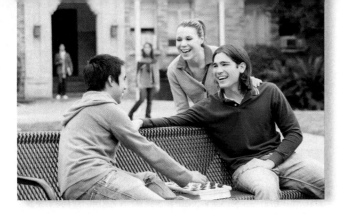

- **Use a firm and pleasant tone.**
- **Don't assume you know what other people are going to say or do:** Let them explain before you react.
- **Think win-win:** Look for a compromise or a way for everyone to get their needs met.

So, if your friends tell you that you're rude, try to adopt a communication style that is assertive instead of aggressive. Assertive people can go far in life for many reasons: They actively seek what they want; they consider others' feelings; and they are willing to work things out so that everyone prospers.

Q | How do you tell if a friendship is worth it?

Relationships don't develop overnight, and they take conscious effort to maintain. But not everyone is meant to be friends. If you find yourself with people who make you feel bad about yourself or who are constantly negative, then they may not be the right people for you. Try to surround yourself with positive, sharing people.

High schools friends often drift apart during and after college. If a relationship fades because the people are changing, then cherish all that you had in the past and wish each other the best for the future. If a relationship is fading because one of the people is not trying, then consider the motivation behind the lack of effort before deciding to work hard to maintain it. Ask yourself these questions regarding both new and established friendships:

- Do you feel that your conversations are more forced than fluid?
- Do you feel the other person truly understands, accepts, and supports you? And do you feel that way toward that person?
- Does spending time with the other person make you feel energized or drained and somewhat depressed?
- Do you include the other person in your life because you cherish his or her company or just to have a bigger social circle?

Listen to your feelings. Ultimately, you're the only one who knows if a relationship is worth keeping. But it's important to have a few special people you can count on in your life. Keep in mind that not everything always goes perfectly in any relationship. Feelings get hurt; people get angry at each other; and sometimes you feel pressured.

These are normal occurrences, yet they should pass quickly if the relationship is healthy overall. If these difficult times happen often or don't seem to go away, it may be time to reevaluate the relationship.

Relationship violence is something that should never happen, not even one time. Violence can be physical, sexual, or psychological, but it is never OK. You should never make light of abuse or try to justify or excuse violent behavior by blaming the victim, or blaming yourself if you are the victim. Respect your friends at all times, express your feelings, and don't compromise when it comes to your own safety. If you or someone you know is in an abusive relationship, contact the Rape, Abuse, and Incest National Network (RAINN) Hotline at 1-800-656-HOPE (4673), the National Domestic Violence Hotline at 1-800-799-SAFE (7233), or your local emergency services at 911.

Healthy Lifestyle Choices: Activity, Diet, and Sleep

The more stress in your life, the more likely you are to make poor health choices. At the same time, the more poor health choices you make, the more stress you are likely to have! Break the cycle and your health will improve while your stress decreases.

Q | Does working out really relieve stress?

PHYSICAL ACTIVITY. Yes! The great thing about exercise and stress is that it doesn't take much activity to reduce your stress level. Although it may take weeks or months to lose weight, you can lose stress in minutes. Exercise bouts as short as ten minutes have been shown to elevate people's moods, and the intensity doesn't need to be too high.[19] A brisk ten-minute walk around the block or on a treadmill can often be an effective mood lifter. Further, people who exercise regularly tend to have a much milder physical stress reaction to typical stressors. See Chapters 3–5 for more on the physical and mental benefits of exercise.

Any amount of physical activity can help. If you're a regular exerciser, you should view your workouts as a means of managing stress, along with all their other health benefits. If you don't currently exercise or exercise only infrequently, try taking a brisk ten-minute walk next time you are feeling particularly stressed. Walking isn't the only exercise that can reduce stress, but it's one of the simplest, especially if you want an immediate de-stressor. If a quick walk isn't possible for you at a time of stress, try the relaxations techniques discussed later in the chapter.

Yoga and t'ai chi, along with Pilates, are all activities that can help manage stress.

- Yoga, described in Chapter 6, involves a series of physical postures and stretches emphasizing balance and breathing control.

- T'ai chi is a martial art that resembles a slow, graceful dance.
- Pilates, described in Chapter 5, includes a series of fluid movements performed in a precise manner, accompanied by specialized breathing techniques and mental concentration.

Although different in their specifics, these activities share certain characteristics: slow, purposeful movements; high levels of concentration; and focused breathing. These traits make them very effective for reducing both acute and chronic stress. However, when you use physical activity as part of a stress management program, the type of activity is not as important as regular participation. Find an activity you like, do it often, and enjoy the benefits.

Q What about t'ai chi for stress?
READ ONLINE

Q Does what I eat affect my stress level?

EATING HABITS. The foods you eat can affect your stress level, for better or worse. A diet that contains a good mix of healthy fats, whole grains, lean protein sources, and fruits and vegetables keeps you healthy overall and can counteract the effects of stress by supporting your immune system and controlling your blood pressure. Eating whole grains and other complex carbohydrates instead of simple sugars can help keep your blood sugar levels steady.

What about foods to avoid or limit? Most people know that caffeine is a stimulant—that's why they consume it! Caffeine may help you stay awake to study, but it will make it more difficult for you to go to sleep, which starts the cycle of reduced sleep and increased stress. Too much caffeine can also make you feel jittery and anxious, very similar to the stress response. Limiting caffeine intake is a good stress-management strategy.

Fried and other fatty foods may also make falling asleep difficult, so it is best to avoid those, especially later in the evening (think late night fast food runs!).

Some people are sensitive to sodium and sugar in their diet, making sleep difficult or creating a feeling of irritability. Try keeping a journal or log that tracks your stress level, your sleeping pattern, and what you are eating or drinking. Look for a pattern linking eating habits and stress. If you reduce or eliminate the offending foods, your stress level will go down.

Q Why do I need sleep? Does it play a role in stress management?

SLEEP. Absolutely. Sleep is essential for optimal wellness, and it is relaxing. Although sleep is critical to our well-being, it tends to be one of the first things neglected when we feel stressed, especially when pressured by time. Make time for sleep! You'll be healthier, and you'll function at a higher physical and mental level when you are awake.

Among adults, sleeping less than six or seven hours a night leads to a host of health problems. College students often make a game of seeing how little sleep they can get, especially around exam time. Sleep deprivation, usually defined as less than about four or five hours in a twenty-four-hour period, makes you function as if you were drunk, so why would you want to take an exam in that condition? Lack of sleep hurts your ability to concentrate and is associated with lower grades. It is linked to increased risk of health problems, in both the short term (colds) and the long term (high blood pressure, blood glucose abnormalities, abdominal fat accumulation).[20] And people who sleep less than six hours or more than nine hours a night are more likely to die prematurely than those who sleep six to eight hours a night.[21]

Periods of high stress are when sleep is the most important—and is the most difficult to obtain. Establishing good sleep habits early in college will serve you well during difficult times. Ideally, strive for a consistent six to eight hours of sleep a night, depending on your personal needs. For some tips, see the box "Getting a Better Night's Sleep."

Q How can I tell if I'm getting enough sleep?

If you feel tired, you're probably not getting enough sleep. If you are getting enough sleep, you should feel rested

Wellness Strategies

Getting a Better Night's Sleep

Maintain a regular sleep schedule. Go to bed and get up at the same time each day of the week. Staying up later than usual and sleeping in on the weekends disrupts your regular sleep schedule. If you try to be consistent for a week, you will be amazed by how much better you start to feel throughout the entire day.

Create a sleep friendly environment. Try to make your bedroom comfortable, quiet, cool, and dark. White-noise generators, fans, air conditioners, and other sources of monotonous, unchanging sound are effective for improving your sleep. Try making your room darker by turning off some of the electrical devices that give off light all night; turn your bright digital clock toward the wall.

Avoid caffeine, alcohol, and nicotine. Caffeine and nicotine are stimulants that take a long time to clear your system; they may double the time it should take you to fall asleep. Alcohol induces sleepiness, but it causes poorer sleep and restlessness later in the night by interfering with the body's sleep cycles. Also, don't eat a large or heavy meal within two or three hours of bedtime.

Establish relaxing bedtime rituals. Reading, listening to soothing music, and taking a warm bath or shower are all ways to help your mind and body associate bedtime with relaxation and peacefulness. Allow yourself time to wind down.

Exercise regularly. Among its many benefits, regular exercise helps you fall asleep and sleep better through the night. Any type of exercise works, especially if it is done regularly and long enough before bedtime. Exercising too late in the day stimulates the body, raising its temperature and making it difficult to fall asleep. However, if you often find yourself lying around watching TV all night, you can try some relaxing yoga or stretching as a way to get ready for bed and relax your mind.

---

during the day and be able to stay focused and attentive even in situations you might describe as boring. You shouldn't feel fatigued or constantly irritable. You should also wake up on your own in the morning, rather than being awakened from a sound sleep by your alarm. If you doze off during the day and can't wake up without a loud alarm, then you probably need more sleep. Take the Epworth Sleepiness Scale to assess your sleep status (http://www.sleepeducation.com/SleepScale.aspx).

Fast Facts

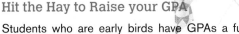

Hit the Hay to Raise your GPA

Students who are early birds have GPAs a full point higher on average than night owls. Students who get up earlier may find it easier to get to class on time and to study. By going to bed earlier, they may also be less likely to drink, party, and engage in other activities that hurt academic performance. If you are a night owl, try slowly shifting your sleep schedule toward that of an early bird. Also, try not to schedule any early-morning classes.

Source: Clay, K., and others. (2008, June 9). *Morningness and eveningness relationship to college GPA.* Research abstract presented at the annual meeting of the Associated Professional Sleep Societies (Abstract 728).

Q Is snoring bad for me or just annoying for other people?

It depends. Snoring is very common. It occurs when tissues in the throat relax during sleep, partially blocking the airway. As air flows past the relaxed tissues, they vibrate and cause harsh sounds. These sounds can be quite loud and make it difficult for others to sleep.

A more serious condition, known as obstructive sleep apnea, is linked to persistent snoring. In apnea, the throat is blocked and the person stops breathing for ten or more seconds. Shifts in blood levels of oxygen and carbon dioxide trigger the body to wake up—the airway opens and the person takes a gasping breath. This typically happens over and over during the course of the night, and although the person may be unaware of it, sleep is significantly disrupted. Sleep apnea can cause severe and persistent daytime sleepiness; it also increases the risk of high blood pressure and other cardiovascular problems.

There are some self-management measures to reduce snoring:

- Lose weight if you are overweight.
- Sleep on your side.
- If you have nasal congestion from a cold or allergies, treat it.
- Avoid alcohol and other sedatives, especially close to bedtime.
- Try over-the-counter nasal strips, which help some people.
- Consider a dental mouthpiece that helps keep airways open during sleep.

Research Brief

Sleep, Stress, and Cortisol

Sleep and stress levels are closely linked. High stress levels upset your sleep, and lack of sleep raises your stress level. Researchers have found that sleep patterns affect levels of stress hormones, especially cortisol. One study followed more than 2,500 adults—information on their sleep was collected, as well as several saliva samples to measure cortisol levels. The researchers found that people who reported short sleep duration or disturbed sleep had higher cortisol levels throughout the day. This finding is important for health, as high cortisol levels are associated with many of the negative long-term health effects of stress. This study provides additional evidence of the importance of sleep for overall wellness.

Source: Kumari, M., Badrick, E., Ferrie, J., Perski, A., Marmot, M., & Chandola, T. (2009). Self-reported sleep duration and sleep disturbance are independently associated with cortisol secretion in the Whitehall II study. *Journal of Clinical Endocrinology and Metabolism, 94*(12), 4801–4809 (http://jcem.endojournals.org/cgi/rapidpdf/jc.2009-0555v1).

---

insomnia A sleep disorder characterized by persistent problems falling asleep or staying asleep.

If these strategies don't reduce snoring, get evaluated by a health-care professional. You can be tested for apnea by wearing monitors at home or in a specialized sleep lab. Treatments for apnea include wearing a pressurized mask during sleep as well as certain types of surgery.

Q | I just can't seem to get to sleep. How can I turn my brain off?

Insomnia is a sleep disorder characterized by persistent difficulty falling asleep or staying asleep, impairing a person's ability to function normally. Many insomniacs complain that they are unable to rest their mind for more than a few minutes at a time, which is usually a sign that the insomnia is due to stress.

Insomnia is more than just difficulty going to sleep. It can also include difficulty returning to sleep in the middle of the night or waking too early in the morning. The pattern of insomnia often is related to the underlying cause. Although psychoactive drugs, hormonal shifts, and mental disorders can all disrupt sleep, the most common causes of insomnia among college students are fear, anxiety, and overall stress.[22] In addition to stress, poor sleep habits and too much noise or light can also affect sleep. Anyone who has ever lived in a residence hall or shared an apartment with three or four roommates knows that this can be a problem!

Because emotional stress is a primary cause of insomnia, finding effective stress reducers can help you sleep better. Stress affects the quality and quantity of sleep, and when we sleep poorly, our stress level the next day often increases. This cycle of poor sleep and increased stress will continue until sleep needs are met, which often requires several nights of quality sleep. Chronic sleep deprivation cannot be made up for by just one or two good nights of sleep.[23]

Try any of the stress-management techniques suggested in this chapter to help reduce your level of stress and improve your sleep. If problems persist, keep a sleep diary of your sleeping and waking times and related information (such as caffeine intake, exercise habits, and stress level), and discuss your sleep problems with a health care professional.

Q Are naps healthy for adults?

READ ONLINE

Spiritual Wellness

Q | Will spirituality make me more or less stressed?

Without an awareness of personal values, our life may be dictated by the demands of others, which is stressful. Having a strong personal belief system makes us more resilient and therefore better able to handle stressful situ-

Fast Facts

Driving While Drowsy

Being awake for twenty hours or more impairs driving ability—judgment, reaction time, performance—as much as being legally drunk. The National Highway Traffic Safety Administration estimates that more than 100,000 crashes each year are caused by drowsy driving, at a cost of $12.5 billion in losses. If you are driving and find yourself yawning, daydreaming, drifting out of your lane, or having trouble focusing or keeping your eyes open, stop and pull over in a safe place for a rest.

Source: National Sleep Foundation. (2010). Facts and stats. *Drowsy Driving.org* (http://drowsydriving.org/about/facts-and-stats).

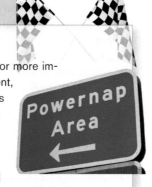

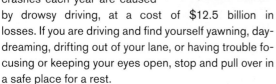

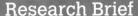

Research Brief

Happiness from Achieving Life Goals? It Depends . . .

Setting goals and then pursuing and attaining them can make people happy and satisfied with their lives. However, it appears that the results of achieving your goals may depend on the type of goals you set.

Researchers followed a group of recent college graduates, evaluating their goals as well as factors such as self-esteem, anxiety, physical signs of stress, and overall satisfaction with life. The group was assessed one year after graduation and then again twelve months after that. What the researchers found was that the individuals whose goals and aspirations were identified as *intrinsic* were happier, less stressed, and more satisfied with their lives than those whose goals were *extrinsic*. Intrinsic goals include having meaningful personal relationships, strong community involvement, and good physical health. Examples of extrinsic goals are achieving a certain level of pay or a certain appearance or image (wealth and good looks). The group

with extrinsic goals, even if they achieved them, reported more negative emotions, more physical symptoms of stress and anxiety, and less satisfaction with their lives.

What explains this pattern? It's possible that striving for extrinsic goals such as wealth and beauty does not satisfy basic psychological needs. Working long hours and worrying about how you compare to others can lead to jealousy and feelings of inadequacy and reduce the time and energy you have for relaxing with friends, engaging in hobbies you love, or volunteering in your community. The take-away message from this study may be that in setting your life goals, you should consider your psychological needs in addition to your material aspirations.

Source: Niemiec, C. P., Ryan, R. M., & Deci, E. L. (2009). The path taken: Consequences of attaining intrinsic and extrinsic aspirations in post-college life. *Journal of Research in Personality, 43*(3): 291–306.

---

spirituality A person's system of beliefs and values, feelings of connectedness to self and others, and experience of finding meaning and purpose in life.

ations. **Spirituality,** although not necessarily religiosity, helps give our lives context. Spirituality has three general components: feeling a connectedness to ourself and to others, developing a system of personal beliefs and values, and finding meaning and purpose in life. For many people, religion and religious practices such as prayer or meditation offer paths to developing spirituality. However, spirituality does not necessarily mean religion, and people can develop spirituality in other ways. Spirituality is personal and subjective; no two people have exactly the same spiritual beliefs, be they religious or not.

Self-discovery is a good way to explore your spirituality. You can begin by thinking about your relationship with yourself and then look to how you nurture relationships with those people important to you. Also consider your beliefs and values—what you think is your purpose in life and what you'd like to accomplish. Ask yourself these questions:

- What are the important relationships in my life?
- Where do I find comfort?
- What gives me hope? Joy?
- What do I believe will happen to me when my physical life ends, and how do I feel about it?

Spirituality has many benefits. Those who regularly engage in spiritual practices (such as communing with nature or meditating) are better able to focus on their personal goals. By knowing what's important, you can focus less on the unimportant things and eliminate stress. Spiritual-

ity also gives you a sense of connectedness and belonging, and it helps keep you from feeling lonely. Knowing your place in the world releases you from the burden of feeling responsible for everything around you. Unburdening yourself then allows you more time to cultivate and nurture meaningful relationships and ultimately lead a healthier life, in all the dimensions of wellness.

Are there any specific steps to take to develop spirituality? Again, this is a highly individual process. These are a few ways to develop spiritually:

- Improve your self-esteem. Try some of the cognitive strategies for stress management described in this chapter, which can also help boost self-esteem.
- Engage in activities that are meaningful to you and allow you to, for example, express your creativity, spend time in nature, or engage in a personal spiritual practice.
- Foster relationships with the people who are important to you.
- Help others. Volunteer your time or return a favor to a friend. Helping others helps you by giving you a different perspective on life and potentially boosting your motivation to achieve. Volunteering can boost your self-esteem and improve your mood.

For most people, spirituality is an ever-changing process of self-exploration. Age and life experiences will certainly make you readjust your spiritual beliefs. Ultimately though, self-exploration will lead to greater personal fulfillment at all stages of life.

Relaxation Techniques

There are specific techniques designed to elicit the relaxation response—the opposite of fight-or-flight. These techniques halt the stress response and allow the body to return to homeostasis. If practiced regularly, the benefits of relaxation techniques can be lasting.

Q | How does a relaxation technique help? On a physical level, what happens?

The **relaxation response** is a physiological state of deep rest that changes the physical and emotional responses to stress.[24] Just as stress causes potentially harmful physiological responses, relaxation causes potentially beneficial ones. It calms the fight-or-flight response and attempts to return the body to normal functioning. Breathing and heart rate slow, muscles relax, and metabolism and blood pressure decrease.

Many techniques and strategies can bring the body back to a state of relaxation. It's important to explore as many as you need to in order to find the one that is most effective for you. Don't give up on a technique after just one try—they can take time to have an impact—and don't assume that what works for a friend or family member will work for you.

Q | What are some ways to calm down in a stressful situation, things that help right away?

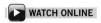

BREATHING AND POSTURE. Try breathing! Most people use only about half of their breathing capacity, at best, and even less when they're under stress. Breathing deeply relaxes muscles, quiets the mind, and gets oxygen into the blood, where it can invigorate all parts of the body, even a tired brain.

Deep breathing, or diaphragmatic breathing, involves filling your lungs by expanding your abdomen rather than your chest. When you breath in, the diaphragm contracts and flattens downward, creating a vacuum that draws in air. When you exhale, the diaphragm returns to its dome shape, pushing air out of the body. You can practice diaphragmatic breathing anywhere: Just rest one hand lightly on your lower abdomen so that you can feel your breath move your body. Breathe in slowly through your nose. Let the air flow into your upper chest and down your spine, filling the diaphragm, and pushing your stomach out a little bit. Then let go of your breath slowly through pursed lips. Allow your lower abdomen to drop, your ribs to pull in, and your chest to drop as you fully expel all the air. This breathing pattern, although physiologically most effective, is uncommon for most of us; typically, we take shallow breaths that expand only the upper chest. Try repeating diaphragmatic breathing a few times,

relaxation response
A physiological state of deep rest that reverses the body's responses to stress.

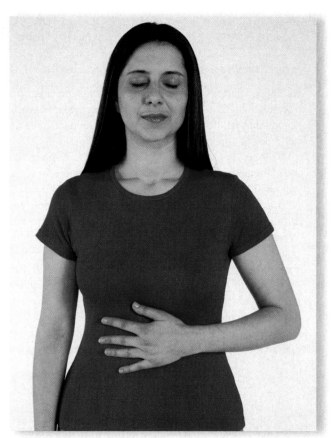

Deep breathing is a technique for inducing the relaxation response that can be used anywhere. Instead of taking shallow breaths that slightly expand your chest, take deep breaths that fill your lungs and expand your abdomen

and next time you are feeling stressed, take a few of these deep breaths, focusing on the movement of your abdomen. You should feel some stress relief in a matter of minutes.

Posture is also important. Good posture radiates ease and confidence and can immediately make you feel better about yourself (it can also make you look slimmer!). Try improving your posture a few times during the day. Then next time you are stressed, stand or sit tall, and you should look and feel better right away.

Q | What's the best way to loosen up my tense muscles?

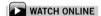

PROGRESSIVE MUSCLE RELAXATION. A general stretching workout can help your muscles relax, but other techniques directly address muscle tension. **Progressive muscle relaxation** (PMR) involves tensing muscles and then actively reducing that tension, while concentrating on your body and not your stressors. Start with a specific muscle group, say, your left calf: Inhale and gently squeeze the calf muscle until you feel some tension and hold it for 6 to 10 seconds. Squeeze gently to avoid

progressive muscle relaxation (PMR) A relaxation method that involves tensing and relaxing muscles in sequence.

soreness or injury. After a few seconds, release the tension and the breath, to allow both physical and emotional relief. Begin each PMR session at either your head or your toes and work in the opposite direction. If time is short, focus on the large muscle groups but be sure to perform the exercises on both sides of your body. If you have time, it is best to practice PMR daily, involving as many muscles as possible, one by one. Even with a brief PMR session, however, you should feel some immediate stress relief.

Q | How does meditation work to reduce stress?

MEDITATION. Meditation, an internal state of relaxed awareness, can be a great way to ease the day's stress. You can practice meditation almost anywhere— at home, school, or work; while commuting; or even while you are out for a walk. Meditation was originally developed to help people deepen their understanding of sacred and mystical life forces. Today, meditation is widely used for relaxation and stress reduction. Meditation can produce a deep state of relaxation and a tranquil mind, and this emotional calming doesn't end with the meditation session.[25] People who meditate regularly can experience long-lasting emotional and physical benefits.

There are many types of meditation, some more formal than others. Some people meditate by focusing on one object or thought, whereas others try to quiet their mind of everything. Don't be intimidated by thinking you aren't mystical enough to meditate or don't know how or why. Prayer and contemplation are examples of using concentration to elicit the relaxation response. Yoga and t'ai chi, discussed earlier, include meditation in their practice, and deep breathing can also be a form of meditation.

Two general categories of meditation are *exclusive meditation* and *inclusive meditation.* To practice exclusive meditation, find a quiet place where you won't be interrupted for at least ten minutes. Exclusive meditation involves focusing on a single word or phrase, while trying to eliminate all other thoughts. You can use any word or phrase that makes you comfortable; it doesn't have to be spiritual or religious. Close your eyes and breathe slowly while repeating your word or phrase. Continue for ten to twenty minutes. Sounds simple, but if you are new to meditation, your thoughts will quickly wander. Once you notice that, refocus and come back to your special word or phrase. So you can relax during meditation, set an alarm to keep your mind from worrying about the time or to wake you should you fall asleep.

Inclusive meditation, also known as mindfulness meditation, allows your mind to wander as you observe your thoughts. The key aspect of this form of meditation is to not judge or react emotionally to your thoughts; just observe them as an outsider might. Inclusive meditation can help reduce negative-thinking patterns and help you realistically reappraise

meditation A broad group of self-directed practices that quiet and focus the mind and relax the body.

potential stressors as less threatening and challenging.

Other meditative techniques that produce relaxation are prayer and sacred chants. Prayer is a widely practiced example of meditation. Most faith traditions use spoken and written prayers. You can pray with your own words or those written by others. Regardless of your specific beliefs, praying can release stress because it is a recognition that help can come from many sources (a higher being, general faith, self-confidence) and that you are not on your own.

Repeating a phrase or sentence that is sacred or meaningful to you, called a *mantra,* can be calming. Find something meaningful to you, something that calms or encourages you (such as "I am capable and strong"). You can say it to yourself quietly or out loud. Although saying it quietly may be necessary at times, it is believed that saying the mantra out loud brings the most fulfillment. Repeating your mantra while walking is a great way to reduce stress. Take a purposeful walk and repeat your mantra, loudly if possible, focusing on the words. Time will pass as you feel your stress going away and your self-confidence increasing, and by the end of the walk, you will feel invigorated.

Q | Is closing my eyes and thinking of the beach really going to help?

VISUALIZATION/MENTAL IMAGERY. For some people, yes. Many people engage in **visualization** for pleasure, without even realizing they are practicing stress reduction. Have you ever imagined yourself being on warm beach, while in reality you were stuck in the middle of winter? Or have you ever thought about what it would feel like to win the lottery? Visualization temporarily removes us from reality, providing a brief respite from the daily grind, some mental rest and relaxation. Practicing visualization is quite simple. You start by finding a quiet spot and making yourself comfortable. Once you are settled, close your eyes and visualize a place you find comfortable, safe, and relaxing. Try to stay focused on your image. Eventually, you will feel like you are actually there, experiencing the sights, sounds, and smells of your image. (Go ahead and put the book down and try it for a few minutes. When you return, you'll feel more focused on what you're reading here.)

Visualization can also be used as a performance booster in sports and other types of activities. Imagine what you would like to happen—hitting a baseball, delivering a great speech, asking a boss for a raise—and use it as a form of mental rehearsal.

Q | I like to listen to music when I'm upset. Does that reduce stress?

OTHER STRATEGIES FOR RELAXATION. For many people, music is a powerful mood elevator, and listening can help anyone relax. When

visualization For stress management, a technique using all the senses to imagine a place or scene that is comfortable, soothing, and relaxing.

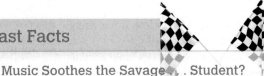

Fast Facts

Music Soothes the Savage . . . Student?

Researchers have found that listening to music that is soothing or that people select for themselves can often reduce anxiety, improve mood, and quiet the physical stress response. These positive changes have been seen among patients in hospital waiting rooms and in students who have just taken a challenging exam! In addition, listening to loud music with a fast tempo increases blood pressure and heart and breathing rates. Pick music to match your mood, level of energy, and level of stress.

you can, get up and dance to your music or sing out loud. It is amazing how quickly your stress level will drop. Other things to try include these:

- *Keep a journal:* Journaling allows you to explore your thoughts and emotions, work through your worries, and revisit the good things that happen in your life. It can increase your awareness of your typical patterns of thinking in response to stressors and be a good problem-solving tool.
- *Read:* Reading a book or some poems, especially when it is by choice and for pleasure, allows you to clear your mind for thirty minutes or so and come back to your routine tasks more invigorated.
- *Get a massage:* Massage can reduce physical discomfort and mental stress.
- *Spend time with a pet:* Pets provide relief from stress and loneliness and their own particular type of social support. Walking and playing with a dog are also opportunities for physical activity.
- *Take a humor break:* Laughter improves both emotional and physical wellness. Find ways to make yourself and those around you laugh more frequently—read or watch cartoons; post funny pictures around your residence or as your computer screensaver; play a silly game.

When Stress Becomes Too Much: Getting Help

Q | My stress is killing me. Should I see someone?

We all have stress in our lives, but for some of us, it may seem overwhelming. Constant or excessive stress can lead to increased anxiety, panic attacks, depression, and in worst-case scenarios, even suicide. Because it can be hard to know when your stress has reached a point that you can no longer deal with it alone, it is better to take action too soon than too late.

Stress becomes dangerous when it interferes with your ability to live a normal life. If you feel out of control or you just don't know what to do, then your stress is becoming a danger to you and you should seek help. Unfortunately, many students don't know where to turn for help, are ashamed of their feelings, or don't think anyone can help them.

Virtually all colleges and universities provide free counseling—a valuable yet underutilized service. The bittersweet irony is that student fees largely pay for this service. Seeking help from the counseling center or calling a stress hotline can help. Even talking with a close friend or family member can help bring you back to a place of greater stability. For many people who are feeling too stressed, talking to someone about their worries can help tremendously. Talking can put worries into perspective, identifying which are controllable and can be addressed and which cannot be controlled and need to be let go of. Although your friends and family may be able to help you with stress, if you're experiencing anxiety attacks, feel you are depressed, or have considered suicide, you need to seek professional help immediately.

Q | When are sad feelings just being "down in the dumps," and when are they serious depression?

Everybody experiences times of feeling sad, blue, or down in the dumps. Ups and downs are normal parts of life. Maybe you didn't turn in a paper on time, or didn't get the work shift you wanted. Maybe you found out the cute person in your class was dating someone else, or maybe you found out your car needs a lot of repair work. These are all situations that can make anyone feel down. Typically, though, these feelings pass in a few hours or days, and we move on. However, when the depressed mood continues for many days or weeks, and especially if it interferes with daily tasks (socializing, parenting, job, school), then you might be suffering from **depression** (Figure 10-4).

depression A psychological disorder characterized by feelings of sadness and hopelessness, loss of interest in activities that were once enjoyable, poor concentration, and physical symptoms such as fatigue, sleeping problems, and poor appetite.

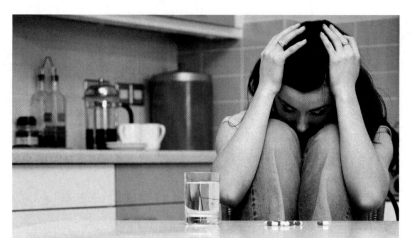

Figure 10-4 **Symptoms of depression and risk factors for suicide.** Not everyone suffering from depression will have all these symptoms. Visit the site for the American Association of Suicidology (http://www.suicidology.org) for more on recognizing and responding to suicide warning signs.

Sources: National Institute of Mental Health. (2010). *Depression* (http://www.nimh.nih.gov/health/topics/depression). Centers for Disease Control and Prevention. (2010). Suicide prevention. *Violence Prevention* (http;//www.cdc.gov/violenceprevention/suicide).

Symptoms of depression

Ongoing sad, anxious, or empty feelings

Feelings of hopelessness

Feelings of guilt, worthlessness, or helplessness

Feeling irritable or restless

Loss of interest in activities or hobbies that were once enjoyable

Feeling tired all the time

Difficulty concentrating, remembering details, or difficulty making decisions

Sleep disturbances: insomnia, waking in the middle of the night, or sleeping all the time

Overeating or loss of appetite

Thoughts of suicide or suicide attempts

Ongoing aches and pains, headaches, cramps, or digestive problems that do not go away

Risk factors for suicide

Previous suicide attempts

History of depression or other mental illness

Alcohol or drug abuse

Family history of suicide or violence

Physical illness

Impulsive or aggressive tendencies

Feeling isolated, cut off from other people

Unwillingness to seek help

fully treated with counseling or medications or both. See the box "Living with . . . Depression" for more information.

Q | What should someone do about a friend who seems depressed or suicidal?

Although we all hope we will never be in this situation, the reality is we may all be there someday. It is very serious when someone appears to be suicidal, and you should not take it lightly. If the threat seems imminent, call 911. If you aren't sure, call, or encourage your friend to call, the National Suicide Prevention Lifeline (1-800-273-TALK). Don't try to talk your friend out of it, unless you are a trained counselor. If you called 911, do your best to keep your friend calm until help arrives. Follow these guidelines: Listen; let your friend express his or her feelings, and don't make any judgments.

If the threat is not imminent, talk to your friend, following the guidelines above: listening, showing empathy, and not judging. It's OK to ask your friend to talk about his or her suicidal thoughts, plans, and timeline. Strongly recommend that your friend seek professional help. Check back with him or her frequently: Did she follow up with a counselor? Is she still harboring suicidal thoughts? Is he taking prescribed medications? Has his mood improved?

Addressing what may be suicidal thoughts in a friend or loved one is difficult, but it must be done. If you misinterpreted your friend's intentions, you risk upsetting him or her with your suspicions. However, the risk of doing nothing is much greater. Don't hesitate to act if you suspect suicidal thoughts.

Unfortunately, many people, especially men, never seek treatment for these symptoms. Maybe they feel they're only temporary ("I'll feel better tomorrow") or that it's a justified feeling ("Everyone feels down when they do badly on an exam"). Maybe they're ashamed ("People in my family don't get depressed"). But depression is a serious illness with serious consequences, including suicide, and it's important to be honest with yourself if you recognize symptoms of depression. Don't just think it will go away; it probably won't. Seeking help is the best thing you can do for yourself and for those around you; depression can be success-

DOLLAR STRETCHER
Financial Wellness Tip

Locate the counseling center on your campus, and investigate its services. It is likely to provide free services to help students manage stress, deal with family problems and relationship issues, and treat depression and other psychological disorders. The center may also offer workshops and self-help resources.

Living with . . .

Depression

Depression is a common and potentially serious illness that can interfere with a person's daily life and relationships. Some people experience bouts of severe symptoms (*major depression*), and others experience long-term but less severe symptoms (*dysthymic disorder*). Depression can run in families, and symptoms usually start between ages 15 and 30. Depression is more common in women than in men, although men have higher rates of suicide.

Overall, about one in twenty Americans report current symptoms of depression, although only about 30 percent of those affected have sought treatment. This is unfortunate, because even in severe cases, depression is a highly treatable condition. The first step for a person experiencing symptoms (see Figure 10-4) is to visit a health care professional for an evaluation. If you're depressed, it is important to realize that feelings of exhaustion and helplessness are part of the illness rather than an accurate reflection of your circumstances. These negative feelings will fade with treatment.

Once diagnosed, depression is typically treated with medication or psychotherapy or both. Antidepressant medications affect levels of neurotransmitters such as serotonin and norepinephrine. Medications affect different people in different ways, so almost everyone needs to try more than one before finding the most effective choice. Psychotherapy can help people change negative patterns of thinking and behaving that contribute to their depression; it can also help them work through problems in personal relationships. Depression symptoms may last or recur, so long-term management of the condition is often needed.

Self-help measures can accompany professional treatment. The National Institute of Mental Health recommends the following:

- Engage in mild physical activity or exercise.
- Go to a movie or sporting event, or engage in another activity that you once enjoyed.
- Participate in religious, social, and other activities.
- Set realistic goals for yourself.
- Break up large tasks into small ones, set priorities, and do only as much as you can.
- Don't isolate yourself, and let others help you; spend time with other people and confide in a trusted friend or relative.
- Expect your mood to improve gradually, not immediately; do not expect to suddenly "snap out of it." During treatment, sleep and appetite may begin to improve before mood.
- Postpone important decisions, such as changing jobs, until you feel better; discuss decisions with others who know you well and have a more objective view of your situation.
- Remember that positive thinking will replace negative thoughts as your depression responds to treatment.

Sources: National Institute of Mental Health. (2010). *Depression* (http://www.nimh.nih.gov/health/topics/depression). Pratt, L. A., & Brody, D. J. (2008). Depression in the United States household population, 2005–2006. *NCHS Data Brief*, No. 7. Hyattsville, MD: National Center for Health Statistics.

Summary

Stressors are all around us, so you need to know how to manage stress, or your physical and emotional reactions to them. Although your body automatically prepares you for physical response, most of the stressors of modern life do not require such a response. If the stress response occurs too often or for extended periods, it can take a serious physical and emotional toll. Factors that affect your response to stressors include personality traits, gender, and typical thinking patterns. Although top sources of stress vary from person to person, common stressors include major life changes, minor daily hassles, relationships, environmental factors, and time, job, and school pressures.

Many techniques can help you manage stress. Some help you change the stressful circumstances (time management, problem solving). Others help maintain your resilience against the effects of stress (relationships, exercise, sleep, healthy diet, spiritual practices). Still others directly induce the relaxation response (meditation, deep breathing, progressive muscle relaxation, visualization). If stress becomes severe or signs of depression occur, seek professional help.

More to Explore

American Psychological Association Help Center
http://www.apa.org/helpcenter/
Benson-Henry Institute for Mind Body Medicine
http://www.massgeneral.org/bhi
Go Ask Alice! Emotional Health
http://www.goaskalice.columbia.edu/Cat4.html
National Institute of Mental Health: Health Topics
http://www.nimh.nih.gov/health/index.shtml
National Sleep Foundation
http://www.sleepfoundation.org
Student Counseling Virtual Pamphlet Collection
http://www.dr-bob.org/vpc

LAB ACTIVITY 10-1 What's Stressing You?

SUBMIT ONLINE

NAME   **DATE**   **SECTION**

This lab includes a checklist of common stressors encountered by many college students. Identifying your stressors is the first step in successful stress management.

Equipment: None

Preparation: None

Instructions

Check each event or situation that you have experienced in the past 12 months.

___ Death of close family member

___ Death of close friend

___ Divorce

___ Marital separation

___ Marriage

___ Pregnancy

___ Miscarriage

___ Birth of a child

___ Parents divorce or remarry

___ Starting or ending an intimate relationship

___ Sexual difficulties

___ Dating problems

___ Change in health of close family member

___ Spouse changing careers or going back to school

___ Major incident with the law

___ Jail term

___ Personal injury or illness

___ Chronic car trouble

___ Holidays or vacation

___ Major dental work

___ Major change in eating habits

___ Major change in sleeping habits

___ Major change in physical activity habits

___ Change in social activities

___ Change in religious activities

___ Change in recreation

___ Change in financial state

___ Change in jobs

___ Change in work hours or responsibilities

___ Trouble with boss at work

___ Trouble getting along with coworkers, classmates, or teammates

___ Change in residence

___ Starting, transferring, or dropping out of college

___ Changing academic majors

___ Dropping a course

___ Failing a course

___ Attempting to get a job or internship

___ Significant personal achievement

Results

Count up the total number of events checked and look for patterns and trends. Are most of your stressors things you have some control over and therefore can change (for example, not getting enough sleep, failing a course, changing eating habits)? Or are your stressors major life events that lie out of your control (such as divorce of parents or a death in the family) and require you to find some effective techniques for coping and relaxation? This lab focuses on the first group, but you should take all your stressors seriously and take steps now to make things better. See Lab Activity 10-2 for more on handling high levels of stress.

Total number of checked events

Number of events that can be eliminated, changed, or improved

Number of events that are out of your control

The more events you check, the more likely you are dealing with unusual amounts of stress. Also, people often don't realize all the stress accumulating in their lives. Although major stressors are easy to recognize (such as divorce and death), the little stressors can add up and have just as damaging an effect on our overall wellness. This list helps you keep track of all your stressors, just as keeping a diary helps you see patterns in your daily life.

Reflecting on Your Results

Are you surprised by the total number of stressful events in your life? Did your responses to this quiz match your impression of how much stress you are dealing with?

Planning Your Next Steps

Everyone has stressors they can eliminate or improve through changes in behavior or thinking patterns. Look at the stressors on the list above that you identified as events or situations that you have some control over. Then consult the chapter for tips and techniques on how you might eliminate one or more of those stressors or reduce their impact on you. Consider time management, social support, realistic goal setting and self-talk, and problem solving. Choose a technique you find interesting and appealing, and try it out for a week. Report on your experiences.

Stress-management technique. Describe specifically what you plan on doing during the week to eliminate or improve a stressor:

Results of trying technique. What effect, if any, did the technique you tried have on your stress level? Do you think it changed how you felt or how you acted regarding the stressors you focused on?

SUBMIT ONLINE

NAME	DATE	SECTION

Do you handle stress well, or do you fly off the handle? How we deal with stress goes a long way toward determining our stress-related health outcomes. Handle it well (use appropriate responses, have good levels of social support, regular sleep and exercise, eat well, and so on), and you are likely to minimize your risk of negative health outcomes. Handle your stress poorly (get angry, hold a grudge, resent others, don't get enough sleep or exercise, overeat, and so on), and you are at greater risk for negative health outcomes. This quiz will help you determine how well you are handling the stress in your life.

Equipment: None

Preparation: None

Instructions
Answer the following questions yes or no.

Yes/No

_____ **1.** Do other people frequently irritate you?

_____ **2.** Are you easily irritated when you can't complete a task?

_____ **3.** Do you notice yourself worrying a lot, especially about things you can't influence?

_____ **4.** Do you normally use alcohol, tobacco, or drugs to relax, especially after a hard day?

_____ **5.** Do you often have trouble falling asleep or sleeping through the night?

_____ **6.** Do you frequently experience an upset stomach, which then keeps you from enjoying your food?

_____ **7.** Are you worried about how others judge you?

_____ **8.** Are you always concerned about passing your classes?

_____ **9.** Do you think you will never graduate, or never get a job if you do graduate?

_____ **10.** Do you struggle with letting others contribute to group projects, instead wishing you could do it all yourself?

Results
Although there is no "right" number of yes or no answers, you should take an careful look at your responses and note any patterns.

_____ TOTAL NUMBER OF YES ANSWERS

If you answered yes to a majority of these questions, then you probably struggle to manage your stress, and others might even see you as someone not so pleasant to be around.

Reflecting on Your Results

Were you surprised by the number of yes answers? Did your responses to this quiz match your impression of how well you handle stress in your life?

Planning Your Next Steps

If you need to work on how you handle stress, look back through this chapter for techniques and tips on managing stress, especially the ones that use physical relaxation. Choose one you find interesting and appealing, and try it out for a week. Report on your experiences.

Stress management technique. Describe specifically what you did during the week:

Results of trying technique. What effect, if any, did the technique you tried have on your stress level? Do you think it changed how you felt or how you acted?

11
Chronic Diseases

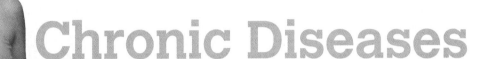

>>> **COMING UP IN THIS CHAPTER**
Learn the major types of cardiovascular disease, cancer, and diabetes › Identify and assess your personal risk factors for these chronic diseases › Become familiar with screening, diagnosis, and treatment options › Take steps to reduce your risk for these diseases

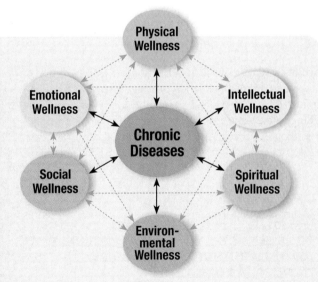

Wellness Connections

How do chronic diseases relate to your overall wellness? Like many of the other topics discussed in this text, the physical wellness component is relatively simple to identify: Chronic diseases have physical signs and symptoms, and these diseases affect our physical functioning. In terms of emotional wellness, the diagnosis of a chronic disease can be devastating, just as test results showing no disease can be a tremendous relief. Even if a chronic disease is in an early stage, the stress of medications, treatments, and lifestyle changes can be overwhelming. It is crucial to seek support from your network of family and friends or other sources of support for people with a chronic disease.

When seeking diagnosis or treatment for chronic diseases, it is also important to make intellectually sound decisions. Second opinions, information from reliable sources, and other critical thinking strategies should be used. Friends and family can help you evaluate your options. Your spiritual wellness is also an important consideration—your values and beliefs may contribute to your treatment options and decisions. Your belief system can also provide comfort and direction.

Environmental factors play a role as well. Was your environment a contributor to your problem? Or can the environment be a part of your solution? Perhaps exploring the beautiful outdoors will help you cope with chronic disease and improve your overall wellness.

Hearing the doctor say *cardiovascular disease, diabetes,* or *cancer* can be very frightening because these chronic diseases sometimes mean death or at least some very difficult times. More than 100 million Americans are living with some form of cardiovascular disease, cancer, or diabetes, and each year, these diseases kill about 1.5 million people, accounting for nearly 70 percent of all U.S. deaths (Table 11-1). Chronic diseases are among the most prevalent and costly of all health problems.

Although many people die from these diseases, it is important to keep in mind that many other people do not—at least not right away. Many forms of cardiovascular disease, diabetes, and, yes, even cancer are treatable and manageable. Perhaps more importantly, these chronic diseases in many instances are preventable diseases. In this chapter, you'll be introduced to the different types of cardiovascular disease, cancer, and diabetes as well as the major risk factors for each. You'll be given opportunities to assess your own disease risk and learn more about common treatment options and prevention measures for each disease.

Cardiovascular Disease

Q | What is cardiovascular disease? How many people die from it?

Cardiovascular disease (CVD) is not a single disease. Rather, it is a broad collection of many diseases that affect the heart (*cardio*) or blood vessels (*vascular*) or both. According to the American Heart Association, approximately 80 million Americans have some form of cardiovascular disease (see Table 11-1). And although deaths due to cardio-

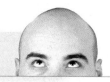

Mind Stretcher
Critical Thinking Exercise

Have you ever thought about your personal risk for cardiovascular disease, cancer, and diabetes? What risk factors do you have? Have you taken any steps to lower your risk for any of these chronic diseases? Why or why not? Are any of your daily health habits influenced by the goal of reducing your future risk of chronic diseases?

vascular disease have declined in the last twenty years, CVD is still responsible for one in every three deaths in the United States.[1]

When working as it should, the heart pumps blood throughout the body, delivering oxygen and nutrients and removing carbon dioxide and cellular waste products via a network of strong and elastic blood vessels. Any problem with the heart or blood vessels decreases the quality of life and increases the risk of death. Chapter 4 described the functioning of a healthy cardiovascular system.

cardiovascular disease (CVD) Any disease that affects the heart (*cardio*) or blood vessels (*vascular*) or both.

coronary artery disease (CAD) Disease of the arteries of the heart characterized by the buildup of fats and other substance and reduction of blood flow.

Types of Cardiovascular Disease

Q | Heart attacks and strokes affect different parts of the body, so why are they always lumped together?

Heart attacks and strokes are both forms of cardiovascular disease (CVD). As mentioned above, CVD is a group of diseases that affect the heart or blood vessels or both. Although a stroke isn't directly related to the heart, it is a result of vascular problems and so it is classified as a form of cardiovascular disease. In fact, stroke is one of the most common types of CVD, responsible for over 100,000 deaths in the United States each year. Other common types of CVD are coronary artery disease, hypertension, heart failure, and peripheral artery disease (Figure 11-1). As you read about the various types of CVD in this section, pay close attention to how they relate to each other. The different types of CVD do not occur in isolation and, unfortunately, having one type of CVD sometimes leads to the development of other types.

Q | What type of cardiovascular disease kills the most people?

CORONARY ARTERY DISEASE. Coronary artery disease (CAD), also sometimes referred to as coronary heart disease (CHD), is the single leading cause of death in

TABLE 11-1 ESTIMATED PREVALENCE AND ANNUAL MORTALITY FROM CARDIOVASCULAR DISEASE, CANCER, AND DIABETES

	PREVALENCE	MORTALITY
CARDIO-VASCULAR DISEASE	81,100,000	830,000
CANCER	11,700,000	570,000
DIABETES	23,500,000	72,500

Sources: American Cancer Society. (2010). *Cancer facts and figures 2010.* Atlanta, GA: American Cancer Society. American Cancer Society. (n.d). Cancer prevalence: What is cancer prevalence? (http://www.cancer.org/cancer/cancerbasics/cancer-prevalence). American Diabetes Association (2010). Diabetes basics: Diabetes statistics (http://www.diabetes.org/diabetes-basics/diabetes-statistics/). American Heart Association. (2010). Cardiovascular disease statistics (http://www.americanheart.org/presenter.jhtml?identifier=4478).

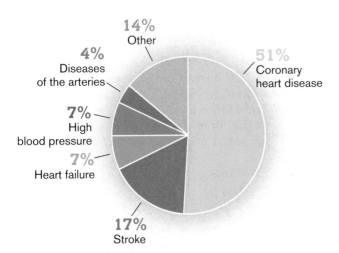

Figure 11-1 Percentage breakdown of U.S. deaths from cardiovascular disease

Source: American Heart Association. (2010). Heart disease and stroke statistics 2010 update: A report from the American Heart Association. *Circulation, 121,* e46–e215.

America. CAD occurs when blood flow in the arteries that feed the heart is inhibited. The most common cause of CAD is **atherosclerosis,** which is the buildup of fats, cholesterol, and other cellular waste products on the lining of the arteries (Figure 11-2). Known as plaque, this buildup narrows the arteries, which reduces blood flow. If the plaque becomes large or it ruptures and creates a clot, the artery may be completely blocked. This is known as an *occlusion.* Atherosclerosis typically begins in childhood

and can worsen with age. It can lead to **arteriosclerosis**—a general hardening, or loss of elasticity, in the arteries.

When atherosclerosis occurs in the coronary arteries—the arteries that supply blood to the heart—the result is coronary artery disease. Atherosclerosis can also affect arteries in other parts of the body. If an artery leading to the brain is affected, the result is a stroke; if an artery in a limb is affected, the condition is called peripheral artery disease. Both of these forms of CVD are described below.

Coronary artery disease often has no symptoms as it develops. When the condition reveals itself, it may be in one of the following ways:

- **Angina pectoris** is chest pain that typically results from reduced blood supply to the heart. The pain often occurs with exercise or stress because the heart isn't receiving enough blood for the demands of increased exertion; the pain quickly subsides with rest. Angina may feel like pressure or a squeezing chest pain that may also radiate to the shoulders, arms, neck, jaw, or back.
- **Heart attack,** also called a myocardial infarction or MI, occurs when the blood supply in one of the coronary arteries is blocked, thus depriving a part of the

atherosclerosis Buildup of plaque in the inner lining of arteries, leading to narrowing, reduction of blood flow, and possible blockage.

arteriosclerosis A chronic disease characterized by abnormal thickening and hardening of the arteries, resulting in loss of elasticity.

angina pectoris Chest pain caused by a reduced blood supply to the heart.

heart attack (myocardial infarction) Damage or death of heart muscle due to insufficient blood supply, usually caused by a blockage in a coronary artery that deprives part of the heart of oxygen.

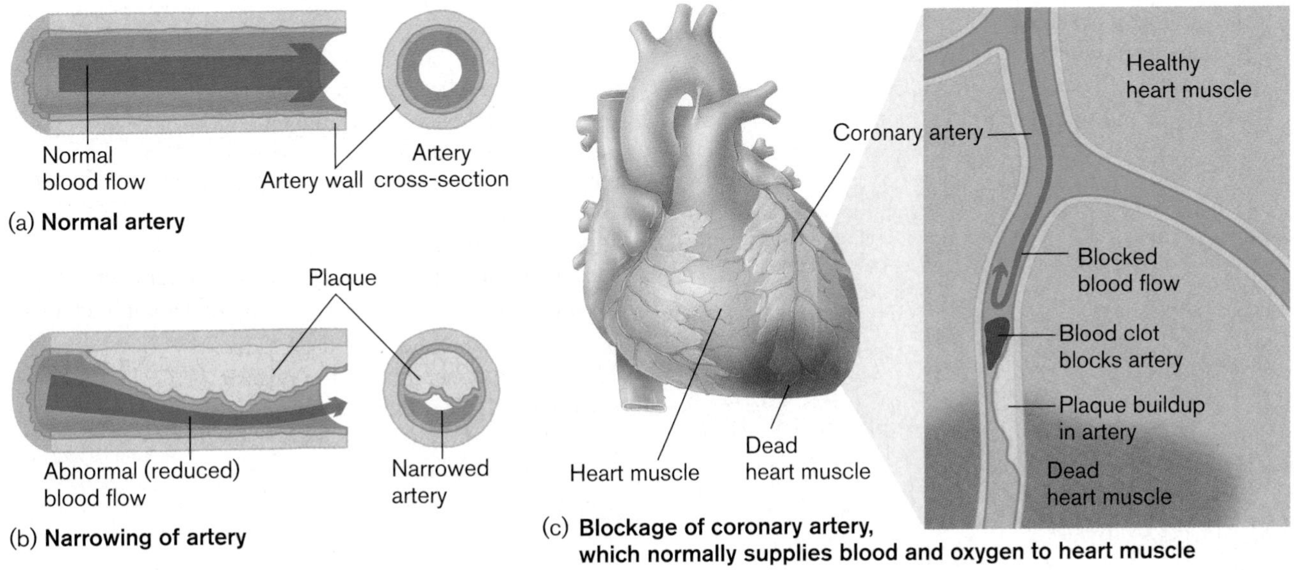

(a) **Normal artery** — Normal blood flow, Artery wall, cross-section, Artery wall

(b) **Narrowing of artery** — Plaque, Abnormal (reduced) blood flow, Narrowed artery

(c) **Blockage of coronary artery, which normally supplies blood and oxygen to heart muscle** — Coronary artery, Heart muscle, Dead heart muscle, Healthy heart muscle, Blocked blood flow, Blood clot blocks artery, Plaque buildup in artery, Dead heart muscle

Figure 11-2 Atherosclerosis and heart attack. Plaque deposits can accumulate and narrow the interior space of an artery, reducing blood flow. If a clot forms and blocks a coronary artery, the result is a heart attack and damage to the heart muscle.

Sources: Adapted from National Heart, Lung, and Blood Institute. (2009). What is atherosclerosis? *Diseases and conditions index* (http://www.nhlbi.nih.gov/health/dci/Diseases/Atherosclerosis/Atherosclerosis_WhatIs.html). NHLBI. (2008). What is a heart attack? *Diseases and conditions index* (http://www.nhlbi.nih.gov/health/dci/Diseases/HeartAttack/HeartAttack_WhatIs.html).

heart of needed oxygen (see Figure 11-2). Unlike angina, the pain associated with a heart attack may occur without exertion, and it doesn't resolve with rest; the pain is also usually more severe than that of angina. Immediate medical attention can help limit the damage to the heart muscle.

- **Arrhythmia** is a change in the normal pattern of the heartbeat. The rhythm may become irregular or too slow or fast. Although some types of arrhythmias are harmless, others prevent the heart from pumping blood effectively and can cause sudden cardiac death. Sudden cardiac death, or **cardiac arrest,** is characterized by a sudden loss of responsiveness, pulse, and blood pressure. It is different from a heart attack, in which the heart usually keeps beating. Cardiac arrest is usually fatal unless treated immediately with CPR or an electrical shock to the heart. Coronary artery disease is a common underlying cause of dangerous arrhythmias.

Risk factors and strategies for preventing coronary artery disease are described later in the chapter.

Q | Is stroke caused by a blocked artery or a burst artery?

STROKE. Either one. **Strokes** are the number-three cause of death in America and are a leading cause of serious disability. A stroke, or "brain attack," occurs when the blood (and oxygen) supply to a part of the brain is suddenly interrupted. If blood flow stops for more than a few seconds, brain cells can die, causing permanent damage (Figure 11-3). There are two major categories of stroke:

- *Ischemic stroke,* in which an artery supplying blood to the brain is blocked by a blood clot. Atherosclerosis is the most common cause of ischemic stroke.
- *Hemorrhagic stroke,* in which a blood vessel bursts, causing blood to leak into the brain. Some people are

An ischemic stroke occurs when a blood vessel supplying the brain becomes blocked, as by a clot.

A hemorrhagic stroke occurs when a blood vessel bursts, leaking blood into the brain.

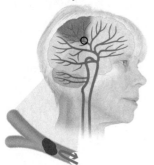 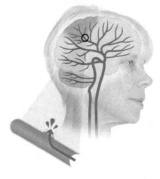

Figure 11-3 Stroke

Source: National Institute of Neurological Disorders and Strokes. (2009). *Stroke: Challenges, progress, and promise.* NIH Publication No. 09-6451.

born with or develop defects in blood vessels that make a hemorrhage more likely to occur.

Sometimes people have **transient ischemic attacks (TIAs),** or "mini-strokes." TIAs are caused by a temporary blockage, and they don't typically cause lasting damage. However, a TIA is a warning sign for a more serious stroke. Strategies for recognizing symptoms of TIAs and strokes are presented later in the chapter.

Q | Can I really get CVD in my arms and legs?

PERIPHERAL ARTERY DISEASE. Yes. As described above, atherosclerosis can occur in arteries anywhere in the body. When it occurs in the limbs, most commonly the legs, the condition is called **peripheral artery disease (PAD).** Many people have mild or no symptoms from PAD, but it can cause leg pain when walking, leg numbness or weakness, and coldness or paleness of the limb. Untreated, PAD can lead to severe infections, causing tissue death and sometimes requiring amputation of the affected limb. Because atherosclerosis in the limbs is typically associated with plaque buildup in other parts of the body, people with PAD are also at increased risk for heart attack and stroke.

Q | If my blood pressure goes up naturally when I exercise, why is high blood pressure so bad?

HIGH BLOOD PRESSURE. Temporary increases in blood pressure are usually fine; consistently high blood pressure is not. Blood pressure refers to the force of blood pushing against the walls of your blood vessels. It is typically reported using two numbers, such as 110/70 mm Hg, with *mm Hg* standing for "millimeters of mercury," the unit used to measure blood pressure. The first, or top, number is the **systolic pressure,** which is the force produced when the heart contracts. The second, or bottom, number is the **diastolic pressure,** which is the force between beats, when the heart is at rest.

Your heart plays a huge role in controlling your blood pressure, and the heart, like any other muscle, typically gets stronger when it is exercised. Consider a comparison to weight lifting. You lift a moderately heavy weight to

arrhythmia Abnormal heart rhythm.

cardiac arrest Sudden temporary or permanent cessation of heartbeat.

stroke Interruption of the blood and oxygen supply to part of the brain; caused by a blocked artery (ischemic stroke) or a ruptured blood vessel (hemorrhagic stroke).

transient ischemic attack (TIA) Temporary blockage of one or more arteries in the brain; doesn't typically cause lasting damage but is a warning sign for a full-blown stroke.

peripheral artery disease (PAD) Damage or dysfunction of arteries in the limbs, most commonly in the legs; usually caused by atherosclerosis and resulting in reduced blood flow.

systolic blood pressure Force of blood on the vessel walls during the contraction of the heart; the top number in a blood pressure reading.

diastolic blood pressure Force of blood on the vessel walls when the heart is at rest (between contractions); the bottom number in a blood pressure reading.

increase muscular strength or endurance, but you would never consider carrying that weight around for extended periods of time. It would be impossible. Your muscles would eventually weaken and you wouldn't be able to carry the weight. The same is true with the heart. The increase in blood pressure that comes with exercise is temporary and strengthens your heart. But sustained high blood pressure, or **hypertension,** leads to weakening of the heart and damage to the blood vessels. (Because your blood pressure can fluctuate, your doctor will likely test you at least three different times before confirming a hypertension diagnosis.)

Sometimes hypertension is a result of other conditions, such as kidney or adrenal gland problems. In these cases, addressing the underlying cause often eliminates the related hypertension. However, in the majority of cases (90–95 percent), the direct cause of hypertension is unknown. There is strong correlation with atherosclerosis and other vascular conditions: As blood vessels affected by atherosclerosis become less elastic, they are less able to expand and thus resist the flow of blood the heart is pumping. Blood pressure increases, straining both the heart and the blood vessels.

As mentioned above, hypertension is one of the more common forms of cardiovascular disease. It is also one of the forms of CVD that can lead to other diseases, including heart attack, stroke, and heart failure.

Q | For blood pressure, how high is too high?

For adults, recommended systolic pressure is less than 120 and diastolic pressure less than 80 (Table 11-2). If your systolic or diastolic blood pressure number is too high, your blood pressure is classified according to that number. It's important for young adults to achieve healthy blood pressure levels because blood pressure tends to rise with age. Luckily, there are many strategies you can adopt to help keep your blood pressure in the healthy range throughout your life.

Although less common, some people have low blood pressure (hypotension), which is classified as a systolic pressure below 90 or diastolic pressure below 60, or both. Consistently low blood pressure can be normal for some and is usually considered a problem only if it causes symptoms such as dizziness or fainting or if it's due to an underlying medical condition. Consistently low blood pressure is different from a sudden drop in blood pressure due to something like bleeding or an allergic reaction; such a drop would be considered dangerous.

Q | Is heart failure the same as a heart attack?

HEART FAILURE. No, but a heart attack can lead to **heart failure.** Heart failure basically means your heart isn't doing its job adequately. It's still pumping, but it isn't able to get enough blood to the body's organs and tissues. This lack of blood supply often leads to shortness of breath, fatigue, and fluid buildup. The fluid buildup can lead to swelling in the ankles or other parts of the body. It can also affect the ability of the kidneys to eliminate fluid, leading to additional swelling as well as fluid buildup in the lungs, which impedes breathing. Heart failure complicated by fluid buildup is referred to as *congestive heart failure.*

Heart failure can develop suddenly or over time. It often results from complications of other forms of cardiovascular disease.

OTHER FORMS OF CARDIOVASCULAR DISEASE. A number of other conditions can also affect cardiovascular health. Some people are born with defects in their heart or major blood vessels; such problems may be repaired with surgery during infancy or may not be discovered until many years later. In other cases, problems may develop as result of infection or underlying atherosclerosis.

Q | What can be done to eliminate a heart murmur?

In most cases, a so-called heart murmur has no ill effects, and no treatment is needed. The diagnosis of

hypertension Sustained high blood pressure.

heart failure A condition in which the heart is unable to pump blood at a sufficient rate or volume, resulting in insufficient blood flow to the organs and tissues and, in some cases, fluid buildup.

TABLE 11-2 BLOOD PRESSURE CLASSIFICATION FOR ADULTS AGE 18 AND OLDER

CATEGORY	SYSTOLIC (TOP NUMBER)		DIASTOLIC (BOTTOM NUMBER)
NORMAL	LESS THAN 120	*AND*	LESS THAN 80
PRE-HYPERTENSION	120–139	*OR*	80–89
HYPERTENSION, STAGE 1	140–159	*OR*	90–99
HYPERTENSION, STAGE 2	160+	*OR*	100+

Source: *Seventh Report of the Joint National Committee on Prevention, Detection, Evaluation and Treatment of High Blood Pressure.* (2003, May). NIH Publication No. 03-52333.

"heart murmur" refers to a variety of conditions involving the valves in the heart. Normally, heart valves work in a coordinated fashion—they open to let blood flow in or out of the heart and then close to stop blood from flowing backward. If a valve doesn't open all the way, blood flow is blocked or reduced. If a valve doesn't close all the way or tightly enough, blood can leak back through the valve in the wrong direction.

Valve problems can result from inherited defects, infections, or heart disease. The most common problem, affecting about 2 percent of adults, is with the mitral valve, located between the left atrium and left ventricle. If the valve is floppy or bulges (prolapses) slightly, a physician listening to the heart may hear a murmur. In most people, *mitral valve prolapse* (MVP) is harmless and requires no treatment or lifestyle changes. People with severe MVP or other more serious valve problems may be treated with medication or surgery. Antibiotics used to be recommended before certain dental and medical procedures for all people with MVP to prevent infection of the heart valve; however, antibiotics are currently recommended for only a small proportion of people with MVP. If you have any questions about your own situation, check with your physician.

Q | What causes varicose veins—and how can I avoid getting them?

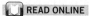 READ ONLINE

Fast Facts

Around the World in What?

- The adult body contains billions of arteries, veins, and capillaries. If all the blood vessels were laid end to end, they would extend about 100,000 miles—enough to encircle the earth four times.

- At any given time, about 70 percent of your blood is in your veins; the rest is in your arteries and capillaries.

- Because the three types of blood vessels carry blood at different pressures, injuries to different blood vessels result in different types of bleeding. Arterial bleeding tends to spurt; capillary bleeding tends to ooze; and venous bleeding tends to be a steady flow.

Sources: Franklin Institute. (2010). Blood vessels. *The human heart* (http://www.fi.edu/learn/heart/vessels/vessels.html). National Cancer Institute. (n.d.). Classification and structure of blood vessels. *SEER Training Modules* (http://training.seer.cancer.gov/anatomy/cardiovascular/blood/classification.html). Community Emergency Response Team. (n.d.). Types of bleeding. *Disaster medical operations principles and guidelines for victim care* (http://www.citizencorps.gov/cert/IS317/medops/medops/ic_04_02_0091.htm).

Assessing Your Risk for Cardiovascular Disease: Factors You Cannot Control

Q | Who is most at risk of getting cardiovascular disease?

Because one in three Americans dies from cardiovascular disease, everyone is at risk in some way and to some degree. However, some people are at much higher risk than others. As a rule, people with a family history of cardiovascular disease (CVD) are more at risk that those without, men are more at risk than women, African Americans are at greater risk than Caucasians, and people over 65 are more at risk than those who are younger. These are not the only factors contributing to CVD risk, and it's extremely important to evaluate which of your risk factors you can change (modify or alter) and which you cannot. This section describes factors over which you have little control, including heredity, age, gender, and ethnicity. The next section describes factors that you can change, such as diet, smoking, alcohol consumption, and stress.

Q | Is there any way you can reverse genetically predisposed heart problems?

HEREDITY/GENETICS. Maybe not entirely reverse—but there are many things you can do. We have long known that people with a family history of cardiovascular disease are more likely than others to develop CVD themselves. That's one of the reasons it's important to know your family health history. Recently, specific genes have been identified that are responsible for some inherited cardiovascular disorders.[2] Types of CVD that may be caused by inherited traits include certain forms of cardiomyopathy (enlarged and weakened heart muscle), arrhythmia, and aneurysm, as well as Marfan's syndrome, a connective tissue disorder that may affect the heart.

Treatment for inherited forms of CVD is the same as for other forms. The advantages to knowing if you have a genetic predisposition for CVD is that you can seek early treatment and prevention of additional forms of CVD, and your family members can be tested for potential CVD problems.

Q | Why does getting older make a person more likely to have CVD?

AGE. According to the American Heart Association, the prevalence of CVD rises with age, from less than 15 percent among those under age 40 to over 70 percent among those over age 60.[3] This is primarily due to wear and tear on the heart and blood vessels. Over time, there are changes in the structure and functioning of the heart and in the ability of blood vessels to relax and contract.[4] These changes contribute to all forms of cardiovascular disease; for example, Figure 11-4 shows the increasing prevalence of high blood pressure with age.

The association between aging and CVD doesn't mean it is inevitable or that older people can't have a healthy heart and live active, productive lives. It just means there is no denying that time and use take a toll.

Q | Why do more men have heart attacks than women?

GENDER. More men develop and die from cardiovascular disease than women—and they do so at younger ages (Figure 11-5). There isn't a single clear reason for this discrepancy. Researchers attribute the differences to a number of factors, including higher rates of smoking, excess alcohol use, and other negative lifestyle choices among men. There may be biological causes as well. Premenopausal women tend to have better cholesterol profiles than men, and although the cause for this is still being studied, increased estrogen levels and other hormonal differences are thought to play a key role.[5] Long

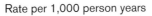
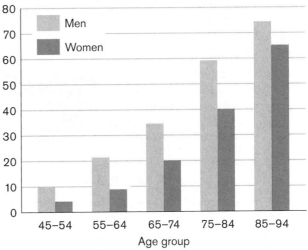

Figure 11-5 **Incidence of cardiovascular disease among adults age 20 and over, by age and sex.** The rates here include coronary artery disease, stroke, heart failure, and PAD.

Source: American Heart Association. (2010). Heart disease and stroke statistics 2010 update: A report from the American Heart Association. *Circulation, 121,* e46–e215.

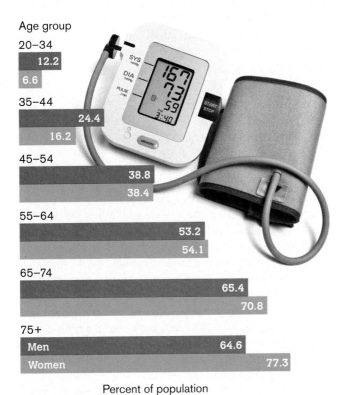

Figure 11-4 **Prevalence of high blood pressure among adults age 20 and over, by age and sex.** The risk of hypertension rises steadily with age. Hypertension is defined as having systolic blood pressure of 140 or over, having diastolic blood pressure of 90 or over, taking antihypertensive medication, or being diagnosed with hypertension twice by a medical professional.

Source: American Heart Association. (2010). Heart disease and stroke statistics 2010 update: A report from the American Heart Association. *Circulation, 121,* e46–e215.

before signs of CVD appear, these hormonal differences affect the cardiovascular system. (See p. 390 for more information on cholesterol.)

It should be noted, however, that although more men have heart attacks, women are more likely to die from them.[6] Because most women have heart attacks later in life, they tend to be sicker and to have more risk factors and other diseases, which can complicate diagnosis and treatment. Certain types of medications also appear to work better in men than in women.

Additional studies are being conducted to determine other possible reasons for the difference in CVD prevalence and mortality among men and women. Studies examining the differences in heart physiology and heart rhythms look promising.

Q | How does ethnicity affect cardiovascular disease? What group or groups are most at risk?

ETHNICITY. Studies have found different rates of CVD and associated risk factors among different ethnic groups. African Americans have a higher prevalence of CVD overall and of high blood pressure and strokes in particular; in fact, African American adults have the highest rate of hypertension in the world.[7] Asian Americans and Latinos have a lower prevalence of heart disease than other groups, and Asian Americans have a significantly lower prevalence of stroke. As a group, American Indians and Alaska Natives have the highest prevalence of stroke.

Reasons for the differences among ethnic groups are complex, but socioeconomic factors as well as significant

Fast Facts

Heart at Work

The smaller the animal, the faster its heart rate: A hummingbird's heart beats about 1,200 times per minute when the bird is feeding, while that of an elephant beats about 30 times per minute.

The human heart beats about . . .

- 70 times per minute
- 100,000 times in one day
- 35 million times in a year
- 2.5 billion times during an average lifetime

The human heart pumps about . . .

- 2,000 gallons of blood in one day
- 700,000 gallons of blood in a year
- 50 million gallons of blood during an average lifetime

Source: NOVA Online. *Amazing heart facts* (http://www.pbs.org/wgbh/nova/heart/heartfacts.html).

differences in modifiable CVD risk factors may play a role. For example, Latinos have a significantly lower rate of smoking than African Americans or Caucasians, but American Indians and Alaska Natives have a higher rate of smoking than other groups. Latinos, African Americans, and American Indians and Alaska Natives have higher rates of diabetes. Rates of leisure-time physical activity are low among all groups but particularly low among Latinas.[8] (These and other modifiable risk factors are discussed in more detail in the prevention section of the chapter.)

There may also be biological differences among the groups. For example, researchers have found higher levels of salt sensitivity among African Americans, meaning their blood pressure goes up in response to salt consumption.[9] These findings have led to a lower recommended sodium intake target for African Americans; see Chapter 8 for more information.

Cardiovascular Disease Prevention

Controllable factors can also affect your risk for cardiovascular disease. Unlike the unchangeable factors of heredity, gender, age, and ethnicity discussed in the previous section, you can modify factors related to your lifestyle in order to reduce your risk of CVD.

Q How can one avoid CV disease and high blood pressure?

You can make lifestyle changes related to your diet; use of tobacco, alcohol, and drugs; and stress. And you can get your blood pressure

and cholesterol levels checked regularly. The lifestyle factors discussed in this section, because they can be changed or modified, are both risk factors and prevention strategies. As is the case with other areas of your health, when it comes to preventing CVD, your lifestyle choices have the greatest impact.

Q Are people who can eat all they want and not gain weight still at risk for cardiovascular disease?

CHOOSE A HEALTHY DIET AND ACTIVITY LEVEL AND CONTROL YOUR WEIGHT. Yes, because body weight and food choices are only part of what affects our risk for cardiovascular disease. Aside from the factors of genes, age, gender, and ethnicity, you're leaving out physical activity. Even for someone who doesn't seem to gain weight, weight maintenance isn't possible unless energy intake is balanced with energy output.

In addition, being physically active directly reduces your risk for CVD. Regular moderate exercise increases cardiovascular capacity by strengthening the heart and improving the elasticity of the arteries. Regular exercise also helps control of cholesterol, high blood pressure, diabetes, and body weight. All these factors combine to reduce CVD risk. See Chapter 4 for more on setting up a program for developing cardiorespiratory fitness.

Q If you have excellent cardiovascular fitness but CVD runs in your family, do you have a greater risk than someone with no family history of CVD?

This is a tough question to answer because to consider only fitness and genetics ignores other important factors that affect risk: How old are the two people? What gender? Do they smoke? How much do they drink? What types of foods do they consume? These factors, along with a number of others, will give a more complete picture of risk. Although an increased level of fitness certainly helps to prevent CVD, it may or may not balance out the other factors.

You are a sum of all of your risk factors—those that can be modified and those that can't—so examining only part of the equation can't give an accurate answer. It's like trying to see the full picture when you've only matched the first couple of pieces in the puzzle.

To assess your overall risk for cardiovascular disease, complete Lab Activity 11-1.

Q What types of foods help prevent cardiovascular disease? Does salt affect CVD?

Yes, salt can affect cardiovascular disease by raising blood pressure in sensitive people. The effect of salt on blood pressure is one of the reasons the Dietary Reference Intakes set a limit for sodium (see Chapter 8). CVD risk can also be affected by fat intake; for heart health, it's recommended that you choose unsaturated fats and limit your intake of saturated and *trans* fats. The best food plan is balanced and moderate: Eat more fiber-rich whole grains, fruits, vegetables, legumes, fat-free and low-fat dairy products, and seafood. Limit excess calorie intake from added sugars, unhealthy fats, cholesterol, and highly processed foods. If you drink alcohol, keep your intake moderate. See Chapters 8 and 9 for more on limiting salt intake and putting together a healthy dietary plan. The DASH diet is especially recommended for people who are salt sensitive or have high blood pressure.

Q If I'm overweight, is my risk a lot higher?

Yes. Added weight puts added stress on the heart. The degree of extra stress depends on how overweight you are—the greater the weight, the greater the stress on the heart. If you're just a few pounds overweight, the stress is not as great. You would, however, still decrease your risk if you lost the extra weight. If you're severely overweight, your risk is considerably higher. The risk for cardiovascular disease increases by about 20 percent in people who are overweight. Among people who are obese, CVD risk goes up 46 percent in men and 64 percent in women.[10]

People with excessive body fat are more likely to develop cardiovascular diseases even if they have no other risk factors. Unfortunately, other risk factors often accompany overweight or obesity. Excess body fat is linked to increased cholesterol and blood pressure levels and increased risk for type 2 diabetes. As described in Chapter 7, people with more abdominal fat (apple shape) are at greater risk than those who carry their excess fat in the hip area (pear shape).

Increased physical activity and a balanced diet are CVD prevention strategies that have a direct effect on overweight and obesity. Remember, however, obesity is a complex condition that may involve genetic and other factors. If you are severely overweight or obese, see your doctor before beginning additional activities or making significant changes to your diet. See Chapters 7 and 9 for more information on evaluating your body composition and setting appropriate goals.

Q Smoking causes cancer, not cardiovascular disease—right?

AVOID TOBACCO. Wrong. Smoking not only increases cancer risk, but it also significantly increases risk for cardiovascular disease. Smokers have twice the risk of heart attack of nonsmokers and are more likely than nonsmokers to die suddenly from heart attacks.[11] Smoking contributes to CVD in a number of ways. Smoking affects fatty buildup in the arteries by negatively affecting good and bad cholesterol levels (more on this below). Smoking also increases heart rate, contributes to arrhythmias, increases blood pressure, reduces the oxygen level in the

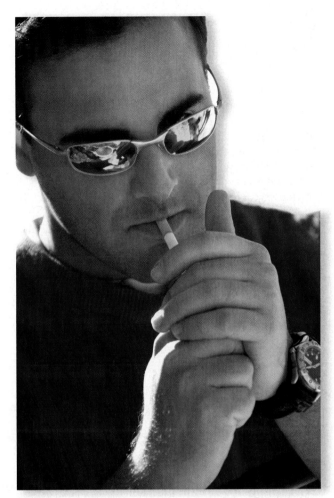

Although most people associate smoking with cancer risk, smoking is also one of the biggest contributors to cardiovascular disease. If you smoke, quit. If you've tried and failed to quit, keep trying.

blood, and may trigger blood clots. Almost all cases of peripheral artery disease occur in smokers, and smokers face greater complications from the disease, including amputations, than do nonsmokers. Smoking also limits the capacity to exercise—which is one of the few things that might help reverse some of smoking's negative effects.

Q How long does it take to recover your cardio fitness after quitting smoking?

The good news is the body slowly begins to heal as soon as someone quits smoking. According to the U.S. Surgeon General, the risk of CVD is reduced by 50 percent after just one year as a nonsmoker.[12] Your cardiorespiratory fitness still has to be developed through aerobic fitness. The length of time to restore it depends on the amount and length of time you smoked as well as the frequency, intensity, and duration of your activities.

See Chapter 13 for more on the effects of smoking and strategies for quitting.

Q | Does alcohol affect cardio-vascular disease? What about other drugs?

KEEP ALCOHOL USE MODERATE AND AVOID DRUGS. The effects of alcohol use can be positive or negative.[13] Research has found an association between moderate alcohol intake and reduced risk of cardiovascular disease. Moderate intake of alcohol is defined as no more than two drinks per day for men or one drink per day for women—with one drink being the equivalent of 12 ounces of beer, 5 ounces of wine, or 1.5 ounces of 80-proof spirits (see Chapter 13).

The underlying cause for the benefit of moderate alcohol consumption is unclear, but alcohol use is associated with a small increase in HDL (good cholesterol). Another possible effect may be reduced clot formation, which can reduce the risk of heart attack and stroke. Some components in grapes and red wine, including flavonoids and resveratrol, have received special attention by researchers; these compounds act as antioxidants and may also relax the blood vessels and reduce blood pressure.[14]

On the other hand, drinking too much alcohol on a regular basis or in binge episodes has many negative cardiovascular effects. It is linked to high blood pressure, heart failure, arrhythmia, stroke, and sudden cardiac death. Excessive alcohol intake can also contribute to obesity because alcohol is relatively high in calories.

Refer to Table 11-3 for information on the effects of selected other drugs on CVD.

Q | Is stress a major factor in cardiovascular disease?

MANAGE STRESS IN HEALTHY WAYS. At this point there is no exact scientific proof of a direct cause-and-effect relationship between stress and cardiovascular disease. However, there are a number of likely possible connections. The acute stress response can raise blood pressure and change heart rhythms, and over time the hormones associated with uncontrolled stress may alter glucose and blood fat levels. However, the strongest link between stress and health may be in how we choose to

TABLE 11-3 DRUGS AND RELATED CARDIOVASCULAR DISEASE COMPLICATIONS

ANABOLIC STEROIDS (NONMEDICAL USE)	Abuse can lower HDL and raise LDL; increase the risk of atherosclerosis, hypertension, stroke, and heart attack; and may also cause blood clots and enlargement of the ventricles of the heart.
CAFFEINE	Probably safe in moderate amounts, according to the American Heart Association. Research studies on the links between caffeine and CVD have yielded conflicting results.
COCAINE	Use can lead to overstimulation of the heart, resulting in increased risk for heart attack, stroke, high blood pressure, heart failure, blood clots, enlargement of the heart, and infections of the heart lining. Further complications may include aneurysm and aortic dissection (splitting of the inner wall of the aorta), both of which can be fatal.
HEROIN	Injection use can cause permanent damage to veins. Users are also more susceptible to blood vessel blockages and blood clots, heart attack, stroke, and infections of the heart lining.
INHALANTS	Some types can cause rapid and irregular heart rhythms, leading to heart failure; other types reduce the oxygen-carrying capacity of the blood and harm the heart muscle.
MARIJUANA	Use increases heart rate and blood pressure and reduces the oxygen-carrying capability of the blood, which can strain the cardiorespiratory system. Marijuana smoke contains some of the same harmful chemicals as cigarette smoke, and research suggests a possible increased risk for heart attack and stroke among heavy users and older users.
METHAMPHETAMINE	Use increases heart rate and blood pressure and damage to blood vessels in the brain. Overdose is linked to heart attack and stroke.

Sources: Adapted from American Heart Association. (2010). *Cocaine, marijuana, and other drugs* (http://www.americanheart.org/presenter.jhtml?identifier=4552). American Heart Association. (2010, May 20). *AHA recommendation: Caffeine* (http://www.heart.org/HEARTORG/GettingHealthy/NutritionCenter/Caffeine_UCM_305888_Article.jsp). National Institute of Drug Abuse. (2010). Inhalant abuse. *Research report series* (http://www.nida.nih.gov/researchreports/inhalants/other.html). National Institute on Drug Abuse. (2010). Marijuana abuse. *Research report series* (http://www.nida.nih.gov/ResearchReports/Marijuana).

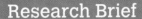

Research Brief

Don't Worry, Be Happy

Researchers have looked at psychological and social influences on cardiovascular disease risk. In one recent large-scale study, adults were followed for ten years and assessed for symptoms of depression, hostility, and anxiety as well as for the expression of positive emotions—happiness, enthusiasm, joy, and contentment. The researchers found that the happiest people had a lower risk of angina and heart attacks compared to those who were moderately happy and, especially, those who were unhappy, anxious, and depressed.

How do positive emotions reduce CVD? Researchers speculate that the happier, more satisfied people may

handle stress better, sleep better, and practice more heart-healthy lifestyle behaviors. All these differences can contribute to better heart health.

What does this mean for you? Along with other established CVD prevention strategies—not smoking, eating right, staying active—try to also do more of the things that make you happy.

Source: Davidson, K. W., Mostofsky, E., & Whang, W. (2010). Don't worry, be happy: Positive affect and reduced 10-year incident coronary heart disease: The Canadian Nova Scotia Health Survey. *European Heart Journal, 31*(9), 1065–1070.

---

manage stress—especially if we do so in a negative way. Without good coping skills or appropriate stress management techniques, people may choose negative outlets for stress such as overeating or increasing tobacco or alcohol use. These actions, in turn, have a direct negative impact on cardiovascular health. See Chapter 10 for more information on finding healthy ways to manage your stress.

Q | How often do I have to get my blood pressure and cholesterol checked?

HAVE REGULAR SCREENINGS. Regular screenings are very important, but blood pressure and cholesterol aren't the only things you should have checked. You should have regular screenings for blood pressure, cholesterol, triglycerides, and diabetes. Regular, however, doesn't mean the same frequency for each of these factors.

- *Blood pressure:* Unless your doctor recommends otherwise, the American College of Physicians recommends that blood pressure be measured in adults every one to two years. Your doctor may recommend a different frequency based on your results.
- *Cholesterol and triglycerides:* For adults over 20, cholesterol should be checked every five years unless your doctor recommends more frequent screening due to high levels or other risk factors.
- *Diabetes:* Screening is recommended for all adults age 45 and

older and for younger people who have risk factors, including overweight.

You can use the results of your screening tests to take appropriate action, if needed, to reduce your risk for CVD.

Q | What can I do to lower my blood pressure?

REDUCE ELEVATED BLOOD PRESSURE. There are many steps you can take to lower your blood pressure if it is high (see the blood pressure classifications in Table 11-2). It's important to address blood pressure even if it's only slightly elevated, in the pre-hypertension range. Young adults with pre-hypertension are more likely to develop atherosclerosis over time than those with healthy blood pressure.[15]

You'll notice blood pressure has been mentioned many times in this chapter—it keeps reappearing because it is so important. First, hypertension is a type of cardiovascular disease. Second, it is a risk factor for other types of CVD. And third, addressing hypertension is a prevention strategy because keeping your blood pressure in check can help prevent CVD and complications from many conditions.

Other prevention strategies described in this section can have a positive affect on blood pressure. Eating a balanced diet that is low in sodium, engaging in regular physical activity, maintaining a healthy weight, limiting alcohol consumption, and avoiding smoking can all help reduce your risk for hypertension. If you can't maintain healthy blood

DOLLAR STRETCHER
Financial Wellness Tip

If you don't have a regular source of medical care, take advantage of free blood pressure screenings. Many campuses and community health departments offer free blood pressure checks, free glucose tests, and other screenings. Check with the campus health center.

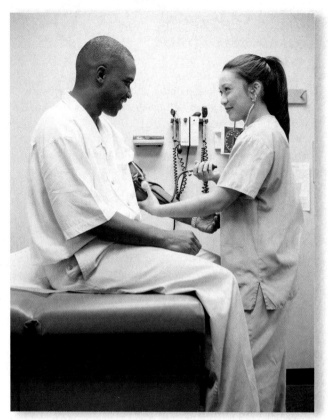

High blood pressure often has no symptoms, but even slightly elevated blood pressure harms the cardiovascular system. Everyone should get their blood pressure checked regularly and take steps to reduce it if it is elevated.

pressure with lifestyle measures, many types of medications are available.

Q | How does the fat in the foods I eat affect my cholesterol levels?

MAINTAIN HEALTHY CHOLESTEROL AND TRIGLYCERIDE LEVELS. Cholesterol and triglycerides are found both in foods and your blood, but the connections between the foods you eat and the fats (lipids) in your blood are complex. **Cholesterol** is a waxy substance that occurs naturally in all cells of the body. It is produced by the liver and obtained in the diet; it is carried by the blood and is used to maintain cell walls and to produce certain hormones. Although it's a needed substance, excess cholesterol can build up on artery walls and increase your risk for cardiovascular disease.

To understand how cholesterol affects your risk for CVD, recall the types of cholesterol that were introduced in Chapter 8:

- **Low-density lipoprotein (LDL)** is known as bad cholesterol because it tends to deposit cholesterol on artery walls, thus limiting blood flow and increasing the risk for CVD.

- **High-density lipoprotein (HDL)** is known as good cholesterol because it carries excess cholesterol back to the liver so it can be eliminated from the body.

You want a low level of LDL and a high level of HDL. **Triglycerides** are another common fat that is found in both foods and the body; high blood levels of triglycerides are also linked to increased CVD risk.

To help assess a person's risk for CVD, blood-fat screening is recommended every five years for adults. It's a blood test, done after 9–12 hours of fasting. The results typically include values for total cholesterol, HDL, LDL, and triglycerides (Table 11-4). Based on the results, your physician may recommend specific lifestyle strategies.

Elevated LDL levels may be caused by genetic factors that affect the liver's production of cholesterol, or they may be the result of excessive intake of dietary cholesterol or, especially, saturated and *trans* fats. (Eating saturated and *trans* fats encourages the body to produce more total cholesterol and LDL; *trans* fats also decrease HDL.)

Triglyceride levels tend to increase with age, but high levels can be found in people of any age. Risk factors for high triglyceride levels include overweight, inactivity, cigarette smoking, excessive alcohol use, and diets very high in carbohydrate. A high level of triglycerides, like elevated cholesterol, appears to facilitate the development of atherosclerosis.

To improve cholesterol and triglyceride levels, the following lifestyle measures are recommended:

- Choose unsaturated fats over saturated and *trans* fats.
- Eat fish, especially oily fish, two or more times per week (see Chapter 8 for more on the omega-3 fatty acids in fish).
- Get recommended amounts of dietary fiber, while keeping intake of refined carbohydrates and added sugars low.
- Avoid excess alcohol consumption.
- Maintain a healthy weight.
- Be physically active.
- Avoid tobacco.

Because elevated cholesterol levels are sometimes genetic, prevention strategies may have a limited effect for some people. But "limited effect" does not mean "no effect," and these strategies are important for overall good health.

It's also important not to wait to address unhealthy cholesterol and triglyceride levels. Young adults may not be likely to have a heart attack within the next few years, but that doesn't

cholesterol A fat, waxy substance produced by the liver and consumed from animal products; excess cholesterol in the bloodstream can be deposited on artery walls.

low-density lipoprotein (LDL) A type of lipoprotein that circulates in the blood and deposits cholesterol on artery walls, increasing the risk of cardiovascular disease; also known as bad cholesterol.

high-density lipoprotein (HDL) A type of lipoprotein that circulates in the blood and carries excess cholesterol back to the liver for elimination from the body; also known as good cholesterol.

triglycerides The most common form of fat in foods and in the body; high blood levels of triglycerides increase risk for CVD.

TABLE 11-4 CHOLESTEROL AND TRIGLYCERIDE CLASSIFICATION

	RISK CATEGORY
TOTAL CHOLESTEROL LEVEL	
LESS THAN 200 MG/DL	Desirable
200–239 MG/DL	Borderline high
240 MG/DL AND ABOVE	High blood cholesterol
LDL CHOLESTEROL LEVEL	
LESS THAN 100 MG/DL	Optimal
100–129 MG/DL	Near or above optimal
130–159 MG/DL	Borderline high
160–189 MG/DL	High
190 MG/DL AND ABOVE	Very high
HDL CHOLESTEROL LEVEL	
LESS THAN 40 MG/DL	A major risk factor for heart disease
40–59 MG/DL	The higher, the better
60 MG/DL AND ABOVE	Considered protective against heart disease
TRIGLYCERIDE LEVEL	
LESS THAN 150 MG/DL	Normal
150–199 MG/DL	Borderline high
200–499 MG/DL	High
500 MG/DL AND ABOVE	Very high

Note: These values apply to healthy adults. For people with heart disease or diabetes, the targets for LDL cholesterol and triglycerides may be lower.

Source: National Heart, Lung, and Blood Institute. (2001). *Third report of the National Cholesterol Education Program Expert Panel on Detection and Evaluation, and Treatment of High Blood Cholesterol in Adults: Executive summary.* NIH Publication No. 01-3670.

mean they can ignore their cholesterol levels. Young adults with unhealthy blood lipid levels are much more likely to have buildup in their arteries when they reach middle age than those without abnormal levels.[16] Don't wait to adopt healthy eating and exercise habits—what you do in your younger years matters.

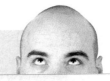

Mind Stretcher
Critical Thinking Exercise

Have you had the recommended screening tests for CVD, cancer, and diabetes? Why or why not? If not, what could you do to make them a priority and obtain them at recommended intervals? Think about what state of change best described you in terms of obtaining recommended screening tests. Develop three appropriate strategies for moving forward in the cycle of change. Refer to Chapter 2 for more information on behavior change.

Q | Why does diabetes affect the heart?

CONTROL DIABETES. People with diabetes are two to four times more likely to develop cardiovascular disease than nondiabetics, and at least 65 percent of people with diabetes die from some form of heart disease or stroke.[17] Over time, elevated blood glucose levels associated with diabetes damage nerves and blood vessels and contribute to atherosclerosis. Diabetes is often accompanied by other CVD risk factors, including hypertension, high lipid levels, and increased weight. Elevated blood glucose levels can harm the cardiovascular system even if they aren't high enough for a diagnosis of full-blown diabetes. High blood glucose levels are one of the five traits that define **metabolic syndrome,** a cluster of medical conditions that puts people at risk for both heart disease and type 2 diabetes. A person who has at least three of the five traits listed in Table 11-5 is classified as having metabolic syndrome.

Following the CVD prevention strategies described earlier will help to reduce your risk for diabetes and metabolic syndrome. Diabetes will be discussed in more detail later in the chapter. For a summary of strategies to protect yourself from CVD, refer to the box "Preventing Cardiovascular Disease."

Symptoms, Diagnosis, and Treatment of Cardiovascular Disease

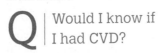

Q | Would I know if I had CVD?

Maybe, but maybe not. Some forms of cardiovascular disease have no visible symptoms. Even if there are some observable symptoms, you may still need further testing to determine whether you have CVD.

metabolic syndrome A group of risk factors linked to overweight and obesity that increase the chance of heart disease, diabetes, and stroke: large waistline, low HDL, and elevated triglycerides, fasting blood sugar, and blood pressure.

TABLE 11-5 METABOLIC SYNDROME*

TRAITS/MEDICAL CONDITIONS	DEFINITION
LARGE WAIST CIRCUMFERENCE	■ 40 inches (102 cm) or more in men ■ 35 inches (88 cm) or more in women
ELEVATED LEVELS OF TRIGLYCERIDES	■ 150 mg/dl or higher **or** ■ Taking medication for elevated triglyceride levels
LOW LEVELS OF HDL (GOOD) CHOLESTEROL	■ Below 40 mg/dl in men ■ Below 50 mg/dl in women ■ **or** taking medication for low HDL cholesterol levels
ELEVATED BLOOD PRESSURE LEVELS	■ 130 mm Hg or higher for systolic blood pressure **or** ■ 85 mm Hg or higher for diastolic blood pressure **or** ■ Taking medication for elevated blood pressure levels
ELEVATED FASTING BLOOD GLUCOSE LEVELS	■ 100 mg/dl or higher **or** ■ Taking medication for elevated blood glucose levels

*Metabolic syndrome is defined as having three or more of the traits/conditions listed.

Source: Grundy, S. M., and others. (2005). Diagnosis and management of the metabolic syndrome: An American Heart Association/National Heart, Lung, and Blood Institute scientific statement. *Circulation, 112,* 2735–2752.

Q Does cardio-vascular disease hurt? Would it affect my everyday activities?

SYMPTOMS. It depends. Different types of cardiovascular disease have different symptoms. Some are painful and some are not. For example, hypertension typically doesn't have any noticeable symptoms, but heart attacks and strokes can be very painful. Other types of CVD, such as heart failure, have longer-lasting complications that may or may not be painful. Shortness of breath or swelling of the legs and ankles, for example, may make day-to-day activities difficult or even painful. Signs of CVD include chest pain, fatigue, shortness of breath, leg pain, palpitations (the sensation of irregular or forceful heartbeat), and lightheadedness and fainting.

Q How can you tell if a person is having a heart attack or a stroke?

Each has clear warning signs that you can learn to recognize—and it's important to react appropriately if you do spot any symptoms. Call 911 or the appropriate emergency number if you detect any of the signs listed in Table 11-6. Prompt treatment can increase the chance of survival and limit the damage caused by the heart attack or stroke. Women may be less likely to believe or recognize they're having a heart attack and more likely to delay treatment. As it is for men, the most common heart attack symptom for women is chest pain or discomfort. But women are somewhat more likely than men to experience other symptoms, including shortness of breath, nausea, and back or jaw pain.

Q When are you supposed to use CPR?

Cardiopulmonary resuscitation, or CPR, is a form of artificial blood circulation and respiration. Basic CPR consists of chest compressions alternated with rescue breathing (mouth-to-mouth respiration) at a ratio of thirty compressions to two breaths. Compression-only CPR, with chest compressions delivered at the rate of one hundred per minute without any rescue breaths, has been found to be an equally effective technique and is now also endorsed by the American Heart Association.[18]

CPR is used for victims of cardiac arrest, or when the heart suddenly stops beating or beats so irregularly that oxygenated blood isn't being pumped to the brain and the rest of the body. Victims typically become suddenly unresponsive and may also stop breathing. If these signs are present, call 911 and then begin CPR right away.

Wellness Strategies

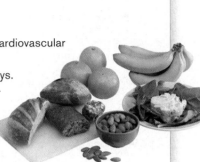

Preventing Cardiovascular Disease

Recognize risk factors that cannot be changed:

Age
Gender
Ethnicity
Family history/heredity

Focus on risk factors that can be changed:

Choose a healthy diet—consider the DASH diet and the following guidelines:

- Eat a variety of nutrient-rich fruits, vegetables, and whole grains.
- Choose unsaturated fats; limit intake of saturated and *trans* fats and dietary cholesterol.
- Eat fish at least twice a week.
- Cut back on foods high in added sugars.
- Choose and prepare foods with little or no salt.

Be physically active.
Control body weight.
Avoid tobacco.
Keep alcohol use moderate.
Avoid drugs harmful to the cardiovascular system.
Manage stress in healthy ways.
Have recommended screening tests.
Take appropriate steps to reduce elevated blood pressure, maintain healthy cholesterol and triglyceride levels, and control diabetes.

CPR doesn't usually restart the heart, but it can temporarily maintain circulation, providing the opportunity for a successful resuscitation while limiting damage to the brain and heart from lack of blood flow. Resuscitation usually requires advanced care with defibrillation. Some locations now have automated external defibrillators (AEDs) designed for use by laypeople. AEDs are relatively simple to use; they automatically detect arrhythmias and deliver an electrical shock, which may correct the heart rhythm.

AEDs can be used in conjunction with CPR, and training for both is available. Most classes can be taken in a single day. Contact a local health care provider, the American Red Cross, or American Heart Association to find a class near you. CPR and use of AEDs are easy skills to learn and could mean the difference between life and death for someone you love.

Q | Can CVD be diagnosed before a person has symptoms?

DIAGNOSIS. Absolutely. Everyone should get recommended screening tests, including those for blood pressure and cholesterol, as well as regular health checkups. CVD

TABLE 11-6 WARNING SIGNS OF HEART ATTACK AND STROKE

HEART ATTACK WARNING SIGNS	STROKE WARNING SIGNS
■ **Chest discomfort:** Most heart attacks involve discomfort in the center of the chest that lasts for more than a few minutes, or goes away and comes back. The discomfort can feel like uncomfortable pressure, squeezing, fullness, or pain.	■ **Sudden numbness** or weakness of face, arm, or leg, especially on one side of the body.
■ **Discomfort in other areas of the upper body:** Can include pain or discomfort in one or both arms, the back, neck, jaw, or stomach.	■ **Sudden confusion,** trouble speaking or understanding.
■ **Shortness of breath:** Often comes along with chest discomfort, but it also can occur before chest discomfort.	■ **Sudden trouble seeing** in one or both eyes.
■ **Other symptoms:** Breaking out in a cold sweat, nausea and vomiting, or light-headedness.	■ **Sudden trouble walking,** dizziness, loss of balance or coordination.
	■ **Sudden severe headache** with no known cause.

Source: National Heart, Lung, and Blood Institute. (n.d.). *Heart attack warning signs* (http://www.nhlbi.nih.gov/actintime/haws/haws.htm). National Institute of Neurological Disorders and Stroke. (2009, June 29). *Brain basics: Preventing stroke* (http://www.ninds.nih.gov/disorders/stroke/preventing_stroke.htm).

TABLE 11-7 TESTS FOR DIAGNOSING AND MONITORING CARDIOVASCULAR DISEASE

ELECTROCARDIOGRAM (ECG OR EKG)	Electrodes are placed on the skin to detect the heart's electrical signals, which are recorded; the test can show problems with heart rate or rhythm and detect underlying damage to the heart.
EXERCISE STRESS TEST	An ECG is performed while the person is exercising on a treadmill or stationary bike; the test monitors the person's response to exercise and detects problems with the cardiovascular system during physical effort.
CORONARY ANGIOGRAPHY	A catheter is threaded though an artery, typically in the leg, and dye is injected into the arteries of the heart; special X-rays are then used to identify blockages. A similar procedure can be done to visualize the brain's blood vessels.
BLOOD TESTS	In addition to checking cholesterol and glucose levels, blood samples can be analyzed for enzymes and proteins in the blood that indicate heart-muscle damage.
CHEST X-RAY	Ionizing radiation creates pictures of the heart, lungs, and blood vessels, which can be used to determine the size and shape of the heart as well as to detect fluid buildup or damage.
ECHOCARDIOGRAM	A small device called a transducer transmits ultrasound waves into the chest, which are converted into computerized images of the heart; the test can show the heart's size, structure, and motion, as well as blood volume and speed and direction of blood flow.
NUCLEAR SCAN OR POSITRON EMISSION TOMOGRAPHIC (PET) SCAN	In both tests, small amounts of radioactive tracer materials are injected into the bloodstream; special imaging equipment monitors blood flow to the heart, how well the heart pumps blood, and whether the heart muscle is damaged.
COMPUTED TOMOGRAPHY (CT) SCAN	A special X-ray machine takes cross-sectional images that are used to create three-dimensional models of organs. Scans can be used to detect problems in blood vessels in both the heart and brain.
MAGNETIC RESONANCE IMAGING (MRI)	A special scanner uses radio waves, magnets, and a computer to create images of organs and tissues; MRIs can evaluate the condition of the heart and blood vessels and detect the presence and size of aneurysms and malformed blood vessels that are potential causes of hemorrhagic stroke.
ELECTROENCEPHALOGRAM (EEG)	Similar to an ECG, electrodes are placed on the scalp, and the electrical activity of the brain is monitored for any indications of problems.

can be diagnosed before you have symptoms, and you can take early steps to control it.

There are many diagnostic tests to recognize and assess problems with the heart and blood vessels. Your physician may conduct multiple tests to rule out other possible causes for your symptoms as well as to confirm a CVD diagnosis. Some of the tests that might be used are described in Table 11-7.

Q What kinds of medicine and help are available?

TREATMENT. A diagnosis of cardiovascular disease can be scary, but many successful forms of treatment are available. Lifestyle changes are always the first line of defense and can be used to both prevent and treat CVD. A variety of medications are available to help when lifestyle changes fall short; the type of medication depends on the type of CVD. Commonly used drugs include those that lower blood pressure or cholesterol, prevent clots from forming, increase the pumping strength of the heart, and relax blood vessels.

Unfortunately, lifestyle changes and medications aren't always successful at controlling CVD. In some cases, surgery or other procedures may be needed. *Coronary angioplasty* is a procedure in which a catheter is inserted into blocked coronary arteries. When the blockages are reached, a small balloon is used to push through the blockage. Often a *stent,* a small wire tube, is inserted to assist in keeping the artery open. If coronary artery blockages are too severe, *coronary bypass surgery* may be needed. During bypass surgery, a blood vessel taken from elsewhere in the body is grafted to the heart producing a bypass, or detour, around the blocked artery, creating a new route for blood flow. If several arteries are blocked, multiple bypasses can be performed.

A *pacemaker* is an electrical device that regulates heart beat for people who have abnormal heart rhythms. The device is typically implanted in the upper chest near the collarbone, using local anesthesia. In most instances, the procedure is considered minor surgery, and patients go home within a day.

If a heart valve malfunction is too severe to treat with medication, open heart surgery may be necessary for *heart valve repair or replacement.* Repairing the valve or valves is the preferred choice but this is not always possible. Replacement valves may be tissue valves (human or animal) or mechanical valves made from plastic or metal.

When the heart can no longer perform its job of getting oxygenated blood to the body's tissues and there is risk for death, a *heart transplant* may be the option. A transplant involves replacing the diseased heart with a healthy heart from a human donor. In the world of cardiology, a heart transplant is now considered a relatively simple operation; annually, more than two thousand Americans receive new hearts.

Fast Facts

Chronic Disease—By the Numbers

The average lifetime probability of developing a chronic disease is fairly high. But remember—these are averages. Your risk could be much higher or lower depending on your personal risk factors, including your lifestyle choices.

Cancer
Men: 1 in 2
Women: 1 in 3

Cardiovascular disease
Men: 2 in 3
Women: 1 in 2

Diabetes
Men: 1 in 3
Women: 2 in 5

Sources: American Heart Association. (2009). *Heart disease and stroke statistics: 2009 update at a glance* (http://www.americanheart.org/downloadable/heart/1240250946756LS-1982%20Heart%20and%20Stroke%20Update.042009.pdf). American Cancer Society. (n.d.). Lifetime risk of developing or dying from cancer. *Cancer basics* (http://www.cancer.org/Cancer/CancerBasics/lifetime-probability-of-developing-or-dying-from-cancer). Centers for Disease Control and Prevention. (2010). Lifetime risk for diabetes mellitus in the United States. *Diabetes public health resource* (http://www.cdc.gov/diabetes/news/docs/lifetime.htm).

Q How likely is it that someone will survive and recover from CVD? Is there a cure for it?

Because one in three Americans dies from some type of cardiovascular disease, it's hard to talk in terms of a cure. However, most people who die from CVD are older. Some younger people do develop and die from CVD, but it's much less common. It's important to realize that many forms of CVD are treatable. Many people not only survive but live long and productive lives when they appropriately manage their CVD.

Cancer

Cancer is common and potentially deadly. In their lifetimes, about one in two men and one in three women will develop some form of cancer. Luckily, there are many things you can do to reduce your risk of developing cancer, and many forms of cancer are very treatable, especially when discovered in the early stages.

Q What is cancer? What is the difference between malignant and benign tumors?

Like cardiovascular disease, **cancer** is not one disease but rather is a broad category of disease. All cancers are characterized by uncontrolled growth of cells.

Typically cells grow and divide in a controlled and orderly fashion, and rates of new cell growth and old cell death are balanced. If a damaging mutation occurs in a cell, under normal circumstances, the cell will either undergo repair or self-destruct.

If something affects this cycle, abnormal cells may grow and reproduce in an uncontrolled manner (Figure 11-6). Mutated cells often divide more quickly than surrounding tissues and may "clump" into masses known as **tumors.** It usually takes many mutations before a cell becomes cancerous and begins to divide uncontrollably.

Most tumors are **benign,** or noncancerous. Benign tumors do not invade other tissues and are typically not harmful unless they interfere with bodily functions. For example, uterine fibroids, which are benign tumors, are relatively common in women of childbearing age. They can vary from the size of a seed to the size of a grapefruit or larger, but they typically don't interfere with day-to-day function. However, benign brain tumors put pressure on sensitive areas of the brain and cause serious symptoms so they typically are removed.

Malignant tumors are known as cancer. Not only can these tumors invade nearby healthy cells and organs,

cancer A group of diseases characterized by uncontrolled growth and spread of abnormal cells.

tumor Mass of cells with no physiological function that arises from uncontrolled cellular growth; may be benign or malignant.

benign Noncancerous.

malignant Cancerous.

Normal cell division and growth control

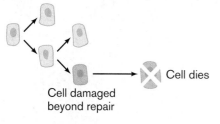

Cell damaged beyond repair

Cell dies

Cancer cell division and loss of growth control

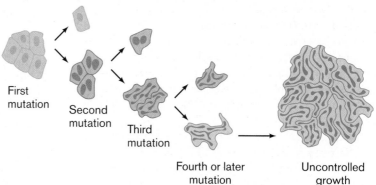

First mutation

Second mutation

Third mutation

Fourth or later mutation

Uncontrolled growth

Figure 11-6 Normal cell division versus cancer cell division. Normal cells divide in a controlled fashion and will self-destruct if they are damaged beyond repair. Cancer usually involves multiple mutations, after which cancer cells will grow and divide uncontrollably.

Source: Adapted from National Cancer Institute. (2009). *Understanding cancer series: Cancer* (http://www. cancer.gov/cancertopics/understandingcancer/cancer/allpages).

metastasis The spread of cancerous cells from the original site to other parts of the body.

they can also **metastasize,** or spread, to other parts of the body through the blood and lymphatic systems. Tumors that have metastasized are known as *secondary tumors,* and the original, or first, tumor is considered the *primary tumor.*

Some benign tumors undergo changes and become malignant. For example, benign tumors in the colon are known as polyps, and they can be easily removed with minor surgery. However, if left in place, polyps can become malignant over time, and colon cancer can invade surrounding tissues and organs and then spread to other parts of the body.

Q | How many Americans have cancer?

The American Cancer Society estimates that nearly 11.4 million Americans with a history of cancer are alive today. This figure includes both people who are currently undergoing treatment and those who are now considered cancer-free.[19] About 1.5 million new cancer cases are diagnosed each year, and cancer claims about 570,000 lives per year, or more than 1,500 a day. Though still large, the number of new cases of cancer occurring each year has begun to decline slightly.

Types of Cancer

Q | How many kinds of cancer are there?

Scientists estimate there are hundreds of types of cancer. Cancers are classified according to the location in the body where they originate and by the kind of tissue or fluid from which they develop. Though some cancers are mixed types, most fall into one of the following general groupings:[20]

- *Carcinoma* arises in skin or in tissues that line or cover internal organs, glands, or other body structures such as breasts, lungs, bladder, skin; it accounts for 80–90 percent of all cancer cases.
- *Sarcoma* arises from connective or supportive tissues such as bone, cartilage, fat, muscle, blood vessels, and tendons; sarcoma is less common than carcinoma but often much more dangerous.
- *Lymphoma and myeloma* originate in the cells of the immune system. There are two major types of lymphoma: Hodgkin lymphoma, characterized by abnormal B cells (those that produce antibodies), and non-Hodgkin lymphomas (all other forms). Myeloma originates in the plasma cells of bone marrow; it is commonly referred to as multiple myeloma because it typically occurs at multiple sites.
- *Leukemia* occurs in the blood-forming tissues of the body such as bone marrow. It is characterized by abnormal white blood cells (needed to fight infection), red blood cells (needed to carry oxygen), and platelets (needed to minimize excessive bruising and bleeding) rather than the solid tumors of most other cancers.
- *Central nervous system cancers* begin in the tissues of the brain or spinal cord.

Q | What is the most common type of cancer? Which type is most severe?

The most frequently diagnosed cancers in the United States are two types of skin cancer—basal cell carcinoma and squamous cell carcinoma—for which 2 million people are treated each year. Because most cases of these cancers are noninvasive and highly curable, they are not included in cancer registries and statistics.

In terms of cancers that are potentially invasive, lung cancer is the leading cause of cancer deaths in both men and

TABLE 11-8 MOST FREQUENTLY DIAGNOSED CANCERS IN THE UNITED STATES, 2010 ESTIMATES

SITE OR TYPE	ESTIMATED NEW CASES	ESTIMATED DEATHS	5-YEAR SURVIVAL RATE, ALL STAGES
LUNG AND BRONCHUS	222,520	157,300	16%
PROSTATE	217,730	32,050	99%
BREAST, FEMALE*	207,090	39,840	89%
COLON AND RECTUM	142,570	51,370	66%
BLADDER	70,530	14,680	79%
MELANOMA	68,130	8,700	91%
NON-HODGKIN LYMPHOMA	65,540	20,210	69%
KIDNEY	58,240	13,040	68%
THYROID	44,670	1,690	97%
UTERUS	43,470	7,950	83%
PANCREAS	43,140	36,800	6%
LEUKEMIA (ALL TYPES)	43,050	21,840	57%
ORAL CAVITY AND PHARYNX	36,540	7,880	61%
LIVER	24,120	18,910	15%
BRAIN	22,020	13,140	35%
OVARY	21,880	13,850	46%

*Male breast cancer is rare, accounting for about 1% of all breast cancers; risk factors include increased estrogen levels, radiation exposure, heavy drinking, and a family history of breast cancer.

Sources: American Cancer Society. (2010). *Cancer facts & figures 2010.* Atlanta, GA: American Cancer Society. National Cancer Institute. (2010). *SEER cancer statistics* (http://seer.cancer.gov/statistics).

women, accounting for about 30 percent of all cancer deaths (Table 11-8). In terms of incidence, lung cancer is followed by prostate cancer in men and breast cancer in women.

Overall, cancer deaths in the United States have decreased slightly in recent years. But some cancers, such as lung, liver, and pancreatic cancers, still have poor survival rates because they are typically diagnosed at an advanced stage. The five-year survival rates for common cancers are shown in Table 11-8.

Assessing Your Risk for Cancer

Q | What are my chances of getting cancer?

Anyone can get cancer. There's no way to tell for sure who will develop cancer or when it might happen, but some general patterns of risks are associated with cancer. Overall cancer risks can be viewed in two ways. *Lifetime risk* is the probability of developing or dying from cancer in your lifetime, and *relative risk* refers to the extent of the relationship between a risk factor and a specific kind of cancer. For example, women in the United States have a one-in-three lifetime risk of developing cancer.[21] A woman who smokes has a relative risk of lung cancer of 12, meaning she is twelve times more likely to develop lung cancer than a nonsmoker.

Specific risk factors, some of which are controllable and some of which are not, are described in the next sections.

Q | If someone in my family has cancer, am I likely to get it too?

HEREDITY/GENETICS. Because cancer is uncontrolled cell growth, and cell growth is controlled by genes, all

Wellness Strategies

The Ups and Downs of Genetic Testing: What You Should Know

Genetic testing is available for some types of cancer, including cancers of the breast, colon, ovary, thyroid, kidney, and prostate. It is also available to screen for genes that increase the risk of CVD and diabetes.

Limitations

- An accurate gene test will indicate if a certain mutation is present. However, having the mutation does not guarantee cancer will develop. Additionally, people without the mutation can still get cancer.
- Current tests look only for the most common mutations; other cancer-causing mutations are not detected. And most cancer cases are not due to inherited mutations.
- There are consequences of determining higher risk for disease, including psychological stress, child-bearing decisions, family communications, and so on.
- The National Cancer Institute identifies the most serious limitation of genetic testing as the lack of "state-of-the-art diagnostics and therapies" to keep up with the identification of mutant genes.

Benefits

- A negative result can provide tremendous relief and eliminate the need for additional frequent and expensive testing.
- A positive result can lead people to take more prudent risk management measures, including lifestyle changes, more frequent testing, and other measures prescribed by their physician.
- Testing is becoming more accurate, and more mutations are being identified. The more we know about genetic mutations, the more we will know about the causes and cures for the various forms of cancer.

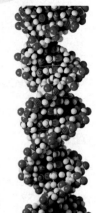

Source: Adapted from National Cancer Institute. Gene testing. *Understanding cancer series* (http://www.cancer.gov/cancertopics/understandingcancer/genetesting).

---

cancers involve some type of genetic mutation (damage). These mutations can take many forms, which is why diseases as different at leukemia and lung cancer are both considered cancers.

Most genetic mutations are random, occurring as a result of a genetic mistake when a cell divides or in response to environmental factors such as sunlight, chemicals, or tobacco. Only about 5–10 percent of all cancers are linked to inherited genetic mutations—those that an individual is born with. As a rule, hereditary cancers tend to occur at an earlier age than those due to other causes.

In evaluating your own risk, consider how many family members have had a particular type of cancer and if any were diagnosed at a young age. Let your health care provider know about any family history of cancer. Depending on your circumstances, earlier or more frequent screenings for particular cancers may be recommended. For some forms of cancer, specific genetic tests are available; see the box "The Ups and Downs of Genetic Testing" for more information.

Q | Is cancer common in young adults? What types of cancer should I worry about now, when I'm 20?

AGE. The likelihood of being diagnosed with cancer increases with age. Although cancer can occur at any age, 78 percent of all cancers are diagnosed in people age 55 or older.[22] Over time, genetic mutations from internal and environmental factors can build up. Increased exposure along with the body's decreasing ability to repair damaged cells makes us more susceptible to cancer as we age. It's important to adopt lifestyle prevention strategies early in life in order to curb susceptibility as much as possible.

Testicular cancer seems to be an exception to cancer incidence increasing with age. Although not a common cancer, with about 8,500 cases and 350 deaths reported annually in the United States, the highest rates of testicular cancer occur in males ages 15–34. Among men in their twenties, this is the most prevalent form of cancer, followed by lymphoma. The most common cancers among women in their twenties are cancers of the thyroid, breast, cervix, and uterus and Hodgkin lymphoma. About 8 percent of cases of melanoma are diagnosed in people under age 35, so skin cancer prevention and awareness is also very important for young adults.

Q | Are men or women more likely to get cancer?

GENDER. It's estimated that half of all men and one third of all women in the United States will develop cancer at some point in their lives. Data gathered to date is inconclusive as to why more men than women are affected. Many researchers theorize the differences are related to lifestyle factors, such as higher rates of smoking and excessive alcohol consumption, as well as greater occupational exposure to dangerous chemicals.

Wellness Strategies

Self-Exams for Cancer

There are several self-exams that can help spot different kinds of cancer, including those that sometimes strike younger people.

■ *Testicular self-exam* can be performed monthly to check for lumps that could indicate early cancer. National Men's Resource Center: Testicular Cancer Awareness Week (http://www.tcaw.org).

■ *Breast self-exam* has both benefits and limitations, and the American Cancer Society recommends it as a non-mandatory option for checking for changes in the breasts. If performed, it should be done carefully and correctly.

American Cancer Society: How to Perform a Breast Self-Exam (http://www.cancer.org/Cancer/BreastCancer/DetailedGuide/breast-cancer-detection)

■ *Skin self-exam* can be performed check for problems; a record such as a body mole map can help determine if changes occur over time. American Academy of Dermatology: Performing a Skin Self-Exam (http://www.aad.org/public/exams/self.html)

In all cases, if you notice anything unusual during a self-exam, have it checked by your health care provider.

Q What group of people is most at risk for cancer?

ETHNICITY. According to the American Cancer Society, the highest incidence of cancer diagnoses and cancer deaths is among African Americans.[23] The death rate for African American females is 17 percent greater than that of white females, and for males, it's 35 percent greater. Other ethnicities have lower cancer rates overall but have higher rates of specific cancers, including those of the cervix, uterus, liver, and stomach. Asian American and Pacific Islander men have the highest rate of liver cancer (twice that of African Americans), and Latinas have the highest rate of cervical cancer.

These disparities can be attributed to a number of reasons. Low income is associated with limited access to health care and insurance. Cultural dietary practices and preferences for early marriage and childbirth affect cancer risk. Genetic factors may also play a role in the more aggressive forms of breast cancer in African American women and the elevated risk of prostate cancer among African American men. For more on cancer disparities, visit the Web sites for the American Cancer Society (http://www.cancer.org) and the National Cancer Institute (http://www.cancer.gov).

Q What's a carcinogen?

EXPOSURE TO CANCER-CAUSING AGENTS. A **carcinogen** is any substance that causes cancer. Carcinogens include solvents, pesticides, asbestos fibers, tobacco smoke, certain hormones and viruses, and radiation from X-rays, radon, sunlight, and tanning lamps or beds.[24] Radiation sources and risks are described in more detail below.

The news often has stories about pollutants in the environment that can cause cancer. Although these risks are real, exposure to environmental chemicals isn't a major cause of cancer for most people—it's responsible for perhaps 2 percent of all cancers.[25] Lifestyle choices and other factors play a much more important role in determining cancer risk. But for people exposed to carcinogens regularly or at relatively high levels because of their jobs—chemical workers and miners, for example—carcinogenic chemicals is a significant risk factor.

carcinogen A substance or agent that causes cancer.

Cancer Prevention

Q Is there a way to keep from getting cancer?

For most people diagnosed with cancer, the precise cause is unknown. Experts believe a combination of controllable and uncontrollable risk factors plays a role. Although you can't do anything about your family history, age, gender, or ethnicity, there are many positive steps you can take to reduce your risk. Your use of tobacco, your diet, your level of physical activity, and the other lifestyle factors discussed below can increase or reduce your risk. See the box "Healthy Choices for Cancer Prevention" for a summary of recommendations.

Tobacco. Cigarettes contain thousands of chemicals, including more that sixty known cancer-causing agents. Smoking leads to 87 percent of lung cancer deaths, most cancers of the larynx, oral cavity, pharynx, esophagus, and bladder, and it contributes to kidney, pancreatic, cervical, and stomach cancers as well as cardiovascular and other diseases. Regular cigar smokers who inhale are exposed to many of the same risks as cigarette smokers. Smokeless tobacco contains twenty-eight known cancer-causing agents and leads to increased risk of oral cancer. Second-hand smoke, also known as environmental tobacco smoke

Research Brief

Indoor Tanning and Melanoma

Ultraviolet rays from tanning beds and lamps are classified as a carcinogen, meaning they cause cancer. How big is the risk? Researchers recently studied over two thousand adults ages 25 to 59 with a history of indoor tanning. They looked at the amount of exposure—total number of hours of tanning—as it related to a diagnosis of melanoma. After controlling for other risk factors for skin cancer, including hair and skin color and freckling, they found a significant association between indoor tanning and melanoma, as shown in the graph.

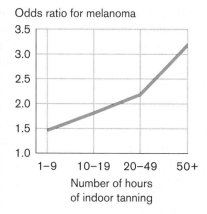

Odds ratio for melanoma

Number of hours of indoor tanning

The take-away from this study is obvious: Avoid indoor as well as outdoor tanning. Ultraviolet radiation from both natural and artificial sources is a carcinogen and increases the risk of cancer.

Source: Lazovich, D., Vogel, R. I., Berwick, M., Weinstock, M. S., Anderson, K. E., & Warshaw, E. M. (2010). Indoor tanning and risk of melanoma: A case-control study in a highly exposed population. *Cancer Epidemiology, Biomarkers & Prevention, 19*(6), 1557–1568.

(ETS), contains more than fifty cancer-causing agents and has been linked to lung cancer, nasal sinus cancer, respiratory infections, and heart disease in exposed nonsmokers. Research findings on marijuana have been mixed, but marijuana smoke contains some of the same chemicals as tobacco smoke and has been implicated in increased risk of certain cancers.[26] For your health and wellness, avoid tobacco in all forms.

Diet, physical activity, and body weight. The American Cancer Society estimated that one-third of all cancer deaths in the United States are due to poor nutrition and physical inactivity, and/or excess body weight. Obesity has been linked to breast, endometrial, colon, kidney, and esophageal cancers. Regular exercise helps control body weight; in addition, physical activity improves bowel functioning and the levels of insulin and other hormones. Certain nutrients and foods have been linked to a lower risk of cancer; although researchers have tried to identify specific nutrients as protective, the best evidence at present supports the consumption of a healthy overall diet. The American Cancer Society recommends a diet rich in plant-based foods, including whole grains, fruits, and vegetables. See Chapter 9 for more on planning a healthy diet.

Alcohol. More than two drinks per day increases the risk of cancers of the mouth, throat, esophagus, larynx, liver, and breast. For women, even just one alcoholic drink per day results in a very small increase in breast cancer risk. Alcohol may have direct effects on body cells, and it can also influence levels of hormones and certain nutrients. Risk increases with the amount of alcohol consumed and with tobacco use in combination with the alcohol.

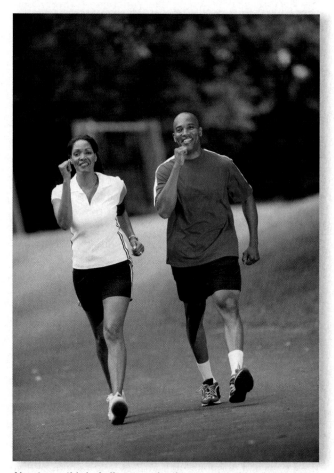

About one-third of all cancer deaths are related to physical inactivity and poor dietary choices. Regular exercise directly reduces the risk of certain cancers, including those of the breast and colon. Exercise also helps maintain healthy body weight, which further reduces cancer risk.

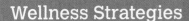

Wellness Strategies

Healthy Choices for Cancer Prevention

- Eat a healthy, balanced diet rich in fruits, vegetables, and whole grains; limit consumption of processed foods and red meats.
- Participate in regular physical activity.
- Avoid smoking, smokeless tobacco, and exposure to secondhand smoke.
- If you drink alcohol, do so in moderation.
- Practice safe sex to avoid infection with HPV and hepatitis B. Get vaccinated if appropriate (see Chapter 12).

- Use appropriate stress-management techniques.
- Avoid unnecessary exposure to medical radiation.
- Avoid unnecessary exposure to the sun, sun lamps, and tanning booths. For times you must be in the sun, protect yourself with appropriate clothing and sunscreen.
- Limit exposure to chemicals and other sources of radiation whenever possible. Always use appropriate safety precautions.

Infectious agents. Infection with human papillomaviruses (HPV) is the primary cause of cervical cancer and may also be linked to other cancers. Chronic infection with hepatitis B can cause liver cancer, and *Helicobacter pylori* infection can cause stomach cancer. Cancers from these viruses and bacteria can be prevented through vaccination, antibiotic treatment, and lifestyle choices that prevent infection.

Radiation. All sources of radiation, including medical X-rays, radioactive substances, and sunlight (see below) are potential carcinogens. Avoid unnecessary medical X-rays and imaging scans; ask how each X-ray or scan will help, and keep a record of all your X-rays to avoid duplication. Be aware that computed tomography (CT) scans use much higher radiation doses than standard X-rays, dental X-rays, and mammography. If radon (a naturally occurring radioactive gas) is a concern where you live, test your residence for radon and take appropriate steps if levels are high. For more on radon, visit the Web site for the Environmental Protection Agency (http://www.epa.gov/radon).

Sunlight, tanning lamps and booths. Ultraviolet (UV) rays from any source—sunlight, sun lamps, or tanning booths—cause early aging of the skin and skin damage that can lead to melanoma, the most dangerous form of skin cancer. Getting a "base tan" isn't healthy and doesn't protect your skin from sun damage—a tan is damage. Use sunscreen when you're outdoors, and don't use tanning lamps or booths. Although people with lighter skin tones are at higher risk for melanoma, darker skin does not eliminate risk. African Americans and Latinos have much lower rates of skin cancer than whites, but when they do develop melanoma, it is usually diagnosed at a more advanced stage and has a lower survival rate.[27]

Stress. Stress activates the body's hormones, which can cause changes in the immune system and the body's ability to protect itself against infection and diseases, including cancer. Though there has been no conclusive evidence that increased stress levels lead directly to cancer; minimizing stress does, of course, have other positive effects on the body.

Chemicals. In the United States, exposure to carcinogenic chemicals on the job is linked to many more cases of cancer than exposure to general environmental pollution is. Workers exposed to asbestos, benzene, cadmium, nickel, and vinyl chloride are at increased risk for a number of cancers. Chemicals and others substances in the home—such as some cleaners, paint and solvents, motor oil, and pesticides—may also increase risk for cancer, although to a lesser degree. Always handle and dispose of hazardous chemicals appropriately.

To identify your personal risk factors as well as strategies for prevention, complete Lab Activity 11-1.

Symptoms, Diagnosis, and Treatment of Cancer

Q How can you look for cancer before it's too late to stop it from spreading?

How you look for cancer depends on the type of cancer. As discussed earlier in the chapter, cancer takes many forms. Some have early warning signs and some do not. Some have screening tests and some do not. In all cases, it's better to detect cancer as early as possible. The best things you can do are to be alert for early warning signs and have preventive screenings as recommended.

Q When am I supposed to get all those cancer tests—and does everyone really need to get them?

EARLY SCREENING. Early cancer screening is critical for everyone. Screening tests performed before any

Practical Prevention

Protecting Your Skin from the Sun

Ultraviolet (UV) radiation can cause sunburn as well as other skin damage. Different types of UV light have different effects on the skin. Ultraviolet B (UVB) radiation has shorter wavelengths and affects primarily the skin's top layer, causing a sunburn you can see. Ultraviolet A (UVA) radiation has longer wavelengths and is more likely to infiltrate deeper into the skin and cause damage that is less immediately obvious—but over time leads to premature aging of the skin. Both UVA and UVB exposure can cause skin cancer.

The best way to avoid damage from UV radiation is to stay out of the sun, especially when the sun is most intense (between 10 a.m. and 4 p.m.). When you are out in the sun, covering up with long sleeves and a hat provides the most protection; special clothing for sun protection is also available. If your skin will be exposed to the sun, use sunscreen—and plenty of it. Here are some tips for choosing and using sunscreen:

■ Choose a sunscreen with an SPF (Sunburn Protection Factor) of 30 or higher, which should block 97 percent of the sun's UVB rays if used correctly. SPF is a relative measure based on sun exposure; a sunscreen with an SPF of 30 should allow skin to be exposed without burning to 30 times more UVB rays than normal.

■ Look for a sunscreen that protects against both UVA and UVB rays—one that is labeled "broad spectrum" or that contains a UVA-blocking ingredient such as ecamsule, avobenzone, titanium dioxide, or zinc oxide. The SPF rating applies only to UVB radiation; as of 2010, the FDA was working on a UVA rating system.

■ Use plenty of sunscreen—most people use too little. The average person needs about 1 ounce to cover the body—that's one quarter of a 4-ounce bottle.

■ Apply sunscreen thirty minutes before you go outside, and then reapply it at least every two hours.

■ If you'll be in the water or if you sweat heavily, use a water-resistant sunscreen.

■ Combination sunscreen and insect-repellant products are less effective, so use a higher SPF and apply it more frequently.

■ Remember that UV rays are not blocked by clouds, and use sunscreen even on cloudy or hazy days.

For more information, visit the Web sites for the Skin Cancer Foundation (http://www.skincancer.org/Sunscreen) and SkinCancerNet (http://www.skincarephysicians.com/skincancernet).

---

symptoms appear can help find cancer in its earliest and most treatable stage. The American Cancer Society recommendations for screening are shown in Table 11-9. Follow these guidelines or more specific guidelines provided by your physician based on your family history and risk factors. Some of the screening tests might not sound fun, but they can help detect early cancers and improve your chances for a long and healthy life.

Q | What are symptoms of cancer?

SIGNS AND SYMPTOMS. The initial stages of cancer often have no symptoms or symptoms that are very general and may indicate a number of other health issues. The acronym CAUTION can help you remember general symptoms to watch for:

- **C**hanges in bowel or bladder habits
- **A** sore that does not heal
- **U**nusual bleeding or discharge
- **T**hickening or lump in the breast or elsewhere
- **I**ndigestion or difficulty swallowing
- **O**bvious change in wart or mole
- **N**agging cough or hoarseness

Also remember to check your skin for the ABCDEs of melanoma; see Figure 11-7. Consult your physician if you experience any of these symptoms.

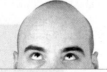

Mind Stretcher
Critical Thinking Exercise

What do you consider to be the major causes of cancer? Do you feel you have the ability to influence your own risk? Why or why not? Has your idea about your level of control over your risk affected your health habits and your choices about screening tests?

TABLE 11-9 AMERICAN CANCER SOCIETY SCREENING GUIDELINES FOR THE EARLY DETECTION OF CANCER IN ASYMPTOMATIC PEOPLE

CANCER SITE	POPULATION	TEST OR PROCEDURE	FREQUENCY
BREAST	Women, age 20+	Breast self-examination	Beginning in their early 20s, women should be told about the benefits and limitations of breast self-examination (BSE). The importance of prompt reporting of any new breast symptoms to a health professional should be emphasized. Women who choose to do BSE should receive instruction and have their technique reviewed on the occasion of a periodic health examination. It is acceptable for women to choose not to do BSE or to do BSE irregularly.
		Clinical breast examination	For women in their 20s and 30s, it is recommended that clinical breast examination (CBE) be part of a periodic health examination, preferably at least every three years. Asymptomatic women aged 40 and over should continue to receive a clinical breast examination as part of a period health examination, preferably annually.
		Mammography	Begin annual mammography at age 40.*
COLORECTAL†	Men and women, age 50+	*Tests that find polyps and cancer:*	
		Flexible sigmoidoscopy,‡ or	Every five years, starting at age 50
		Colonoscopy, or	Every 10 years, starting at age 50
		Double-contrast barium enema (DCBE),‡ or	Every five years, starting at age 50
		Tests that mainly find cancer: Fecal occult blood test (FOBT) with at least 50% test sensitivity for cancer, or fecal immunochemical test (FIT) with at least 50% test sensitivity for cancer‡§ or	Annual, starting at age 50
		Stool DNA test (sDNA)‡	Interval uncertain, starting at age 50
PROSTATE	Men, age 50+	Prostate-specific antigen test (PSA) with or without digital rectal exam (DRE)	Asymptomatic men who have at least a 10-year life expectancy should have an opportunity to make an informed decision with their health care provider about screening for prostate cancer after receiving information about the uncertainties, risks, and potential benefits associated with screening. Men at average risk should receive this information beginning at age 50. Men at higher risk, including African American men and men with a first degree relative (father or brother) diagnosed with prostate cancer before age 65, should receive this information beginning at age 45. Men at appreciably higher risk (multiple family members diagnosed with prostate cancer before age 65) should receive this information beginning at age 40.
CERVIX	Women, age 18+	Pap test	Cervical cancer screening should begin approximately three years after a woman begins having vaginal intercourse, but no later than 21 years of age. Screening should be done every year with conventional Pap tests or every two years using liquid-based Pap tests. At or after age 30, women who have had three normal test results in a row may get screened every two to three years with cervical cytology (either conventional or liquid-based Pap test) alone, or every three years with an HPV DNA test plus cervical cytology. Women 70 years of age and older who have had three or more normal Pap tests and no abnormal Pap tests in the past 10 years and women who have had a total hysterectomy may choose to stop cervical cancer screening.
ENDOMETRIAL	Women, at menopause	At the time of menopause, women at average risk should be informed about risks and symptoms of endometrial cancer and strongly encouraged to report any unexpected bleeding or spotting to their physicians.	
CANCER-RELATED CHECKUP	Men and women, age 20+	On the occasion of a periodic health examination, the cancer-related checkup should include examination for cancers of the thyroid, testicles, ovaries, lymph nodes, oral cavity, and skin, as well as health counseling about tobacco, sun exposure, diet and nutrition, risk factors, sexual practices, and environmental and occupational exposures.	

*Beginning at 40 age, annual clinical breast examination should be performed prior to mammography.

†Individuals with a personal or family history of colorectal cancer or adenomas, inflammatory bowel disease, or high-risk genetic syndromes should continue to follow the most recent recommendations for individuals at increased or high risk.

‡Colonoscopy should be done if test results are positive.

§For FOBT or FIT used as a screening test, the take-home multiple sample method should be used. A FOBT or FIT done during a digital rectal exam in the doctor's office is not adequate for screening.

Source: American Cancer Society. (2010). *Cancer facts & figures 2010.* Atlanta, GA: American Cancer Society.

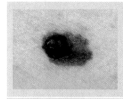

Asymmetry:
The two halves of the mole don't match

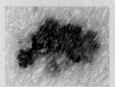

Border:
The borders are uneven and edges may be scalloped or notched

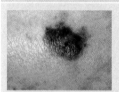

Color:
The mole has a variety of colors—different shades of brown, tan, or black or even red, blue, or another color

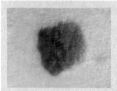

Diameter:
A size larger than a pencil eraser (1/4 inch or 6 mm)

Evolving:
Changing in size, shape, color, elevation, or another trait, or any new symptom such as bleeding, itching, or crusting

Figure 11-7 ABCDEs of melanoma. Most of the spots and growths on your skin are harmless, but atypical moles can be the first sign of serious skin cancer. If any of your moles have or develop the characteristics shown here, see your physician.
Source: Skin Cancer Foundation. (2010). *Warning signs: The ABCDEs of melanoma* (http://www.skincancer.org/the-abcdes-of-melanoma.html).

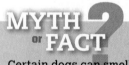
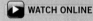

MYTH or FACT?

Certain dogs can smell cancer.

▶ WATCH ONLINE

Q What tests will a doctor do to figure out if a symptom really means cancer?

DIAGNOSIS. There is no single test to diagnose cancer. Depending on the type of cancer suspected, one or more of the following tests may be used to diagnose cancer and monitor its progress:

- *Biopsy:* Removal of a tissue sample so that the cells can be examined under a microscope for abnormalities.
- *Imaging procedures:* X-rays, magnetic resonance imaging (MRI), computed tomography (CT), ultrasound, and other high-tech scans are used to produce visual images of abnormal masses or sites of unusual chemical activity.

- *Tumor marker and other lab tests:* Measurement of specific substances in the blood, urine, or tissues that tend to occur in high levels with certain cancers. DNA testing may also be used to look for specific genetic mutations.

Q What does it mean when they say someone has stage IV cancer?

When someone is diagnosed with cancer, both the type of cancer and stage of development will be identified. There are a number of staging systems, but staging is typically based on factors such as the size and location of the tumor, the number of lymph nodes involved, and whether the disease has metastasized (spread) to a distant location in the body. A stage of I, II, III, or IV will be designated, with stage I indicating early stage cancer and stage IV indicating an advanced cancer that has spread. Stage 0 is sometimes used to describe cancer that is found only in the layer of cells in which it began; this is also known as *in situ* (Latin for "in its place") cancer. Figure 11-8 shows the different stages in cancer.

The prognosis, or projected outcome, for survival typically decreases as the stage increases. For example, in stage I colon cancer, the tumor is small and localized and the potential for successful treatment is high. On the other hand, in stage IV colon cancer, the malignant cells have spread to the lymph nodes and other tissues and organs, and treatment is likely to be more complicated and less successful.

Q Once someone has cancer, what's the best way to treat it?

TREATMENT. The type of cancer as well as the stage of the cancer will help determine the most effective type of treatment. The person's age, health, and lifestyle are also taken into account. Although we tend to think of cancer treatments as being used for the sole purpose of curing cancer, sometimes treatments are used to keep cancer from spreading or simply to relieve cancer symptoms. The most common cancer treatments are chemotherapy, radiation, and surgery, and often more than one treatment type is used.

Q How do chemotherapy and radiation treat cancer?

Chemotherapy is the use of drugs to kill cancer cells or to inhibit their growth. Often it is a combination of drugs that may be administered intravenously, inserted into a body cavity, or taken orally in pill form. Chemotherapy is considered a systemic treatment because it circulates through the blood to other parts of the body in order to also reach secondary tumors. More than 50 percent of people diagnosed with cancer are treated with

chemotherapy Treatment involving the use of chemical agents (drugs) to kill cancer cells.

Time →

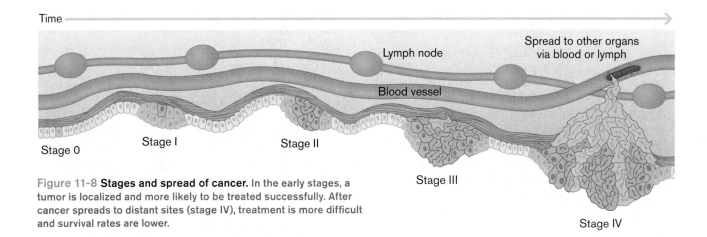

Spread to other organs via blood or lymph

Lymph node

Blood vessel

Stage 0

Stage I

Stage II

Stage III

Stage IV

Figure 11-8 Stages and spread of cancer. In the early stages, a tumor is localized and more likely to be treated successfully. After cancer spreads to distant sites (stage IV), treatment is more difficult and survival rates are lower.

radiation therapy The use of high-energy rays to kill or damage cancer cells to keep them from growing or spreading; also known as radiation.

some type of chemotherapy. Because chemotherapy typically targets all rapidly dividing cells, including non-cancerous ones, its side effects include nausea, hair loss, and anemia.

Radiation therapy, commonly referred to as radiation, is the use of high-energy rays to kill or damage cancer cells in an attempt to keep them from growing or spreading. Unlike chemotherapy, radiation is a local rather than a systemic treatment. Therapy may be administered externally—by a machine aiming radiation directly at the tumor site—or in-

ternally by implanting a small amount of radioactive material in or near the tumor. Radiation is not typically used for cancers that have spread; it may be used alone or in conjunction with chemotherapy or other types of treatment.

Surgery is also used for cancer treatment. It is the oldest form of cancer treatment and, like radiation, is a local treatment. Surgery can serve a number of purposes. It can be preventive, removing suspicious cells before they turn cancerous. It can be curative, entirely removing an early-stage cancerous growth, along with surrounding tissue. If the entire primary tumor cannot be surgically removed or if the cancer is suspected of having spread, surgery is usually combined with other treatment methods.

Q | Besides chemo and radiation, what cancer treatments are available?

[📖] **READ ONLINE**

Diabetes

Diabetes is a serious chronic condition that affects a growing number of Americans. It's estimated that 24 million people have diabetes, although many are unaware of their condition.

Q | What is diabetes?

Typically referred to simply as *diabetes,* **diabetes mellitus** is a metabolic disorder characterized by problems with the body's production or use of insulin. Much of the food you eat is converted to glucose by your digestive system. Glucose is the body's main source of fuel and is transported via the bloodstream to cells throughout the body, which use it for growth and energy production. Glucose requires two things to enter a cell: *glucose transporters,* which are the doorways

diabetes mellitus A disorder of carbohydrate metabolism characterized by inadequate production or use of insulin, leading to elevated blood glucose levels.

Fast Facts

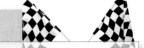

The Promise of Prevention

Controlling risk factors improves quality of life and increases life expectancy. Researchers calculated the gains in life expectancy from reducing the prevalence of just four key risk factors: smoking, high systolic blood pressure, elevated fasting plasma glucose, and excess body fat (BMI).

Gains in Life Expectancy (Years)		
	Men	Women
Systolic blood pressure	1.5	1.6
Body mass index	1.3	1.3
Fasting plasma glucose	0.5	0.3
Smoking	2.5	1.8
Overall gain	4.9	4.1

Source: Danaei, G., Rimm, E. B., Oza, S., Kulkarni, S. C., Murray, C. J., and others. (2010). The promise of prevention: The effects of four preventable risk factors on national life expectancy and life expectancy disparities by race and county in the United States. *PLoS Medicine, 7*(3), e1000248.

insulin A hormone produced and secreted by the pancreas that circulates in the blood and enables glucose absorption by cells.

hyperglycemia Excessively high blood glucose levels; also known as high blood sugar.

hypoglycemia Abnormally low blood glucose levels; also known as low blood sugar.

in cell walls that glucose can pass through, and **insulin,** a hormone produced by the pancreas. In normal metabolism, when glucose enters the bloodstream, the pancreas responds by pumping out insulin. The insulin binds to receptors on a cell wall, signaling the glucose transporter to open and allow glucose to pass into the cell. Once most glucose is absorbed, the pancreas stops releasing insulin, and blood levels of both insulin and glucose are fairly low.

In diabetes, the pancreas does not produce enough insulin or the body's cells do not respond appropriately to the insulin that is produced. When this happens, glucose builds up in the bloodstream because it cannot be transported into cells, a condition called *high blood sugar,* or **hyperglycemia.** Eventually, blood glucose levels are so high that the excess glucose is excreted in the urine. In addition, because the cells can't obtain sufficient glucose, the body loses its main source of energy.

Q | What's bad about high blood sugar?

Prolonged hyperglycemia damages nerves, blood vessels, and other organs. Symptoms of hyperglycemia include increased thirst, frequent urination, headaches, blurred vision, weight loss, fatigue, and stomach and intestinal problems. Left untreated, hyperglycemia can lead to a life-threatening condition called *ketoacidosis,* also sometimes referred to as diabetic ketoacidosis (DKA). When elevated levels of glucose remain in the blood rather than being absorbed and utilized by the cells, the cells call on the body to release another form of fuel. The body shifts to "starvation mode" and begins to break down fats for fuel—which does not break down quite as efficiently as glucose. This "burning" of fat produces a harmful acidic by-product known as ketones, which can eventually build up to toxic levels in the blood.

Over the long-term, diabetes is associated with many serious complications, including higher rates of cardiovascular disease and lower life expectancy (Figure 11-9).

Q | Can blood sugar be too low?

When the amount of glucose in the blood rises, the pancreas produces more insulin in an attempt to push the additional glucose to the cells. This increased push can leave the glucose levels in the blood low, a condition commonly referred to as low blood sugar or **hypoglycemia.** Most cases of hypoglycemia occur in people with diabetes and are related to inaccurate use of glucose-lowering medications or irregular eating patterns. Though

Eyes	Changes in vision; damage to the small blood vessels in the eyes; blindness
Skin	Problems ranging from rashes and blisters to bacterial and fungal infections
Mouth	Bleeding gums and frequent oral infections
Stomach	Delayed stomach emptying, leading to heartburn, nausea, and vomiting
Heart and blood vessels	Increased risk of hypertension, atherosclerosis, heart attack, stroke, and peripheral artery disease
Bladder	Urinary tract infections and bladder problems
Sexual function	Erectile dysfunction in men; problems with sexual response and vaginal lubrication in women
Kidney	Damage that, if severe, requires treatment with dialysis (artificial cleaning and filtering of the blood with a specialized machine) or kidney transplant
Lower legs and feet	Nerve and blood vessel damage leading to poor circulation, infections, and sores that don't heal; in severe cases amputation may be required, and diabetics are eight times more likely to have a lower limb amputated than those without diabetes

Figure 11-9 Possible complications of diabetes

hypoglycemia can occasionally be caused by hormone deficiencies or other medical conditions such as cancer, it is relatively rare in healthy adults and children older than 10. The primary danger of hypoglycemia is to the brain: Without glucose, brains cells die, which can cause permanent brain damage or, in severe cases, death. Symptoms of hypoglycemia can include confusion, dizziness, pounding heart or racing pulse, pale skin, sweating, weakness, poor concentration, and loss of consciousness.

Q | How many people have diabetes?

Overall, an estimated 23.6 million Americans, or about 8 percent of the population, have diabetes, yet more than

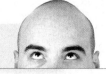

Mind Stretcher
Critical Thinking Exercise

Has anyone in your family had serious heart disease, cancer, or diabetes? How did it affect their life? How did it affect your perception of your own risk and the importance of prevention measures to you?

one-quarter of them—nearly six million people—don't know it.[28] Diabetes is more common in older adults. Less than 1 percent of Americans under 21 years of age have diabetes, but the number of diabetes cases continues to grow among children and teens.

Types of Diabetes

Q | Are some kinds of diabetes more dangerous than others?

There are three primary types of diabetes: type 1, type 2, and gestational. **Type 1 diabetes** can occur at any age but appears most often in children and young adults under the age of 20. Type 1 diabetes is considered an autoimmune disease because it is usually caused by the body's own immune system attacking and destroying the insulin-producing cells of the pancreas. These cells, called beta cells, are then unable to produce any insulin. Without insulin, glucose quickly builds up in the bloodstream and cells start dying from lack of an energy source. Type 1 diabetes is fatal within days or weeks if not treated.

Type 2 diabetes, which develops more slowly, is the most common type of diabetes and accounts for 90–95 percent of all diagnosed diabetes cases in the United States.[29] In type 2 diabetes, cells don't respond properly to insulin, a condition called *insulin resistance.* When glucose enters the bloodstream, the pancreas does release insulin. However, due to problems with insulin receptors or glucose transporters, glucose is unable to enter cells. The pancreas may pump out more insulin to help overcome the resistance, and some amount of glucose is absorbed—but levels of both glucose and insulin in the blood rise. The pancreas can't produce extra insulin indefinitely, so glucose levels in the blood increase further (Figure 11-10).

When the signs of high blood-glucose levels are first recognized during pregnancy, the diagnosis is **gestational diabetes.** This type of diabetes affects about 3–8 percent

type 1 diabetes Form of diabetes characterized by little or no insulin secretion; an autoimmune disease that occurs when the immune system destroys the insulin-producing cells of the pancreas.

type 2 diabetes The most common form of diabetes, characterized by impaired insulin use by the cells and, in some cases, insufficient insulin production.

gestational diabetes The form of diabetes in which high blood glucose levels occur during pregnancy.

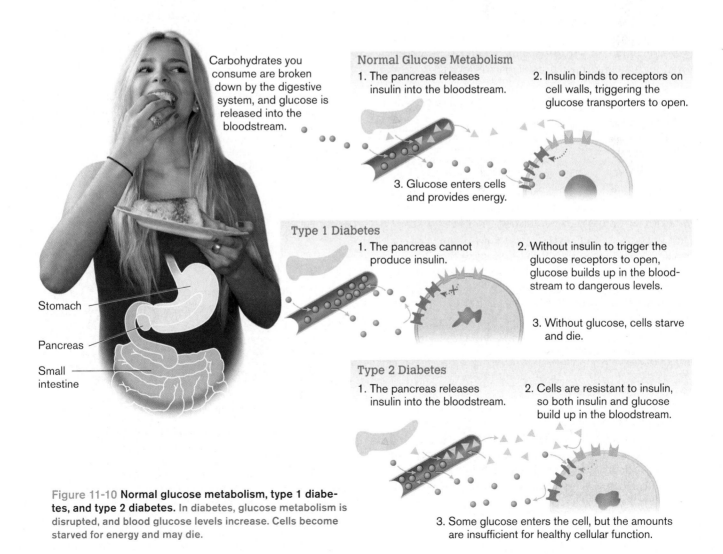

Carbohydrates you consume are broken down by the digestive system, and glucose is released into the bloodstream.

Stomach
Pancreas
Small intestine

Normal Glucose Metabolism
1. The pancreas releases insulin into the bloodstream.
2. Insulin binds to receptors on cell walls, triggering the glucose transporters to open.
3. Glucose enters cells and provides energy.

Type 1 Diabetes
1. The pancreas cannot produce insulin.
2. Without insulin to trigger the glucose receptors to open, glucose builds up in the bloodstream to dangerous levels.
3. Without glucose, cells starve and die.

Type 2 Diabetes
1. The pancreas releases insulin into the bloodstream.
2. Cells are resistant to insulin, so both insulin and glucose build up in the bloodstream.
3. Some glucose enters the cell, but the amounts are insufficient for healthy cellular function.

Figure 11-10 **Normal glucose metabolism, type 1 diabetes, and type 2 diabetes.** In diabetes, glucose metabolism is disrupted, and blood glucose levels increase. Cells become starved for energy and may die.

pre-diabetes A condition characterized by blood glucose levels that are above normal but not yet high enough to be classified as diabetes.

of pregnant women in the United States.[30] Gestational diabetes typically occurs late in pregnancy and is a result of pregnancy's many hormone changes and how those changes affect insulin production and absorption. If not managed properly, gestational diabetes can cause problems for both mother and baby, including growth abnormalities and chemical imbalances after birth. Babies born to mothers with gestational diabetes may be large, leading to more complicated births. Gestational diabetes usually disappears after the birth of the baby, but women with gestational diabetes are at increased risk of developing type 2 diabetes after pregnancy.

Q | Can you have high blood sugar without having diabetes?

Before developing type 2 diabetes, people often have a condition called **pre-diabetes,** also known as impaired glucose tolerance. It is estimated that 54 million Americans have blood glucose levels that are higher than normal but not yet high enough to be classified as diabetes. People with pre-diabetes can suffer from many of the same complications as those with full-blown diabetes, so it is important to take action if your blood glucose is elevated even slightly above normal. See the section on diagnosis below for more information about glucose levels.

Assessing Your Risk for Diabetes

Q | What causes diabetes?

Different types of diabetes have different causes. Type 1 diabetes is an autoimmune condition; it is suspected that the primary triggers are genetic and viral, but doctors don't yet know the exact causes. This makes pinpointing specific risk factors difficult. However, we do know that type 1 diabetes develops most often in children, occurs about equally in males and females, and is highest among non-Hispanic whites.[31]

The direct causes of type 2 diabetes are also unknown, but due the greater numbers of people with type 2 diabetes, more research has been conducted about it. Anyone can get type 2 diabetes, but according to the National Institutes of Health, those most at risk are people with one or more of the following characteristics:[32]

- age 45 or older
- overweight or obesity
- not physically active
- a family history of diabetes
- high blood pressure or high cholesterol
- gestational diabetes—diabetes during pregnancy—or gave birth to a baby weighing more than 9 pounds
- blood glucose levels that are higher than normal but not high enough for diabetes

- African American, American Indian, Asian American, Pacific Islander, or Latino
- polycystic ovary syndrome—a hormonal condition that leads to irregular or absent ovulation
- dark, thick, velvety skin around the neck or in the armpits
- blood vessel problems affecting the heart, brain, or legs

To assess your risk for diabetes, complete Lab Activity 11-1.

Q | If both my dad and my grandfather have diabetes, will I get it too?

Not necessarily—though you are at higher-than-average risk for developing diabetes. A family history of diabetes, which you obviously can't change, is a risk factor for getting the disease. However, if you take a look at the other risk factors for diabetes, you'll notice most of them are related to lifestyle choices. Making positive choices in these areas can help you delay, and even prevent, the onset of diabetes.

Q | I keep hearing that more and more people are getting diabetes. Why is that?

As a nation, we are becoming bigger, fatter people, and as mentioned above, obesity is a key risk factor for type 2 diabetes (Figure 11-11). The impact of overweight on diabetes risk is greater for people who develop obesity at a relatively young age. Obesity promotes insulin resistance, leading to difficulties in

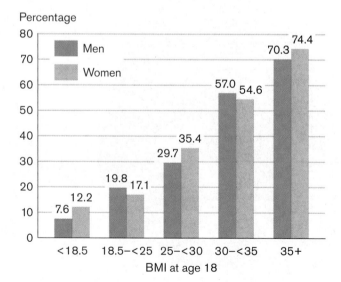

Figure 11-11 **Lifetime risk of diabetes by BMI at age 18. A person who is overweight or, especially, obese at age 18 has a very high lifetime risk for developing type 2 diabetes. Excess body fat is one of the key risk factors for diabetes.**

Source: Narayan, K. M. V., and others. (2007). Effect of BMI on lifetime risk for diabetes in the U.S. *Diabetes Care, 30*(6), 1562–1566.

glucose regulation and thus diabetes. At any age, however, excess body fat increases the risk for diabetes. Lifestyle choices related to diet and exercise are key diabetes prevention strategies, because they can help people achieve and maintain a healthy weight.

Diabetes Prevention

Q | Can diabetes be prevented?

Yes, there are many things you can do to prevent diabetes. Like CVD and cancer, diabetes has some risk factors that can't be changed and others that you can change. Diabetes also has many of the same prevention strategies as CVD and cancer: good dietary choices and a regular exercise program to maintain a healthy weight, control cholesterol, and protect against vascular diseases. Because smoking can raise cholesterol and blood pressure as well as blood glucose levels, avoiding smoking also aids in the prevention of diabetes.

Q | Does eating too much sugar cause diabetes?

No, not directly. Eating excess sugar, or anything in excess, can lead to obesity, which is a risk factor for diabetes. But the sugar itself does not cause diabetes. Diabetes is a disease related to genetics and a variety of lifestyle choices, as described above.

For someone who has diabetes, a recommended dietary plan may include specific goals and limits for carbohydrate intake, because foods that contain carbohydrates raise blood glucose levels. And as described in Chapter 8, some carbohydrate-rich foods are healthier choices than others. Choose mostly whole grains and unprocessed carbohydrates; limit intake of added sugars and processed grains.

Symptoms, Diagnosis, and Treatment of Diabetes

Q | How would I know if I had diabetes? What are the symptoms?

SYMPTOMS. Diabetes cannot be observed directly, and many of the symptoms of early diabetes are subtle. That helps explain why millions of Americans with diabetes are unaware of their condition. Symptoms you can watch for including the following:

- Increased thirst
- Increased hunger after eating
- Dry mouth

- Frequent urination
- Unexplained weight loss or weight gain
- Fatigue
- Blurred or decreased vision
- Numbness or tingling in hands or feet
- Slow-healing sores or cuts
- Itching of the skin, most often around the vaginal or groin area
- Frequent yeast infections
- Impotency
- Loss of consciousness (in rare cases)

Many of these symptoms aren't specific to diabetes, but if you experience one or more of them, you should discuss it with your health care provider.

Q | Do I need to be tested for diabetes even if I don't have any symptoms?

DIAGNOSIS. Possibly. The American Diabetes Association recommends that all adults over the age of 45 should be tested, and the tests should be repeated at least every three years. However, if you are at higher risk, as indicated by the risk factors above, earlier or more frequent tests may be recommended, especially if symptoms appear. Discuss any symptoms or concerns with your health care provider.

Q | How do doctors test for diabetes?

Usually through a blood test. Three different tests are used to diagnose diabetes and pre-diabetes (Figure 11-12). If any of these tests indicates elevated glucose levels, a repeat test will be done for confirmation:

- *A1C test,* which provides an estimate of average blood glucose levels over the preceding two to three months
- *Fasting plasma glucose test (FPG),* which measures blood glucose after an eight-hour fast
- *Oral glucose tolerance test (OGTT),* which measures glucose at set intervals following ingestion of glucose-containing fluids

	A1C	Fasting plasma glucose (FPG)	Oral glucose tolerance test (OGTT)
Diabetes	≥6.5%	≥126 mg/dl	≥200 mg/dl
Pre-diabetes	5.7%–6.4%	100–125 mg/dl	140–199 mg/dl
Normal	<5.7%	<100 mg/dl	<140 mg/dl

Figure 11-12 Criteria for diagnosing diabetes. The numbers for the A1C test refer to the average plasma glucose concentration. The numbers for the other two tests refer to the milligrams of glucose per deciliter of blood.

Source: American Diabetes Association. (2010). Position statement: Standards of medical care in diabetes—2010. *Diabetes Care, 33*(suppl 1), S11–S61.

Living with . . .

Type 2 Diabetes

With proper management, people with type 2 diabetes can live long, productive lives. Managing your blood sugar is key. Here are four very important management steps:

Regular exercise: Be active at least thirty minutes on most days. Even brisk walking four or five times a week can help a great deal in controlling blood sugar. Physical activity can also help in reducing weight and blood pressure, improving cholesterol levels, and preventing heart and blood flow problems.

Regular eating habits: It is important to realize that you don't have to completely eliminate sugar from your diet. However, carbohydrates, no matter the form, have the most dramatic affect on blood sugar. For this reason you need to plan meals and snacks carefully. In order to keep blood sugar levels from fluctuating too much, you should eat something every three or four hours.

All meals and snacks should include carbohydrates but in limited amounts. Your dietitian can help you work out a carb-counting method that is appropriate for you, but a general rule of thumb is 15–30 grams per snack and 45–75 grams per meal. Overall, meals should follow general dietary principles. The American Diabetes Association's "Create Your Plate" plan is one approach:

- Draw an imaginary line down the middle of the plate; divide one side again so that you have three sections on the plate.
- Fill the largest section with nonstarchy vegetables such as broccoli, carrots, tomatoes, green beans, mushrooms, peppers, cabbage, and salad greens.
- Fill one of the smaller sections with starchy foods such as whole grains, rice, pasta, cooked beans, potatoes, and corn.
- Fill the other smaller section with meat or meat substitutes such as fish, seafood, lean meats, chicken or turkey without skin, or tofu.
- Add a glass of nonfat or low-fat milk, yogurt, or a small roll as well as a piece of fruit.

Blood glucose testing: Careful blood sugar monitoring is important to help you know when your diabetes is under control and when it isn't. Your doctor or diabetes educator will help you select and learn to use a testing device. The best times to check your levels are before meals and before bed. (In the beginning, your doctor may have you check your levels more often as well as keep a diet log.) Always keep a record of your blood glucose. This will serve as a reference in the event you have unexpected symptoms.

Medication: Take any prescription medications as directed.

Management of type 2 diabetes is a team effort. Contact a local diabetes education expert or visit a reputable diabetes education Web site for information anytime. See your doctor regularly and always report any changes or concerns. For more information, visit the Web site of the American Diabetes Association (http://www.diabetes.org) and the Centers for Disease Control and Prevention Diabetes Public Health Resource (http://www.cdc.gov/diabetes).

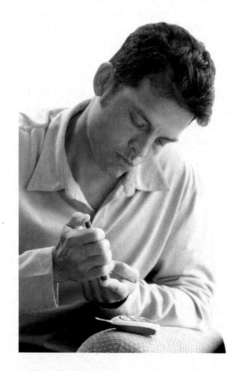

Wellness Strategies

Lifestyle Strategies for Chronic-Disease Risk Reduction

- Engage regularly in physical activity, preferably every day.
- Eat a balanced diet that is rich in fruits, vegetables, whole grains, and healthy fats and low in saturated and *trans* fats, cholesterol, added sugars, refined foods, and salt.
- Don't smoke or use other forms of tobacco, and avoid secondhand smoke. If you do smoke, quitting is one of the best things you can do to reduce your risk of chronic disease.
- Consume alcohol only in moderation.
- Communicate your family health history to your health care provider.

If you already have severe symptoms, your doctor may also order a urinalysis to help determine if you have additional complications that need to be treated. Because there is no cure for diabetes, a diagnosis can be scary. The good news is that in most instances diabetes can be successfully treated and managed.

Q I have a friend who has to give herself shots. Does everyone with diabetes have to do this?

TREATMENT. No. People with type 1 diabetes require daily insulin, which is usually administered in the form of regular self-injections, although some people use an insulin pump, a small computerized device that injects a constant dose of insulin. The pump is typically strapped to the waist area and has a small tube with a needle that is inserted and taped to the stomach. A newer inhaled form of insulin may be used along with other forms of insulin in order to decrease the number of injections needed and to help people with problems controlling blood glucose levels.

Many people with type 2 diabetes can manage their condition with oral medications and lifestyle strategies such as a healthy eating plan, regular exercise, and maintenance of a healthy weight. A number of types of oral medications are available. Some lower blood glucose levels by stimulating the pancreas to release more insulin, and others improve glucose absorption by cells. These may be prescribed individually or in combination. Some people with type 2 diabetes also need to take insulin.

Most physicians prefer to manage gestational diabetes with lifestyle changes, although insulin may be needed in some cases.

DOLLAR STRETCHER
Financial Wellness Tip

If you have diabetes, don't pay extra for special diabetic foods. They usually offer no special benefit to people with diabetes, and they can be quite expensive. Follow the dietary guidelines given to you by your health care provider.

Q What about all those ads for "diabetes supplies"? Besides taking medication, what does someone with diabetes have to do?

With all types of diabetes, self-management is crucial. People with diabetes should work with their physicians and other health care professionals to develop an appropriate and manageable plan for diet, exercise, and medication. It is also important to learn how and when to accurately self-test glucose levels in order to get the optimum benefits from the diet, exercise, and medication regime. Another essential part of self-management is to watch for signs of diabetes complications and report any changes or concerns to the appropriate health care provider without delay. See the box "Living with . . . Type 2 Diabetes" for more information.

Putting It All Together for Chronic Disease Prevention

As you can see from reviewing the information in the chapter on cardiovascular disease, cancer, and diabetes, these conditions are common but there are many strategies you can adopt to help reduce your risk. And many of these strategies are the same for all three groups of diseases. See the box "Lifestyle Strategies for Chronic-Disease Risk Reduction" for a summary.

Summary

Although chronic diseases are often associated with older age, everyone is susceptible. Modifiable risk behaviors are responsible for much of the incidence of chronic disease, and you can reduce your risk by making good choices related to tobacco use, nutrition, physical activity, and alcohol use. What you do as a young adult is a critical factor in whether or when you develop a chronic disease and how severe its effects will be.

Cardiovascular disease, cancer, and diabetes can be scary but, in many instances, they are quite manageable. Understanding the nature of each disease and knowing your risk factors for them is crucial, as is having regular screenings. If a disease is present, early detection and appropriate treatment or management are essential. Maintaining healthy lifestyle habits as well as a support network of friends and family are vital to maintaining or regaining your health.

More to Explore

American Cancer Society
http://www.cancer.org

American Diabetes Association
http://www.diabetes.org

American Heart Association
http://www.americanheart.org

CDC Chronic Disease Prevention and Health Promotion
http://www.cdc.gov/chronicdisease

National Cancer Institute
http://www.cancer.gov

National Heart, Lung, and Blood Institute
http://www.nhlbi.nih.gov

National Institute of Diabetes and Digestive and Kidney Diseases (NIDDK)
http://www.niddk.nih.gov

SUBMIT ONLINE

NAME	DATE	SECTION

Risk factors for the major chronic diseases that affect Americans have been clearly identified. In this lab, you'll complete online risk assessments for CVD, cancer, and diabetes and then reflect on your results. Save your assessment results for future reference and to discuss with your health care provider.

Equipment

- Computer with Internet access
- Printer (optional); you can also save your assessment results to a file on your computer

Preparation: None

Instructions

Complete each of the following online risk assessments, save or print your results, and enter your information in the chart that appears in the Results section below.

- American Heart Association: My Life Check
  http://www.mylifecheck.heart.org
  In the Results section below, record your score (out of 10) and list areas where your rating for "Where You Are Now" was not excellent.

- MD Anderson Cancer Center: Cancer Risk Check
  https://www3.mdanderson.org/publicedu/prevention/index.cfm?pagename=index
  In the Results section below, note any factors—controllable or uncontrollable—that are identified as placing you at elevated risk for cancer. The top section of the report may identify cancers for which your age or ethnicity are risk factors.

- American Diabetes Association: Diabetes Risk Test
  http://www.diabetes.org/diabetes-basics/prevention/diabetes-risk-test/
  In the Results section below, record the assessment of your current risk for diabetes. Note areas the tool identifies as risk factors that may increase your future risk of diabetes.

Results

Record key components of the results of each of your assessments. For each category of chronic disease, list at least three risk factors you have. These can be anything identified by the assessment—age, blood pressure, tobacco use, activity level, diet, and so on. For each risk factor you list, indicate whether it is modifiable.

ASSESSMENT	RISK FACTORS	MODIFIABLE?
Cardiovascular disease Overall score: ☐ / 10	1. 2. 3.	☐ yes ☐ no ☐ yes ☐ no ☐ yes ☐ no
Cancer	1. 2. 3.	☐ yes ☐ no ☐ yes ☐ no ☐ yes ☐ no

(continued)

ASSESSMENT	RISK FACTORS	MODIFIABLE?
Diabetes Current risk:	1.	☐ yes ☐ no
	2.	☐ yes ☐ no
	3.	☐ yes ☐ no

Reflecting on Your Results

What commonalities do you see among your modifiable risk factors? What risk factors do you have that raise your risk for more than one chronic disease?

Planning Your Next Steps

Choose one specific modifiable risk factor identified by the assessments you completed. Set a goal for change, and then list three strategies for achieving your goal. (If you have no modifiable risk factors, focus on strategies for addressing an uncontrollable risk factor—for example, obtaining age-appropriate screening tests.)

Are the modifiable risk factors you identified ones you were already aware of? Do the results of these assessment tests make you think more seriously about making changes? Why or why not?

Give it a shot—take action today to lessen your disease risk. If one approach doesn't work, try another until you experience success. Once you've successfully changed a risk factor, try working on another. Reassess yourself periodically to see the effect your actions have on your disease risk.

Up for the challenge? Write a date for reassessment here and then record a reminder on your own calendar.

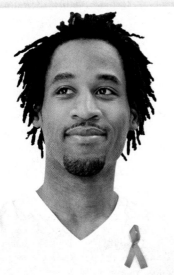

12
Infectious Diseases

Wellness Connections

How do infectious diseases relate to your overall wellness? If you're a young adult, they are probably one of the most obvious causes of temporary illness and discomfort in your life. Physical wellness is diminished in the short term by even minor infections, such as head colds. However, good physical wellness and intellectually sound health choices can help protect you from infections. Are you using your critical thinking skills to try to avoid and to safely treat infectious diseases? Do you wash your hands regularly? Are your immunizations up-to-date?

Emotional, social, and spiritual wellness, especially as they affect your stress levels, can make you less susceptible to infections, or more. Along with intellectual wellness, these wellness dimensions also influence the decisions you make about sexual behavior, which in turn affect your risk for contracting a sexually transmitted infection. How are your communication and relationship skills? If you're sexually active, do you always practice safer sex?

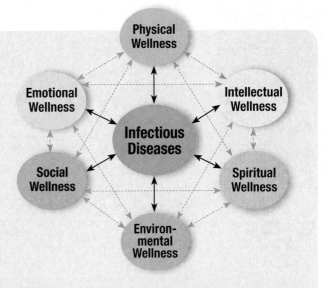

Your environment also plays an important role in your risk for infection. Water and food can spread infectious diseases, as can insects and rodents. You can help by promoting environmental wellness and by preparing for emergencies, such as natural disasters that cause a breakdown of the public health measures that protect us from many infections that plagued past generations.

As described in Chapter 1, infectious diseases were the leading cause of death in the United States before 1900, and they remain a leading killer worldwide. Although U.S. death rates have dropped dramatically, infectious diseases are still a major cause of illness and lost work and school time. This chapter provides an introduction to infectious diseases, including those that are sexually transmitted. You'll learn how to recognize and treat common diseases—and most importantly, how to prevent them.

Infection and Immunity

An **infectious disease** is one that can be passed among people. Common infections include colds, flu, bronchitis, mononucleosis, and the many sexually transmissible infections. Some infections are easy to catch and relatively mild; others are much more serious—but often more difficult to catch.

Pathogens

Q | What causes infectious diseases?

Infections are caused by **pathogens,** disease-causing agents that can be passed among people. Pathogens fall into a number of categories (Figure 12-1). Most pathogens are tiny, including the viruses and

infectious disease A disease that is transmissible from person to person through direct or indirect means; infection refers to invasion and multiplication of an organism; symptomatic disease follows if the body cannot quickly eliminate the pathogen.

pathogen A specific causative agent of infectious disease; examples include virus, bacteria, protozoa, and fungi.

	Pathogen	Effects	Diseases
	Viruses Tiny microbes consisting of one or more molecules of DNA or RNA surrounded by a protein coat	Viruses can enter and take over body cells, using them to rapidly produce more copies of the virus while at the same time damaging or destroying the cells.	Common cold, influenza, mononucleosis, hepatitis, cold sores, genital herpes, HIV/AIDS, genital warts, measles, mumps, rabies, polio
	Bacteria Single-celled organisms that may be in the shape of rods, balls, or spirals	Bacteria may secrete toxins or enzymes that destroy cells or interfere with cell functioning.	Lyme disease, pneumonia, peptic ulcers, tuberculosis, boils, toxic shock syndrome, strep throat, meningitis, gonorrhea
	Fungi A primitive form of plant that may be single- or multi-celled	Fungi may release enzymes that destroy cells.	Yeast infections, thrush, athlete's foot, jock itch, certain types of pneumonia and meningitis
	Protozoa Microscopic single-celled animals that can live independently of a host	In the human body, protozoa may release toxins and enzymes that destroy cells or interfere with their functioning.	Malaria, giardia, toxoplasmosis, African sleeping sickness
	Prions Specific types of abnormal proteins	Prions accumulate in the central nervous system and cause degenerative diseases.	Bovine spongiform encephalopathy ("mad cow disease"), Creutzfeldt-Jakob disease
	Helminths Parasitic worms that live in or on a host	Worms compete with body cells for nutrients and can block blood and lymph vessels or the digestive tract.	Tapeworm infection, pinworm infection, hookworm infection, swimmer's itch
	Ectoparasites Complex organisms that may live in or on a host's skin	Infestations may cause local irritation; in some cases, ectoparasites also transmit other types of pathogens.	Lice, scabies, ticks, fleas

Figure 12-1 **Pathogens, effects, and associated diseases**

bacteria that cause many familiar infections; these are often referred to as microbes or microorganisms. However, infections can also be caused by larger organisms, including lice and parasitic worms, although these infections may also be referred to as infestations.

It's important to note that many microbes live in a healthy human body and are needed to keep the body functioning normally. For example, your intestines contain types of bacteria that help digest food, destroy disease-causing microbes, and provide needed vitamins. However, even these helpful organisms can cause illness if their numbers become unbalanced or if they gain entry into a part of the body that is normally microbe-free. For example, healthy people usually carry *Staphylococcus aureus* bacteria on their skin and in their nasal passages without suffering any illness. But *S. aureus* can cause a number of different diseases if it enters the body through a cut or sore. Similarly, antibiotics can kill friendly bacteria in the mouth, which allows fungi to grow out of control and cause a disease known as thrush.

In some cases, it's important to distinguish between *infection,* meaning a disease-causing organism invades your body and starts to multiply, and *disease,* meaning you're experiencing obvious signs and symptoms. In some cases, you can have an infection—and be capable of transmitting the responsible pathogen to someone else—without ever experiencing symptoms. Your body may also be able to destroy an infectious agent before it ever causes symptoms, meaning you had an infection but not a disease. An infectious disease with symptoms occurs when your body's defenses cannot quickly and completely fight off an invading pathogen.

Q | Why are some infections more serious than others?

Many factors determine the severity of an infectious disease. Pathogens vary in their *virulence*—their innate ability to cause intense or severe symptoms. The viruses responsible for colds typically cause only mild, temporary infections affecting the upper respiratory system; the viruses that cause AIDS and smallpox, on the other hand, usually cause severe symptoms. Pathogens can also infect different parts of the body; for example, a bacterial infection confined to a small area of skin is likely to be less severe than an infection by the same bacteria if it gains access to the bloodstream and therefore the entire body. The amount of the pathogen you are initially exposed to can also have an impact—it's easier for your body to destroy a smaller number of pathogens.

And of course, your health status is also important. Just because a pathogen is present doesn't mean you'll become ill. Think about the times you've been around someone who was sick but you didn't become ill yourself. Many pathogenic organisms are present on and in your body at all times, but if the agent isn't too virulent, and if your own resistance is strong, then you won't become ill. A strong immune system can fight off more infectious agents than a

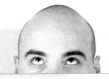
weak one. Some groups of people are at more risk for serious effects from infections, including infants, older adults, and pregnant women; infections that pose little risk to a healthy adult may be dangerous to people in these groups.

The Cycle of Infection

Q | How do you actually catch an infectious disease?

In order for an infectious disease to occur, a pathogen must gain entry into a host's body and start to replicate and cause symptoms. The transmission of an infection requires (1) a source of pathogens, (2) a susceptible host, and (3) a mode of transmission. Whether a person gets a disease depends on the relationship among these three factors.

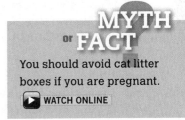
MYTH or FACT?
You should avoid cat litter boxes if you are pregnant.
▶ WATCH ONLINE

- **Source of pathogens:** Infectious agents can come from another person, an animal, water, or even soil. The environment that supports a pathogen's survival and growth is called its *reservoir,* and reservoirs often contain a large community of the pathogen. For many common infectious diseases, the reservoirs are the bodies of people who are already infected. Many disease-causing organisms can survive only a short time once they leave their usual reservoir or host.

- **Susceptible host:** People are more susceptible to infection if their immune system is weak or one of their natural physical defenses is compromised—such as by a cut in the skin. For example, very young children, older adults, and people with underlying health problems are all more susceptible to infections. Factors such as stress, smoking, use of antibiotics or other drugs, and vaccination history all affect a person's risk of infection.

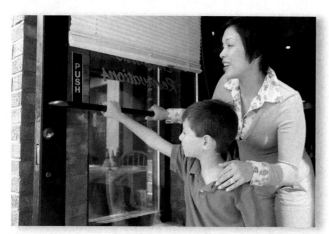

Many viruses and bacteria can be easily transmitted through direct and indirect contact. You can pick up pathogens by shaking hands or by touching shared surfaces such as door-knobs and keyboards.

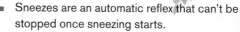

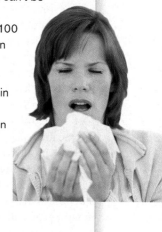
- **Mode of transmission:** Understanding how pathogens are transmitted can help you identify ways to break the cycle. To cause an infection, a pathogen must exit its reservoir and then reach and enter a new host. There are different modes of transmission: direct and indirect contact, inhalation, and contact with a disease *vector* such as a mosquito or tick. Different pathogens have different typical modes of transmission. People can transfer pathogens from their hands, mouth, or genitals by coming into direct contact with another person—through touching, kissing, or sexual activity. Sexually transmitted infections such as chlamydia, gonorrhea, and herpes are usually transmitted through direct con-tact. Injection drug use can also directly transmit a pathogen into the bloodstream of a new host.

The viruses that cause the common cold may be trans-mitted directly or indirectly. If a person with a cold sneezes onto her hand and her phone, a potential new host could pick up the virus from shaking her hand or borrowing her phone—and then touching his own eyes or nose and trans-ferring the virus.[1]

The flu virus is most often transmitted through inhala-tion: A person sneezes or coughs, and the virus is sprayed into the air in tiny droplets, which other people can breath in. These droplets can also land on surfaces in the environ-ment. Although some pathogens die quickly after leaving their hosts, cold and flu viruses are viable after many hours on surfaces such as desks and doorknobs.[2] Indirect contact can also occur when a person ingests contaminated water or food.

Finally, some pathogens are transmitted through insect or animal vectors. Malaria is an example of a vector-borne disease. A mosquito picks up the protozoa by biting an in-fected person and then can pass the protozoa on to the next person it bites. Lyme disease is another example of an infec-tion transmitted through an insect vector. The Lyme disease bacterium normally lives in mice and other small animals, but it is transferred to humans through the bite of a tick.

How do the pathogens enter the new host? Typically, they enter through any of the body's natural openings (mouth, nose, genitals, and so on), as well as through cuts and scrapes on the surface of the skin.

The Body's Defenses

Q | Do I start out with any re-sistance to disease?

Each of us is born with a specific capacity to resist certain diseases, but there is little consistency from one person to the next. This is why some people seem to never get colds, some peo-ple who have inhaled tuberculosis bacteria never get the disease, and some people do not become sick in the midst of an epidemic. Scientists are still trying to determine the exact causes for differences in disease resistance. Some of it seems to be present from birth, yet it remains to be de-termined how much of our resistance is inherited and how much is determined by factors such as age, illness, and nu-tritional status.

We all have built-in defenses against infectious dis-eases. Physical barriers are the first line of protection. Your skin is your body's largest organ, and most patho-gens cannot get through your skin unless it is damaged in some way. Thus, you are more likely to get an infection if your skin has been scraped, cut, or burned, or if passage

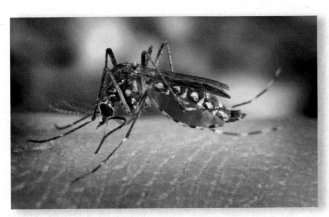

Your skin provides an effective physical barrier, but pathogens can be transmitted through cuts, scrapes, and burns, and via injection drug use or the bites of certain animal or insect vectors. Female mosquitoes can penetrate the skin and potentially transmit infections such as malaria and West Nile virus.

through the skin is aided by something like an injection or a bite from a mosquito.

Many of the openings in the human body—mouth, nostrils, eyelids, lungs, and genitals—are lined with mucous membranes. Although these linings seem delicate, they provide significant protection by secreting mucus that traps pathogens. The hairs in your nose and ears also trap many pathogens. Any foreign substances that enter the lungs may be expelled through the cough reflex or by the actions of hairlike cilia in your lungs that help push particles up and out.

Just as damage to the skin increases your risk of infection, so does damage to these other physical barriers. One reason that smoking increases your risk of infection is that it destroys the cilia in the lungs. If you have a sexually transmitted infection that causes sores or blisters, you are more likely to contract another infection. For example, having genital warts or herpes infection increases your risk for contracting HIV infection.[3]

Your body also has chemical barriers to pathogens. Your digestive tract contains acids, proteins, enzymes, and friendly bacteria that can all discourage the entry and spread of pathogens. Substances in tears can dissolve the outer coating of certain bacteria. Vaginal secretions normally produce a slightly acidic environment, which encourages the growth of some microbes and discourages the growth of others.

You can help out your body's physical defenses through actions such as washing your hands and limiting contact with objects and surfaces used by a person who is ill.

The Immune System

Q How do I develop my immunity?

Your immunity can come from several sources. Your **immune system** comes into play if a pathogen gets through the physical and chemical barriers. Your immune system is a complex network of specialized organs, tissues, and cells that defends the body from disease-causing microbes and helps repair damaged tissue. A complete description of the immune system and the immune response is beyond the scope of this text, but here are a few key concepts to keep in mind:

- Immune cells constantly circulate through your body, ready to recognize foreign substances and take action. All cells carry protein markers on their surface; protein markers on pathogens, known as **antigens,** are recognized as being foreign and trigger the immune response.
- Some cells of the immune system respond to the damage and toxins a pathogen produces. They move to the site of the infection, "eat" the invading microbes, and destroy infected body cells. Pain and swelling at the site of an infection are often the result of the body's battle to keep the infection from spreading.
- If an infection persists or spreads, other cells of the immune system produce large numbers of **antibodies.** These specialized proteins bind to the pathogen's specific antigen and help mark it for destruction.
- The fever (elevated body temperature) that often accompanies an infection can help speed up parts of the immune response. It may also make the host a less hospitable environment for the pathogen. Fevers of 100°F or less are usually not harmful and don't need to be treated.
- For certain pathogens, once you've been exposed, the body produces specialized "memory" cells. These cells are able to recognize the antigen associated with the pathogen and respond quickly if you ever become infected with the same microbe again. In this way, you can essentially become immune to the pathogen—if you are infected, your body will quickly kill the pathogens and no disease will develop.

In addition to the natural immunity that develops after an infection, you can also acquire immunity without actually experiencing the infection. This occurs following a vaccination (see p. 420) or through direct injection of antibodies. Babies can also temporarily acquire immunity from their mothers through breast-feeding, because breast milk contains protective maternal antibodies.[4]

Q What causes swollen lymph glands?

Swollen lymph glands, also called lymph nodes, usually indicate an active immune response to an infection.

immune system A complex network of organs, tissues, and cells that produce the immune response and defend the body from disease-causing agents.

antigen Protein molecules on the surface of infectious agents that the immune system recognizes as foreign, triggering the immune response.

antibody Molecule produced by the immune system that binds to a specific antigen, marking it for destruction.

Your lymph glands are part of the **lymphatic system,** a collection of vessels and organs that carry out several different functions in the body. Lymph vessels pick up fluid lost from capillaries and return it to the circulatory system. The lymph vessels are similar to blood vessels, but to move fluid, they rely on compression from muscle contractions rather than the pumping action of the heart.

The lymphatic system also plays a key role in the defense against invading pathogens. The spleen, thymus, and bone marrow help produce and activate infection-fighting cells. Lymph vessels transport fluid containing foreign material and cellular debris to lymph nodes for disposal. The lymph nodes are located at intervals throughout the body; they contain many immune cells, which during an infection ingest and destroy invading pathogens.

The lymph nodes that most often become swollen are those in your neck, armpits, and groin. The location of a swollen gland can provide clues to the source or location of an infection. The swelling usually subsides within a few days, but it can take up to several weeks after an infection has cleared for lymph nodes to return to normal size.

The Role of Immunizations

Q | Do vaccines weaken my immune system?

No. **Vaccines** strengthen your immune system by preparing your body to fight infection. They create immunity against infections you haven't had. Vaccines are made from killed, weakened, or incomplete pathogens. They work by exposing the body to foreign antigens from the microbe, which the immune system responds to by producing antibodies. Vaccines do not cause the infectious disease, but they do prime your body to respond to the pathogen if you are ever infected. A vaccine may also include an inactive version of a bacterial toxin so that the body can develop a defense against it.

No vaccine is completely effective, and some people have a stronger immune response to a vaccine than others. The effects of some vaccines fade so that regular booster shots are needed to maintain immunity. Figure 12-2 shows the immunizations recommended for U.S. adults; for additional information and the recommendations for children, visit the "Vaccines and Immunizations" page of the Centers for Disease Control (http://www.cdc.gov/vaccines).

Stages and Patterns of Infectious Diseases

Q | Can all infections be cured?

No. There are different kinds of infections, and the ones most likely to resolve on their own or be cured quickly with treatment are **acute infections,** which are characterized by a short duration and a fairly typical series of stages (Figure 12-3):

- *Incubation:* Time between infection with the pathogen and the first appearance of symptoms. The immune system is able to stop some infections during this stage and clear the pathogen from the body, meaning no disease develops.
- *Prodrome:* Initial appearance of general signs and symptoms of illness. An individual might begin to feel unwell.
- *Illness:* Signs and symptoms of the specific infection develop and become more severe.
- *Convalescence:* Acute symptoms of the infection subside. The time required for recovery depends on the severity of the infection and the underlying health of the individual.

These stages occur for many infectious diseases, including the common cold. However, infections can follow other patterns. In a **chronic infection,** the illness persists or recurs over a long period. Hepatitis can become a chronic liver infection, slowly causing cirrhosis or liver cancer. Up to 10,000 Americans die from chronic hepatitis each year.[5] HIV infection can be a chronic progressive disease, meaning the infection persists and often worsens over time, with more and more of the virus produced in the body.

In a **latent infection,** the pathogen lies dormant in the body but retains the ability to replicate. Illness can recur if immunity weakens due to aging, poor health habits, hormonal imbalance, or another infection. Chicken pox is an example of a latent infection: People can harbor the virus throughout their life without experiencing symptoms. But at some later point, if immunity weakens, they can develop shingles, a painful infection of the nerves.

DOLLAR STRETCHER
Financial Wellness Tip

Wash your hands often and thoroughly to prevent illnesses that can be costly in terms of both time and money. You don't need fancy soaps or chemicals; plain old soap and water is just as effective. If you use liquid soap, get a refillable dispenser that squirts out just enough soap for a single use.

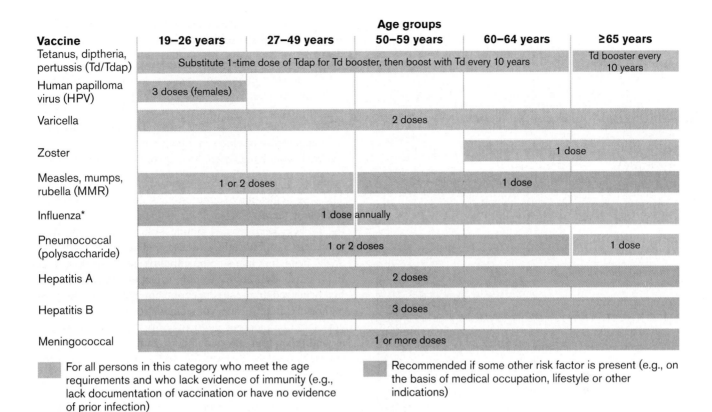

Vaccine	19–26 years	27–49 years	50–59 years	60–64 years	≥65 years
Tetanus, diptheria, pertussis (Td/Tdap)	Substitute 1-time dose of Tdap for Td booster, then boost with Td every 10 years				Td booster every 10 years
Human papilloma virus (HPV)	3 doses (females)				
Varicella	2 doses				
Zoster				1 dose	
Measles, mumps, rubella (MMR)	1 or 2 doses		1 dose		
Influenza*	1 dose annually				
Pneumococcal (polysaccharide)	1 or 2 doses				1 dose
Hepatitis A	2 doses				
Hepatitis B	3 doses				
Meningococcal	1 or more doses				

Age groups

For all persons in this category who meet the age requirements and who lack evidence of immunity (e.g., lack documentation of vaccination or have no evidence of prior infection)

Recommended if some other risk factor is present (e.g., on the basis of medical occupation, lifestyle or other indications)

In 2010, the CDC recommended that all persons 6 months and older receive the seasonal influenza vaccine for the 2010–2011 season.

Figure 12-2 Recommended immunizations for adults. For more information and additional recommendations, visit http://www.cdc.gov/vaccines.

Sources: Centers for Disease Control and Prevention. (2010). Recommended adult immunization schedule—United States, 2010. *Morbidity and Mortality Weekly Report, 59*(1), 1–4. Centers for Disease Control and Prevention. (2010). Prevention and control of influenza with vaccines. *Morbidity and Mortality Weekly Report, 59*, 1–62.

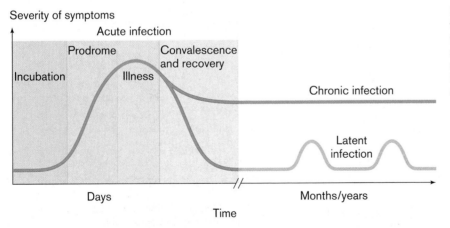

Figure 12-3 Stages and patterns of infections. Acute infections follow a typical four-stage pattern and usually resolve in days or weeks. Chronic infections persist over a longer period, whereas latent infections can recur if an individual's immunity weakens.

Prevention and Treatment of Infectious Diseases

Q | **How can I keep from getting sick?**

Your two best strategies for preventing infectious diseases are to keep pathogens out of your body and to maintain a strong immune system.

What can you do to avoid infectious agents? Your best defense is hand washing—do it often and do it thoroughly (Figure 12-4). If soap and water aren't available, use an alcohol-based hand sanitizer. Many common infectious diseases are transmitted through touch: An infected person transfers microbes directly (handshake) or indirectly (doorknob) to your hands. When you touch your eyes, nose, or mouth, the pathogen gains access to your body. Studies

When to wash

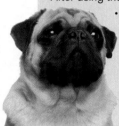

- Before and after preparing food
- Before and after eating food
- After using the toilet
  - After changing diapers or cleaning up a child who has used the toilet
  - Before and after tending to someone who is sick
  - After blowing your nose, coughing, or sneezing
  - After handling an animal or animal waste
  - After handling garbage
  - Before and after treating a cut or wound

How to wash

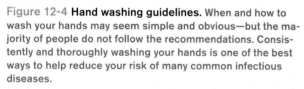

- Wet your hands with clean running water and apply soap
- Use warm water if it is available
- Rub hands together to make a lather and scrub all surfaces
- Continue rubbing hands for 20 seconds; if you need a timer, hum the "Happy Birthday" song from beginning to end twice
- Rinse hands well under running water
- Dry your hands using a paper towel or air dryer; if possible, use your paper towel to turn off the faucet

When using hand sanitizer

- If soap and water are not available, use alcohol-based gel (at least 60% alcohol) to clean hands
- Apply product to the palm of one hand, using the amount of product indicated on the label
  - Rub hands together
  - Rub the product over all surfaces of hands and fingers until hands are dry

Figure 12-4 Hand washing guidelines. When and how to wash your hands may seem simple and obvious—but the majority of people do not follow the recommendations. Consistently and thoroughly washing your hands is one of the best ways to help reduce your risk of many common infectious diseases.

Source: Centers for Disease Control and Prevention. (2010). *Clean hands save lives* (http://www.cdc.gov/cleanhands).

the one who is sick and sneezing or coughing, you can help stop the spread of infections by keeping your germs to yourself:

- Cover your mouth and nose with a tissue when you cough or sneeze.
- Throw out your used tissue.
- If you don't have a tissue, cough or sneeze into your upper sleeve or elbow, not your hands.
- Wash your hands often; if soap and water are not available, use an alcohol-based hand rub.

These strategies may sound obvious, but many people do not follow them.

To help keep your immune system strong, practice good self-care. Eat right, exercise, and get plenty of sleep.[8] Avoid behaviors like smoking and excessive drinking that hurt your body's ability to fight infection. Never inject illicit drugs; contaminated injection equipment can transmit pathogens directly into your bloodstream. If you plan to get a tattoo or piercing, go to a facility that is clean and has a good reputation; ask about sterilization practices and be sure to follow the instructions you're given on caring for your skin.

Also pay special attention to emotional wellness: High levels of stress and poor mental health are associated with higher rates of infectious diseases (Figure 12-5).[9] On the flip side, many of the strategies to reduce stress also help boost the immune system. For example, a study that looked at stress levels, humor, and immune function found that laughing at a humorous video reduced stress and improved the activity of immune cells.[10] Your emotional wellness can have a powerful effect on how well your body responds to infec-

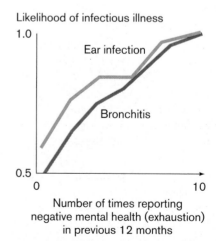

Figure 12-5 Mental health and risk of infectious disease in college students. Students who reported negative mental health—feelings of depression, anxiety, exhaustion, or hopelessness—also experienced higher rates of infectious disease.

Source: Adams, T. B., Wharton, C. M., Quilter, L., & Hirsch, T. (2008). The association between mental health and acute infectious illness among a national sample of 18- to 24-year-old college students. *Journal of American College Health, 56*(6), 657–663.

have linked good hand hygiene with reduced rates of upper respiratory and gastrointestinal illnesses.[6] However, most college students do not follow recommendations for hand washing.[7] Remember to wash your hands often—it works!

For infections like influenza that are transmitted through airborne droplets, your best strategy is to avoid people who are sneezing and coughing or stand at least three feet away—six or more feet is even better. If you're

Research Brief

Hand Hygiene and Illness Rates in College Students

Most people, college students included, do not follow the recommendations for hand washing: They don't wash at all the recommended times or for the recommended duration. But does it really make a difference? Researchers recently studied students in four college residence halls, comparing a study group and a control group. For the study group, alcohol-gel hand-sanitizer dispensers were installed in every room, bathroom, and dining hall. The groups were followed for eight weeks and compared in terms of hand-hygiene behavior, symptom and illness rates, and absenteeism from class.

What did the researchers find? The study group showed improvements over the control group in all areas.

- Improved hand-hygiene practices: both hand washing frequency and the use of hand sanitizers were significantly higher in the study group; the increase in hand washing was thought to be due to increased awareness of the importance of hand hygiene.

- Reduced symptoms of upper respiratory illness: for example, students in the study group were 15% less likely to experience sore throat and stuffy nose and 30% less likely to develop cough or fever.
- Reduced rates of illness: the study group showed a 20% improvement in illness rate.
- Fewer missed school/work days: the study group missed 40% fewer days than the control group.

This study clearly showed the power of just a little more attention to hand hygiene. If you'd like to be sick less often and miss fewer days of school and work due to upper respiratory illness, wash your hands!

Source: White, C., Kolble, R., Carlson, R., et al. (2003). The effect of hand hygiene on illness rates among students in university residence halls. *American Journal of Infection Control, 31*(6), 364–370.

---

tion. See the box "Keeping Yourself Well" for a summary of actions you can take to help support your immune system.

Q | I'm confused about antibiotics—when do they really work?

Antibiotics are powerful medications that have saved many lives. At the same time, they are often misused, which can also lead to problems. Antibiotics primarily fight bacterial infections, although they may also be prescribed for certain conditions caused by fungi and parasites. They act by killing bacteria or preventing them from reproducing. They don't work against any infections caused by viruses, including colds, flu, and most sore throats and coughs. Sometimes a person with a viral infection will develop a secondary bacterial infection as a complication; antibiotics may be prescribed to destroy the bacteria, but they won't treat the initial viral infection.

Most bacteria die when exposed to antibiotics, but some develop resistance to the drug's effects. If these resistant bacteria spread, they are more difficult to treat. Every time you take antibiotics, you increase the chances that some bacteria in your body will develop

resistance.[11] So, it's important to take antibiotics no more often than necessary. In addition, when antibiotics are prescribed for an infection, you should take them for the recommended duration—not just until your symptoms disappear. Stopping treatment too soon can allow an infection to return and also contributes to the development of resistance.

antibiotic A compound that is used to treat bacterial infections by killing the bacteria or inhibiting its growth.

Although beneficial, antibiotics also have side effects, including upset stomach, diarrhea, and, in women, vaginal yeast infections. Some antibiotics can also impair the functioning of the liver or kidneys.

Q | How are infections treated?

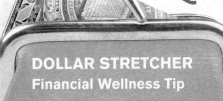

DOLLAR STRETCHER
Financial Wellness Tip

Treat minor infections at home—you don't need to pay for a doctor visit or antibiotics, which don't treat viral infections like colds and flu. For upper respiratory infections, rest and drink plenty of warm liquids. If symptoms are bothersome, try inexpensive, generic medications.

Treatment depends on the type of pathogen, the severity of the infection, and the person's underlying health status. Many minor infections don't need to be treated—your immune system can successfully eliminate the pathogen. If symptoms are uncomfortable during the acute phase the illness, over-the-counter medications are available to relieve nasal congestion, body aches, and other minor symptoms. If your symptoms are

Wellness Strategies

Keeping Yourself Well

- Get regular, moderate exercise.
- Eat a healthy diet.
- Get plenty of sleep.
- Control stress.
- Don't smoke, avoid secondhand smoke, and consume alcohol moderately, if at all.
- Wash your hands frequently and thoroughly.
- Don't rub your eyes, touch your nose, or eat with your fingers without washing your hands first.
- Avoid people with obvious signs of illness.
- Clean shared environmental surfaces (desks, phones, doorknobs), especially if you live or work with someone who is ill.

- Handle and prepare foods safely (see Chapter 9).
- Avoid disease carriers like mosquitoes, ticks, and rodents. To protect yourself from insect bites, wear long pants and long-sleeved shirts when you hike or work outdoors; you can also apply an insect repellent (for more information, visit http://www.nlm.nih.gov/medlineplus/insectbitesandstings.html).
- Abstain from sex or consistently practice safer sex.
- Don't inject drugs.
- Keep immunizations up to date.
- Stock an emergency kit to use in case of a breakdown in public health services, such as after a natural disaster (for advice about kits, visit http://www.ready.gov).

---

unusually severe or your illness persists, check with your health care provider.

Antimicrobial drugs exist for several categories of pathogens. For bacterial infections, antibiotics may be prescribed (see above). Specific antiviral drugs are available for few infections, including herpes, hepatitis, influenza, and HIV. Similarly, there are drugs that specifically target fungal and protozoal infections.

Infectious Diseases on Campus

For college students, even minor infectious diseases can impact academic performance. Students should also be alert to signs and symptoms that may indicate more serious conditions.

Colds and Influenza

Q | How do you tell if you have a cold or the flu?

Colds and **influenza** ("the flu") are both caused by viruses and have some of the same symptoms, but there are differences (Table 12-1). Influenza is the more serious disease, although colds are more common and probably responsible for more lost days at school and on the job than any other infectious disease. For all the misery a cold can cause, in the vast majority of cases it will resolve without treatment—and nothing you do will shorten its duration.

There are hundreds of viruses that can cause the common cold. They are thought to be transmitted primarily by indirect contact—you touch a contaminated surface or object and then rub your eyes. Cold viruses can enter the body through the mucous membrane of the eyes. It takes about 48 hours from the time of exposure for symptoms to appear, and colds generally last two to seven days. Weather doesn't affect your risk for a cold, although being forced indoors into more crowded conditions increases your chance for exposure. Cold viruses pass easily from person to person. Colds are more frequent in children, becoming fewer with age. Complications are fairly unusual but are more likely among older adults.

Influenza viruses are more likely to be transmitted through respiratory droplets that infected people release when they cough, sneeze, or talk. People with influenza can probably pass the virus to others up to about six feet away. They are contagious and able to infect others beginning about a day before symptoms develop and up to five to seven days after becoming ill.[12] Symptoms of influenza usually come on suddenly and typically include fever, body aches, and severe fatigue. The flu typically lasts longer than a cold. It also carries a greater risk of serious complications, including pneumonia, bronchitis, and sinus and ear infections. Older adults, pregnant women, young children, and people with chronic medical conditions are more likely to have serious problems. Thousands of Americans die from influenza and its complications every year.

Q | Why is there a new flu vaccine every year?

Most cases of the flu are caused by influenza A and influenza B viruses. Influenza A viruses are further divided into subtypes based

influenza A highly infectious respiratory disease caused by an influenza virus; the "flu."

TABLE 12-1 IS IT A COLD OR THE FLU?

SYMPTOM	COLD	FLU
FEVER	Rare	Usual; high (100°–102°F or higher); lasts 3–4 days
HEADACHE	Rare	Common
GENERAL ACHES, PAINS	Slight	Usual, often severe
FATIGUE, WEAKNESS	Sometimes	Usual; can last up to 2–3 weeks
EXHAUSTION	Never	Usual; typically at the beginning of the illness
STUFFY NOSE	Common	Sometimes
SNEEZING	Usual	Sometimes
SORE THROAT	Common	Sometimes
CHEST DISCOMFORT, COUGH	Mild to moderate	Common; can be severe
COMPLICATIONS	Sinus congestion, middle-ear infection, worsening of asthma symptoms	Bronchitis, pneumonia; worsening of chronic conditions; can be life-threatening

Source: National Institute of Allergy and Infectious Diseases. (2008). *Is it a cold or the flu?* (http://www.niaid.nih.gov/topics/Flu/understandingFlu/Pages/publications.aspx).

on proteins on their surface (H and N); recall the H1N1 virus that caused a flu *pandemic* (worldwide outbreak of disease) in 2009–2010. Influenza viruses continually change over time—sometimes slightly, sometimes significantly—and when they do, the immune system no longer recognizes the new version of the virus. Any immunity to other strains you had from past infections or vaccinations no longer protects you. So, the flu vaccine is reformulated every year to target the strains most likely to be circulating.

Infectious Mononucleosis

Q | Does mono only come from kissing?

Epstein-Barr virus (EBV), a member of the **herpes** family of viruses, is the pathogen that causes infectious mononucleosis, or "mono." It is transmitted via saliva, which is how it got nicknamed the "kissing disease." Although it can be transmitted through kissing, any activity that brings someone in contact with the saliva of an infected person can transfer the virus—for example, sharing a drinking glass. The primary symptoms are fever, sore throat, swollen glands, and fatigue; some people also develop a swollen spleen. Serious complications

are rare, but the fatigue associated with the infection can sometimes last for several months. People who develop an enlarged spleen will be advised to avoid certain physical activities as well as contact sports to reduce the risk of rupturing the spleen.

By age 40, it's estimated that 95 percent of American adults have been infected with EBV.[13] Not everyone develops symptoms, but EBV is a latent infection, so the virus remains dormant in the body (see p. 420). The infection can reactivate, but it usually causes no symptoms even though it can be passed on to someone else. Because the virus can be carried in the saliva of otherwise healthy people, transmission is nearly impossible to prevent.

Meningitis

Q | Which is the infection that causes stiff neck?

You are probably thinking of **meningitis,** which is inflammation of the membranes that surround the brain and spinal

herpes A family of viruses that includes those responsible for chicken pox, cold sores, mononucleosis, and genital herpes; herpes viruses have the ability to establish lifelong latent infections.

meningitis Inflammation of the meninges, the membranes that surround the brain and the spinal cord.

Wellness Strategies

Starve a Fever, Feed a Cold?

Although popularized by Mark Twain, this old adage—and its exact opposite—dates back to the 1500s. Today's medical experts will tell you that neither of these is prudent advice, but it is hard for many to turn away from medical myths. Your body always needs energy, regardless of the type of infection, so make sure to eat to satisfy your appetite. Even though the common cold has no cure, there are treatments that can make the suffering more tolerable. Many of these strategies are also good for home treatment of influenza.

- Drink plenty of liquids: Water, juice, clear broth, or warm lemon water with honey help loosen congestion and prevent dehydration. Avoid alcohol.
- Rest: Colds can tire you out, but influenza is especially associated with severe fatigue and body aches.
- Try a saltwater gargle: Dissolve 1/2 teaspoon salt in 8 ounces of warm water and gargle to temporarily relieve a sore or scratchy throat.
- Try saline nasal spray: Over-the-counter saline nasal sprays can combat stuffiness and congestion. Avoid or limit use of nasal decongestant sprays, which can lead to a worsening of symptoms when the medication is discontinued.
- Use over-the-counter cold medicines cautiously: Decongestants may relieve some of your symptoms but will not shorten the length of your cold; some also have side effects including drowsiness and upset stomach. Choose single-ingredient products, and don't exceed the rec-

ommended dosages. Antihistamines may provide some relief from cold symptoms, but they are more appropriate for treating allergies.

- Use pain relievers cautiously: Aspirin, acetaminophen, or ibuprofen can all reduce a fever and bring some relief from the aches and pains, but they won't make your symptoms go away any faster. Aspirin and ibuprofen can cause stomach irritation, and if taken for a long period or in higher-than-recommended doses, acetaminophen can be toxic to your liver. Talk to your doctor before giving acetaminophen to children, and don't give aspirin to children or teens because of the risk of Reye's syndrome, a rare but potentially fatal disease.
- Limit or avoid over-the-counter cough medicines: Don't take a cough suppressant if you have a productive cough. Soothing your throat with warm liquids and throat lozenges and humidifying the air in your residence can be more effective than any drugs. (The Food and Drug Administration recommends that nonprescription cough medicines *not* be given to children under age 2.)

And remember, antibiotics are not effective at treating viral infections like colds and the flu.

---

cord. Symptoms in adults typically include high fever, severe headache, stiff neck, and sensitivity to bright light. The most common cause is a viral infection, and viral meningitis usually resolves on its own after about 7–10 days. However, bacterial meningitis, which has the same symptoms, is a much more severe infection that can lead to disability or even death. Anyone experiencing meningitis symptoms needs to see a physician immediately (Table 12-2); if treated early with antibiotics, bacterial meningitis can be cured.

Bacterial Skin Infections

Q | What's MRSA?

The acronym MRSA stands for methicillin-resistant *Staphylococcus aureus*. It's a type of staph bacteria that is resistant to many antibiotics and therefore difficult to treat. MRSA used to be a common cause of hospital-acquired pneumonia and

bloodstream infections, but it is now also a major cause of skin infections outside medical settings. Risk factors for the spread of MRSA include close skin-to-skin contact, skin cuts or abrasions, crowded living conditions, and contaminated items and surfaces. Places where these risk factors are common include athletic facilities, dormitories, military barracks, and daycare centers. See the box "Avoiding Infections from the Gym" for more information.

Skin infections usually start out as red, swollen, painful lumps; they may initially look like pimples, boils, or insect bites. If the infection spreads, you may also become generally ill with fever, swollen glands, and so on. If you experience these symptoms, you should contact your health care provider for a diagnosis and appropriate treatment; MRSA skin infections require professional treatment. Skin infections can also be caused by other pathogens, including *Streptococcus* bacteria. Athlete's foot, herpes, and impetigo are all examples of other common skin infections.

TABLE 12-2 COMMON INFECTIONS: SYMPTOMS AND TREATMENTS

ILLNESS (PATHOGEN)	SYMPTOMS	HOME TREATMENT	WHEN TO SEEK MEDICAL CARE
COMMON COLD (over 200 different viruses)	Runny nose, nasal congestion, mild cough, sore throat, low-grade fever, sneezing	Usually resolves on its own; fluids, rest, and over-the-counter medications to treat symptoms; avoid alcohol and tobacco	Worsening symptoms after third day, difficulty breathing, stiff neck
INFLUENZA (influenza A or B virus)	Sudden-onset fever, extreme fatigue, headache, body aches, cough	Usually resolves on its own; same home treatment as for colds; prescription antivirals available	Difficulty breathing, severe headache or stiff neck, confusion, fever lasting more than 3 days; new, localized pain in ear, chest, sinuses; people at high risk for complications should contact a health care provider if they develop flu symptoms
BRONCHITIS (different viruses or bacteria)	Cough that may start out dry and later produce mucus; sore throat, fever	Usually resolves on its own; same home treatment as for colds	Shortness of breath, high fever, shaking chills (signs of pneumonia); wheezing and cough that last more than 2 weeks; people at high risk for complications should check with a health care provider
MONONUCLEOSIS (Epstein-Barr virus)	High fever, swollen glands, severe sore throat, fatigue; nausea, vomiting, and loss of appetite can occur	Usually resolves on its own; rest, fluids; avoid contact sports until symptoms resolve due to risk of spleen rupture	Fever lasting more than 3 days; symptoms lasting longer than 7–10 days; severe abdominal pain (possibly indicating ruptured spleen)
MENINGITIS (several different viruses or bacteria)	High fever, stiff and painful neck, headache; vomiting, sleepiness, confusion, seizures	Requires medical evaluation; if determined to be a viral infection, home treatment to relieve symptoms is appropriate	Immediately; bacterial meningitis requires treatment with antibiotics to avoid serious or deadly complications
STREP THROAT (*Streptococcus* bacteria)	Sudden-onset sore throat and fever; swollen glands; red and white pus on tonsils; absence of cold symptoms	A visit to health care provider is appropriate; saltwater gargles, throat lozenges, over-the-counter medications to treat symptoms	Strep throat is treated with antibiotics to reduce duration of symptoms and risk of complications
BACTERIAL SKIN INFECTION (*Staphylococcus aureus* or *Streptococcus*)	Skin sore or rash; red, swollen, warm, and painful areas of skin; if infection spreads, general symptoms of fever, chills, swollen glands	A visit to health care provider is appropriate; warm compresses; keep infected area clean and dry; topical antibiotics if advised by health care provider	Bacterial skin infections are usually treated with antibiotics; stay alert for worsening symptoms or infection on the face
URINARY TRACT INFECTIONS (different bacteria)	Cloudy, bloody, or strong-smelling urine; frequent urination; pain or burning with urination; low fever; pain in lower abdomen	Requires medical evaluation; drink plenty of water; in women, drinking cranberry juice has been shown to help prevent but not treat urinary tract infections	Bacterial urinary tract infections are usually treated with antibiotics; stay alert for worsening symptoms, which may indicate the infection has spread to the kidneys

Wellness Strategies

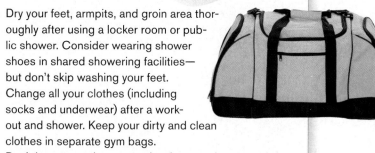

Avoiding Infections from the Gym

Skin infections in athletes are very common and can also affect recreational athletes and anyone who works out at a gym. Here are some steps you can take to reduce your risk:

- Ask your gym or exercise facility about its cleaning procedures—what is cleaned and how often? Does it provide cleansers and wipes for people to use?
- If facility exercise mats aren't cleaned between each class, bring your own exercise mat, and clean your mat after each workout.
- Use clothing or a towel to act as a barrier between exercise equipment and your bare skin; if you use a towel, wash it after each workout.
- If you have any skin abrasions or cuts, cover them with a sterile bandage.
- Wash your hands before and after working out; hand hygiene is important in all settings.
- Shower after a workout. Wash all parts of your body, including your feet. Athletes in sports with high rates of skin infection should wash with antibacterial cleanser.

- Dry your feet, armpits, and groin area thoroughly after using a locker room or public shower. Consider wearing shower shoes in shared showering facilities—but don't skip washing your feet.
- Change all your clothes (including socks and underwear) after a workout and shower. Keep your dirty and clean clothes in separate gym bags.
- Don't borrow or share water bottles, towels, razors, bar soap, deodorant, or other personal hygiene items.
- If you notice any symptoms, see a doctor, follow the recommended treatment, and don't go back to the gym until the doctor says your infection is no longer contagious.

Sources: Zinder, S. M., Basler, R. S. W., Foley, J., Scarlata, C., & Vasily, D. B. (2010). National Athletic Trainers' Association position statement: Skin diseases. *Journal of Athletic Training, 45*(4), 411–428. American Academy of Family Physicians. (2009). *Tinea infections: Athlete's foot, jock itch, and ringworm* (http://familydoctor.org/online/famdocen/home/common/infections/common/fungal/316.html).

Sexually Transmitted Infections

Sexually transmitted infections (STIs) are among the most common types of infections in the United States, with an estimated 19 million new cases each year (Table 12-3). About half of all new infections occur among people ages 15–24. STIs are primarily spread through person-to-person sexual contact—vaginal, oral, or anal sex—although some can also be transmitted in other ways. Some STIs can be easily treated and cured, but others are chronic, incurable, and even life threatening. All STIs are preventable.

Q | Do women get more STIs than men?

Yes, women are more likely to have STIs and more likely to experience serious complications from them. Transmission of many STIs, including genital herpes and HIV, is more likely to occur from an infected male to his female partner than from an infected female to her male partner. Approximately one in five women between 14 and 49 has genital herpes infection compared with one in nine men in the same age group.[14] Young women are also more likely than older women to contract STIs and to experience serious effects; the cervix of young women is covered with cells that are especially susceptible to STIs.

sexually transmitted infection (STI) An infection that is primarily spread through person-to-person sexual contact.

Most STIs affect both men and women, but in many cases, they cause more severe problems in women, including infertility. Having an STI during pregnancy can cause early labor, infection of the uterus, and in some cases dangerous infections in the baby.

Q | Do STIs show up immediately?

Not necessarily. Many sexually transmitted infections are asymptomatic, meaning people are unaware they are infected and can pass the infection on to others. Some STIs have very minor symptoms that can be overlooked or mistaken for other conditions. It's important to realize that anyone who is sexually active can have an STI—even if they've never had any signs or symptoms of disease. It doesn't matter who you are, it's what you do that counts.

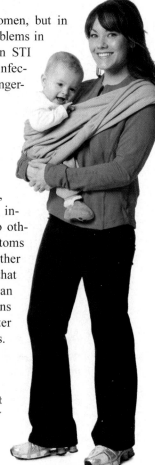

Women are more likely than men to contract sexually transmitted infections and to suffer serious complications from them. Infants can also be at risk for contracting infections from their mothers during pregnancy, childbirth, and breast-feeding.

TABLE 12-3 STIs IN THE UNITED STATES: A SNAPSHOT

	ESTIMATED ANNUAL INCIDENCE	ESTIMATED PREVALENCE*	OUTLOOK IF DIAGNOSED
TRICHOMONIASIS	7.4 million	n/a	Curable with antibiotics
HPV INFECTION	6.2 million	20 million	Vaccine-preventable; incurable but often resolves on its own; can cause cancer
CHLAMYDIA	2.8 million	1.9 million	Curable with antibiotics
GENITAL HERPES	1.6 million	45 million	Chronic and incurable; treatments can reduce symptoms and outbreaks
GONORRHEA	700,000	n/a	Curable with antibiotics
SYPHILIS	60,000	n/a	Curable with antibiotics
HIV INFECTION	56,000	1.1 million	Chronic and potentially fatal; treatable but incurable
HEPATITIS B	43,000	1.25 million	Vaccine-preventable; incurable but often resolves on its own; can cause fatal liver disease

*Because viral STIs can be persistent and incurable, the number of currently infected people capable of transmitting the infection (prevalence) greatly exceeds the annual number of new cases (incidence).

Sources: Centers for Disease Control and Prevention. (2010). Fact sheet: HIV in the United States (http://www.cdc.gov/hiv/resources/factsheets/us.htm). Centers for Disease Control and Prevention. (2010). HCV FAQs for health professionals (http://www.cdc.gov/hepatitis/HCV/HCVfaq.htm). Weinstock, H., Berman, S., & Cates, W. (2004). Sexually transmitted diseases among American youth: Incidence and prevalence estimates, 2000. *Perspectives on Sexual and Reproductive Health, 36*(1), 6–10. Additional data from the Kaiser Family Foundation and the Guttmacher Institute.

Trichomoniasis

Q | What's the most common sexually transmitted infection?

In terms of new cases each year, **trichomoniasis,** or "trich," is the most common. The protozoa *Trichomonas vaginalis* causes vaginal infections in women and infections of the urethra (urine canal) in men. Most infected women have symptoms such as vaginal discharge and painful urination, but most infected men do not have symptoms. Trichomoniasis is diagnosed with lab tests and treated with prescription medication. If a woman develops trichomoniasis, she and her partner both need to be treated because it's likely he is infected even if he has no symptoms. Treatment should be completed before resuming sexual activity. Trichomoniasis has two serious complications if untreated: It significantly increases the risk of HIV transmission, and, in pregnant women, it can lead to premature labor and delivery.

Chlamydia

Q | How often should I get checked for chlamydia?

Annual screening for **chlamydia** is recommended for sexually active women 25 years of age and younger, as well as older women with risk factors (many sex partners or a new sex partner). Testing is also recommended for pregnant women.

Chlamydia is caused by *Chlamydia trachomatis,* a bacterium that can be transmitted during vaginal, oral, or anal sex or from an infected mother to her baby during childbirth. About 70 percent of those who are infected have no symptoms, but among those who do, abnormal discharge from the vagina or penis and pain while urinating are most common.

Untreated, chlamydia can cause serious infections of the fallopian tubes in women and the urethra and epididymis (curved tube on the back of the testicle) in men. People infected through oral sex may have symptoms in the throat.

Chlamydia can be treated with antibiotics, but reinfection is possible—and even likely, if a woman's partner isn't also treated. In women, untreated chlamydia is a leading cause of serious and permanent damage to the reproductive organs, which can lead to infertility. Infected infants may develop pneumonia and eye infections that can potentially cause blindness.

Gonorrhea

Q | Can a person really get gonorrhea from oral sex?

Yes, unprotected oral sex can transmit the infection, although it's not as common as infection of the reproductive

trichomoniasis Sexually transmitted infection caused by the protozoa *Trichomonas vaginalis.*

chlamydia Sexually transmitted infection caused by the bacterium *Chlamydia trachomatis.*

Fast Facts

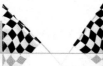

No, Not Really: Top STI Myths

Myth: If someone has an STI, you can tell because you can see the signs.

Fact: Many STIs have no signs or symptoms; someone without any symptoms can have an STI and transmit it to a partner.

Myth: Only people who have a lot of sex partners get STIs.

Fact: Anyone who has sexual contact of any kind can contract an STI.

Myth: You can't get an STI from oral sex.

Fact: The pathogens that cause STIs can enter the body through tiny cuts or tears in the mouth or in some cases through skin-to-skin contact with an infected area or sore.

Myth: Once you've had a particular STI, you can't get it again.

Fact: You do not become immune to STIs such as chlamydia and gonorrhea, so you can contract them multiple times. Infections such as herpes and HIV are chronic and incurable.

Myth: You can't get an STI if you're on the pill.

Fact: Birth control pills do not protect against STIs.

Myth: Douching helps prevent STIs.

Fact: Douching increases the risk for several STIs as well as pelvic inflammatory disease. Douching alters the balance of organisms that live in the vagina in harmful ways and can also force pathogens to go from the vagina higher up into the reproductive system.

the infection can be cured with antibiotics, treatment does not reverse the damage, and re-infection is possible.

Pelvic Inflammatory Disease (PID)

Q | If I have chlamydia, does that mean I also have PID?

Not necessarily, but you are at risk. **Pelvic inflammatory disease (PID)** is infection and inflammation of the uterus, ovaries, fallopian tubes, and other reproductive organs in women. It is usually the result of untreated chlamydia or gonorrhea; douching and use of an intrauterine device (IUD) can also increase the risk of PID.[16]

In PID, bacteria move up from the vagina and infect other reproductive organs. The infection may have no initial symptoms, or there may be severe symptoms, including sudden onset of fever and pain. Signs can include vaginal discharge, painful urination or intercourse, pain in the lower abdomen, and irregular menstrual bleeding.

PID damages the reproductive organs, and the resulting scar tissue can cause chronic pelvic pain, tubal (ectopic) pregnancy, and infertility from blocked fallopian tubes. More than 1 million women are treated for PID each year, and many others have the condition but don't know it. Each year, an estimated 100,000 women become infertile and more than 150 women die from PID.[17] Infertility is more likely to occur if you have prolonged or repeated bouts of PID.

If you think you have pelvic inflammatory disease, see your physician immediately: Early treatment with antibiotics can limit the damage and long-term complications. As with other sexually transmitted diseases, a woman's sex partners also need to be treated.

Syphilis

Q | How many stages of syphilis are there?

There are four separate but sometimes overlapping stages to **syphilis.** The disease is caused by the bacterium *Treponema pallidum,* which can be transmitted through infected skin and mucous membranes in the genitals, lips, mouth, or anus. Syphilis can also be passed from a pregnant woman to her infant during pregnancy, causing a disease called congenital syphilis.

Primary syphilis is the first stage, characterized by the appearance of a painless sore, called a chancre, at the point of infection. The sore is full of bacteria that can be transmitted to others, but it may go unnoticed. A chancre usually disappears within about three to six weeks regardless of whether the infection is treated.

or urinary tract. Among young women, as many as 10–25 percent of infections may be in the throat.[15] **Gonorrhea** is a bacterial infection caused by *Neisseria gonorrhoeae.* It is spread through contact with the penis, vagina, mouth, or anus; it can also be spread from mother to baby during delivery. Most women have no symptoms, and those who do may have nonspecific symptoms that are mistaken for a bladder or vaginal infection. Men can also be asymptomatic, although sometimes discharge and painful urination occur.

As with chlamydia, untreated gonorrhea can damage a woman's reproductive organs and cause infertility and chronic pelvic pain. In men, an untreated infection can damage the epididymis and also potentially lead to infertility—although this is less likely than in women. If transmitted to an infant during childbirth, the bacteria can cause dangerous infections of the blood, joints, and eyes.

Gonorrhea can be treated with antibiotics, but many strains of the bacteria have developed resistance, which can make treatment more difficult. Although

gonorrhea Sexually transmitted infection caused by the bacterium *Neisseria gonorrhoeae.*

pelvic inflammatory disease (PID) Infection of the reproductive system in women, typically caused by untreated chlamydia or gonorrhea; can result in reproductive system damage and infertility.

syphilis A multistage sexually transmitted infection caused by the bacterium *Treponema pallidum.*

TABLE 12-4 PREVALENCE OF HERPES SIMPLEX VIRUS TYPE 2 AS MEASURED BY BLOOD TESTS*

	PREVALENCE (%)
TOTAL	16.2%
AGE GROUP (YEARS)	
14–19	1.4%
20–29	10.5%
30–39	19.6%
40–49	26.1%
REPORTED NUMBER OF LIFETIME SEX PARTNERS	
1	3.9%
2–4	14.0%
5–9	16.3%
≥10	26.7%

*Over 80% of those whose blood test was positive for HSV 2 had never received a diagnosis of genital herpes.

Source: Centers for Disease Control and Prevention. (2010). Seroprevalence of herpes simplex virus type 2 among persons aged 14–49 years—United States, 2005–2008. *Morbidity and Mortality Weekly Report, 59*(15), 456–459.

genital herpes A chronic or latent sexually transmitted infection caused by the herpes simplex virus (HSV) and characterized by genital sores.

Secondary syphilis develops two to ten weeks later. The most common symptom is a non-itchy skin rash, usually on the palms of the hands and soles of the feet. Other signs include swollen lymph glands, headache, fatigue, sore throat, and hair loss. Symptoms of secondary syphilis usually disappear with or without treatment, although they may recur.

Latent syphilis develops in people who haven't been treated. Symptoms of the disease disappear, but the bacteria remains in the body. Early in the latent stage a person can still infect others, but this risk fades over time.

A small percentage of people with latent syphilis go on to develop the fourth stage, *tertiary syphilis*. In this stage, the syphilis bacteria damages major organs and can cause mental illness, heart disease, blindness, and death.

During pregnancy, syphilis can cause miscarriage, premature birth, stillbirth, and infant death. Babies born with congenital syphilis may have birth defects, seizures, development delays, and other problems. Syphilis can be cured with antibiotics in all stages, but organ damage cannot be reversed. A fetus can be cured in the womb if the mother is treated early enough in the pregnancy.

Genital Herpes

Q | Does everyone have herpes?

No, not everyone. But the infection is very common, and the majority of infected

people don't know their status (Table 12-4). **Genital herpes** can be caused by herpes simplex virus type 1 (HSV 1) or type 2 (HSV 2), but in most cases HSV 2 is responsible. HSV 1 more often infects the lips and mouth, causing cold sores, but it can cause genital herpes if transmitted through

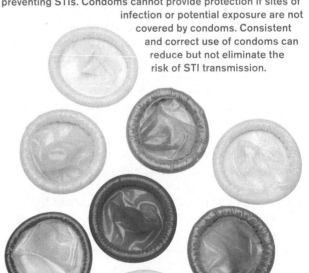

Latex condoms provide an essentially impermeable barrier to particles the size of STI pathogens and are highly effective in preventing STIs. Condoms cannot provide protection if sites of infection or potential exposure are not covered by condoms. Consistent and correct use of condoms can reduce but not eliminate the risk of STI transmission.

Living with . . .

Genital Herpes

Finding out you have genital herpes can be a shock—and you may feel angry and ashamed as well as worried about rejection. Remember that genital herpes is a very common infection and that although challenging, it can be successfully managed. In healthy adults, genital herpes usually doesn't cause any serious health problems. For most people, outbreaks become less frequent over time—perhaps four to five outbreaks during the first year after diagnosis and then fewer after that. Some helpful strategies for managing genital herpes include the following:

- Follow your physician's advice for managing the infection. Take all prescribed medications, even if the symptoms go away.
- Maintain a healthy lifestyle and manage stress to support your immune system and reduce outbreaks (see p. 422).
- Be aware of potential triggers for outbreaks, which can vary from person to person. For example, some people

find outbreaks linked to certain other illnesses or to hormonal changes associated with the menstrual cycle.

- Avoid sexual activity when you feel an outbreak coming on or have symptoms. But remember, you can transmit the infection even if you have no symptoms.
- During an outbreak, keep the sores clean and dry; if you touch a sore, wash your hands thoroughly. Wear loose-fitting cotton underwear and don't wear pantyhose; heat and moisture can slow healing.
- Use latex condoms during sex. Used consistently and correctly, condoms are effective at significantly reducing the risk of spreading herpes; however, since they don't cover all potentially infectious areas, they do not completely eliminate risk.
- Tell your sexual partners so that they can be tested for herpes. Inform any new partners before you have sex.
- Find a counselor or a support group—in person or online.

---

human papillomavirus (HPV) infection A sexually transmitted viral infection that can cause genital warts and cellular changes that lead to cervical and other cancers; can be a chronic infection.

oral sex. HSV 2 can also infect the mouth. Overall, about 50–80 percent of American adults have oral herpes (primarily from HSV 1), and about 20 percent have genital herpes (primarily from HSV 2).

Most people contract genital herpes by having sex or close skin-to-skin contact with an infected person. The main symptom of herpes is sores at the site where the virus entered the body. The sores may start with a tingling feeling, erupt as red bumps, and then develop into small blisters or painful open sores. Some people also experience fever, headache, muscle aches, swollen glands, and other genital or urinary symptoms.

In most people, HSV is a latent infection; the virus remains in nerve cells for life and can become active and cause outbreaks several times a year. Recurrences often include visible sores and symptoms, but the virus can also be active without causing any signs. Although transmission of the virus is more likely when obvious sores are present, people with genital herpes can transmit the virus even if they have no symptoms and no idea they are infected.

There is no treatment or cure for genital herpes. There are antiviral drugs that help treat symptoms and prevent or reduce outbreaks. Using these drugs reduces but does not eliminate the chance of passing herpes to sexual partners. Because HSV can pass from mother to fetus and harm the baby, pregnant women who have herpes or whose sex partners have herpes should develop a plan with their physician to reduce the risk of the baby being infected. Having herpes

also increases the likelihood of contracting HIV from an infected partner.

Genital Warts (HPV Infection)

Q | Do genital warts go away?

For many people, genital warts clear up over time. However, they can become a chronic infection or have other serious effects. Genital warts are caused by **human papillomavirus (HPV) infection.** However, many people have genital HPV infection without having genital warts. There are more than one hundred types of HPV, many of which are harmless. Of those that are sexually transmitted, some types cause genital warts and some can cause changes in cells that can lead to cancer of the cervix, vulva, vagina, penis, or anus. Genital warts can also cause problems during pregnancy; in rare cases, infants born to infected mothers can develop warts in their throats.

HPV infection is very common and easily transmitted through skin-to-skin contact. Close to 30 percent of young women acquire HPV from their first male sex partner, and that within three years of becoming sexually active, 50 percent of women have been infected.[18] Males are also infected at a high rate: In a two-year study of heterosexually active male university students, 62 percent of the study participants acquired new HPV infections.[19]

For many people, genital HPV infection has no symptoms. But even in these cases, complications can develop, and the virus can be transmitted to sexual partners. When warts do appear, they may be raise or flat, small or large;

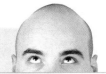

they can appear anywhere on, in, or around the genitals. Women may unknowingly have warts on their cervix. Genital warts do not turn into cancer; the types of HPV that cause warts are different from those that cause cancer. However, an individual can be infected with both types.

There are treatments for visible genital warts, including creams, laser treatment, and freezing or burning; sometimes warts disappear without treatment. However, there is no treatment for the underlying viral infection. Because the virus remains in the body, warts can come back after treatment.

In about 90 percent of cases, the body's immune system clears HPV within two years of infection. But not all cases clear up, and because the infection can have no symptoms, it is difficult to determine who is and is not capable of transmitting it.

The primary complication of HPV infection is cervical cancer. The cellular changes associated with cervical cancer can be detected with regular Pap tests, which are recommended for all women starting within three years after they become sexually active.

Genital HPV infection is one of the two sexually transmitted viruses for which vaccines are available. There are two vaccines (Cervarix and Gardasil) that protect against the types of HPV that cause about 70 percent of cervical cancers. Gardasil also protects against the types of HPV that cause about 90 percent of cases of genital warts. The vaccines are recommended for all females when they are 11 or 12 as well as females between 13 and 26 who haven't already been fully vaccinated. Gardasil is also licensed for use in males ages 9 to 26 for the prevention of genital warts. The vaccines do not treat established HPV infections.

Along with the vaccine, consistent condom use can also protect against HPV infection.[20] However, condoms do not provide complete protection because not all skin surfaces that can carry the virus are covered by a condom. See the box "Preventing Sexually Transmitted Infections" for additional strategies.

Viral Hepatitis

Q | Are herpes and HIV the only incurable STIs?

No. Along with HPV infection, some forms of **viral hepatitis** can also develop into chronic, incurable infections. Hepatitis is inflammation of the liver, and the three most common causes are the following:

■ *Hepatitis A virus (HAV),* which is usually transmitted through contaminated food and water. Hepatitis A usually resolves on its own, and a vaccine is available. There are about 25,000 U.S. cases per year.

Mind Stretcher
Critical Thinking Exercise

Do you feel comfortable about having a frank discussion with a new partner about your sexual histories? Under what circumstances do you feel such a discussion would be appropriate or inappropriate? Develop several statements you could use to bring up the subject of STIs and safer sex with a potential sex partner.

■ *Hepatitis B virus (HBV),* which is transmitted through semen, vaginal fluids, blood, and saliva. Hepatitis B is described in more detail below.

■ *Hepatitis C virus (HCV),* which is primarily transmitted through blood. Most new U.S. infections occur through injection drug use. Hepatitis C leads to chronic infection in about 85 percent of those who are infected.

Hepatitis B is most commonly transmitted through sex with an infected partner, through contact with the blood of an infected person, or from a mother to infant during childbirth. Hepatitis is more easily transmitted than HIV and some other bloodborne infections, so there is some risk of infection from sharing razors or toothbrushes with an infected person. However, the virus isn't transmitted through shaking hands, coughing, or sharing utensils. There are about 43,000 new cases each year (see Table 12-3).

Symptoms of acute hepatitis B may include jaundice (yellowing of the skin and whites of the eyes), abdominal pain, nausea or vomiting, dark urine, and fatigue. The acute phase may last from several weeks to up to six months. There is no specific treatment for hepatitis B infection other than good self-care. In some people, the virus remains in the body after the acute stage of the infection, causing chronic disease. People with chronic hepatitis may exhibit no symptoms, but some develop serious and potentially fatal liver damage or liver cancer.

viral hepatitis Inflammation of the liver caused by infection with one of the hepatitis viruses; can become a chronic infection.

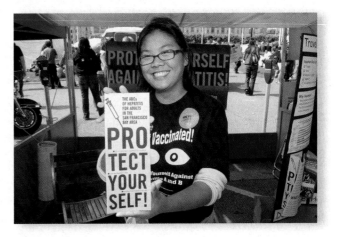

Wellness Strategies

Preventing Sexually Transmitted Infections

You can lower your risk of getting an STI with the following steps. The steps work best when used together. No single strategy can protect you from every single type of STI.

- **Don't have sex.** The surest way to keep from getting any STI is to practice abstinence. This means not having vaginal, oral, or anal sex. Keep in mind that some STIs, such as genital herpes, can be spread without having intercourse.
- **Be faithful.** Having a sexual relationship with one partner who has been tested for STIs and is not infected is another way to lower your risk of getting infected. Be faithful to each other. This means you only have sex with each other and no one else.
- **Limit your number of sex partners.** Choose partners who have also had few sex partners. The fewer partners you have, the less likely you are to encounter someone who is infected with an STI. Keep in mind, however, that even people with only one lifetime sexual partner can have an STI.
- **Use condoms correctly and every time you have sex.** Use condoms from the very start to the very end of each sex act and with every sex partner. A male latex condom offers the best protection. You can use a male polyurethane condom if you or your partner has a latex allergy. For vaginal sex, women should use a female condom if their partner won't wear a condom. For oral or anal sex, use a male latex condom. A dental dam might also offer some protection from some STIs.
- **Know that some methods of birth control—such as birth control pills, shots, implants, and diaphragms—will not protect you from STIs.** If you use one of these methods, be sure to also use a condom correctly *every time* you have sex.

- **Talk with your sex partners about STIs and using condoms before having sex.** It's up to you to set the ground rules and to make sure you are protected.
- **Don't assume you're at low risk for STIs if you're a woman who has sex only with women.** Some common STIs are spread easily by skin-to-skin contact. Also, most women who have sex with women have had sex with men, too.
- **Talk frankly with your doctor and each sex partner about any STIs you or your partner has or has had.** Talk about symptoms, such as sores or discharge. Try not to be embarrassed. Your doctor is there to help you with any and all health problems.
- **Have regular exams—get tested and insist your partners do, too.** Ask your doctor if you should be tested for STIs and how often you should be retested. Testing for many STIs is simple and often can be done during a checkup. The sooner an STI is found, the easier it is to treat.
- **Get vaccinated against HPV.** If you're age 26 or younger, ask if vaccination is appropriate for you.
- **Be alert for symptoms.** If you experience any genital or urinary symptoms, see your doctor. Don't have sex until you and your partners complete treatment.
- **Avoid using drugs or drinking too much alcohol.** These activities may lead to risky sexual behavior, such as not wearing a condom.

Source: National Women's Health Information Center. (2009). Overview. *Sexually Transmitted Infections* (http://www.womenshealth.gov/faq/sexually-transmitted-infections.cfm). Centers for Disease Control and Prevention. (2010). What patients should know when they are diagnosed with genital warts (http://www.cdc.gov/hpv/Signs-Symptoms.html).

There is a vaccine to prevent hepatitis B. It is routinely given to all infants and is also safe for children and adults.

HIV Infection and AIDS

In the United States, someone is infected with HIV every 10 minutes, and someone dies from HIV/AIDS every 45 minutes.[21] Worldwide, the statistics are even more dramatic, with 7,400 people infected every day, half of them under age 25.[22] Although medications developed to treat the infection have dramatically extended survival and greatly improved quality of life, HIV/AIDS remains an enormous global challenge.

HIV is not equally distributed across the population in the United States. Men have higher rates of HIV infection than women (Figure 12-6). Although African Americans make up about 13 percent of the U.S. population, they account for about half of all new HIV cases. However, it's important to remember that anyone can be infected with HIV. Recent surveys indicate that nearly 40 percent of young adults engage in high-risk HIV behavior.[23]

Q | Is there a difference between HIV and AIDS?

Yes. **Human immunodeficiency virus (HIV)** is the infectious agent that causes **acquired immune deficiency syndrome (AIDS).** HIV is a

human immunodeficiency virus (HIV) The virus that causes HIV infection and AIDS; infects and destroys cells of the immune system.

acquired immune deficiency syndrome (AIDS) A disease of the immune system characterized by a severe reduction in the number of CD4+ cells, leaving an individual susceptible to other infections and diseases; the final stage of HIV infection.

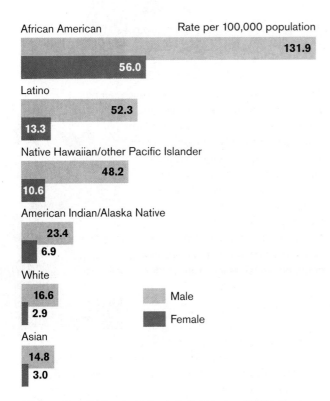

Figure 12-6 Estimated rates of diagnosis of HIV infection among U.S. adults and adolescents, by sex and race/ethnicity

Source: Centers for Disease Control and Prevention. (2010). Diagnoses of HIV infection and AIDS in the United States and dependent areas. *HIV Surveillance Report, 2008, 20* (http://www.cdc.gov/hiv/topics/surveillance/resources/reports).

pathogen, and AIDS is the late stage of HIV infection—a chronic infection that slowly destroys the body's immune system. People with HIV may look and feel healthy, experiencing no symptoms, for years after the initial infection. However, the virus is active in their body, infecting and destroying immune system cells as it reproduces. The specific type of blood cell that HIV destroys is called a CD4+ T cell, which is critical for the body to fight infection. Over time, HIV levels increase and CD4+ T cell levels decrease, leaving people less able to fight off other diseases and infections. Measurement of CD4+ T cell counts indicate the progress of the infection and aid in treatment decisions.

If damage to the immune system is severe, a person develops AIDS. This final stage of HIV infection is diagnosed when he or she develops an opportunistic infection—an infection a person without HIV infection would be unlikely to contract—or has a dangerously low number of CD4+ T cells. Prior to the development of treatments, people progressed from HIV infection to AIDS within a few years. With the new medications, people may live years or even decades with HIV infection without developing AIDS.

Q Where in the world is HIV/AIDS the biggest problem? 🔲 **READ ONLINE**

Q Do condoms really help prevent HIV infection?

TRANSMISSION AND SYMPTOMS. Yes. Use of condoms does not completely eliminate risk, but it greatly reduces the transmission of HIV.[24] Most problems with condom effectiveness relate to improper or inconsistent use. HIV is found in blood, semen, and vaginal secretions and can be transmitted by sharing of these body fluids. According to the Centers for Disease Control and Prevention, HIV is spread primarily in the following ways:[25]

- Not using a condom when having sex with a person who has HIV. All unprotected sex with someone who has HIV contains some risk. However, unprotected anal sex is riskier than unprotected vaginal sex. Unprotected oral sex can also be a risk for HIV transmission, but it is a much lower risk than anal or vaginal sex.
- Having multiple sex partners or the presence of other sexually transmitted infections (STIs) can increase the risk of infection during sex. As described earlier in the chapter, any breaks in the skin or mucous membranes can allow a virus to pass more easily into the body.
- Sharing needles, syringes, other equipment, or rinse water used to prepare illicit drugs for injection.
- Being born to an infected mother—HIV can be passed from mother to child during pregnancy, birth, and breast-feeding.

Among American adolescents and adults, the three most common modes of transmission are male-to-male sexual contact, heterosexual contact, and injection drug use (Figure 12-7). Less commonly, HIV may be transmitted

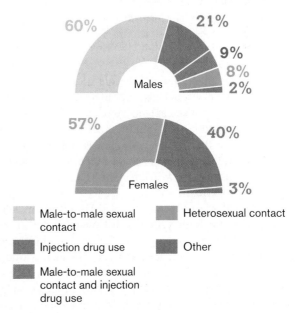

Figure 12-7 Transmission routes among U.S. adults and adolescents diagnosed with AIDS

Source: Centers for Disease Control and Prevention. (2010). Diagnoses of HIV infection and AIDS in the United States and dependent areas. *HIV Surveillance Report, 2008, 20* (http://www.cdc.gov/hiv/topics/surveillance/resources/reports).

Wellness Strategies

Using Condoms the Right Way for STI Prevention

Why Condoms Fail: The failure of condoms to protect against STI transmission usually results from inconsistent or incorrect use, rather than product failure.

- Inconsistent or nonuse can lead to STI acquisition because transmission can occur with a single sex act with an infected partner.
- Incorrect use diminishes the protective effect of condoms by leading to condom breakage, slippage, or leakage. Incorrect use more commonly entails a failure to use condoms *throughout* each entire sex act, from start (of sexual contact) to finish (after ejaculation).

How to Use a Condom Consistently and Correctly:

- Use a new condom for every act of vaginal, anal, and oral sex throughout the *entire* sex act (from start to finish).
- Before any genital contact, put the condom on the tip of the erect penis with the rolled side out.
- If the condom does not have a reservoir tip, pinch the tip enough to leave a half-inch space for semen to collect. Holding the tip, unroll the condom all the way to the base of the erect penis.
- After ejaculation and before the penis gets soft, grip the rim of the condom and carefully withdraw. Then gently pull the condom off the penis, making sure that semen doesn't spill out.
- Wrap the condom in a tissue and throw it in the trash where others won't handle it.
- If you feel the condom break at any point during sexual activity, stop immediately, withdraw, remove the broken condom, and put on a new condom.

- Ensure that adequate lubrication is used during vaginal and anal sex, which might require water-based lubricants. Oil-based lubricants (such as petroleum jelly, shortening, mineral oil, massage oils, body lotions, and cooking oil) should not be used because they can weaken latex, causing breakage.
- Do not use condoms lubricated with the spermicide nonoxynol-9; it can cause irritation and increase the risk of getting an STI from an infected partner.

For more instructions on using condoms, as well as advice on talking to a partner about condoms and safer sex, visit the Web site for the American Social Health Association (http://www.ashastd.org/condom/condom_overview.cfm). For information on the use of condoms for pregnancy prevention—including combining condoms with other contraceptive methods and using over-the-counter emergency contraception in case of condom breakage—visit the Web sites for the American College of Obstetricians and Gynecologists' publications (http://www.acog.org/publications/patient-education) and Planned Parenthood (http://www.plannedparenthood.org).

Source: Centers for Disease Control and Prevention. (2010). *Male latex condoms and sexually transmitted diseases* (http://www.cdc.gov/condomeffectiveness/brief.html).

to health care workers through needle sticks. Before HIV blood tests, people could also be infected from a blood transfusion or organ transplant; however, the risk is now extremely small due to rigorous screening. HIV cannot survive outside the human body and is not transmitted through air, water, or insect bites; there are no documented cases of transmission through saliva, tears, sweat, or closed-mouth kissing.

To prevent the transmission of HIV infection, take steps to avoid or limit your risk behaviors. Refer to the box on p. 434 on preventing STIs for specific guidelines. Abstain from sex or practice safer sex consistently. Many people know what safer sex behaviors are but don't consistently practice them. Think about your own behavior, and if you act in risky ways, ask yourself why. In addition, if you inject drugs, get counseling and treatment; using clean needles and syringes reduces the risk of transmission, but it's much better to stop drug use and avoid all the associated

risks. If you have a risky sexual encounter and believe you were exposed to HIV, see your health care provider immediately. In some cases, HIV medications can prevent infection if they are started shortly after exposure to the virus.

Q Do any methods of birth control besides condoms help with STIs?

🔲 READ ONLINE

Q What are symptoms of HIV and AIDS?

Most people infected with HIV are asymptomatic, although some develop nonspecific symptoms during the acute phase of the initial infection: fever, headache, fatigue, muscle aches, and enlarged lymph nodes. These symptoms typically resolve with no treatment and may be attributed to influenza or an-

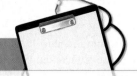

Research Brief

Unprotected Sex: How Do College Students Explain Their Behavior?

By the time young adults get to college, most have received vast amounts of information about the consequences of unprotected sex in terms of both pregnancy and STIs. Despite a lot of knowledge about the risks, many young adults still fail to consistently practice safer sex. How do they explain this inconsistency? In a recent study, researchers asked a group of young adults to keep diaries for several weeks to track their condom use and non-use during intercourse. Once the diaries were complete, the students were interviewed to explore their decision making.

Less than 25 percent of the students used condoms or oral contraceptives consistently. Most who did use condoms saw them as a means of preventing pregnancy rather than preventing disease. Their explanations for their risky behaviors fell into several categories:

- *Biased evaluation of risk:* Students equated the degree of closeness and intimacy they felt for their partner with reduced risk for STIs.
- *Biased evaluation of evidence:* Students believed that since their pattern of behavior (unsafe sex) had not in the past resulted in pregnancy or an STI, it must not be very risky.
- *Endorsement of poor alternatives:* Some students justified their choice to not use condoms with the use of an

alternative prevention strategy—even though they recognized the alternative as a poor one (withdrawal, counting on luck).

- *False justifications:* Despite stating a strong desire to avoid STIs and pregnancy, students weighted short-term benefits of not using a condom as more important than the long-term negative consequences.
- *Dismissing or ignoring risk:* Some students felt invulnerable to the negative outcomes that other people might experience ("it won't happen to me"), and others felt that the negative outcomes could be easily solved (abortion, drug treatment).

Do any of these explanations or rationalizations sound familiar to you? What would you say to yourself or a peer to dispute these false beliefs? If you engage in unprotected sex, examine your own attitudes carefully. Challenge yourself—and others—to acknowledge the personal risks you face, and commit yourself to taking steps to reduce those risks.

Source: O'Sullivan, L. F., Udell, W., Montrose, V. A., Antoniello, P., & Hoffman, S. (2010). A cognitive analysis of college students' explanations for engaging in unprotected sexual intercourse. *Archives of Sexual Behavior, 39,* 1121–1131.

---

other minor illness. During this early acute phase, people are extremely infectious.

After the acute phase is over, any symptoms that occurred resolve. Although the virus remains in the body, replicating and destroying CD4+ T cells, infected people exhibit no symptoms and likely are completely unaware of the infection. However, they are capable of infecting others.

During the late stages of HIV infection, when the immune system has been severely weakened, people may experience a variety of symptoms. These include rapid weight loss, extreme fatigue, prolonged swelling of lymph nodes, sores in the mouth or genitals, and neurological disorders. The opportunistic infections that can occur in people with full-blown AIDS include pneumonia, cancer, liver disease, and many types of otherwise unusual viral, fungal, protozoan, and bacterial infections.

Q | Do you have to wait six months to find out if you have HIV?

TESTING AND TREATMENT. In most cases, no, although standard blood tests for HIV aren't accurate immediately following infection. These tests detect HIV

antibodies, and it takes time for the immune system to produce enough antibodies to be detected by the test. In most cases, the body produces sufficient antibodies for detection within two to eight weeks following infection (the average is 25 days); 97 percent of infections can be detected within three months.[26] That means there is a small chance that it will take longer than three months—and in very rare cases up to six months—to get an accurate test result.

When you get a conventional test, it may take one or two weeks to get your results from the lab. However, some sites also offer rapid HIV testing, which provides results in twenty to thirty minutes. A positive HIV antibody test must be verified by a second test. More expensive tests that directly test for the presence of the virus in the body are available but are not typically used for screening purposes.

Current federal guidelines recommend HIV testing for every American ages 13 to 64 as part of routine medical care.[27] For anyone at high risk, yearly testing is recommended. Despite these guidelines, it's estimated that as many as one in five Americans with HIV are unaware of their status. If diagnosed early, an infected individual can get appropriate treatment and limit the spread of the virus to others. Routine testing is especially important for pregnant women. Babies born to untreated women with HIV infection have about a 25 percent chance of catching HIV; with treatment, the risk drops to about 2 percent.

Q | How long until someone with HIV dies?

With treatment, people can survive many years or even decades with HIV infection. The success of treatment depends on many factors, including an individual's underlying health status and how early in the course of infection treatment begins. Over thirty antiviral drugs are available to treat HIV infection. These medications do not cure the infection or eliminate the virus from the body, but they do suppress the virus, sometimes to undetectable levels. A person being treated for HIV must take antiviral drugs continuously; he or she can still transmit the virus, but the risk is much lower. The medications can have side effects, sometimes serious, and HIV can also become resistant to particular medications.

Researchers have worked for many years to design a vaccine, but HIV poses significant challenges. It directly attacks the immune system—the very cells that need to be activated by a vaccine. In addition, HIV frequently mutates to produce new strains. Although a vaccine remains elusive, there has been some success in developing microbi-

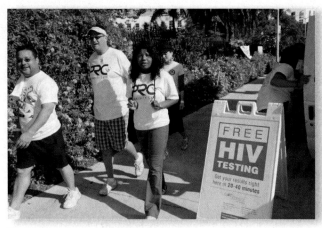

The CDC recommends HIV testing at least once for all Americans ages 13 to 64 as part of routine medical care. For anyone at high risk, annual testing is appropriate.

cides that can be applied to the vagina prior to intercourse to help reduce the risk of transmission.[28] Microbicides may be particularly beneficial for women around the world who aren't able to negotiate mutual monogamy or condom use with their partners.

With no vaccine or cure on the horizon, it's important for everyone to take HIV prevention seriously.

Summary

Infectious agents are all around us and impossible to avoid. Fortunately, the body has many physical and chemical barriers to keep pathogens out and a complex immune system to tackle those microbes that do gain entry. Many infections are relatively mild and cause few problems in healthy individuals. For those that are more serious, many can be cured with medications and self-care. You can help limit the impact of infectious disease by engaging in wellness behaviors that support your immune system and by taking steps to avoid the transmission of pathogens. It's also important to keep your vaccinations up to date.

Although colds, influenza, and similar infections can be challenging to avoid, infections that are sexually transmitted have clear prevention strategies. Not having sex prevents all STIs, and if you are sexually active, you can greatly reduce your risk by using condoms and maintaining a mutually monogamous relationship with your partner. If diagnosed early, the bacterial STIs can be treated before any serious com-

plications occur. The viral STIs are incurable, but there are vaccines for both HPV and hepatitis. HIV/AIDS is the most serious STI, and although treatments have improved, it remains an incurable and life-threatening infection.

More to Explore

American Social Health Association
  http://www.ashastd.org
Centers for Disease Control and Prevention
  http://www.cdc.gov
Joint United Nations Programme on HIV/AIDS
  http://www.unaids.org
MedlinePlus: Infectious Diseases
  http://www.nlm.nih.gov/medlineplus/infections.html
National Institute of Allergy and Infectious Diseases
  http://www.niaid.nih.gov

🖥 **SUBMIT ONLINE**

NAME	**DATE**	**SECTION**

Equipment: None

Preparation: None

Instructions
Indicate whether each statement is true for you always, sometimes, or never; and fill in the additional information. Any statement for which you don't check "always" indicates an area where you could change your behavior to help reduce your risk for infectious diseases.

Avoiding Pathogens

Always   Sometimes   Never

_____ _____   _____   I frequently wash my hands with soap and water for at least 20 seconds.

_____ _____   _____   I don't rub my eyes, touch my nose, or eat with my fingers without first washing my hands.

_____ _____   _____   When soap and water aren't available, I use alcohol-based hand sanitizer.

If these statements aren't always true for you, describe your typical hand hygiene practices:

_____ _____   _____   I avoid close contact with people who have colds, flu, or other infectious diseases transmitted via touch or respiratory droplets.

_____ _____   _____   I avoid disease carriers such as mosquitoes, ticks, and rodents. To avoid insect disease vectors, I use insect repellant and/or wear long sleeves and pants when necessary.

_____ _____   _____   I never inject drugs (except if medically prescribed).

_____ _____   _____   I follow food safety recommendations (see Chapter 9), including keeping foods at safe temperatures, not thawing foods on the counter, thoroughly cleaning all equipment, and using a food thermometer to check that foods are cooked to a safe temperature.

_____ _____   _____   I have a kit prepared in case of emergencies that disrupt sanitation and other public health services.

Supporting Your Immune System

Always   Sometimes   Never

_____ _____   _____   I exercise regularly.

_____ _____   _____   I eat a healthy diet.

_____ _____   _____   I get plenty of sleep.

_____ _____   _____   I manage my stress.

_____ _____   _____   I don't smoke, and I avoid secondhand smoke.

_____ _____   _____   I consume alcohol moderately, if at all.

_____ _____   _____   My immunizations are up to date, including recommended booster shots.

Check your immunization status against the recommendations in Figure 12-2 and note any vaccines recommended for you that you haven't had.

Assessing Your Risk for Sexually Transmitted Infections

Complete one of the following online assessments for STI risk. Then briefly comment on the experience.

The Body: http://www.thebody.com/surveys/sexsurvey.html

STD Wizard: http://www.stdwizard.org

Were you surprised by any of the questions or the results? Did you identify any risk areas that you had been unaware of?

Assessing Your Recent Experiences with Infectious Diseases

To help further identify infectious disease risks in your life, list and describe your three most recent infections. Note the symptoms and duration of your illness, and speculate on how you think you acquired the infection. For each, note one strategy you think might have reduced your risk for contracting the infection or lessened its effects on you.

Reflecting on Your Results

Are you doing all you can to prevent infectious diseases? Note at least three areas in which you could improve your behavior to reduce your risk. Then comment on what you think is holding you back. For example, if you know you should wash your hands more often, why don't you?

Planning Your Next Steps

Choose one behavior that you could change to help reduce your risk for infectious diseases, and develop at least three concrete strategies for making the change. For example, would putting hand washing reminders in your bathroom or hand sanitizer in your backpack help improve your hand hygiene?

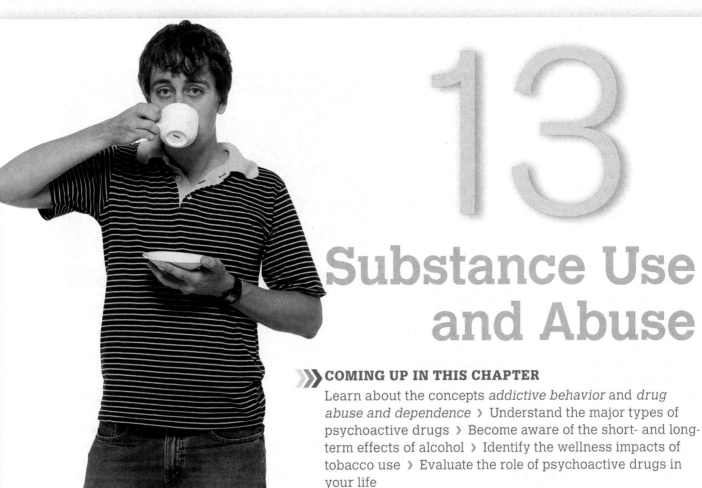

13

Substance Use and Abuse

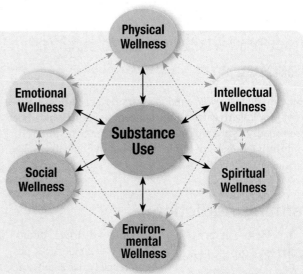

>> **COMING UP IN THIS CHAPTER**

Learn about the concepts *addictive behavior* and *drug abuse and dependence* › Understand the major types of psychoactive drugs › Become aware of the short- and long-term effects of alcohol › Identify the wellness impacts of tobacco use › Evaluate the role of psychoactive drugs in your life

Wellness Connections

How does substance use and abuse relate to your overall wellness? For wellness, you need to be in control of your choices and behavior, and dependence means you're not in control. Do you want a habit to control you? Your physical wellness can be profoundly affected by the choices you make related to alcohol, tobacco, and other drugs, which can cause both short- and long-term problems. Good physical and emotional wellness—enough sleep, and effective stress management strategies—eliminate some of the underlying triggers for substance use. Attention to emotional and spiritual wellness is also key: Is your behavior compatible with your values, goals, and ethical beliefs? Are you using tobacco, alcohol, or other drugs to manage stress, emotional pain, or anxiety?

Your intellectual wellness and functioning can be significantly harmed in the short term by many drugs. Your critical thinking skills don't work when you're intoxicated! Make sound choices about substance use and abuse based on a critical evalua-

tion of the risks and costs of your behavior in terms of your goals for your life. Social and environmental wellness factors are also important: What potentially addictive behaviors do you see in your family and friends? What aspects of your environment support or hinder your ability to stick with your goals related to substance use? What can you do to encourage responsible attitudes and behaviors in those around you?

The use of **drugs,** chemical substances that can alter the structure or function of the body, is widespread in the United States. People use powerful drugs for medical reasons: to prevent or treat chronic and infectious diseases as well as to reduce unpleasant symptoms. Used correctly, many drugs can improve health and wellness.

However, many Americans also use drugs for other reasons and in other ways—some potentially dangerous. When we think about abuse or addiction, we usually consider **psychoactive drugs,** those that affect a person's state of mind or consciousness by altering the functioning of the brain. Psychoactive drugs have both immediate and long-term effects on wellness. In the short term, use of many psychoactive drugs leads to **intoxication,** meaning the person is mentally affected by the actions of the chemical. Depending on the drug, in an intoxicated state, people may feel excited or relaxed, their mood may be altered, and their physical and mental functioning will be impaired—in unpredictable or dangerous ways. Drugs can also have serious effects on all the wellness dimensions when used over the long term.

This chapter introduces the general concept of addiction. It also reviews the basics of drug use, misuse, abuse, and dependence as applied to the most commonly used psychoactive drugs in the United States.

Understanding Addictive Behaviors

Although the term *addiction* is most often used in the context of psychoactive drugs, the concept of addiction can be more broadly applied to other behaviors. In general terms, an **addictive behavior** is one that is out of control and has a serious effect on a person's life.

Defining Addiction

Q | How do you know if someone is addicted to something? What does that mean?

In relation to drugs, addiction, or dependence, has been precisely defined by the American Psychiatric Association (see p. 445). Drug dependence typically involves changes in brain chemistry that have physical, mental, and behavioral effects. But some of these same effects have been seen in other behaviors, such as gambling, shopping, or use of the Internet and other electronic communications.[1] Some characteristics that are generally associated with addictive behaviors include the following:[2]

- *Preoccupation:* Spending a great deal of time thinking about and engaging in the behavior

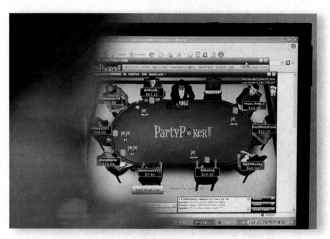

Addiction is most closely associated with use of psychoactive drugs, but any behavior that becomes the focus of a person's life and interferes with day-to-day activities is potentially addictive.

- *Loss of control:* Feeling unable to stop or cut back on the behavior
- *Craving or compulsion:* Having an obsessive, compelling need to engage in the behavior on a regular basis
- *Reinforcement:* Engaging in the behavior provides feelings of pleasure or reduces feelings of anxiety or distress in the short term
- *Negative consequences:* Experiencing significant negative consequences but continuing the behavior nevertheless

Generally speaking, it isn't the amount of time spent on a behavior that is used to define an addiction; rather, it is the effect of the behavior on a person's life. An addiction is something that pulls a person away from other important things—relationships, school and job responsibilities—and becomes the dominant focus of his or her life (see Lab Activity 13-1). The individual's health and finances may suffer, and there can also be legal problems. Despite the negative consequences, an addicted person feels out of control and unable to stop. Associated emotions may include anxiety, guilt, humiliation, hopelessness, and fear. An addiction severely impairs overall functioning and wellness.

Developing Addiction

Q | Why do some people develop addictions?

There is no real consensus on why addiction develops in one person and not another. Multiple factors are involved, including the following:

drug A chemical substance that alters the structure or function of the body.

psychoactive drug A drug that alters a person's state of mind or consciousness.

intoxication The state of being mentally affected by a drug.

addictive behavior A behavior or habit that is out of control and has a serious effect on the person's life; characterized by craving and compulsive use.

- *Genes and biology:* Researchers are working to identify genes and receptors that make some people more susceptible. Gender and underlying physical and emotional health also play a role. For drugs, it's thought that genetics may account for 40–60 percent of a person's vulnerability to addiction.[3]
- *Exposure:* Early and frequent exposure to a behavior or substance can increase the risk for addiction.
- *Environment:* Factors such as parental behavior, chaotic or abusive home life, and peer and community attitudes are additional influences.
- *Nature of the behavior or substance:* Behaviors or drugs that cause a rapid change in feelings—a sudden but very brief rush of pleasurable feelings—may be inherently more addicting.

Q | How long does it take to become addicted to something?

It varies, but addictions don't occur overnight. At first, the behavior may not be at all harmful. Yet over time, there is an increasing desire to engage in the behavior, ultimately resulting in loss of control and negative consequences. In some cases, there is a pattern of escalation, in which a person must take more and more of a substance or engage in a behavior more frequently or for longer periods in order to experience the expected positive result. Over time, an addict has to engage in the behavior just to feel normal.

Just as it takes time to become addicted, it also takes time to effectively treat an addiction. In fact, for some people it can take a lifetime of treatment. Treating an addiction is difficult and usually requires an individual treatment plan developed by an experienced health care professional. Psychologists, psychiatrists, and licensed counselors are often involved in treatment for addiction. Relapses are common—for example, when a former smoker or alcoholic goes back to smoking or excessive drinking. Although treatment success rates are relatively low, many people do succeed in breaking addictions and developing healthier lifestyles. And relapse rates for addiction are similar to those for other chronic medical conditions like diabetes and high blood pressure. Anyone who experiences loss of control over a behavior—whether or not it involves drugs—should seek early treatment.

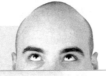

Mind Stretcher
Critical Thinking Exercise

Have you ever had a pattern of behavior that you thought might be an addiction? If so, what led you to think you might be addicted to a particular substance or behavior? What do you think is the difference between an addiction and a habit?

Psychoactive Drugs

There are many different and overlapping ways to group and describe drugs and drug use. Substances may be classified as prescription drugs, over-the-counter drugs, or dietary supplements, depending on how they are sold and regulated. Drugs may also be grouped according to their effects, such as antibiotics, stimulants, and sleeping aids. In terms of abuse and addiction, psychoactive drugs are the category of most concern—those drugs that alter mental functioning. Psychoactive drugs may be legal or illegal, depending on whether they have legitimate medical uses (for example, painkillers or tranquilizers) or are classified as legal for use by adults (for example, alcohol or tobacco). Misuse or abuse of any drug, legal or illegal, can have serious effects.

Q | What are the most common drugs being used?

Among legal psychoactive drugs, the answer is caffeine, alcohol, and tobacco. Among drugs classified as illegal, the most widely used substance is marijuana (Table 13-1). It's important to note that the proportion of people who've tried a drug during their lives is much higher than the percentage of current users. Although close to half of Americans over age 12 have used an illicit drug at least once in their lives, only about 9 percent are current users, with *current* defined as use in the past month. The vast majority of Americans do not use illicit drugs.

Men are more likely to use psychoactive drugs than women, and rates of use peak among young adults (Figure 13-1). People who are unemployed are more likely to use drugs than those with either full-time or part-time employment. Overall rates of drug use haven't changed substantially over the years, although use of particular drugs rises and falls. Alcohol use among people under age 21 is relatively high—a concern not only because of the immediate risks of intoxication but also because early exposure is associated with greater likelihood of long-term problems. Geographically, the upper Midwest has the highest rates of overall alcohol use and binge drinking, and the Southeast has the highest rates of tobacco use.[4] If you believe TV and the movies, you might think Seattle has the highest rate of caffeine use based on all the coffee shops. However, caffeine isn't just from coffee (don't forget soda, energy drinks, and supplements), and rates of caffeine use are high everywhere.

drug misuse Intentional or unintentional use of a medication in ways other than directed or intended.

Drug Misuse, Abuse, and Dependence

Q | Is all drug abuse addiction?

No. Different, but related, patterns of drug use can be problematic. **Drug misuse** is the intentional or unintentional use

TABLE 13-1 USE OF PSYCHOACTIVE DRUGS IN THE UNITED STATES

	PERCENTAGE OF PEOPLE AGE 12 AND OLDER REPORTING USE		
	LIFETIME	PAST YEAR	PAST MONTH
ALCOHOL	82.8	66.8	51.9
TOBACCO (ALL FORMS)	69.1	33.1	27.7
CIGARETTES	64.6	27.5	23.3
SMOKELESS TOBACCO	17.8	4.8	3.4
CIGARS	35.8	10.5	5.3
ANY ILLICIT DRUG	47.1	15.1	8.7
MARIJUANA	41.5	11.3	6.6
NONMEDICAL USE OF PSYCHOTHERAPEUTICS*	20.6	6.4	2.8
COCAINE	14.5	1.9	0.7
INHALANTS	8.9	0.8	0.2
ECSTASY	5.7	1.1	0.3
LSD	2.5	0.3	0.1
HEROIN	1.5	0.2	0.1

*Includes nonmedical use of prescription pain relievers, tranquilizers, sedatives, or stimulants.

Source: Substance Abuse and Mental Health Services Administration. (2010). *Results from the 2009 National Survey on Drug Use and Health.* Rockville, MD: Office of Applied Studies, Substance Abuse and Mental Health Services Administration.

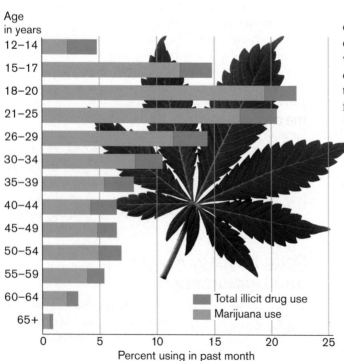

Age in years: 12–14, 15–17, 18–20, 21–25, 26–29, 30–34, 35–39, 40–44, 45–49, 50–54, 55–59, 60–64, 65+

■ Total illicit drug use
■ Marijuana use

Percent using in past month (0, 5, 10, 15, 20, 25)

of a medication in ways other than directed or indicated, regardless of whether harm results. Examples of drug misuse would be taking twice the dose of a painkiller because the first dose wasn't effective or giving your prescription sleeping pills to someone else to try.

Drug abuse is any use of a drug that increases the risk of problems for the user or others—problems with physical health, safety, interpersonal relationships,

drug abuse A harmful pattern of drug use that persists despite negative consequences; may involve continual or intermittent use of a drug.

Figure 13-1 Percent of people age 12 and older who reported any illicit drug use and marijuana use in the past month. Rates of drug use are highest among young adults and then fall among older age groups. Marijuana use accounts for most of the illicit drug use in the United States.

Source: Substance Abuse and Mental Health Services Administration. (2010). *Results from the 2009 National Survey on Drug Use and Health.* Rockville, MD: Office of Applied Studies, Substance Abuse and Mental Health Services Administration.

drug addiction (dependence) A chronic disease characterized by compulsive, ongoing use of a drug despite serious consequences.

legal status, or meeting school and job responsibilities. The problems may stem from the type or amount of the drug used or the situation in which it is used. Drug abuse generally encompasses the use of any illegal drug or the use of a medication with the intent of altering consciousness. Examples of drug abuse are taking LSD or a prescription stimulant in order to get high, smoking marijuana and then missing a class, or drinking alcohol before driving.

Drug addiction or **dependence** is a more serious disorder usually characterized by ongoing use of a drug and many of the characteristics of addictive behaviors described earlier in the chapter. The American Psychiatric Association (APA) defines drug dependence as behavior meeting three or more of the following seven criteria:[5]

1. *Tolerance:* A person requires increased amounts of a drug to achieve the desired effect or has a markedly reduced response to use of the same amount.
2. *Withdrawal:* A person develops significant physical and cognitive symptoms when use of the drug stops or is reduced. For example, a long-time heavy alcohol user may experience nausea, vomiting, and tremors when the concentration of alcohol in the body drops.
3. *Difficulty setting and keeping to limits on drug use:* A person uses more of a drug or uses the drug for a longer period than he or she originally intended.
4. *Inability to cut down on drug use:* A person wants to cut down or regulate drug use but is unable to do so.
5. *Time and focus on drug use:* A person spends a great deal of time obtaining and using the drug or recovering from its effects.
6. *Activities given up due to drug use:* A person reduces or stops his or her involvement or participation in important activities, including school, work, hobbies, and family and recreational activities.
7. *Continued use despite problems:* A person continues to use the drug despite recognizing that it is causing physical, psychological, and other problems.

People who develop tolerance and withdrawal are considered to be physically dependent on the drug. This means their body chemistry has adapted to the presence of the drug. It's important to note, however, that a person can be addicted to a drug based on psychological dependence alone, without a physical addiction.

Q | How do drugs change how a person's brain works?

Most psychoactive drugs alter the function of neurons. Some drugs are chemically similar to the brain's natural chemical messengers (neurotransmitters) and so they can activate neurons, telling them to send messages. Other drugs trigger large increases in neurotransmitters.

Many drugs act on the brain's reward system.[6] Under normal conditions, when we engage in a life-sustaining activity such as eating, the brain's reward center is activated—we feel good and therefore motivated to engage in the same behavior again. Drugs can also stimulate the brain's reward center—but with many times the normal amount of neurotransmitters. This reaction is much greater in magnitude and lasts longer than the response experienced to normally rewarding behaviors.

With ongoing drug use, the brain adjusts to high levels of a drug and changes its functioning; usually this means less activation of the reward center under normal circumstances. Without the drug, users feel depressed and unable to enjoy activities that they used to find enjoyable. They need the drug just to bring neurotransmitter levels and brain activity back to normal. This is how tolerance develops.

Figure 13-2 summarizes key information about major groups of psychoactive drugs, including their health effects. In the following sections, we'll briefly review selected psychoactive drugs of special concern to college students, including marijuana. Later in the chapter, we'll take a closer look at two widely used pyschoactive drugs that impair health and wellness: alcohol and tobacco.

Caffeine

Caffeine, a relatively mild central nervous system stimulant, is the most widely used psychoactive drug. When people think of caffeine, they tend to think of coffee. But caffeine is also found in tea, soft drinks, energy drinks, dietary supplements, and some over-the-counter medications. Its stimulant effects are not as powerful as those from amphetamines and cocaine, but users of caffeine can both develop tolerance and experience withdrawal, the hallmarks of physical dependence on a drug.

Q | What is caffeine, and how does it keep me awake?

On the most basic level, caffeine is a pure white crystalline powder that is very bitter. Chronic caffeine drinkers, however, will tell you what it is: the boost they need to get their day started. Caffeine is found naturally in coffee beans, leaves of the tea bush, kola nuts, and other plant sources. The decaffeination process is how the most pure form of caffeine is made, so thanks to all you decaf drinkers!

The reason caffeine is so good at keeping you alert is that it affects the action of the neurotransmitter adenosine, which typically makes people feel sleepy. Caffeine can bind to adenosine receptors in the brain, thereby blocking the effects of adenosine. Caffeine also enhances the action of epinephrine in the body. Together these effects result in increased heart rate and physical arousal as well as a sense of mental alertness. When consumed at higher-than-usual levels, caffeine disrupts sleep patterns and also acts as a

Category and representative drugs	Street names	Potential short-term (intoxication) effects	Potential health consquences
CNS depressants		Reduced pain and anxiety, feeling of well-being, lowered inhibition, slowed pulse and breathing, lowered blood pressure, poor concentration, loss of consciousness	Fatigue; confusion; impaired memory, judgment, coordination; respiratory depression and arrest; addiction
Alcohol	Booze, brewskies, cold one, hooch, hard stuff, sauce	Also: slurred speech, mood changes	
Barbiturates (sedatives)	Barbs, reds, red birds, yellows, yellow jackets	Also: sedation, drowsiness	Also: depression, fever, irritability, poor judgment, dizziness, slurred speech, life-threatening withdrawal
Benzodiazepines (tranquilizers)	Candy, downers, forget-me pill, roofies, sleeping pills, tranks	Also: sedation, drowsiness	Also: dizziness
Methaqualone	Ludes, quad, quay	Also: euphoria	Also: slurred speech, poor reflexes, coma
Gamma hydroxy butyrate (GHB)	G, Georgia home boy, grievous bodily harm, liquid ecstasy	Also: drowsiness, nausea	Vomiting, headache, loss of consciousness, loss of reflexes, seizures, coma, death
CNS stimulants		Increased heart rate, blood pressure, metabolism; feelings of exhilaration and energy, increased mental alertness	Rapid or irregular heartbeat, nervousness, insomnia, reduced appetite, weight loss, heart failure, stroke, seizures, liver damage
Amphetamine	Uppers, black beauties, speed, crosses, hearts, truck drivers	Also: rapid breathing, hallucinations	Also: tremor, loss of coordination, irritability, anxiety, impulsivity, aggressiveness, restlessness, panic, paranoia, delerium, psychosis, tolerance, addiction
Cocaine, crack cocaine	Blow, bump, C, candy, Charlie, coke, crack flake, rock, snow, toot	Also: increased body temperature	Also: chest pain, respiratory failure, stroke, seizure, nausea, panic attacks, headaches, malnutrition
MDMA	Ecstasy, X, XTC, Adam, Eve, beans, clarity	Mild hallucinogenic effects, increased tactile sensitivity, empathetic feelings	Impaired memory and learning, hyperthermia, renal failure, cardiac and liver toxicity
Methamphetamine	Crank, crystal, chalk, glass, ice, speed	Also: aggression, violence, psychotic behavior	Also: impaired memory and learning, cardiac and neurological damage, tolerance, addiction
Ritalin	JIF, MPH, R-ball, Skippy		
Opioids (Narcotics)		Pain relief, euphoria, drowsiness, lethargy, apathy, inability to concentrate, nausea	Nausea, constipation, confusion, sedation, respiratory depression and arrest, tolerance, addiction, unconsciousness, coma, death
Heroin	Brown sugar, dope, H, junk, skag, skunk, smack, white horse	Also: staggering gait	
Morphine	M, Miss Emma, monkey, white stuff	Also: staggering gait	
Synthetic opioids (codeine, oxycodone)	Oxycotton, oxycet, hillbilly heroin, percs, demmies	Also: staggering gait	

Category and representative drugs	Street names	Potential short-term (intoxication) effects	Potential health consequences
Cannabinoids		Euphoria, slowed thinking and reaction time, confusion, anxiety, impaired balance and coordination	Frequent respiratory infections, impaired lung function, cough, impaired memory and learning, increased heart rate, anxiety, panic attacks, sperm abnormalities, tolerance, addiction
Marijuana	Dope, ganja, grass, pot, joint, herb, Mary Jane, reefer, skunk, weed		Also: chronic bronchitis
Hashish	Broom, gangster, hash, hemp		
Inhalants	Laughing gas, poppers, snappers, whippets	Stimulation, loss of inhibition, slurred speech, loss of motor coordination, loss of consciousness, nausea, vomiting, headache	Cramps, weight loss, muscle weakness, memory impairment, hearing loss, bone marrow damage, depression, damage to cardiovascular and nervous systems, sudden death
Hallucinogens		Altered states of perception and feeling, nausea	Persisting perception disorder (flashbacks)
LSD	Acid, boomers, blotter, dots, yellow sunshines	Also: increased body temperature, heart rate, blood pressure, loss of appetite, sleeplessness, tremors, numbness, weakness	Also: impaired memory and learning, cardiac and neurological damage, tolerance, addiction
PCP	Angel dust, hog, love boat, ozone, peace pill, rocket fuel, wack	Also: increased heart rate and blood pressure, impaired motor function, panic, aggression, violence	Also: memory loss, numbness, nausea, vomiting, loss of appetite, depression

Figure 13-2 Effects of commonly abused classes of psychoactive drugs

Sources: Adapted from National Institute on Drug Abuse. (2007). Commonly abused drugs (http://www.drugabuse.gov/drugpages/drugsofabuse.html). Adapted from National Institute on Drug Abuse. (2007). Selected prescription drugs with potential for abuse (http://www.drugabuse.gov/DrugPages/PrescripDrugsChart.html).

diuretic (increasing the rate of urination). It is important to note that although caffeine may give the impression of promoting alertness in someone who is intoxicated from alcohol or other drugs, caffeine does not reduce the effects of other psychoactive drugs. Consuming an energy drink with alcohol doesn't make a person any less intoxicated.

Caffeine has other physical effects as well. It causes an increase in the secretion of stomach acid, which can potentially cause heartburn and indigestion. Adenosine is a vasodilator, meaning it causes blood vessels to relax and open; so caffeine acts in the opposite way, as a vasoconstrictor, causing blood vessels to close and constrict. This effect is the reason for the use of caffeine in some headache medications. Constricted blood vessels decrease the throbbing blood flow to the head that is thought to be the cause of some headaches.

Q | What has the most caffeine? The top sources of caffeine for American adults are coffee, soft drinks and energy drinks, and tea. These drinks vary in the amount of caffeine they provide (Table 13-2), and it can be hard to judge how much caffeine you are actually taking in. Researchers estimate that close to 90 percent of all Americans age 2 and older consume some caffeine, with rates highest among young and middle-aged adults.[7] Average consumption is about 200–250 mg per day, which is considered a moderate level. Some individuals consume much more.

Q | Is caffeine good for sports? Many athletes use caffeine, and studies have shown some benefit for performance in events requiring long-term endurance, short-term high-intensity effort, and repeated bouts of effort.[8] However, the effects of caffeine are variable and influenced by individual sensitivity to caffeine, timing of ingestion, previous consumption patterns, and other factors. Not everyone obtains a benefit or the same degree of benefit. The International Olympic Committee banned caffeine use among athletes in 1962, but caffeine was removed from its banned substances list in 2004. The National Collegiate Athletic Association does set a limit on caffeine consumption as measured through urine testing; the level is set to allow ordinary levels of caffeine consumption but to ban high intake levels.

TABLE 13-2 COMMON SOURCES OF CAFFEINE

	SERVING SIZE	CAFFEINE (MG)
COFFEE, DRIP BREWED	6 oz.	60–150
COFFEE, INSTANT	6 oz.	50–90
COFFEE, ESPRESSO	1 oz.	30–50
TEA, BREWED	6 oz.	40–80
ENERGY DRINKS	8 oz.	50–180
SOFT DRINKS	12 oz.	20–70
CHOCOLATE, MILK	1 oz.	2–15
CHOCOLATE, DARK	1 oz.	5–35
CANDY, DARK CHOCOLATE–COATED COFFEE BEANS	10 pieces	120
VIVARIN/DEXATRIM	1 tablet	200
NODOZ	1 tablet	100
ANACIN	1 tablet	32

Sources: International Food Information Council Foundation. (2008). *IFIC review: Caffeine and health: Clarifying the controversies.* Washington, DC: IFIC. U.S. Department of Agriculture, Agricultural Research Service. (2009). *USDA national nutrient database for standard reference,* Release 22. Nutrient Data Laboratory Home Page (http://www.ars.usda.gov/ba/bhnrc/ndl).

Q | Is caffeine addictive? Is it really all that bad?

Yes, caffeine can be addictive in that caffeine users develop tolerance and will experience withdrawal if their intake drops. People who habitually consume caffeine need the drug to return to a normal level of alertness and to reduce withdrawal symptoms, which include headache, irritability, anxiety, loss of concentration, and fatigue. These withdrawal symptoms mean that caffeine users have a consistent incentive to maintain their intake.

For most people, the equivalent of about two cups of coffee a day is considered a moderate and safe caffeine intake. This is based on the recommendation of no more than about 1.4 mg of caffeine per pound of body weight, or about 200 mg of caffeine a day for someone who weighs 150 pounds (see Table 13-2). Moderate caffeine intake is associated with a number of positive health effects, including a reduced risk of type 2 diabetes.[9]

As described above, high levels of intake can have adverse effects. In the short term, someone may experience nervousness, restlessness, muscle twitching, rambling flow of thoughts and speech, facial flushing, gastrointestinal disturbance, and problems sleeping. A high dose of caffeine can also affect heart rate and rhythm, which is potentially dangerous for people with underlying cardiovascular dis-

ease. However, moderate caffeine consumption has not been associated with adverse effects in those with heart disease.

The unpleasant effects of high doses of caffeine may be one reason why most caffeine users stick to fairly moderate intakes. To avoid problems, take care not to consume an excessive amount of caffeine. Check labels on beverages, supplements, and over-the-counter drugs. There is a wide range of caffeine content in different products, and you may unknowingly consume a much larger dose than you expect. One other thing to consider is cost—depending on your choices, a caffeine habit can be expensive!

Marijuana

Q | If marijuana is just a plant, then how is it a drug?

Marijuana is a plant—it's a mixture of leaves, flowers, stems, and seeds of the hemp plant, *Cannabis sativa.* But this plant contains a psychoactive chemical, delta-9-tetrahydrocannabinol, more commonly known as THC. Marijuana is most often smoked, which allows THC to pass very rapidly from the lungs, into the bloodstream, and then into the brain. It causes intoxication, which can last several hours. Like many psychoactive drugs, it affects the brain's reward system, causing a euphoric high. It also

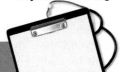

Research Brief

Marijuana Use and College Students

Rates of use of marijuana among college students are relatively high, with many students reporting occasional or even regular use. Aside from the potential legal consequences, how does marijuana use affect students? Researchers recently looked at cannabis-related problems among a group of over 1,200 first-year college students. They found a high rate of problems associated with marijuana use, including problems with academic work as well as health and safety. Among students who had used cannabis five or more times in the past year, the most prevalent marijuana-related problems were the following:

- 40.1% had trouble with concentration after being high
- 24.3% placed themselves at risk for physical injury
- 18.6% drove while high
- 13.9% missed class
- 8.4% had problems with friends
- 3.0% got into trouble for a housing violation due to drug use

Among these students, regular marijuana use was also more strongly linked with abuse and dependence than occasional use was—but even occasional use was associated with problems. These research findings demonstrate that college students who use marijuana are at risk for problems even if they don't meet all the criteria for abuse and dependence.

Marijuana use by students		
	Five or more times in past year	Six or more times in past month
Abuse criteria		
Regularly used and put self in physical danger	24.3	42.1
Continued use despite problems with family/friends	10.6	19.4
Serious problems at home, work, or school	7.6	15.0
Repeated trouble with the law	2.3	4.3
Dependence criteria		
Great deal of time spent related to drug use	32.6	60.7
Tolerance	27.0	51.4
Giving up important activities	14.4	25.9
Continued use despite knowledge of problems	12.3	21.4
Unsuccessful efforts to cut down	10.1	26.4
Consuming larger amounts than intended	9.3	20.1

Source: Caldeira, K. M., Arria, A. M., O'Grady, K. E., Vincent, K. B., & Wish, E. D. (2008). The occurrence of cannabis use disorders and other cannabis-related problems among first-year college students. *Addictive Behaviors, 33,* 397–411.

---

affects the areas of the brain involved in memory, thinking, concentration, coordination, movement, and sensory and time perception.[10]

Q | How does smoking marijuana affect the body?

In the short term, marijuana use produces physical, cognitive, emotional, and behavioral effects. The physical changes include an increase in heart rate, dilation of the blood vessels in the eyes (causing bloodshot eyes), reduction of the blood's capacity to carry oxygen, and enlargement of the bronchial passages. These effects impair exercise performance and may increase short-term risk of a heart attack.[11] Marijuana use also disrupts motor coordination and balance and slows reaction time. In terms of cognitive functioning, it impairs judgment, attention, the ability to form new memories, and the ability to quickly shift focus from one topic to another. These cognitive effects can last for days or even weeks after the period of intoxication, making learning difficult. A daily marijuana user is likely to be operating with reduced cognitive and intellectual functioning. Some users also experience more dramatic intoxication effects, including hallucinations, delusions, and loss of personal identity.

Taken together, the changes associated with marijuana use affect a person's ability to drive safely, and marijuana intoxication is associated with increased risk of being in a crash and causing a crash.[12] Further, driving under the influence of both alcohol and marijuana is greater than the risk of driving under the influence of either drug alone.[13]

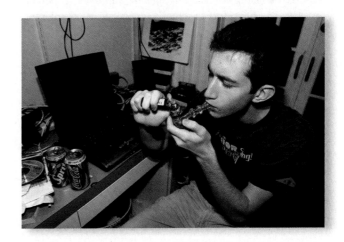

Long-term effects of habitual use of marijuana are more difficult to study. For example, it's hard to say if marijuana is better or worse than cigarettes for your health. We know that tobacco users have enormously high rates of lung cancer, yet the evidence on long-term marijuana use is less conclusive. This is in part because of its illegal status, meaning it is much more difficult to track users and identify negative outcomes. Also because it is illegal, people are less likely to be lifetime users, in contrast to many cigarette smokers, and are also likely to smoke smaller amounts of marijuana (fewer joints than cigarettes). However, like tobacco smoke, marijuana smoke does contain carcinogenic chemicals, and frequent users of marijuana may experience problems like daily cough, excess mucus production, more frequent acute respiratory illnesses, and a heightened risk of chronic lung disease.[14]

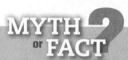

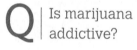

Marijuana gives you the munchies.

▶ WATCH ONLINE

Chronic marijuana use has also been linked to a number of mental health problems, including increased rates of anxiety, depression, suicidal ideation, and schizophrenia. At the present time, the strongest evidence links marijuana use and schizophrenia and related disorders.[15] Marijuana can also disrupt sleep patterns.

Q | Is marijuana addictive?

Yes, long-term marijuana abuse can lead to addiction. Problems controlling and stopping marijuana use are most prevalent in people who start using the drug in their teens. Similar to other drugs, long-term abusers trying to quit complain of withdrawal symptoms, including irritability, sleeplessness, decreased appetite, anxiety, and drug craving. Withdrawal symptoms typically start and peak within a few days, but tend to subside within one or two weeks following drug cessation.[16] Marijuana is responsible for about 15 percent of all admissions to drug treatment facilities in the United States. A worrisome trend is that more than 50 percent of all marijuana treatment patients reported abusing the drug by age 14, and over 90 percent by age 18. Therefore, virtually everyone in the United States admitted for marijuana treatment began abusing the drug prior to the age of 18.[17]

Ecstasy (MDMA)

Q | Are there problems associated with Ecstasy?

Yes, like all psychoactive drugs, it is associated with potential problems. Ecstasy, also known by the acronym for its chemical name, MDMA, is associated with raves and dance clubs. It has properties of both stimulants

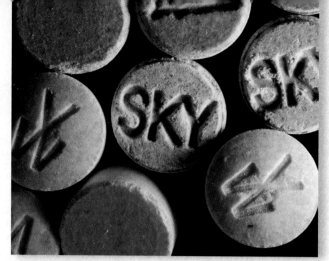

Ecstasy has both stimulant and hallucinogenic effects. It may be particularly dangerous when consumed with alcohol because it increases alertness and can mask the intoxicating effects of alcohol.

and hallucinogens and it affects several neurotransmitters, producing feelings of stimulation, emotional warmth, and well-being, as well as distortions in the user's sense of time and sensory perception. Less positive effects include nausea, involuntary teeth clenching, muscle cramps, and blurred vision.

MDMA increases heart rate and blood pressure; it also increases body temperature, which in rare cases can lead to dehydration and kidney failure. In 2010, there were two known clusters of Ecstasy overdoses associated with large-scale raves in Los Angeles and San Francisco, resulting in several deaths.[18] MDMA also significantly reduces mental abilities, including information processes and memory formation. Some research has also found that heavy use of Ecstasy can cause damage to specific types of nerve cells in the brain. The drug can be addictive in some people.

The effects can be hard to quantify because as an unregulated street drug, MDMA is often sold in tablets that contain other drugs such as methamphetamine and caffeine. Users also often mix MDMA with other drugs, especially alcohol. The combination of alcohol and Ecstasy may be particularly dangerous because the stimulant effect of MDMA makes an alcohol-intoxicated person feel more alert—even though her or his motor skills are significantly impaired by alcohol.[19] The concern is that a person taking this combination of drugs will drive while impaired due to a false sense of alertness.

Nonmedical Use of Prescription Drugs

Q | Are oxycodone and other drugs like that still a problem in the United States?

Yes, the nonmedical use of prescription drugs remains a problem, in part because these drugs are often readily accessible at home. The most commonly abused prescription drugs are opioid pain relievers like Vicodin and OxyContin, followed by tranquilizers, stimulants, and sedatives. Although viewed by some people as safer options because they aren't street drugs, prescription drugs can be dangerous or even deadly when not used as indicated. Deaths due to overdoses on opioid drugs now represent more than a third of all poisoning deaths each year—more than 14,000 deaths annually.[20] The risks from these drugs are also greater when they are combined with alcohol or other drugs.

If you or someone you know has a problem with any type of psychoactive drug, get help. Resources can be found by visiting the Web site for the Substance Abuse and Mental Health Services Administration (http://www.samhsa.gov) or calling its telephone hotline (800-662-HELP).

Alcohol

In the past month, about half of all Americans age 12 and over consumed alcohol at least one time. People use alcohol to relax, unwind, and decrease inhibitions. Alcohol consumption is widely accepted and may be a part of social gatherings and celebrations. But drinking can be beneficial or harmful, depending on the situation, the individual's age and health status, and how much is consumed. Although most Americans drink moderately or not at all, problem drinking affects everyone.

National laws regulate the use of alcohol, primarily for health and safety reasons, but not a day goes by where these regulations aren't violated, intentionally or not. Rates of drinking and driving are still remarkably high; alcohol is frequently purchased for, supplied to, or consumed by under-age individuals; and many people regularly consume more alcohol than their bodies can tolerate. Although the legal drinking age is 21, people between 12 and 20 consume almost 20 percent of all alcohol consumed in the United States.[21] And although people who drink heavily and frequently represent only 7 percent of the population, they drink 45 percent of all the alcohol.[22]

Excessive or unsafe alcohol consumption has many serious consequences: Drunk drivers routinely kill others and themselves, and alcohol abuse frequently plays a role in domestic violence, sexual abuse, unintended pregnancies, firearm injuries, and boating accidents. Regularly drinking too much alcohol leads to a host of health problems, including the risk for alcoholism. As described in Chapter 1, researchers estimate that alcohol is responsible for 85,000 deaths in the United States per year.

Alcohol can surely provide short-term pleasure and even excitement. However, a wise person recognizes that these transient pleasures come with real and significant risks. For wellness, you need to balance the risks and benefits of alcohol use and make wise choices. For you, that could be not using alcohol or choosing to use it only moderately and in situations that don't place yourself or others at risk.

Alcoholic Beverages and Drinking Patterns

Q | What counts as a drink?

The psychoactive, intoxicating substance found in all alcoholic beverages is **ethyl alcohol,** commonly referred to just as *alcohol.* The National Institute on Alcohol Abuse and Alcoholism (NIAAA) defines one drink as the amount of a beverage that contains 0.6 ounce (14 grams) of pure alcohol. The concentration of alcohol varies in different beverages; see Figure 13-3. One drink is the equivalent of 12 ounces of beer, 5 ounces of table wine, or a 1.5-ounce shot of 80-proof distilled liquor. The term *proof* refers to the alcohol content of hard liquor. Proof is twice the percentage of alcohol in a beverage; so, for example, a 100-proof liquor is 50 percent alcohol by volume. An additional helpful measurement is the number of drinks in a typical container:

- Regular bottle (750 ml) of table wine = 5 drinks
- Half-pint bottle (200 ml) of 80-proof spirits = 4½ drinks
- A fifth (750 ml) of 80-proof spirits = 17 drinks

Q | Is recreational drinking safe?

Whether or not "recreational" drinking is safe depends on the amount and the circumstances. The National Institute on Alcohol Abuse and Alcoholism (NIAAA) has defined a daily and a weekly limit for what is called a low-risk drinking pattern (Figure 13-4). The limits are lower for women than for men because women tend to be smaller, to have higher levels of body fat, and to absorb alcohol more quickly due to lower activity of alcohol-metabolizing enzymes in the stomach; together, these differences mean that a woman will have a higher blood alcohol concentration than a man who consumes the same amount of alcohol. Men and women who stay within both

ethyl alcohol The intoxicating psychoactive drug found in alcoholic beverages; also called *alcohol.*

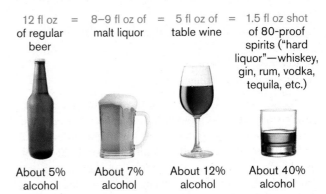

| 12 fl oz of regular beer | = | 8–9 fl oz of malt liquor | = | 5 fl oz of table wine | = | 1.5 fl oz shot of 80-proof spirits ("hard liquor"—whiskey, gin, rum, vodka, tequila, etc.) |

About 5% alcohol   About 7% alcohol   About 12% alcohol   About 40% alcohol

Figure 13-3 A standard drink. Each drink contains about 0.6 ounce of alcohol.

Source: National Institute on Alcohol Abuse and Alcoholism. (2010). *Rethinking drinking: Alcohol and your health.* NIH Pub. No. 10-3770.

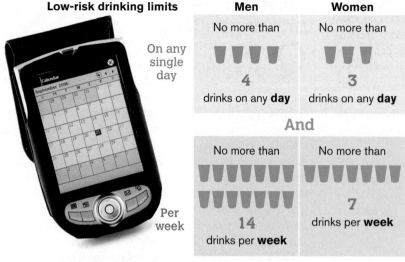

Low-risk drinking limits

Men
No more than
4 drinks on any **day**

Women
No more than
3 drinks on any **day**

On any single day

And

No more than
14 drinks per **week**

No more than
7 drinks per **week**

Per week

To stay low-risk, keep within **both** the single-day **and** the weekly limits.

Figure 13-4 Low-risk drinking limits
Source: National Institute on Alcohol Abuse and Alcoholism. (2010). *Rethinking drinking: Alcohol and your health.* NIH Pub. No. 10-3770.

limits for alcohol consumption have much lower rates of alcohol abuse and alcoholism than those who exceed one or both of them.

However, it's important to note that low-risk drinking does not eliminate risk. Even within these limits, drinkers can have problems—especially if they drink quickly, drink unsafely, have underlying health problems, or have had problems with alcohol use in the past. For example, consuming up to the number of drinks representing the daily limit in a very short period of time can lead to intoxication. For health and safety, some people need to drink less or not at all. People who should never drink include the following:

- Women who are pregnant or trying to become pregnant
- People who plan to drive or engage in other activities that require alertness and skill
- People taking certain over-the-counter or prescription medications
- People with medical conditions that can be made worse by drinking
- Recovering alcoholics
- People younger than age 21

People who exceed the limits recommended by the NIAAA are either at great risk for alcohol abuse or alcoholism or have already developed a problem with alcohol. The majority of adults either don't drink or drink at low-risk levels, but a substantial number of Americans have drinking patterns that place themselves and others at risk (Figure 13-5). Heavy drinkers who haven't yet developed a serious alcohol-related problem can reduce their risk of

harmful effects by cutting back. For people with alcoholism or a serious alcohol problem, quitting is the safest strategy.

Q | What is meant by binge drinking?

Binge drinking is consuming a significant number of drinks—five or more for men and four or more for women—in a relatively short period of time (usually within two hours). Binge drinking causes intoxication and brings blood alcohol concentration up to an unsafe level (see the next section for more on BAC). Binge drinking is a problem on college campuses, where students may party sporadically but heavily.

Students who frequently engage in binge drinking are much more likely to drive after drinking, to be injured, to engage in unplanned or unprotected sex, to miss classes and get behind in school work, and to argue with their friends (Figure 13-6). Non-drinking students are also affected by their bingeing peers: They experience property damage, unwanted sexual advances, verbal insults, physical violence, and interrupted sleep or studies. Binge drinking is the cause of most alcohol-related deaths among college students—from alcohol overdose and injuries.

Short-Term Effects of Alcohol Use

The immediate effects of alcohol are determined by **blood alcohol concentration (BAC),** which directly relates to the degree of intoxication. BAC depends on the amount of alcohol consumed and on individual factors including gender and body weight, the rate of alcohol consumption, and whether the person has eaten.

binge drinking Becoming intoxicated by consuming several drinks (five or more for men or four or more for women) in a short period (two hours or less).

blood alcohol concentration (BAC) A measure of intoxication; the amount of alcohol in the blood in terms of weight of alcohol per unit volume of blood, expressed as a percentage.

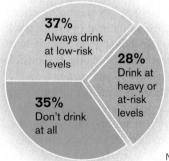

37% Always drink at low-risk levels

28% Drink at heavy or at-risk levels

35% Don't drink at all

Figure 13-5 Alcohol use by U.S. adults
Source: National Institute on Alcohol Abuse and Alcoholism. (2010). *Rethinking drinking: Alcohol and your health.* NIH Pub. No. 10-3770.

Percent reporting an alcohol-related injury

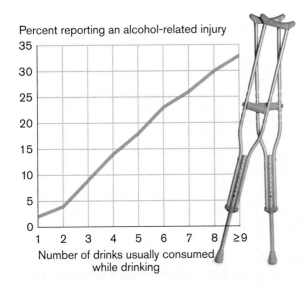

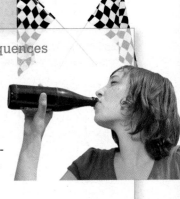

Figure 13-6 Drinking and injury rates among college students. Alcohol-related injuries are much more common among students whose typical drinking pattern fits the definition of binge drinking.

Source: Wechsler, H., and Nelson, T. F. (2008). What we have learned from the Harvard School of Public Health College Alcohol Study: Focusing attention on college student alcohol consumption and the environmental conditions that promote it. *Journal of Studies on Alcohol and Drugs, 69*(4), 481–490.

Q | I'm a big guy. Can my blood alcohol level really go up a lot?

BLOOD ALCOHOL CONCENTRATION (BAC). Yes, depending on how much and how fast you drink. A larger person can drink more than a smaller one before becoming significantly impaired, but any alcohol consumption has an effect (Table 13-3). The higher your BAC, the greater the impairment in motor skills, judgment, and behavior. BAC is also the measure used for defining drunk driving: The legal blood alcohol limit is 0.08% for anyone over 21 years. For those under age 21, zero tolerance laws are in effect, and a BAC of 0.02% or higher is considered above the legal limit for this age group.

Q | What should I eat before drinking to keep my BAC down?

The best way to keep your BAC in the safe range is to drink slowly and limit the amount of alcohol you consume. Factors that can affect BAC include the contents of your stomach, the rate of consumption, the type of beverage, and body weight.

Gender also plays a role. As described earlier, women tend to absorb more alcohol then men and take longer to break down and remove alcohol from the body. This is largely due their smaller body size and higher fat percentage, which both increase absorption. Females also produce

Fast Facts

College Drinking Consequences

College students spend over $5 billion a year on alcohol, more than they spend on textbooks, soft drinks, tea, milk, juice, and coffee combined. Each year, the following numbers of students experience these negative consequences from alcohol use:

1,825	Die from alcohol-related injuries, including motor vehicle crashes.
3,360,000	Drive under the influence of alcohol.
600,000	Are injured while under the influence of alcohol.
700,000	Are assaulted by another student who has been drinking.
400,000	Have unprotected sex while intoxicated.
150,000	Develop an alcohol-related health problem.
110,000	Are arrested for an alcohol-related violation such as public drunkenness or driving under the influence.
100,000	Have sex while too intoxicated to know if they consented.
100,000	Are victims of alcohol-related sexual assault, including date rape.

In addition:

25%	Experience academic consequences of drinking, including missing classes, falling behind, doing poorly on exams or papers, and receiving lower grades overall.
5%	Are involved with the police or campus security as a result of their drinking.

Sources: National Institute on Alcohol Abuse and Alcoholism. (2010). A snapshot of annual high-risk college drinking consequences. *College Drinking* (http://www.collegedrinkingprevention.gov/StatsSummaries/snapshot.aspx). See also data collected by the College Alcohol Health Study (http://www.hsph.harvard.edu/cas).

less of the alcohol-metabolizing enzyme and therefore absorb about 30 percent more alcohol into their bloodstream than men.

Food taken along with alcohol tends to result in both a lower peak BAC and a more gradual increase in BAC. Because alcohol is absorbed most efficiently in the small intestine, anything that prevents or inhibits alcohol from moving there will slow the increase in BAC. With food in the stomach, the valve at the bottom of the stomach will

TABLE 13-3 EFFECTS OF DIFFERENT LEVELS OF BLOOD ALCOHOL CONCENTRATION

BLOOD ALCOHOL CONCENTRATION (%)	TYPICAL EFFECTS
0.01–0.05	Sense of well-being, relaxation, loss of inhibitions; reduced ability to perform two tasks at the same time; impaired judgment and alertness
0.06–0.10	Pleasure, emotional arousal, numbness of feelings, nausea, sleepiness; impaired memory, self-control, motor coordination, and visual tracking
0.11–0.20	Mood swings, anger, mania, sadness, loss of balance; exaggerated emotions and inappropriate social behavior; nausea and vomiting; impaired reasoning, concentration, information processing, and depth perception
0.21–0.30	Aggression, depression, reduced response to pain and stimulation, stupor, slurred speech, inability to stand or walk; loss of temperature regulation and bowel and bladder control
0.31–0.40	Unconsciousness, slowed heart rate, difficulty breathing, coma; death possible from respiratory paralysis
0.41 AND ABOVE	Coma, death

Sources: Adapted from National Highway Traffic Safety Administration. (2005). *The ABCs of BAC*. DOT HS Publication 809 844. BCS/National Institute on Alcohol Abuse and Alcoholism. (2003). *Understanding alcohol: Investigations into biology and behavior*. NIH Pub. No. 04-4991.

close in order to hold food in, keeping alcohol there also. Alcohol can still be absorbed from the stomach, but much more slowly. There is no conclusive evidence that any specific type of food in the stomach will dramatically alter the rate of alcohol absorption. However, it is important to eat something—don't drink alcohol on an empty stomach.

Q | If you drink too much, is sleeping it off the best strategy? Coffee doesn't work, right?

You are correct that coffee doesn't help sober a person up. Neither do cold showers or fresh air. To sober up, you must wait for your body to absorb and metabolize all the alcohol you've consumed. BAC generally peaks 30–90 minutes after drinking. The rate of metabolism varies with the individual, but it generally takes about two hours per drink for the body's BAC to return to zero.[23] Thus, if you consume three drinks in an hour, it will take about six hours for your body to completely absorb and metabolize all the alcohol.

"Sleeping it off" isn't a good strategy if you have consumed a significant amount of alcohol. People who drink rapidly can consume a fatal dose of alcohol before exhibiting signs of intoxication, and their BAC can continue to rise even after they have passed out. In this situation, someone who appears to be sleeping may actually be unconscious and at risk for fatal respiratory failure. See the box "Handling an Alcohol Emergency" for more information on what to do in cases of suspected alcohol overdose ("alcohol poisoning").

Q | How bad is drinking and driving?

DRINKING AND DRIVING. Very bad. In 2008 alone, almost 12,000 people died in motor vehicle crashes involving a drunk driver; this is more than 30 percent of all annual traffic fatalities in the United States.[24] The risk of being involved in a crash goes up dramatically with increasing BAC, but driving skills are impaired even at relatively low BACs (Figure 13-7). The effects of alcohol on driving skills are particularly dramatic for young adults, who tend to have less driving experience and higher rates of risky driving overall. Males are also more likely to be involved in alcohol-related motor vehicle crashes than females.

Drinking and driving also carries significant legal penalties and financial costs. The cost varies by location

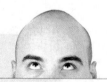

Mind Stretcher
Critical Thinking Exercise

Have you ever said or done anything under the influence of alcohol or other drugs that you regretted later? What were the consequences, and how did you deal with them? Did you change your behavior so it didn't happen again? Do you think it is right to excuse or discount things people say or do while intoxicated?

Wellness Strategies

Handling an Alcohol Emergency

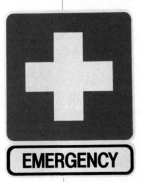

A fatal dose of alcohol depresses the nerves that control involuntary actions like breathing and the gag reflex. It is common for someone who drank excessive alcohol to vomit because alcohol is an irritant to the stomach. There is then the danger of choking on vomit, which could cause death by asphyxiation in a person who is not conscious because of intoxication. Never assume that someone who drinks heavily and falls asleep is OK and can be left alone.

What can happen to someone with alcohol poisoning who goes untreated?

- Victim chokes on his or her own vomit
- Breathing slows, becomes irregular, or stops
- Heart beats irregularly or stops
- Hypothermia (low body temperature)
- Hypoglycemia (too little blood sugar) leads to seizures
- Untreated severe dehydration from vomiting can cause seizures, permanent brain damage, or death

What are signs and symptoms of alcohol poisoning?

- Mental confusion, stupor, coma, or person appears to be sleeping but cannot be wakened
- Vomiting
- Seizures
- Slow breathing (fewer than eight breaths per minute)
- Irregular breathing (10 seconds or more between breaths)
- Hypothermia (low body temperature), bluish skin color, paleness

What should I do if I suspect someone has alcohol poisoning?

- Be aware that a person who has passed out may die; don't wait for all the symptoms to be present before you act. Do not assume that the person will sleep it off or would prefer not to be disturbed.
- If there is any suspicion of an alcohol overdose, call 911 for help. Don't try to guess the level of drunkenness.
- Roll the person on his or her side to lesson the risk of choking on vomit.
- Tell the ambulance driver or medical personnel if you believe that other drugs were also ingested.

Don't be afraid to seek medical help for a friend who has had too much to drink. Don't worry that your friend may become angry or embarrassed. Always be safe, not sorry.

Source: Adapted from National Institute on Alcohol Abuse and Alcoholism. (2010). Facts about alcohol poisoning. *College Drinking* (http://www.collegedrinkingprevention.gov/OtherAlcoholInformation/factsAboutAlcoholPoisoning.aspx).

and situation (first versus repeat offense), but even if you don't hit anyone or anything, you can expect the following expenses:

- Bail
- Cost of towing and storing your vehicle
- Court and lawyer fees, fines
- Cost of alcohol education classes
- License reinstatement fees
- Increased insurance premiums for many years

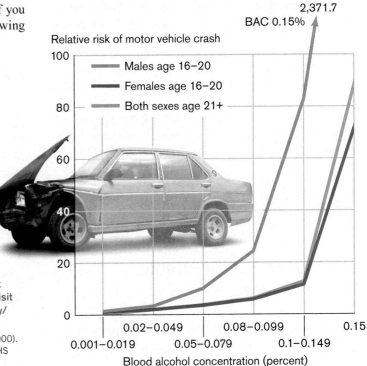

Figure 13-7 Risk of motor vehicle crashes, by sex, age, and blood alcohol concentration. The risk of being in an alcohol-related vehicle crash goes up dramatically with increasing BAC, but even a low level of alcohol increases risk. Crash risk is especially high for young adults, especially young males. Never drink and drive. To estimate your blood alcohol concentration, visit the BAC calculator at http://www.dot.wisconsin.gov/safety/motorist/drunkdriving/calculator.htm

Source: Data from National Highway Traffic Safety Administration. (2000). *Relative risk of fatal crash involvement by BAC, age, and gender.* DOT HS 809 050.

Costs often exceed $10,000. You will also lose time at work and school and possibly lose your job. Some jobs require a vehicle and some companies will not hire people with open court cases or criminal records.

Q | **Why is our drinking age so high?**

    READ ONLINE

Q | **What exactly is a hangover?** HANGOVERS. Besides miserable? A hangover is the body's way of telling you that you drank too much. Most people who drink to intoxication can expect a hangover to follow. Symptoms may last from eight to twenty-four hours and include the following symptoms:[25]

- Fatigue, lethargy, weakness, thirst
- Headache and muscle aches
- Nausea, vomiting, painful or upset stomach
- Decreased sleep, disturbed sleep patterns
- Sensitivity to light and sound, vertigo
- Depression, irritability, anxiety
- Decreased attention and concentration
- Tremor, sweating, and increased heart rate and blood pressure

Hangover symptoms may be due in part to the direct effects of alcohol, which can cause mild dehydration, electrolyte imbalance, gastrointestinal upset, low blood sugar, and sleep disturbances. A habitual drinker may experience symptoms of alcohol withdrawal after drinking stops. Different alcoholic beverages also contain other ingredients that may also contribute to hangover symptoms.

The best approach to hangovers is to avoid them—by not drinking to intoxication. The only thing that actually cures a hangover is time. Strategies for treating hangover symptoms include replacing lost fluids by drinking nonalcoholic beverages, eating (if possible), and resting. Soup is a good choice for replacing depleted electrolytes. If you take a pain reliever, don't choose acetaminophen because it can cause liver damage when combined with alcohol. Also keep in mind that hangovers are linked to reduced cognitive functioning and motor skills, so avoid driving or engaging in other potentially risky activities until your hangover symptoms subside.[26]

Q | **How many calories do I consume if I drink 5–7 drinks on two nights per week?**   READ ONLINE

Long-Term Health Effects of Alcohol Use

In addition to the immediate effects related to intoxication, alcohol use over an extended period also impairs health and wellness. Alcohol use during pregnancy has long-lasting effects as well.

Q | **How is the liver affected by drinking alcohol?** The liver is the main site of alcohol metabolism in the body, and even moderate drinkers can experience liver damage:

- *Fatty liver:* This condition, characterized by liver cells swollen with fat and water, can usually be reversed if alcohol use stops.
- *Hepatitis:* As described in Chapter 12, inflammation of the liver is often due to a viral infection, but it can also be caused by alcohol use. In some cases, hepatitis can lead to liver failure, liver cancer, and death.
- **Cirrhosis:** In this incurable disease, liver cells are replaced with scar tissue and the liver can no longer function. Liver transplantation is the only treatment.

The liver is not the only organ affected by chronic alcohol use—nearly every body system is involved (Figure 13-8). Heavy drinking, particularly over time, can damage the heart and lead to high blood pressure, cardiomyopathy (enlarged and weakened heart), congestive heart failure, and stroke. Heavy drinking also puts more fat into the circulatory system, raising your triglyceride level, which increases your risk of heart disease.

Q | **Is drinking alcohol good for my heart?** Possibly. Moderate alcohol consumption, defined as one to two drinks per day for men and about one per day for women, has been reported to decrease the incidence of cardiovascular disease as well as all-cause mortality. This is known as a J-curve response because nondrinkers have a slightly higher rate of CVD and premature death than moderate drinkers, but people who drink more than moderate amounts of alcohol have an increasingly greater risk of death.

The potential positive effects of alcohol are still being studied. One potential benefit is that moderate drinkers tend to have higher levels of beneficial HDL (good cholesterol) than nondrinkers. Moderate alcohol consumption also appears to decrease the stickiness of blood cells called platelets, reducing the formation of clots that can potentially cause heart attacks and strokes.

Not all the news about moderate drinking is good, however. For women, moderate drinking raises the risk of breast cancer. Anyone with a family or personal history of alcohol abuse also needs to take special care. And occasional binges on top of moderate intake undoes any benefit from moderate drinking. You need to evaluate the role of alcohol in your life based on your own personal risk factors and situation.

Q | **During pregnancy, how much alcohol is too much?**

No level of alcohol intake has been proven safe during pregnancy. The

cirrhosis A liver disease in which cells are replaced by fibrous scar tissue; can be caused by excessive long-term alcohol use.

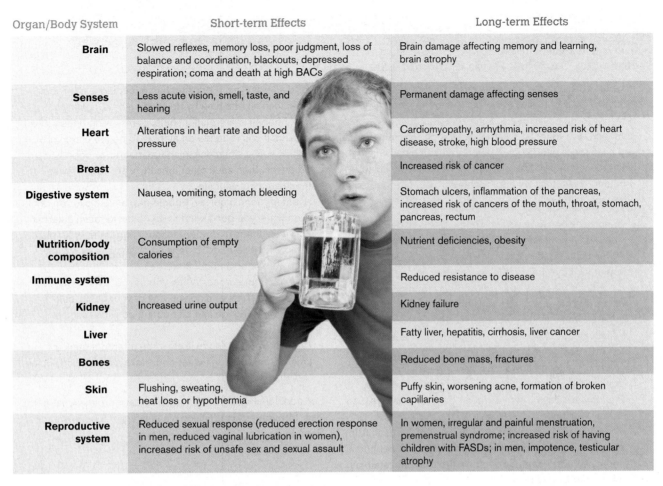

Organ/Body System	Short-term Effects	Long-term Effects
Brain	Slowed reflexes, memory loss, poor judgment, loss of balance and coordination, blackouts, depressed respiration; coma and death at high BACs	Brain damage affecting memory and learning, brain atrophy
Senses	Less acute vision, smell, taste, and hearing	Permanent damage affecting senses
Heart	Alterations in heart rate and blood pressure	Cardiomyopathy, arrhythmia, increased risk of heart disease, stroke, high blood pressure
Breast		Increased risk of cancer
Digestive system	Nausea, vomiting, stomach bleeding	Stomach ulcers, inflammation of the pancreas, increased risk of cancers of the mouth, throat, stomach, pancreas, rectum
Nutrition/body composition	Consumption of empty calories	Nutrient deficiencies, obesity
Immune system		Reduced resistance to disease
Kidney	Increased urine output	Kidney failure
Liver		Fatty liver, hepatitis, cirrhosis, liver cancer
Bones		Reduced bone mass, fractures
Skin	Flushing, sweating, heat loss or hypothermia	Puffy skin, worsening acne, formation of broken capillaries
Reproductive system	Reduced sexual response (reduced erection response in men, reduced vaginal lubrication in women), increased risk of unsafe sex and sexual assault	In women, irregular and painful menstruation, premenstrual syndrome; increased risk of having children with FASDs; in men, impotence, testicular atrophy

Figure 13-8 Potential effects of alcohol use on the body

Centers for Disease Control and Prevention recommend that women should not drink alcohol if they are pregnant, if they are planning to become pregnant, or if they are sexually active and do not use effective birth control. Drinking increases the risk of miscarriage and premature delivery, and it can cause a range of lifelong disorders in infants, known as **fetal alcohol spectrum disorders (FASDs)**. Infants and children with FASDs may have abnormal facial features, low body weight, shorter-than-average height, poor coordination, poor memory, difficulty paying attention, speech and language delays, poor reasoning and judgment skills, low IQ, and problems with the heart, kidneys, or bones.

Although there is no cure for FASDs, early intervention can help. FASDs are also 100 percent preventable. The more a pregnant woman drinks, the bigger the risk, but no level of alcohol consumption is considered completely safe during pregnancy.

Alcohol Abuse and Alcoholism

Q | How exactly is alcohol abuse classified?

There are a number of ways to define and classify serious problems with alcohol. The APA definitions for substance abuse and dependence are often applied to alcohol.[27] **Alcohol abuse** is a pattern of drinking that results in harm to one's health, interpersonal relationships, and ability to succeed at school or work. Characteristics of alcohol abuse include the following:

- Failure to fulfill major responsibilities at work, school, or home
- Drinking in dangerous situations, such as drinking while driving or operating machinery
- Legal problems related to alcohol, such as being arrested for drunk driving or for physically hurting someone while drunk
- Continued drinking despite ongoing relationship problems that are caused or worsened by drinking

Long-term alcohol abuse can turn into **alcohol dependence,** also known as alcohol addiction and alcoholism. The signs and symptoms of this chronic disease include a strong craving for alcohol, an inability to limit drinking, and

fetal alcohol spectrum disorders (FASDs) A range of birth defects that can occur in infants exposed to alcohol before birth.

alcohol abuse A pattern of drinking that is harmful to health, results in behavior that is harmful to others, or impairs the ability to meet school, work, and family responsibilities.

alcohol dependence Chronic, pathological use of alcohol despite repeated and serious consequences; usually characterized by tolerance and withdrawal; also known as *alcoholism.*

Wellness Strategies

Reducing Your Risk for Alcohol Problems

Is your drinking pattern high risk? If you're considering changing your drinking, you need to decide whether to cut down or to quit. Discuss options with a doctor, a friend, or someone else you trust. Quitting is strongly recommended if you have tried cutting down before but can't stay within the limits you set or if you have symptoms of an alcohol disorder. If cutting down may be appropriate for you, here are some strategies to try:

- *Keep track of how much you drink.* Use a paper notebook or enter notes in a mobile phone notepad or personal digital assistant. Making note of each drink before you drink it may help you slow down when needed.
- *Count and measure your drinks.* Away from home, it can be hard to keep track, especially with mixed drinks, and at times, you may be getting more alcohol than you think. With wine, you may need to ask the host or server not to top off a partially filled glass.
- *Set goals.* Decide how many days a week you want to drink and how many drinks you'll have on those days. Plan to have days when you don't drink, and always plan to stay within the low-risk limits.
- *Pace and space.* When you do drink, pace yourself. Sip slowly. Have no more than one standard drink per hour, and make every other drink a nonalcoholic one, such as water, soda, or juice.
- *Include food.* Don't drink on an empty stomach. Eat some food so the alcohol will be absorbed into your system more slowly.

- *Find alternatives.* If drinking has occupied a lot of your time, then fill free time by developing new, healthy activities, hobbies, and relationships, or renewing ones you've missed. If you've relied on alcohol to be more comfortable in social situations, manage moods, or cope with problems, then seek other, healthy ways to deal with those areas of your life.
- *Avoid triggers.* If certain people or places make you drink even when you don't want to, try to avoid them. If certain activities, times of day, or feelings trigger the urge, plan something else to do. If drinking at home is a problem, keep little or no alcohol there.
- *Plan to handle urges.* When you cannot avoid a trigger and an urge hits, remind yourself of your goals, call a buddy, or engage in a distracting activity, such as exercise.
- *Know your "no."* You're likely to be offered a drink at times when you don't want one. Have a polite, convincing "no, thanks" ready.

For additional information and to locate professional help, visit http://rethinkingdrinking.niaaa.nih.gov/ToolsResources/Resources.asp.

Source: Adapted from National Institute on Alcohol Abuse and Alcoholism. (2010). *Rethinking drinking: Alcohol and your health.* NIH Pub. No. 10-3770.

---

continued use despite repeated and serious physical, psychological, and/or interpersonal problems. Alcoholics also experience physical dependence on alcohol—with tolerance to alcohol's effects and withdrawal if they stop drinking.

If you are wondering about your own drinking habits or those of someone you know, compare your pattern of consumption to the low-risk drinking pattern illustrated in Figure 13-4. Lab Activity 13-1 provides additional assistance in identifying alcohol problems. See also the suggestions in the box "Reducing Your Risk for Alcohol Problems."

Q | Is alcoholism inherited?   Alcoholism does tend to run in families; however, environmental and social influences also seem to be important contributors. Children of alcoholic parents are at greater risk of also developing alcoholism but not all of them do, and people can develop alcoholism even though no one else in their family has a drinking problem. Environmental factors that affect risk include the influence of friends, stress levels, and the ease of obtaining alcohol. If alcoholism does

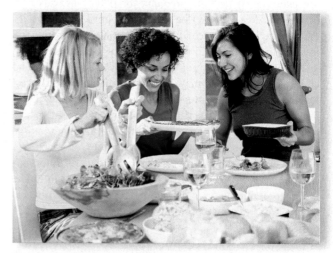

Low-risk drinking means avoiding intoxication. Men should limit their intake to no more than four drinks on any day and no more than fourteen drinks in a week. Women should limit their intake to no more than three drinks on any day and no more than seven drinks in a week. If you exceed the low-risk drinking limits, you can improve your health, safety, and well-being by cutting down or quitting drinking.

run in your family, monitor your use of alcohol and your responses to it carefully.

Q | Can alcoholism be treated?

Alcoholism can be treated, but it cannot be cured. As with any other chronic disease, some treatments are more effective than others. Regardless, it is important to remember that many people relapse before achieving long-term sobriety. Relapses are common and do not mean that a person has failed or cannot eventually recover from alcoholism. If a relapse occurs, it is important to try to stop drinking again and to get whatever help is needed to abstain from alcohol. A key resource is the Center for Substance Abuse Treatment (1-800-662-HELP), which provides information about treatment programs in local communities. Support groups including Alcoholics Anonymous (AA), Al-Anon (for friends and family members in an alcoholic person's life), and Alateen (for children of alcoholics) are also available in most communities.

Tobacco

According to the Centers for Disease Control and Prevention (CDC), tobacco use remains the leading cause of preventable death in the United States, contributing to over 400,000 deaths each year and resulting in almost $100 billion in direct medical costs. Lung cancer, heart disease, and emphysema are just a few of the health problems linked with tobacco use and secondhand smoke.

Given the tremendous health risks associated with tobacco use, it might seem remarkable that 20 percent of adults in the United States still choose to use this product. Youth and adolescent use continues to exceed that of adults, and typically, anyone who starts using tobacco prior to 21 years of age is more likely to continue using for many years to come. Tobacco companies spend about $15 billion annually on advertising and marketing, emphasizing the excitement, allure, and prosperity that can come from using their products. Conversely, local and national public health organizations spend less than a tenth of that amount combating all these myths and trying to protect the public's health.

Quitting tobacco is one of the most difficult health behavior changes, which is another reason why tobacco use continues. In a recent survey, 42 percent of all cigarette smokers had stopped smoking for at least one day during the preceding twelve months. This is a good indication of two interesting points: first is the strong desire by current smokers to quit, and second is the difficulty of quitting.[28]

Prevalence and Patterns of Use

Q | Everyone knows smoking is dangerous, so how many people are still doing it?

Overall, about 20 percent of U.S. adults are current smokers (Table 13-4). Rates vary across different population groups

as defined by gender, ethnicity, and educational attainment. Although many college students report having tried cigarettes, only a small percentage are regular smokers. In fact, college graduates (bachelors degree or higher) smoke at less than half the rate of those with less education.

One interesting trend in smoking rates is that between the ages of 18 and 64 years, there is no significant difference in the rate of people smoking, but after age 65, the proportion of smokers sharply declines. Considering that the average lifespan in the United States is about 78 years, and that smokers lose about ten years off of their lives,

TABLE 13-4 PATTERNS OF SMOKING AMONG U.S. ADULTS

	PERCENT WHO ARE CURRENT SMOKERS		
	MEN	WOMEN	TOTAL
AGE			
18–24	28.0	15.6	21.8
25–44	26.5	21.5	24.0
45–64	24.5	19.5	21.9
≥65	9.5	9.5	9.5
RACE/ETHNICITY (AGE ≥18)			
White	24.5	19.8	22.1
Black	23.9	19.2	21.3
Hispanic	19.0	9.8	14.5
American Indian/ Alaska Native	29.7	n/a	23.2
Asian	16.9	7.5	12.0
EDUCATION LEVEL (AGE ≥25)			
Less than a high school diploma			29.9
High school diploma or GED			28.1
Some college			22.1
Bachelor's degree or higher			8.6
TOTAL	23.5	17.9	20.6

Sources: Centers for Disease Control and Prevention. (2010). Vital signs: Current cigarette smoking among adults aged ≥ 18 years—United States, 2009. *Morbidity and Mortality Weekly Report, 59*(35), 1135–1140. National Center for Health Statistics. (2009). Summary health statistics for U.S. adults: National Health Interview Survey, 2008. *Vital and Health Statistics,* Series 10, No. 242.

maybe the rates are much lower after age 65 because many chronic smokers simply don't live this long.

In spite of the statistics, smoking doesn't start after high school. In fact, most lifetime smokers start well before they turn 18, often due to various types of exposure, influence, and peer pressure.[29]

Tobacco and Nicotine

Nicotine, a naturally occurring chemical in tobacco, is both a poison and a highly addictive psychoactive drug. Nicotine affects many parts of the body, including the brain, heart, and circulatory system. During pregnancy, nicotine freely crosses the placenta. One of the beauties of nicotine (especially if you are a major tobacco company) is that it can produce pleasurable effects that make the user want more.

Q Other than nicotine, what exactly is in a cigarette? Cigarette smoke contains over 4,000 chemicals and more than fifty known carcinogens, or cancer-causing compounds. There are at least another four hundred toxins in a typical cigarette. It's hard to believe so much can fit in such a small product! Nicotine and carbon monoxide are probably the most well-known ingredients in tobacco smoke, but others include formaldehyde, ammonia, hydrogen cyanide, arsenic, and pesticides. Some of the other chemicals in tobacco may also contribute to its addictive potential.

One cigarette additive of particular concern is menthol, which gives a sensation of coolness in the mouth, throat, and lungs—and may also mask the harshness of cigarette smoke. Menthol may make it easier for new smokers to start and for experienced smokers to smoke more and inhale more deeply. Use of menthol cigarettes is highest among young people who have recently started to smoke and among African Americans.

Q What makes someone start smoking? Although there are many reasons a person may choose to start smoking, it is difficult to point out one of them as most important. Peer pressure and exposure to smoking (parents, siblings, relatives, and friends) make people more likely to try smoking. Advertisers target young people, who may see smoking as a way to rebel or show their independence. Also, certain demographic features are more predictive of starting and continuing cigarette smoking. Lower educational attainment is strongly associated with smoking (see Table 13-4). The best way to keep children and adolescents from starting smoking is to model nonsmoking behavior. If they aren't exposed to smoking, they are much less likely to be tempted.

nicotine Poisonous, addictive psychoactive drug in tobacco.

Q Why is it so hard to quit? As stated earlier, almost half of all smokers try quitting at least once a year—if not more often. Quitting smoking has been studied by behavioral scientists for decades. The one fact they continue to find is that quitting smoking is hard. It's unusual for chronic smokers to quit on their first attempt.

Like many other psychoactive drugs, nicotine activates the reward system of the brain and so provides a pleasurable response. Nicotine's effects occur rapidly when the drug is smoked, but they also wear off quickly. To maintain the drug's pleasurable effects and prevent withdrawal, a user seeks to continue dosing at regular intervals. Smokers who are addicted to nicotine often report that the first cigarette in the morning is the one they crave the most and that seems the strongest or "best."

Use of tobacco leads to tolerance of nicotine's effects. If users stop or reduce tobacco use, their withdrawal symptoms include depression, irritability, anxiety, difficulty concentrating, and craving for nicotine. Dependence is also often supported by behavioral factors. The rituals associated with smoking—handling and lighting cigarettes, being in certain locations or with certain people—can make quitting more difficult.

Nicotine is a stimulant, causing an increase in physical arousal (heart rate and blood pressure) and mental alertness. Some people associate smoking with a reduction in stress, but the only stress that smoking reduces is the stress of nicotine withdrawal. The short-term effects of smoking on the body are summarized in Figure 13-9.

Effects of Smoking

Cigarettes kill more Americans than alcohol, motor vehicle crashes, suicide, HIV infection, homicide, and illegal drugs combined. Most people understand that smoking causes cancer and heart disease, but it also affects the skin, senses, hormones, and reproductive system.

Q What are the biggest health problems caused by smoking? The list of problems caused by smoking is a long one. Smoking is responsible for 90 percent of all lung cancer deaths in men, 80 percent of all lung cancer deaths in women, and 90 percent of all deaths from chronic obstructive lung disease (chronic bronchitis and emphysema).[30] In addition to lung cancer, smoking also causes cancers of the mouth, throat, pancreas, stomach, cervix, uterus, and kidney. Smoking reduces bone density and increases the risk of fractures.

Compared with nonsmokers, smokers are two to four times more likely to have coronary heart disease or a stroke. Smoking reduces the amount of oxygen in the blood, straining the cardiorespiratory system. Smoking

Brain
Nicotine reaches the brain within 10 seconds, triggering the reward center of the brain and causing overall nervous system stimulation; effects peak in about 10 minutes

Lungs
Smoke increases mucus production, thickens mucus, and damages cilia, preventing them from filtering foreign particles; chemicals from smoke damage cells in the lungs and are absorbed into the bloodstream and circulated throughout the body

Stomach
Smoking causes heartburn and ulcers, interferes with the absorption of several vitamins

Liver
Liver converts glycogen to glucose, increasing blood sugar levels

Kidneys
Nicotine inhibits the production of urine

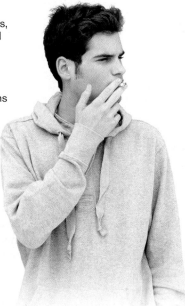

Nose
Tar and toxins in smoke irritate nasal membranes, dull sense of smell

Mouth and throat
Tar and toxins in smoke irritate membranes, dull taste buds, stain teeth, cause raspy voice and bad breath

Heart and blood vessels
Nicotine increases heart rate and blood pressure and constricts blood vessels; less oxygen is delivered to cells; platelets become stickier; blood fat levels are adversely affected

Reproductive system
Smoking reduces fertility in men and women; causes impotence in men and irregular menstruation in women; in pregnant women, nicotine and tobacco chemicals pass through the placenta to the fetus

Skin
Tobacco smoke dries and damages the skin; nicotine reduces blood flow to the skin

Figure 13-9 Short-term effects of smoking

narrows blood vessels, raises blood pressure, damages arteries, and contributes to unhealthy blood fat levels. All of these effects increase the risk of cardiovascular disease.

As you'd expect, smoking is also terrible for the respiratory system: It damages airways and alveoli in the lungs. It increases both the volume of mucus produced in the lungs and its thickness. At the same time, smoking destroys the cilia, which would normally move the mucus and trapped foreign material up and out of the body. The result of more and thicker mucus and lack of functional cilia is the dreaded "smoker's cough."

Smoking damages quality of life and shortens lives.

Q | Is it true smokers get wrinkles faster? Yes. Smoke in the environment dries the skin's surface. Smoking also reduces the amount of blood flow to the skin, thereby depleting the skin of oxygen and essential nutrients. These factors lead to an increase in wrinkles; smokers in their 40s often have as many facial wrinkles as nonsmokers in their 60s. In addition to accelerate wrinkling, prolonged smoking causes discoloration of the fingers and fingernails on the hand used to hold cigarettes. Smoking also yellows the teeth and causes halitosis, or bad breath.

Q | Can smoking control your weight? Many people are under the belief that smoking can help control body weight, and BMI tends to be lower in current smokers and higher in ex-smokers when compared with nonsmokers.[31] Although a slightly lower BMI might sound appealing, re-

call that smokers also develop chronic diseases and die prematurely. In addition, smokers tend to have unhealthy body fat distributions, with more fat stored in the torso (the "apple" shape)—the more cigarettes smoked, the greater the waist-to-hip ratio.[32]

Nicotine is a stimulant, so smokers burn slightly more calories. About 80 percent of smokers do gain some weight when they quit, an average of less than 10 pounds. They may gain weight because they feel hungrier (smoking dulls taste buds) and because they are burning calories at a normal, nondrugged rate. Most health experts recommend that smokers focus first on quitting—that is the most important step for health and wellness. Once you've quit, your body will adjust to life without nicotine. Most weight tends to be gained in the first six months after quitting; after that, many people start to lose the weight they gained as they adjust to being an ex-smoker.

Q | Will smoking affect me in sports? Yes! Tobacco affects athletic performance because it lowers maximal oxygen consumption and reduces lung function.[33] There is a misconception that chewing tobacco is better than smoking it because there is no smoke inhalation. Wrong. All forms of tobacco contain nicotine, which is not only addictive but also narrows blood vessels, which puts additional strain on the heart. Smoking causes problems with the lungs too, possibly even slowing lung growth, and it reduces the amount of oxygen in the blood available to muscles during activity. If you want to perform well on the court or in the field, you should consider quitting or not starting in the first place.

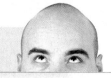

Mind Stretcher
Critical Thinking Exercise

Consider your smoking behavior: Are you a current smoker, an ex-smoker, or a lifetime nonsmoker? If you were ever a regular smoker, what were your reasons for starting to smoke and for continuing with the habit? If you quit, what were your reasons for doing so and what quitting techniques worked for you? If you never smoked, what were your reasons for that choice? Did you ever feel pressure to smoke? If so, how did you resist that pressure?

Q | **Will smoking mess with me getting pregnant?**

Yes, smoking appears to reduce fertility in both men and women. It also increases the risk of ectopic pregnancy, miscarriage, and preterm labor. Ultimately, smoking lowers your chances of conceiving by as much as 40 percent.[34] Smoking can also have serious effects on infants, including premature birth, low birth weight, and death. Nicotine and carbon monoxide reduce the supply of oxygen to the developing baby, which can have devastating effects on growth and development. Babies born to smoking mothers also have higher rates of asthma, attention deficit hyperactivity disorder (ADHD), and learning problems—and they are more likely to become smokers themselves.[35]

Other Forms of Tobacco Use

Q | Are light or low-tar cigarettes better for me?

No. Although cigarettes marketed as "light" or "low-tar" may contain less nicotine and tar, researchers have found that smokers usually compensate for these differences by inhaling more deeply, taking more puffs, or smoking more cigarettes. The National Cancer Institute has concluded that light cigarettes provide no benefit to smoker's health, and that smokers who use light cigarettes remain at high risk for developing smoking-related cancers and other chronic health problems. There is no such thing as a safe cigarette, and the way to reduce the risk of smoking-related diseases is to quit. Beginning in 2010, a new federal law bans the use of the words *light, mild,* and *low* on tobacco products.

DOLLAR STRETCHER
Financial Wellness Tips

Any form of substance use can hurt your bank balance. If you need additional incentive to cut back or quit, try calculating the weekly or monthly cost of your habit. Include not just how much you spend on the product—coffee and other caffeinated drinks, beer, cigarettes, and so on—but other costs as well (such as lost work time due to hangover, tooth-whitening products for nicotine-stained teeth).

Q | I know some athletes who use a water pipe. Is that a safer way to smoke?

No. Hookahs, or water pipes, have recently become more popular among college students, particularly athletes, who are less likely than other students to smoke standard cigarettes.[36] The flavored tobacco smoke from the water pipe tends to be less irritating to the throat than cigarette smoke, giving the impression of greater safety. However, studies comparing the two have found that water pipe use is associated with similar nicotine levels, greater carbon monoxide levels, and significantly more smoke exposure.[37]

Q | Smokeless isn't so bad, right?

Wrong. Smokeless tobacco is not a safe substitute for smoking cigarettes, as these products can also cause cancer and lead to nicotine addiction. The nicotine in smokeless tobacco is absorbed through the mucous membranes in the mouth when a user places a piece of chewing tobacco or a pinch of snuff between the cheek and gum. Use of smokeless tobacco causes *leukoplakia* (precancerous lesions in the mouth), gum recession, bone loss around the teeth, tooth decay, and bad breath. The most serious risk, though, is cancer of the mouth and pharynx. Oral cancer rates can be as much as fifty-fold higher for chronic snuff dippers compared with people who do not use tobacco.

Smokeless tobacco use leads to nicotine addiction. People who use dip eight to ten times a day are exposing themselves to the amount of nicotine in thirty to forty cigarettes. This may be one reason it is so hard to quit using smokeless products.

Q | What about cigars? You don't really inhale the smoke.

Although it's true most cigar smokers don't inhale the smoke, that doesn't protect them from the nicotine or other chemicals in a cigar. Some cigars have the amount of nicotine in an entire pack of cigarettes, and nicotine and other chemicals are absorbed more slowly through the mucous membranes. Because of the differences in how they are smoked, cigar smokers usually have lower rates of lung cancer than cigarette smokers but higher rates of cancers of the mouth and throat. Cigar smokers can also become dependent on nicotine. If a cigar smoker does inhale the smoke, he or she is at increased risk for both lung cancer and chronic respiratory disease. Cigar smoking isn't safe.

Environmental Tobacco Smoke

Q | Is secondhand smoke really as bad as everyone says?

Secondhand smoke is estimated to kill up to 70,000 nonsmokers per year—which seems pretty bad![38] It causes about 3,000 deaths from lung cancer, 62,000 deaths from heart disease, and nearly 3,000 infant deaths from sudden infant death syndrome (SIDS). Secondhand smoke is also referred to as **environmental tobacco smoke (ETS)** and consists of **sidestream smoke** and **mainstream smoke.** Sidestream smoke comes directly from lighted tobacco products, such as cigarettes, cigars, and pipes. Mainstream smoke is the smoke exhaled by smokers.

Environmental tobacco smoke is classified as a "known human carcinogen," meaning it causes cancer. In addition to cancer, heart disease, and SIDS, exposure to environmental tobacco smoke is linked to these diseases and conditions:

- Bronchitis, pneumonia, and ear infections in children
- Exacerbation of asthma and other chronic respiratory problems in children
- Low birth weight
- Increased risk of cervical cancer

Despite restrictions on where people can smoke, secondhand smoke exposure is common among nonsmokers. Based on an analysis of a blood marker for smoke exposure, the CDC estimates that 88 million nonsmokers are exposed to secondhand smoke,[39] with the highest rates of exposure among children ages 4–11 years. There is no risk-free level of secondhand smoke exposure, and it's likely that future research will identify even more negative effects from exposure to ETS.

Quitting Tobacco

Q | Why should I quit? I don't want to gain weight.

environmental tobacco smoke Smoke that enters the atmosphere from being exhaled by a smoker and by the burning end of a cigarette, cigar, or pipe; also called *secondhand smoke.*

sidestream smoke Smoke that enters the atmosphere from the burning end of a cigarette, cigar, or pipe.

mainstream smoke Smoke that enters the atmosphere by being exhaled by a smoker.

Quitting smoking brings with it tremendous health improvement—some would even say lifesaving! Even if you do gain weight, the small amount gained (5–10 pounds on average) poses much less of a health risk than the cigarettes you used to smoke. And you can always work to lose the weight. Quitting smoking reduces your risk for heart disease, cancer, stroke, chronic lung diseases, and many other health problems. Women who stop smoking before pregnancy or very early in the pregnancy dramatically reduce their

Behavior Change Challenge
Video Case Study

▶ WATCH ONLINE **Meet James**

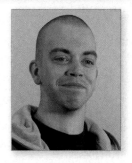

James is a 25-year-old college student who plans to join the Army. He's been a smoker for nine years and wants to quit smoking before boot camp. He also doesn't want to smoke around his young daughter. He doesn't smoke very many cigarettes a day, but he finds it difficult to quit. In his efforts to change, he is challenged by his stressors as well as by the other smokers in his life. Watch the video to learn more about James and his quit-smoking plan. As you watch the video, think about the following questions:

- Do you think James has enough motivation and specific strategies for his program to be successful?
- What can you learn from James's experience that will help you in your own behavior-change efforts? What strategies that he adopted can you use or adapt for your own program?

risk of having a low-birth-weight baby. People who quit by their 30s may avoid most tobacco-related health risks. However, even smokers who quit after age 50 substantially reduce their risk of dying early. It is never too late to quit smoking!

Although long-term health improvements are critical, consider some of these immediate benefits of quitting:[40]

- Your breath, clothes, and hair will smell better.
- Your sense of smell will return, and food will taste better.
- Your fingers and fingernails will slowly appear less yellow.
- Your stained teeth will slowly become whiter.
- Your children will be less likely to start smoking themselves.
- It will be easier and cheaper to find an apartment.
- You will miss fewer work days, or you may have an easier time getting a job.
- The constant search for a place to smoke when you're out will be over.
- Friends will be more willing to be in your car or home.
- Your dating prospects will become much wider, because 80 percent of the population does not smoke.
- You will have more money (one-pack-per-day smokers spend around $1,800 per year on cigarettes).

Q | What are the most effective ways of quitting smoking?

Quitting smoking is difficult, but millions of Americans have done it. It may require multiple attempts before you are successful. Smokers often relapse due to stress and withdrawal symptoms. Some smokers quit on their own, but others do better with support. A number of techniques have been shown to be effective:

- Talking with a doctor, who can provide advice and assistance
- Counseling, either individual or group sessions or via the telephone (call 1-800-QUIT-NOW)
- Behavioral strategies, such as setting goals, planning techniques for overcoming urges, and so on
- Medications

In addition, review the general behavior-change strategies from Chapter 2. Identify your stage of change, and choose techniques for change that are most likely to be helpful for you.

Q | Are all these patches, gums, etc., really worth it to try and help me quit?

Yes, medications can help people quit. The patches and gums you often see advertised are types of nicotine-replacement therapy, which provide a dose of nicotine to help reduce unpleasant feelings of withdrawal. Nicotine-replacement therapy doubles the rates of success. Nicotine chewing gum, lozenges, and skin patches are available over the counter; you need a prescription to buy the nicotine inhaler or nasal spray. These products do not completely eliminate nicotine withdrawal because they provide a smaller dose of nicotine at a slower rate. They do reduce cravings and withdrawal symptoms. Depending on the product, you may slowly reduce the amount you are using until you are completely nicotine-free. Two other prescription medications approved for smoking cessation—bupropion (Zyban) and varenicline (Chantix)—work by affecting neurotransmitter levels and provide no nicotine.

An additional challenge for people trying to quit is breaking the habit of putting or having something in their mouth most of the time. Often cigarettes are replaced by food, which is one of the reasons why weight gain often accompanies quitting. Therefore, finding a healthy way to occupy your hands and mouth (chewing gum, toothpicks, and so on) may also aid in the quitting process.

Regardless of the quitting method used, regular telephone contact seems helpful. After the attempt to quit has begun, weekly or monthly telephone calls from a health professional or loved one to support the attempt have proven quite successful in helping people maintain a smoke-free life. The online Smokefree.gov program includes many additional tips for putting together a step-by-step quitting program.

Fast Facts

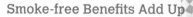

Smoke-free Benefits Add Up

Some health benefits begin almost immediately too, but every week, month, and year without tobacco use only improves your health.

- **Within 20 minutes of quitting,** your blood pressure and pulse rate drop to normal and the temperature of your hands and feet increases to normal.
- **Within 8 hours of quitting,** your blood carbon-monoxide levels drop and your blood oxygen levels increase, both to normal levels.
- **Within 24 hours of quitting,** your risk of a sudden heart attack decreases.
- **Within 48 hours of quitting,** nerve endings begin to regenerate and your senses of smell and taste begin to return to normal.
- **Within 2 weeks to 3 months of quitting,** your circulation improves and walking becomes easier; your lung function increases by up to 30 percent.
- **Within 1 to 9 months of quitting,** your energy typically increases and symptoms like coughing, nasal congestion, fatigue, and shortness of breath improve. You will have fewer illnesses, colds, and asthma attacks. You will gradually no longer be short of breath during everyday activities.
- **Within 1 year of quitting,** your risk of coronary heart disease is half that of someone still using tobacco.
- **Within 5 years of quitting,** your risk of dying from lung cancer decreases by nearly 50 percent compared to one-pack-per-day smokers; your risk of cancer of the mouth is half that of a tobacco user.
- **Within 10 years of quitting,** your risk of dying from lung cancer is similar to that of someone who never smoked; precancerous cells are replaced with normal cells; your risk of stroke is lowered, possibly to that of a nonsmoker; your risk of cancer of the mouth, throat, esophagus, bladder, kidney, and pancreas all go down.

Source: MedlinePlus.gov. (2009). *Making the decision to quit tobacco* (http://www.nlm.nih.gov/medlineplus/ency/article/002032.htm).

If you smoke, now is the time to start thinking about quitting. The first few weeks and months are usually the most difficult. But by planning ahead to cope with difficult situations and triggers, you can succeed. Quitting smoking is one of the best things you can ever do for health and wellness.

Q | If tobacco is so bad, what is our government doing about it? **READ ONLINE**

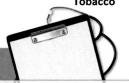

Research Brief

Medications for Smoking Cessation

Is there any one best strategy for quitting smoking? Probably not, as everyone is different. Researchers have been studying different medications, alone and in combination, to determine which are associated with the best outcomes.

One recent study looked at how medications for smoking cessation worked in the real world. Smokers were recruited during routine visits to their primary care physicians; they were offered free medication plus counseling via a quit line. The more than 1,300 participants were divided into five groups and followed for six months.

Therapy	6-month abstinence rate
Bupropion	16.8%
Nicotine lozenge	19.9%
Nicotine patch	17.7%
Nicotine patch plus lozenge	26.9%
Buproprion plus nicotine lozenge	29.9%

This study suggests that combinations of medications may be most effective at helping smokers quit. The nearly 30 percent abstinence rate achieved by the top group in the study is a good result, indicating that combinations of medication along with phone counseling can be an effective program for many smokers who are trying to quit.

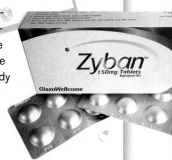

Source: Smith, S. S., McCarthy, D. E., Japuntich, S. J., et al. (2009). Comparative effectiveness of five smoking cessation pharmacotherapies in primary care clinics. *Archives of Internal Medicine, 169*(22), 2148–2155.

Summary

Substance use and abuse in the United States is a problem that has been around for generations and is not likely to go away anytime soon. Legal psychoactive drugs—such as alcohol, tobacco, and caffeine—play a major but paradoxical role in our country's economy: Although many communities depend on the income from these products to boost their economy in the short term, they also have to bear the long-term social costs of addiction, crime, morbidity, and mortality.

People use psychoactive substances for many reasons. In the short term, drug use carries risks ranging from missing class or doing something you later regret to intoxication, overdose, and death. Regular use also carries the risk of dependence. The effects of tobacco use are well known and include chronic disease and premature death for both smokers and the people around them.

Any substance or behavior that becomes the most important thing in someone's life detracts from wellness. The best way to prevent a drug problem is to never misuse or abuse drugs. Prescription drugs should be used strictly as intended and prescribed. Legal drugs like alcohol and caffeine should be used in moderation, and tobacco and illicit drugs should be avoided at all times. If you experience a problem with a behavior or drug—use that has gotten out of control—seek help.

More to Explore

Alcoholics Anonymous
   http://www.aa.org
Center for Internet Addiction
   http://www.netaddiction.com
Narcotics Anonymous
   http://www.na.org
National Council on Problem Gambling
   http://www.ncpgambling.org
National Institute on Alcohol Abuse and Alcoholism
   http://www.niaaa.nih.gov
National Institute on Drug Abuse
   http://www.drugabuse.gov
Smokefree.gov
   http://www.smokefree.gov
Substance Abuse and Mental Health Services Administration
   http://www.samhsa.gov

SUBMIT ONLINE

NAME	DATE	SECTION

Equipment: None

Preparation: None

Part 1: AUDIT Questionnaire for Alcohol Use

Instructions

For each question, give yourself the point total that corresponds to the answer that best describes your behavior.

QUESTIONS	0	1	2	3	4	
1. How often do you have a drink containing alcohol?	Never	Monthly or less	2 to 4 times a month	2 to 3 times a week	4 or more times a week	
2. How many drinks containing alcohol do you have on a typical day when you are drinking?	1 or 2	3 or 4	5 or 6	7 to 9	10 or more	
3. How often do you have 5 or more drinks on one occasion?	Never	Less than monthly	Monthly	Weekly	Daily or almost daily	
4. How often during the last year have you found that you were not able to stop drinking once you had started?	Never	Less than monthly	Monthly	Weekly	Daily or almost daily	
5. How often during the last year have you failed to do what was normally expected of you because of drinking?	Never	Less than monthly	Monthly	Weekly	Daily or almost daily	
6. How often during the last year have you needed a first drink in the morning to get yourself going after a heavy drinking session?	Never	Less than monthly	Monthly	Weekly	Daily or almost daily	
7. How often during the last year have you had a feeling of guilt or remorse after drinking?	Never	Less than monthly	Monthly	Weekly	Daily or almost daily	
8. How often during the last year have you been unable to remember what happened the night before because of your drinking?	Never	Less than monthly	Monthly	Weekly	Daily or almost daily	
9. Have you or someone else been injured because of your drinking?	No		Yes, but not in the last year		Yes, during the last year	
10. Has a relative, friend, doctor, or other health care worker been concerned about your drinking or suggested you cut down?	No	Yes, but not in the last year			Yes, during the last year	
					Total	

Results

A total score of 8 or more indicates a strong likelihood of hazardous or harmful alcohol consumption. Even if you score below 8, if you are having drinking-related problems with your academic performance, job, relationships, or health, or with the law, you should consider seeking help. Briefly describe any problems you've experienced as a result of drinking alcohol. In addition, compare your drinking pattern to the low-risk pattern described in Figure 13-4 in the chapter.

Part 2: Addictive Behavior Checklist

Instructions

Some addictive behaviors are easier to recognize than others, and some people don't notice signs that a behavior is out of control in some way. Below is a checklist of actions, thoughts, and feelings that can be associated with addictive behaviors. Choose a behavior to evaluate. Recall that many different types of behaviors can become addictive—from exercise to eating, gambling to video games, sex to shopping. Check any of the following statements that are true for you in relation to the behavior you are evaluating.

Behavior: _____

_____ I engage in this behavior fairly often.

_____ I have been engaging in this behavior for a long time.

_____ I engage in this behavior when I am stressed, worried, frustrated, angry, or in emotional pain.

_____ After engaging in this behavior, I feel bad inside—angry, guilty, or disappointed with myself.

_____ I sometimes feel panicky, restless, or irritable if I haven't engaged in the behavior in a while.

_____ I often find myself distracted from other things because I am thinking about or planning to engage in this behavior.

_____ I often reward myself with this behavior.

_____ When I engage in this behavior, I tend to lose track of time.

_____ I now engage in this behavior more often and/or for longer periods of time than I used to in order to get any satisfaction from it.

_____ I often tell myself I can stop this behavior at any time, yet I keep doing it.

_____ This behavior takes me away from healthier activities.

_____ I am often secretive about this behavior; I hide the behavior and/or lie about it to others.

_____ This behavior often leads to problems for myself and/or others.

_____ I've had others tell me this behavior is not good for me.

_____ I've lost some friends because of my involvement with this behavior.

_____ My life would be better without this behavior or if this behavior were more under control.

Results

The more items you check, the greater the chance that your behavior is a problem for you. If your answers suggest a problem, seek help from your school's counseling center or another health care provider. Professional addiction counselors can help you identify triggers, develop healthier strategies for dealing with stress and difficult emotions, and eliminate addictive behaviors.

Reflecting on Your Results

Were you surprised by the results of the AUDIT screening or by the number of yes answers on the addictive behavior checklist? Did your responses match your own impression of the role that alcohol use or other behaviors play in your life? What, if anything, in the results concerns you?

Planning Your Next Steps

If the results of these tests indicate that you could benefit from changing your behavior, state your goal for change and list at least three concrete strategies you plan to try.

Source: AUDIT test: Saunders, J. B., et al. (1993, June). Development of the Alcohol Use Disorders Identification Test (AUDIT): WHO collaborative project on early detection of persons with harmful alcohol consumption—II. *Addiction, 88,* 791–804.

Afterword: Wellness for Life

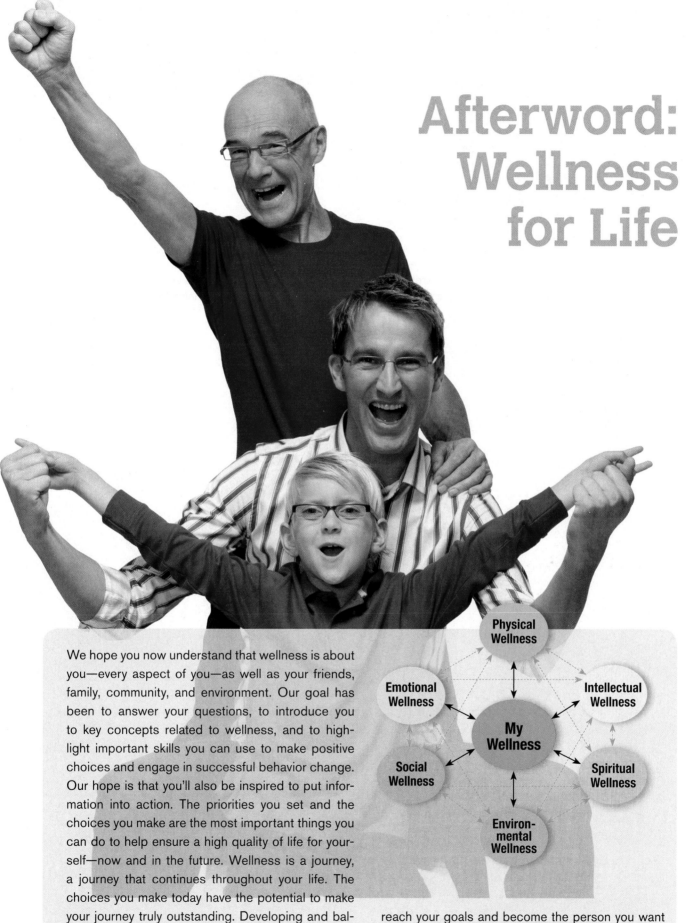

We hope you now understand that wellness is about you—every aspect of you—as well as your friends, family, community, and environment. Our goal has been to answer your questions, to introduce you to key concepts related to wellness, and to highlight important skills you can use to make positive choices and engage in successful behavior change. Our hope is that you'll also be inspired to put information into action. The priorities you set and the choices you make are the most important things you can do to help ensure a high quality of life for yourself—now and in the future. Wellness is a journey, a journey that continues throughout your life. The choices you make today have the potential to make your journey truly outstanding. Developing and balancing all the dimensions of wellness will help you reach your goals and become the person you want to be. We wish you a safe and wonderful journey.

Diagram labels

- Physical Wellness
- Emotional Wellness
- Intellectual Wellness
- My Wellness
- Social Wellness
- Spiritual Wellness
- Environmental Wellness

LAB ACTIVITY A-1 Wellness Reflection: How Far Have You Come?

SUBMIT ONLINE

NAME	DATE	SECTION

Equipment: None

Preparation: None

Instructions

Reflect on your experiences during your wellness course by answering the following questions.

Wellness Knowledge and Attitudes: What are some of the most surprising and relevant things you've learned about fitness and wellness? Have you learned any new skills in terms of critical analysis or consumer choices? Has what you've learned had an impact on your attitudes toward wellness? On your choices? If so, how?

Wellness Behaviors: Think about all your wellness-related behaviors. Are you more aware of them now? Are you more likely to think before you act? Have any of your habits changed during your wellness course? How and why? If possible, repeat Lab Activity 1-1 to see if your score has changed.

Lifestyle Changes: Have you engaged in a behavior-change program of any kind? If so, describe the goals and progress of your program, including the strategies you used and the key challenges you encountered. In addition, describe how you felt about the process and the change you tried to make. How successful were you? How did your efforts make you feel? Do you think you'll stick with your new behavior after the class is over? Why or why not?

Dimensions of Wellness: Think about your status for each of the wellness dimensions. What are your wellness strengths and weaknesses? How has your evaluation changed since the beginning of the course? Review the results of Lab Activity 1-2 if you completed it, and indicate what wellness strengths you've added and whether you would raise any of your wellness dimension scores.

Where Will You Go from Here? What are your major goals and aspirations? Where do you see yourself ten years in the future?

How does your current lifestyle match up to the image you have for your future? How will your current wellness strengths and positive behaviors help you achieve your goals? Could any of your current habits hold you back? List both your key strengths and positive behaviors and the areas where you need to improve. Make plans now to support your positive behaviors and make changes in any negative ones.

References

CHAPTER 1

1. American College Health Association (ACHA). (2009). *American College Health Association national college health assessment II: Reference group executive summary fall 2009.* Baltimore, MD: ACHA.

2. Ibid.

3. World Health Organization (WHO). (1948). Preamble to the constitution of the World Health Organization. *Official Records of the World Health Organization, 2,* 100.

4. Bouchard, C., Shephard, R. J., & Stephens, T. (1994). *Physical activity, fitness, and health: International proceedings and consensus statement.* Champaign, IL: Human Kinetics.

5. U.S. Department of Health & Human Services. (2008). *2008 physical activity guidelines for Americans.* ODPHP Publication No. U0036.

6. National Center for Health Statistics (NCHS). (2010). United States life tables, 2006. *National Vital Statistics Reports, 58*(21).

7. Central Intelligence Agency (CIA). (2010). *The world factbook online.* Retrieved from https://www.cia.gov/library/publications/the-world-factbook/index.html

8. Centers for Disease Control and Prevention (CDC). (1999). Ten great public health achievements—United States, 1900–1999. *MMWR, 48*(12), 241–243.

9. U.S. Census Bureau. (2009). National population estimates for the 2000s. Retrieved from http://www.census.gov/popest/national/asrh/2007-nat-res.html

10. National Center for Health Statistics (NCHS). (2009). Deaths: Leading causes for 2005. *National Vital Statistics Reports, 58*(8).

11. Molla, M. T., Madans, J. H., Wagener, D. K., & Crimmins, E. M. (2003). *Summary measures of population health: Report of findings on methodological and data issues.* Hyattsville, MD: National Center for Health Statistics.

12. National Center for Health Statistics (NCHS). (2009). *DATA 2010: The Healthy people 2010 database,* February 2009 edition. Retrieved from http://wonder.cdc.gov/data2010

13. Peeters, A., Barendregt, J. J., Willekens, F., Mackenbach, J. P., Al Mamun, A., & Bonneaux, L. (2003). Obesity in adulthood and its consequences for life expectancy: A life-table analysis. *Annals of Internal Medicine, 138*(1), 24–32.

14. Centers for Disease Control and Prevention (CDC). (2009). State-specific smoking-attributable mortality and years of potential life lost—United States, 2000–2004. *MMWR, 58*(02), 29–33

15. National Center for Health Statistics (NCHS). (2008). Deaths: Final data for 2005. *National Vital Statistics Reports, 56*(10).

CHAPTER 2

1. Rotter, J. B. (1966). Generalized expectancies for internal versus external control of reinforcement. *Psychological Monographs,* 80.

2. Roden, J. (2004). Revisiting the health belief model. *Nursing and Health Sciences, 6,* 1–10.

   Taylor, S., and others. (2000). Psychological resources, positive illusions, and health. *American Psychologist, 55,* 99–109.

   Peterson, C. (1999). Personal control and well-being. In D. Kahneman, E. Diener, & N. Schwartz (Eds.), *Well-being: The foundations of hedonic psychology.* New York, NY: Russell Sage Foundation.

   Myers, D. G., & Diener, E. (1995). Who is happy? *Psychological Science, 6,* 10–18.

3. UICC (Union Internationale contre le Cancer). (2008). *Population survey of cancer-related beliefs and behaviours.* Retrieved from http://www.cancervic.org.au/site/browse.asp?ContainerID=uicc-program3

4. Harvard Center for Cancer Prevention. (1996). Harvard reports on cancer prevention; Vol. 1. Human causes of cancer. *Cancer Causes and Control, 7*(suppl 1).

5. Scheier, M. F., & Carver, C. S. (1992). Effects of optimism on psychological and physical well-being: Theoretical overview and empirical update. *Cognitive Therapy and Research, 16,* 201–228.

   Carver, C., & Scheier, M. (2002). Optimism. In C. R. Snyder & S. J. Lopez (Eds.), *Handbook of positive psychology.* New York, NY: Oxford University Press.

   Peterson, C. (2000). The future of optimism. *American Psychologist, 55,* 44–55.

6. Bandura, A. (1977). Self-efficacy: Toward a unifying theory of behavioral change. *Psychological Review, 84,* 191-215.

   Bandura, A. (1997). *Self-efficacy: The exercise of control.* New York: Freeman.

7. Pekmezi, D., Jennings, E., & Marcus, B. H. (2009). Evaluating and enhancing self-efficacy for physical activity. *ACSM's Health & Fitness Journal, 13*(2), 16–21.

8. Bandura, A. (1977). *Social learning theory.* Englewood Cliffs, NJ: Prentice-Hall.

   Bandura, A. (1997). *Self-efficacy: The exercise of control.* New York: Freeman.

9. Ashford, S., Edmunds, J., & French, D. P. (2010, May). What is the best way to change self-efficacy to promote lifestyle and recreational physical activity? A systematic review with meta-analysis. *British Journal of Health Psychology, 15*(2), 265–288.

10. Maddux, J. (2002). Self-efficacy: The power of believing you can. In C. R. Snyder & S. J. Lopez (Eds.), *Handbook of positive psychology.* New York, NY: Oxford University Press.

11. Williams, S. (1995). Self-efficacy, anxiety, and phobic disorders. In J. E. Maddux (Ed.), *Self-efficacy, adaptation, and adjustment: Theory, research, and application.* New York, NY: Plenum.

    Maddux, J. (2002). Self-efficacy: The power of believing you can. In C. R. Snyder & S. J. Lopez (Eds.), *Handbook of positive psychology.* New York, NY: Oxford University Press.

12. Michie, S., Abraham, C., Whittington, C., McAteer, J., & Gupta, S. (2009). Effective techniques in healthy eating and physical activity interventions: A meta-regression. *Health Psychology, 28*(6), 690–701.

    Artinian, N. T., and others. (2010). Interventions to promote physical activity and dietary lifestyle changes for cardiovascular risk factor reduction: A scientific statement from the American Heart Association. *Circulation, 122,* 406–441.

13. Baumeister, R. F., & Scher, S. J. (1988). Self-defeating behavior patterns among normal individuals: Review and analysis of common self-destructive tendencies. *Psychological Bulletin, 104,* 3–22.

14. Prochaska, J. O., Redding, C. A., & Evers, K. E. (2008). The transtheoretical model and stages of change. In K. Glanz, B. K. Rimer, & K. Viswanath (Eds.). *Health behavior and health education: Theory, research, and practice* (4th ed.). San Francisco, CA: Jossey-Bass.

15. Prochaska, J., Norcross, J., & Diclemente, C. (1994). *Changing for good.* New York, NY: Morrow.

    Prochaska, J. O., Redding, C. A., & Evers, K. E. (2008). The transtheoretical model and stages of change. In K. Glanz, B. K. Rimer, & K. Viswanath (Eds.), *Health behavior and health education: Theory, research, and practice* (4th ed.). San Francisco, CA: Jossey-Bass.

    Hayden, J. (2009). *Introduction to health behavior theory.* Boston, MA: Jones and Bartlett.

16. Sheldon, K. M., & Kasser, T. (1998). Pursuing personal goals: Skills enable progress, but not all progress is beneficial. *Personality and Social Psychology Bulletin, 24,* 1319–1331.

    Sheldon, K. M., & Elliot, A. J. (1999). Goal striving, need satisfaction, and longitudinal well-being: The self-concordance model. *Journal of Personality and Social Psychology, 76,* 482–497.

17. Cantor, N., & Sanderson, C. A. (1999). Life task participation and well-being: The importance of taking part in daily life. In D. Kahneman, E. Diener, & N. Schwartz (Eds.), *Well-being: The foundations of hedonic psychology.* New York, NY: Russell Sage Foundation.

18. Locke, E. A. (2002). Setting goals for life and happiness. In C. R. Snyder & S. J. Lopez (Eds.), *Handbook of positive psychology.* New York: Oxford University Press.

19. Prochaska, J., Norcross, J., & Diclemente, C. (1994). *Changing for good.* New York, NY: Morrow.

CHAPTER 3

1. U.S. Department of Health & Human Services. (2008). *2008 physical activity guidelines for Americans.* ODPHP Publication No. U0036. Rockville, MD: Office of Disease Prevention and Health Promotion.

2. Physical Activity Guidelines Advisory Committee. (2008). *Physical Activity Guidelines Advisory Committee report, 2008.* Washington, DC: U.S. Department of Health and Human Services.

   Franco, O. H., Laet, C. D., Peeters, A., Jonker, J., Mackenbach, J., & Nusselder, W. (2005). Effects of physical activity on life expectancy with cardiovascular disease. *Archives of Internal Medicine,* 2355–2360.

   Sisson, S. B., Camhi, S. M., Church, T. S., Tudor-Locke, C., Johnson, W. D., & Katzmarzyk, P. T. (2010). Accelerometer-determined steps/day and metabolic syndrome. *American Journal of Preventive Medicine, 38*(6), 575–582.

3. Lacy, A. C., & Hastad, D. N. (2007). *Measurement and evaluation in physical education and exercise science.* San Francisco, CA: Benjamin Cummings.

4. Ibid.

5. American College of Sports Medicine. (2009). *ACSM's resource manual for guidelines for exercise testing and prescription* (6th ed.). Baltimore, MD: Lippincott Williams & Wilkins.

6. Ibid.

7. Tudor-Locke, C., Hatano, Y., Pangrazi, R. P., & Kang, M. (2008). Revisiting "How many steps are enough?" *Medicine and Science in Sports and Exercise, 40*(7 Suppl.), S537–S543.

   Marshall, S. J., and others. (2009). Translating physical activity recommendations into a pedometer-based step goal: 3000 steps in 30 minutes. *American Journal of Preventive Medicine, 36*(5), 410–415.

8. American College of Sports Medicine. (2009). *ACSM's resource manual for guidelines for exercise testing and prescription* (6th ed.). Baltimore, MD: Lippincott Williams & Wilkins.

9. American College of Sports Medicine. (2009). *ACSM's guidelines for exercise testing and prescription* (8th ed.). Baltimore, MD: Lippincott Williams & Wilkins.

10. Heckert, P. A. (n.d.). Night running walking safety tips. *Suite101.com.* Retrieved from http://walkingrunning.suite101.com/article.cfm/night_running_walking_safety_tips

11. Congeni, J. A. (2004, December). Sports and exercise safety. *Teens Health.* Retrieved from http://www.kidshealth.org/teen/food_fitness/exercise/sport_safety.html

12. American Academy of Orthopaedic Surgeons. (2007). *Selecting home exercise equipment.* Retrieved from http://orthoinfo.aaos.org/topic.cfm?topic=a00415

13. International Health, Racquet & Sportsclub Association. (2009). *About the industry.* Retrieved from http://cms.ihrsa.org/index.cfm?fuseaction=Page.viewPage&pageId=18735&nodeID=15

14. MayoClinic.com. (2007, February 16). *How to choose a fitness center.* Retrieved from http://www.mayoclinic.com/health/fitness/SM00027

15. MayoClinic.com. (2007, June 29). *Summer exercise: How to keep cool in hot weather.* Retrieved from http://www.mayoclinic.com/health/exercise/HQ00316

16. MayoClinic.com. (2007, November 1). *Exercise and cold weather: Stay motivated, fit and safe.* Retrieved from http://www.mayoclinic.com/health/fitness/HQ01681

17. Ibid.

18. U.S. Department of Health & Human Services. (2008). *2008 physical activity guidelines for Americans.* ODPHP Publication No. U0036. Rockville, MD: Office of Disease Prevention and Health Promotion.

19. Cheung, K., Hume, P., & Maxwell, L. (2003). Delayed onset muscle soreness: Treatment strategies and performance factors. *Sports Medicine, 33*(2), 145–164.

   Zainuddin, Z., Newton, M., Sacco, P., & Nosaka, K. (2005). Effects of massage on delayed-onset muscle soreness, swelling, and recovery of muscle function. *Journal of Athletic Training, 40*(3), 174–180.

CHAPTER 4

1. U.S. Department of Health and Human Services. (1996). *Physical activity and health: A report of the Surgeon General.* Atlanta, GA: U.S. Department of Health and Human Services, Public Health Service, Centers for Disease Control and Prevention, National Center for Chronic Disease Prevention and Health Promotion.

2. Fox, S. M., & Haskell, W. L. (1970). The exercise stress test: Needs for standardization. In M. Eliakim & H. N. Neufeld (Eds.), *Cardiology: Current topics and progress* (pp. 149–154). New York, NY: Academic Press.

3. Lanteri, C. J., & Sly, P. D. (1993). Changes in respiratory mechanics with age. *Journal of Applied Physiology, 74,* 369–378.

4. Morton, D. P., & Callister, R. (2002). Factors influencing exercise-related transient abdominal pain. *Medicine and Science in Sports and Exercise, 34*(5), 756–766.

5. Leon, A. S., Franklin, B. A., Costa, F., Balady, G. J., Berra, K. A., Stewart, K. J., Thompson, P. D., Williams, M. A., & Lauer, M. S. (2005). Cardiac rehabilitation and secondary prevention of coronary heart disease: An American Heart Association scientific statement from the Council on Clinical Cardiology (Subcommittee on Exercise, Cardiac Rehabilitation, and Prevention) and the Council on Nutrition, Physical Activity, and Metabolism (Subcommittee on Physical Activity), in collaboration with the American Association of Cardiovascular and Pulmonary Rehabilitation. *Circulation, 111*(3), 369–376.

6. Bouchard, C., An, P., Rice, T., Skinner, J. S., Wilmore, J. H., Gagnon, J., Perusse, L., Leon, A. S., & Rao, D. C. (1999). Familial aggregation of VO₂max response to exercise training: Results from the HERITAGE Family Study. *Journal of Applied Physiology, 87*(3), 1003–1008.

7. Reybrouck, T., & Fagard, R. (1999). Gender differences in the oxygen transport system during maximal exercise in hypertensive subjects. *CHEST, 115*(3), 788–792.

8. Thompson, W. R., Gordon, N. F., & Pescatello, L. S. (Eds.). (2009). *ACSM guidelines for exercise testing and prescription* (8th ed., pp. 84–86). Baltimore, MD: Lippincott Williams & Wilkins.

9. Thompson, W. R., Gordon, N. F., & Pescatello, L. S. (Eds.). (2009). *ACSM guidelines for exercise testing and prescription* (8th ed., p. 190). Baltimore, MD: Lippincott Williams & Wilkins.

10. McArdle, W. D., Katch, F. I., & Katch, V. L. (2006). *Essentials of exercise physiology* (3rd ed., p. 453). Baltimore, MD: Lippincott Williams & Wilkins.

11. American College of Sports Medicine. (2004). Position stand: Exercise and hypertension. *Medicine & Science in Sports & Exercise, 36,* 533–553.

12. U.S. Department of Health and Human Services. (2008). Chapter 2: Physical activity has many health benefits. *2008 physical activity guidelines for Americans.* Retrieved from http://www.health.gov/paguidelines/guidelines/default.aspx#toc

13. Blair, S. N., Kohl, H. W., III, Paffenbarger, R. S., Jr., Clark, D. G., Cooper, K. H., & Gibbons, L. W. (1989). Physical fitness and all-cause mortality. A prospective study of healthy men and women. *Journal of the American Medical Association, 262*(17), 2395–2401.

14. Klem, M. L., Wing, R. R., McGuire, M. T., Seagle, H. M., & Hill, J. O. (1997). A descriptive study of individuals successful at long-term maintenance of substantial weight loss. *American Journal of Clinical Nutrition, 66,* 239–246.

15. Franklin, B. (2004). MeritCare Speaker Series, Moorhead, MN.

16. American College of Sports Medicine. (2009). Position stand: Appropriate physical activity intervention strategies for weight loss and prevention of weight regain for adults. *Medicine & Science in Sports & Exercise, 41*(2), 459–471.

17. American College of Sports Medicine. (2009). *Resource manual to accompany guidelines for exercise testing and prescription* (6th ed.). Baltimore, MD: Lippincott Williams & Wilkins.

18. American College of Sports Medicine. (1998). Position stand: The recommended quantity and quality of exercise for developing and maintaining cardiorespiratory and muscular fitness and flexibility in healthy adults. *Medicine & Science in Sports & Exercise, 30*(6), 975–991.

19. Thompson, W. R., Gordon, N. F., & Pescatello, L. S. (Eds.). (2009). *ACSM guidelines for exercise testing and prescription* (8th ed., pp. 166–167). Baltimore, MD: Lippincott Williams & Wilkins.

   U.S. Department of Health and Human Services. (1996). *Physical activity and health: A report of the Surgeon General.* Atlanta, GA: U.S. Department of Health and Human Services, Public Health Service, Centers for Disease Control and Prevention, National Center for Chronic Disease Prevention and Health Promotion.

   American College of Sports Medicine. (2009). Position stand: Exercise and physical activity for older adults. *Medicine & Science in Sports & Exercise, 41*(7), 1510–1530.

   U.S. Department of Health and Human Services and U.S. Department of Agriculture. (2005). *Dietary guidelines for Americans* (6th ed.). Washington, DC: U.S. Government Printing Office.

20. U.S. Department of Health & Human Services. (2008). *2008 physical activity guidelines for Americans*. ODPHP Publication No. U0036. Rockville, MD: Office of Disease Prevention and Health Promotion.

21. Thompson, W. R., Gordon, N. F., & Pescatello, L. S. (Eds.). (2009). *ACSM guidelines for exercise testing and prescription* (8th ed., pp. 166–167). Baltimore, MD: Lippincott Williams & Wilkins.

22. Swain, D. P., Leutholtz, B. C., King, M. E., Haas, L. A., & Branch, J. D. (1998). Relationship between % heart rate reserve and % VO_2 reserve in treadmill exercise. *Medicine & Science in Sports & Exercise, 30*(2), 318–321.

23. U.S. Department of Health and Human Services. (1996). *Physical activity and health: A report of the Surgeon General*. Atlanta, GA: U.S. Department of Health and Human Services, Public Health Service, Centers for Disease Control and Prevention, National Center for Chronic Disease Prevention and Health Promotion.

24. Nieman, D. C. (2003). Current perspective on exercise immunology. *Current Sports Medicine Reports, 2*(5), 239–242.

CHAPTER 5

1. Centers for Disease Control and Prevention. (2010). *Growing stronger—Strength training for older adults*. http://www.cdc.gov/physical activity/growingstronger/why/index.html.

2. Andersen, J. L., Schjerling, P., & Saltin, B. (2000). Muscle, genes, and athletic performance. *Scientific American, 283*(3), 49–55.

3. Suter, E., Herzog, W., Sokolosky, J., Wiley, J. P., & MacIntosh, B. R. (1993). Muscle fiber type distribution as estimated by cybex testing and by muscle biopsy. *Medicine and Science in Sport and Exercise, 25*(3), 363–370.

4. Janssen, I., Heymsfield, S. B., Wang, Z., & Ross, R. (2000). Skeletal muscle mass and distribution in 468 men and women aged 18–88 years. *Journal of Applied Physiology, 89,* 81–88.

    Abe, T., Kearns, C. F., & Fukunaga, T. (2003). Sex differences in whole body skeletal muscle mass measured by magnetic resonance imaging and its distribution in young Japanese adults. *British Journal of Sports Medicine, 37,* 436–440.

5. Kraemer, W. J., Nindl, B. C., Ratamess, N. A., Nicholas, A., Gotshalk, L. A., Volek, J. S., & Hakkinen, K. (2004). Changes in muscle hypertrophy in women with periodized resistance training. *Medicine and Science in Sports Exercise, 36,* 697–708.

6. Beunen, G., & Thomis, M. (2006). Gene driven power athletes? Genetic variation in muscular strength and power. *British Journal of Sports Medicine, 40,* 822–823.

7. Quinn, E. (2009). Body composition—Body fat—Body weight: Learn why body weight and body fat are not always an indication of health. *About.com Sports Medicine.* http://sportsmedicine.about.com/od/fitnessevalandassessment/a/Body_Fat_Comp.htm.

8. Baumgartner, R. N., Heymsfield, S. B., & Roche, A. F. (1995). Human body composition and the epidemiology of chronic disease. *Obesity Research, 3*(1), 73–95.

9. Sui, X., LaMonte, M. J., Laditka, J. N., Hardin, J. W., Chase, N., Hooker, S. P., & Blair, S. N. (2007). Cardiorespiratory fitness and adiposity as mortality predictors in older adults. *Journal of the American Medical Association, 298*(21), 2507–2516.

10. Baumgartner, R. N., Heymsfield, S. B., & Roche, A. F. (1995). Human body composition and the epidemiology of chronic disease. *Obesity Research, 3*(1), 73–95.

11. Häkkinen, K. J. (1989). Neuromuscular and hormonal adaptations during strength and power training. A review. *Sports Medicine and Physical Fitness, 29*(1), 9–26.

12. Kelley, G. (1996). Mechanical overload and skeletal muscle fiber hyperplasia: A meta-analysis. *Journal of Applied Physiology, 81*(4), 1584–1588.

13. Carmelli, D., & Reed, T. (2000). Stability and change in genetic and environmental influences on hand-grip strength in older male twins. *Journal of Applied Physiology, 89,* 1879–1883.

    Tiainen, K., Sipilä, S., Alen, M., Heikkinen, E., Kaprio, J., Koskenvuo, M., & Rantanen, T. (2004). Heritability of maximal isometric muscle strength in older female twins. *Journal of Applied Physiology, 96,* 173–180.

    Bouchard, C., An, P., Rice, T., Skinner, J. S., Wilmore, J. H., Gagnon, J., & Rao, D. C. (1999). Familial aggregation of VO_2 max response to exercise training: Results from the HERITAGE Family Study. *Journal of Applied Physiology, 87*(3), 1003–1008.

14. Stewart, C. E. H., & Rittweger, J. (2006). Adaptive processes in skeletal muscle: Molecular regulators and genetic influences. *Journal of Musculoskeletal and Neuronal Interactions, 6*(1), 73–86.

15. Poehlman, E. T., Denino, W. F., Beckett, T., Kinaman, K. A., Dionne, I. J., Dvorak, R., & Ades, P. A. (2002). Effects of endurance and resistance training on total daily energy expenditure in young women: A controlled randomized trial. *Journal of Clinical Endocrinology Metabolism, 87*(3), 1004–1009.

    Hunter, G. R., Wetzstein, C. J., Fields, D. A., Brown, A., & Bamman, M. M. (2000). Resistance training increases total energy expenditure and free-living physical activity in older adults. *Journal of Applied Physiology, 89*(3), 977–984.

16. Hass, C. J., Feigenbaum, M. S., & Franklin, B. A. (2001). Prescription of resistance training for healthy populations. *Sports Medicine, 31*(14), 953–964.

17. Scully, D., Kremer, J., Meade, M. M., Graham, R., & Dudeon, K. (1998). Physical exercise and psychological well-being: A critical review. *British Journal of Sports Medicine, 32*(2), 111–120.

18. Singh, N. A., Stavrinos, T. M., Scarbek, Y., Galambos, G., Liber, C., & Fiatarone Singh, M. A. (2005). A randomized controlled trial of high versus low intensity weight training versus general practitioner care for clinical depression in older adults. *Journals of Gerontology: Biological Sciences, 60*(6), 768–776.

19. Evans, W. J., Meredith, C. N., Cannon, J. G., Dinarello, C. A., Frontera, W. R., Hughes, V. A., et al. (1985). Metabolic changes following eccentric exercise in trained and untrained men. *Journal of Applied Physiology, 61,* 1864–1868.

20. American College of Sports Medicine (ACSM). (2010). *Guidelines for exercise testing and prescription* (8th ed.). New York, NY: Lippincott Williams & Wilkins.

21. Ibid.

22. Fridén, J., Kjorell, U., & Thornell, L.-E. (1984). Delayed muscle soreness and cytoskeletal alterations: An immunocytological study in man. *International Journal of Sports Medicine, 5,* 15–18.

    Fridén, J., & Lieber, R. L. (1992). The structural and mechanical basis of exercise-induced muscle injury. *Medicine and Science in Sport and Exercise, 24,* 521–530.

    Connolly, D. A. J., Sayers, S. P., & McHugh, M. P. (2003). Treatment and prevention of delayed onset muscle soreness. *Journal of Strength and Conditioning Research, 17*(1), 197–298.

    Fridén, J., & Lieber, R. L. (1992). The structural and mechanical basis of exercise-induced muscle injury. *Medicine and Science in Sport and Exercise, 24,* 521–530.

23. Häkkinen, K. J. (1989). Neuromuscular and hormonal adaptations during strength and power training. A review. *Sports Medicine and Physical Fitness, 29*(1), 9–26.

24. Baker, K. R., Nelson, M. E., Felson, D. T., Layne, J. E., Sarno, R., & Roubenoff, R. (2001). The efficacy of home-based progressive strength training in older adults with knee osteoarthritis: A randomized controlled trial. *The Journal of Rheumatology, 28*(7), 1655–1665.

25. Kloubec, J. A. (2010). Pilates for improvement of muscle endurance, flexibility, balance, and posture. *Journal of Strength and Conditioning Research, 24*(3), 661–667.

    Caldwell, K., Harrison, M., Adams, M., Quin, R. H., & Greeson, J. (2010). Developing mindfulness in college students through movement-based courses: Effects on self-regulatory self-efficacy, mood, stress, and sleep quality. *Journal of American College Health, 58*(5), 433–442.

26. Cordain, L. (1998). Does creatine supplementation enhance athletic performance? *Journal of the American College of Nutrition, 17*(3), 205–206.

    Greenhaff, P. L. (1995). Creatine and its application as an ergogenic aid. *International Journal of Sport Nutrition, 5,* S100–S110.

    Greenhaff, P. L., Casey, A., Short, A. H., Harris, R. C., Soderlund, K., & Hultman, E. (1993). Influence of oral creatine supplementation on muscle torque during repeated bouts of maximal voluntary exercise in man. *Clinical Science, 84,* 565–571.

27. Alén, M., & Komi, P. V. (1984). Changes in neuromuscular performance and muscle fiber characteristics of elite power athletes self-administering androgenin and anabolic steroids. *Acta Physiologica Scandanavia, 122,* 535–544.

    Hickson, R. C., & Kurowski, T. G. (1986). Anabolic steroids and training. *Clinics in Sports Medicine, 5*(3), 461–469.

CHAPTER 6

1. Weppler, C. H., & Magnusson, S. P. (2010). Increasing muscle extensibility: A matter of

increasing length or modifying sensation? *Physical Therapy, 90*(3), 438–449.

Gajdosik, R. L., Allred, J. D., Gabbert, H. L., & Sonsteng, B. A. (2007). A stretching program increases the dynamic passive length and passive resistive properties of the calf muscle-tendon unit of unconditioned younger women. *European Journal of Applied Physiology, 99*(4), 449–454.

2. Ben, M., & Harvey, L. A. (2009). Regular stretch does not increase muscle extensibility: A randomized controlled trial. *Scandinavian Journal of Medicine and Science in Sport, 20*(1), 136–144.

3. Sharman, M. J., Cresswell, A. G., & Riek, S. (2006). Proprioceptive neuromuscular facilitation stretching: Mechanisms and clinical implications. *Sports Medicine, 36*(11), 929–939.

Law, R. Y., Harvey, L. A., Nicholas, M. K., Tonkin, L., DeSousa, M., & Finniss, D. G. (2009). Stretch exercises increase tolerance to stretch in patients with chronic musculoskeletal pain: A randomized controlled trial. *Physical Therapy, 89*(10), 1016–1026.

4. Smith, L. L., Burnet, S. P., & McNeil, J. D. (2003). Musculoskeletal manifestations of diabetes mellitus. *British Journal of Sports Medicine, 37,* 30–35.

5. Steultjens, M. P., Dekker, J., van Baar, M. E., Oostendorp, R. A., & Bijlsma, J. W. (2000). Range of joint motion and disability in patients with osteoarthritis of the knee or hip. *Rheumatology, 39*(9), 955–961.

6. Battié, M. C., Levalahti, E., Videman, T., Burton, K., & Kaprio, J. (2008). Heritability of lumbar flexibility and the role of disc degeneration and body weight. *Journal of Applied Physiology, 104*(2), 379–385.

7. Park, S. K., Stefanyshyn, D. J., Loitz-Ramage, B., Hart, D. A., & Ronsky, J. L. (2009). Changing hormone levels during the menstrual cycle affect knee laxity and stiffness in healthy female subjects. *British Journal of Sports Medicine, 37*(3), 588–598.

8. American College of Sports Medicine. (2009). *ACSM's guidelines for exercise testing and prescription.* Philadelphia, PA: Lipincott Williams & Wilkins.

9. Araujo, C., & Araujo, D. (2005). Does flexibility always decrease with aging? An 18-year follow-up in 10 women. *Medicine and Science in Sports and Exercise, 37*(5), S234–S235.

10. Thacker, S. B., Gilcrest, J., Stroup, D. F., & Kimsey, C. D., Jr. (2004). The impact of stretching on sports injury risk: A systematic review of the literature. *Medicine and Science in Sports and Exercise, 36*(3), 371–378.

11. Caplan, N., Rogers, R., Parr, M. K., & Hayes, P. R. (2009). The effect of proprioceptive neuromuscular facilitation and static stretch training on running mechanics. *Journal of Strength and Conditioning Research, 23*(4), 1175–1180.

12. Kokkonen, J., Nelson, A. G., Eldredge, C., & Winchester, J. B. (2007). Chronic static stretching improves exercise performance. *Medicine and Science in Sports and Exercise, 39*(10), 1825–1831.

13. Thacker, S. B., Gilcrest, J., Stroup, D. F., & Kimsey, C. D., Jr. (2004). The impact of stretching on sports injury risk: A systematic review of the literature. *Medicine and Science in Sports and Exercise, 36*(3), 371–378.

Woods, K., Bishop, P., & Jones, E. (2007). Warm-up and stretching in the prevention of muscular injury. *Sports Medicine, 37*(12), 1089–1099.

Jamtvedt, G., Herbert, R. D., Flottorp, S., and others. (2009). A pragmatic randomised trial of stretching before and after physical activity to prevent injury and soreness. *British Journal of Sports Medicine.* Retrieved from http://bjsportmed.com/content/early/2010/06/20/bjsm.2009.062232.full.pdf

14. Thacker, S. B., Gilcrest, J., Stroup, D. F., & Kimsey, C. D., Jr. (2004). The impact of stretching on sports injury risk: A systematic review of the literature. *Medicine and Science in Sports and Exercise, 36*(3), 371–378.

15. Jamtvedt, G., Herbert, R. D., Flottorp, S., and others. (2009). A pragmatic randomised trial of stretching before and after physical activity to prevent injury and soreness. *British Journal of Sports Medicine.* Retrieved from http://bjsportmed.com/content/early/2010/06/20/bjsm.2009.062232.full.pdf

Small, K., McNaughton, L., & Matthews, M. (2008). A systematic review into the efficacy of static stretching as part of a warm-up for the prevention of exercise-related injury. *Research in Sports Medicine, 16*(3), 213–231.

16. Malliaropoulos, N., Papalexandris, S., Papalada, A., & Papacostas, E. (2004). The role of stretching in rehabilitation of hamstring injuries. *Medicine and Science in Sports and Exercise, 36*(5), 756–759.

17. Cristopoliski, F., Barela, J. A., Leite, N., Fowler, N. E., & Rodacki, A. L. (2009). Stretching exercise program improves gait in the elderly. *Gerontology, 55*(6), 614–620.

Menz, H. B., Morris, M. E., & Lord, S. R. (2005). Foot and ankle characteristics associated with impaired balance and functional ability in older people. *Journal of Gerontology: Biological Sciences, 60,* 1546–1552.

18. Carlson, C. R., Collins, F. L., Jr., Nitz, A. J., Sturgis, E. T., & Rogers, J. L. (1990). Muscle stretching as an alternative relaxation training procedure. *Journal of Behavior Therapy and Experimental Psychiatry, 21*(1), 29–38.

19. Schwellnus, M. P., Drew, N., & Collins, M. (2008). Muscle cramping in athletes—Risk factors, clinical assessment, and management. *Clinics in Sports Medicine, 27*(1), 183–194.

20. American College of Sports Medicine. (2009). *ACSM's guidelines for exercise testing and prescription.* Philadelphia, PA: Lipincott Williams & Wilkins.

21. Fletcher, I. M. (2010). The effect of different dynamic stretch velocities on jump performance. *European Journal of Applied Physiology, 109*(3), 491–498.

22. Mitchell, U., Myrer, J., Hopkins, J., Hunter, I., Feland, J., Hilton, S., and others. (2006). Reciprocal inhibition, successive inhibition, autogenic inhibition, or stretch perception alteration: Why do PNF stretches work? *Medicine and Science in Sports and Exercise, 38*(5), S66–S67.

23. American College of Sports Medicine. (2009). *ACSM's guidelines for exercise testing and prescription.* Philadelphia, PA: Lipincott Williams & Wilkins.

24. Ibid.

25. U.S. Department of Health and Human Services. (2008.) *2008 physical activity guidelines for Americans.* ODPHP Publication No.

U0036. Rockville, MD: Office of Disease Prevention and Health Promotion.

26. Fernández-de-Las-Peñas, C., Cuadrado, M. L., & Pareja, J. A. (2007). Myofascial trigger points, neck mobility, and forward head posture in episodic tension-type headache. *Headache, 47*(5), 662–672.

27. Eltayeb, S., Staal, J. B., Hassan, A., & de Bie, R. S. (2009). Work related risk factors for neck, shoulder and arms complaints: A cohort study among Dutch computer office workers. *Journal of Occupational Rehabilitation, 19*(4), 315–322.

28. National Institute of Neurological Disorders and Stroke. (2010). Low back pain fact sheet. Retrieved from http://www.ninds.nih.gov/disorders/backpain/detail_backpain.htm.

29. Shiri, R., Karppinen, J., Leino-Arjas, P., Solovieva, S., & Viikari-Juntura, E. (2010). The association between smoking and low back pain: A meta-analysis. *American Journal of Medicine, 123*(1), 87.e7–87.e35.

30. Chou, R., Qaseem, A., Snow, V., and others. (2007). Diagnosis and treatment of low back pain: A joint clinical practice guideline from the American College of Physicians and the American Pain Society. *Annals of Internal Medicine, 147*(7), 478–491.

CHAPTER 7

1. Stehno-Bittel, L. (2008). Intricacies of fat. *Physical Therapy: Diabetes Special Issue, 88*(11), 1265–1278.

2. Hackney, K. J., Engels, H. J., & Gretebeck, R. J. (2008). Resting energy expenditure and delayed-onset muscle soreness after full-body resistance training with an eccentric concentration. *Journal of Strength and Conditioning Research, 22,* 1602–1609.

Paschalis, V., Nikolaidis, M. G., Theodorou, A. A., and others. (2010, May 27). A weekly bout of eccentric exercise is sufficient to induce health-promoting effects. *Medicine and Science in Sports and Exercise,* epub ahead of print.

3. Spaulding, K. L., Arner, E., Westermark, P. O., and others. (2008). Dynamics of fat cell turnover in humans. *Nature, 453*(7196), 783-787.

Jo, J., Gavrilova, O., Pack, S., and others. (2009). Hypertrophy and/or hyperplasia: Dynamics of adipose tissue growth. *PLoS Computational Biology, 5*(3), e1000324.

4. Bouchard, C. (1991). Heredity and the path to overweight and obesity. *Medicine and Science in Sports and Exercise, 23*(3), 285–291.

Bray, M. S. (2008). Implications of gene-behavior interactions: Prevention and intervention for obesity. *Obesity, 16*(3), S72–S78.

5. Herbert, A., Gerry, N. P., McQueen, M. B., and others. (2006). A common genetic variant is associated with adult and childhood obesity. *Science, 312*(5771), 279–283.

6. Frayling, T. M., Timpson, N. J., Weedon, M. N., and others. (2007). A common variant in the FTO gene is associated with body mass index and predisposes to childhood and adult obesity. *Science, 316*(5826), 889–894.

7. Rampersaud, E., Mitchell, B. D., Pollin, T. I., and others. (2008). Physical activity and the association of common FTO gene variants with body mass index and obesity. *Archives of Internal Medicine, 168*(16), 1791–1797.

Ruiz, J. R., Labayen, I., Ortega, F. B., and others. (2010). Attenuation of the effect of the FTO rs9939609 polymorphism on total and central body fat by physical activity in adolescents: The HELENA study. *Archives of Pediatric and Adolescent Medicine, 164*(4), 328–333.

8. Wells, J. (2007). Sexual dimorphism of body composition. *Best Practices & Research Clinical Endocrinology & Metabolism, 21*(3), 415–430.

9. Muralidhara, D. (2009). Body composition in subjects of different age and body mass index. *Journal of Physiological and Biomedical Sciences, 22*(1), 23–28.

10. U.S. Department of Health and Human Services. (2009). Mean percentage body fat by age group and sex—National Health and Nutrition Examination Survey, United States, 1999–2004. *MMWR Weekly, 57*(552), 1383. Retrieved from http://www.cdc.gov/mmwr/preview/mmwrhtml/mm5751a4.htm

    Wells, J. (2007). Sexual dimorphism of body composition. *Best Practices & Research Clinical Endocrinology & Metabolism, 21*(3), 415–430.

11. Westcott, W. (2009). ACSM strength training guidelines: Role in body composition and health enhancement. *ACSM's Health & Fitness Journal, 13*(4), 14–22.

12. Mott, J. W., Wang, J., Thorton, J. C., Allison, D. B., Heymsfield, S. B., & Pierson, R. (1999). Relationship between body fat and age in four ethnic groups. *American Journal of Clinical Nutrition, 69*, 1007–1013.

13. Ibid.

14. Knutson, K. L., & Van Cauter, E. (2008). Associations between sleep loss and increased risk of obesity and diabetes. *Annals of the New York Academy of Science, 1129*, 287–304.

    Cappuccio, F. P., Taggart, F. J., Kandala, N. B., Currie, A., Peile, E., Stranges, S., & Miller, M. A. (2008). Meta-analysis of short sleep duration and obesity in children and adults. *Sleep, 31*(5), 619–626.

15. George, S. A., Khan, S., Briggs, H., & Abelson, J. L. (2010). CRH-stimulated cortisol release and food intake in healthy, non-obese adults. *Psychoneuroendocrinology, 35*(4), 607–612.

    Epel, E., Lapidus, R., McEwen, B., & Brownell, K. (2001). Stress may add bite to appetite in women: A laboratory study of stress-induced cortisol and eating behavior. *Psychoneuroendocrinology, 26*, 37–49.

    Epel, E., McEwen, B., & Lupien, S. (2000). Cortisol reactivity to repeated stress as a function of fat distribution: Effects on cognition. *Psychoneuroendocrinology, 25*(1), S32.

16. Larson, N. I., Story, M. T., & Nelson, M. C. (2009). Neighborhood environments: Disparities in access to healthy foods in the U.S. *American Journal of Preventive Medicine, 36*(1), 74–81.

    Ford, P. B., & Dzewaltowski, D. A. (2008). Disparities in obesity prevalence due to variation in the retail food environment: Three testable hypotheses. *Nutrition Review, 66*(4), 216–228.

17. American Institute for Cancer Research. (2009). *New estimate: Excess body fat alone causes over 100,000 cancers in U.S. each year.* Retrieved from http://www.aicr.org/site/News2?abbr=pr_&page=NewsArticle&id=17333&news_iv_ctrl=1102

18. Stehno-Bittel, L. (2008). Intricacies of fat. *Physical Therapy: Diabetes Special Issue, 88*(11), 1265–1278.

19. Lewis, C. E., and others. (2009). Mortality, health outcomes, and body mass index in the overweight range. A Science Advisory from the American Heart Association. *Circulation, 119*, 3263–3271.

20. American College of Sports Medicine. (2007). Position stand: The Female Athlete Triad. *Medicine and Science in Sports and Exercise, 39*(10), 1867–1882.

21. Benardot, D. (2006). *Advanced sports nutrition.* Champaign, IL: Human Kinetics.

22. Meyers, P., & Biocca, F. (1992). The elastic body image: An experiment on the effect of advertising and programming on body image distortions in young women. *Journal of Communication, 42*(3), 108–133.

23. Razak, F., Anand, S. S., Shannon, H., and others. (2007). Defining obesity cut points in a multiethnic population. *Circulation, 115*(16), 2111–2118.

    World Health Organization. (2010). BMI classification. *Global database on body mass index.* http://apps.who.int/bmi/index.jsp?introPage=intro_3.html

24. Schneider, H. J., Friedrich, N., Klotsche, J., and others. (2010). The predictive value of different measures of obesity for incident cardiovascular events and mortality. *Journal of Clinical Endocrinology and Metabolism, 95*(4), 1777–1785.

25. Ashwell, M. (2009). Obesity risk: Importance of waist-to-height ratio. *Nursing Standard, 23*(41), 49–54.

26. Horowitz, J., & Klein, S. (2000). Lipid metabolism during endurance exercise. *American Journal of Clinical Nutrition, 72*(2), 558S–563S.

    Irving, B., Davis, C., Brock, D., Weltman, J., Swift, D., Barrett, E., Gaesser, G., & Weltman, A. (2008). Effect of exercise training intensity on abdominal visceral fat and body composition. *Medicine & Science in Sport & Exercise, 40*(11), 1863–1872.

27. U.S. Department of Health & Human Services. (2008). *2008 physical activity guidelines for Americans.* ODPHP Publication No. U0036.

28. Wing, R. R., & Phelan, S. (2005). Long-term weight loss maintenance. *American Journal of Clinical Nutrition, 82*(1), 222S–225S.

CHAPTER 8

1. Dietary Guidelines Advisory Committee. (2010). *Report of the Dietary Guidelines Advisory Committee on the dietary guidelines for Americans, 2010.* Retrieved from http://www.cnpp.usda.gov/DGAs2010-DGACReport.htm

2. U.S. Department of Agriculture, Agricultural Research Service. (2009). *USDA national nutrient database for standard reference,* Release 22. Retrieved from Nutrient Data Laboratory home page, http://www.ars.usda.gov/ba/bhnrc/ndl

3. Dietary Guidelines Advisory Committee. (2010). *Report of the Dietary Guidelines Advisory Committee on the dietary guidelines for Americans, 2010.* Retrieved from http://www.cnpp.usda.gov/DGAs2010-DGACReport.htm

4. Marriott, B., Olsho, L., Hadden, L., & Connor, P. (2010). Intake of added sugars and selected nutrients in the United States, National Health and Nutrition Examination Survey (NHANES) 2003–2006. *Critical Reviews in Food Science and Nutrition, 50*, 228–258.

    Welsh, J. A., Sharma, A., Abramson, J. L., Vaccarino, V., Gillespie, C., & Vos, M. B. (2010). Caloric sweetener consumption and dyslipidemia among U.S. adults. *JAMA, 303*(15), 1490–1497.

    Jalal, D. I., Smits, G., Johnson, R. J., & Chonchol, M. (2010). Increased fructose associates with elevated blood pressure. *Journal of the American Society of Nephrology, 21*(9), 1543–1549.

5. Dietary Guidelines Advisory Committee. (2010). *Report of the Dietary Guidelines Advisory Committee on the dietary guidelines for Americans, 2010.* Retrieved from http://www.cnpp.usda.gov/DGAs2010-DGACReport.htm

    Fardet, A. (2010). New hypotheses for the health-protective mechanisms of whole-grain cereals: What is beyond fibre? *Nutrition Research Reviews, 23*(1), 65–134.

6. Foster-Powell, K., Holt, S., & Brand-Miller, J. (2002). International table of glycemic index and glycemic load values: 2002. *American Journal of Clinical Nutrition, 76*, 5–56.

7. Dietary Guidelines Advisory Committee. (2010). *Report of the Dietary Guidelines Advisory Committee on the dietary guidelines for Americans, 2010.* Retrieved from http://www.cnpp.usda.gov/DGAs2010-DGACReport.htm

8. World Health Organization. (2003). Obesity and overweight. *Global strategy on diet, physical activity, and health.* Retrieved from http://www.who.int/dietphysicalactivity/publications/facts/obesity/en/

9. Ibid.

10. Dietary Guidelines Advisory Committee. (2010). *Report of the Dietary Guidelines Advisory Committee on the dietary guidelines for Americans, 2010.* Retrieved from http://www.cnpp.usda.gov/DGAs2010-DGACReport.htm

11. Bijkerk, C. J., de Wit, N. J., Muris, J. W., Whorwell, P. J., Knottnerus, J. A., & Hoes, A. W. (2009). Soluble or insoluble fibre in irritable bowel syndrome in primary care? Randomised placebo controlled trial. *British Medical Journal, 339*, 606–609.

12. Dahm, C. C., and others. (2010). Dietary fiber and colorectal cancer risk: A nested case-control study using food diaries. *Journal of the National Cancer Institute, 102*(9), 614–626.

13. American Dietetic Association. (2009). Position of the American Dietetic Association: Vegetarian diets. *Journal of the American Dietetic Association, 109*(7), 1266–1282.

14. National Academies, Institute of Medicine, Food and Nutrition Board. (2005). *Dietary reference intakes for energy, carbohydrate, fiber, fat, fatty acids, cholesterol, protein, and amino acids (macronutrients).* Washington, DC: National Academies Press.

    American College of Sports Medicine, American Dietetic Association, and Dietitians of Canada. (2009). Position stand: Nutrition and athletic performance. *Medicine and Science in Sports and Exercise, 41*(3), 709–731.

15. Hoffman, J. R., & Falvo, M. J. (2004). Protein—Which is best? *Journal of Sports Science and Medicine, 3,* 118–130.

Martin, W. F., Armstrong, L. E., & Rodriguez, N. R. (2005). Dietary protein intake and renal function. *Nutrition & Metabolism, 2*(25), n.p.

Frank, H., and others. (2009). Effect of short-term high-protein compared with normal-protein diets on renal hemodynamics and associated variables in healthy young men. *American Journal of Clinical Nutrition, 90*(6), 1509–1516.

16. Dietary Guidelines Advisory Committee. (2010). *Report of the Dietary Guidelines Advisory Committee on the dietary guidelines for Americans, 2010.* Retrieved from http://www.cnpp.usda.gov/DGAs2010-DGAC Report.htm

17. National Cancer Institute, Risk Factor Monitoring and Methods Branch. (2010). *Food sources.* Retrieved from http://riskfactor.cancer.gov/diet/foodsources/

18. Abumweis, S. S., Barake, R., & Jones, P. J. (2008, August 18). Plant sterols/stanols as cholesterol lowering agents: A meta-analysis of randomized controlled trials. *Food and Nutrition Research.*

19. Lukert, B. P., Carey, M., McCarty, B., Tiemann, S., Goodnight, L., Helm, M., and others. (1987). Influence of nutritional factors on calcium-regulating hormones and bone loss. *Calcified Tissue International, 40*(3), 119–125.

20. Harnack, L., Stang, J., & Story, M. (1999). Soft drink consumption among U.S. children and adolescents: Nutritional consequences. *Journal of the American Dietetic Association, 99*(4), 436–441.

National Cancer Institute, Risk Factor Monitoring and Methods Branch. (2010). *Food sources.* Retrieved from http://riskfactor.cancer.gov/diet/foodsources/

21. Tucker, K. L., Morita, K., Qiao, N., Hannan, M. T., Cupples, L. A., & Kiel, D. P. (2006). Colas, but not other carbonated beverages, are associated with low bone mineral density in older women: The Framingham osteoporosis study. *American Journal of Clinical Nutrition, 84*(4), 936–942.

McGartland, C., and others. (2003). Carbonated soft drink consumption and bone mineral density in adolescence: The Northern Ireland Young Hearts project. *Journal of Bone Mineral Research, 18*(9), 1563–1569.

22. Dietary Guidelines Advisory Committee. (2010). *Report of the Dietary Guidelines Advisory Committee on the dietary guidelines for Americans, 2010.* Retrieved from http://www.cnpp.usda.gov/DGAs2010-DGAC Report.htm

23. Bronstein, A. C., Spyker, D. A., Cantilena, L. R., Jr., Green, J. L., Rumack, B. H., & Heard, S. E. (2008). Annual report of the American Association of Poison Control Centers' National Poison Data System (NPDS): 25th annual report. *Clinical Toxicology, 46*(10), 927–1057.

24. USDA Food and Nutrient Laboratory. (2010). *USDA database for the oxygen radical absorbance capacity (ORAC) of selected foods, Release 2.* Beltsville, MD: USDA.

International Food Information Council Foundation. (2009, October 15). Functional foods fact sheet: Antioxidants. *Food Insight.* Retrieved from http://www.foodinsight.org/Resources/Detail.aspx?topic=Functional_Foods_Fact_Sheet_Antioxidants

25. Dietary Guidelines Advisory Committee. (2010). *Report of the Dietary Guidelines Advisory Committee on the dietary guidelines for Americans, 2010.* Retrieved from http://www.cnpp.usda.gov/DGAs2010-DGAC Report.htm

26. Lippi, G., Franchini, M., Favaloro, E. J., & Targher, G. (2010). Moderate red wine consumption and cardiovascular disease risk: Beyond the "French paradox." *Seminars in Thrombosis and Hemostasis, 36*(1), 59–70.

Desch, S., and others. (2010). Effect of cocoa products on blood pressure: Systematic review and meta-analysis. *American Journal of Hypertension, 23*(1), 97–103.

27. Dietary Guidelines Advisory Committee. (2010). *Report of the Dietary Guidelines Advisory Committee on the dietary guidelines for Americans, 2010.* Retrieved from http://www.cnpp.usda.gov/DGAs2010-DGAC Report.htm

28. Ibid.

29. Office of Dietary Supplements, National Institutes of Health. (2009). *Dietary supplement fact sheet: Vitamin D.* Retrieved from http://ods.od.nih.gov/factsheets/vitamind.asp

30. Dietary Guidelines Advisory Committee. (2010). *Report of the Dietary Guidelines Advisory Committee on the dietary guidelines for Americans, 2010.* Retrieved from http://www.cnpp.usda.gov/DGAs2010-DGAC Report.htm

31. Drewnowski, A. (2010). The Nutrient Rich Foods Index helps to identify healthy, affordable foods. *American Journal of Clinical Nutrition, 91*(4), 1095S–1101S.

CHAPTER 9

1. Dietary Guidelines Advisory Committee. (2010). *Report of the Dietary Guidelines Advisory Committee on the dietary guidelines for Americans, 2010.* Retrieved from http://www.cnpp.usda.gov/DGAs2010-DGAC Report.htm

2. Guenther, P. M., Dodd, K. W., Reedy, J., & Krebs-Smith, S. M. (2006). Most Americans eat much less than recommended amounts of fruits and vegetables. *Journal of the American Dietetic Association, 106*(9), 1371–1379.

3. Ruxton, C. H. S., Gardner, E. J., & Walker, D. (2006). Can pure fruit and vegetable juices protect against cancer and cardiovascular disease too? A review of the evidence. *International Journal of Food Sciences and Nutrition, 57*(3/4), 249–272.

4. Goldstone, A. P., de Hernandez, C. G. P., Beaver, J. D., Muhammed, K., Croese, C., Bell, G., and others. (2009). Fasting biases brain reward systems towards high-calorie foods. *European Journal of Neuroscience, 30,* 1625–1635.

Wyatt, H. R., Grunwald, G. K., Mosca, C. L., Klem, M. L., Wing, R. R., & Hill, J. O. (2002). Long-term weight loss and breakfast in subjects in the National Weight Control Registry. *Obesity Research, 10*(2), 78–82.

5. American Dietetic Association. (2009). Position of the American Dietetic Association: Vegetarian diets. *Journal of the American Dietetic Association, 109,* 1266–1282.

6. Ibid.

7. Dietary Guidelines Advisory Committee. (2010). *Report of the Dietary Guidelines Advisory Committee on the dietary guidelines for Americans, 2010.* Retrieved from http://www.cnpp.usda.gov/DGAs2010-DGAC Report.htm

8. National Heart, Lung, and Blood Institute. (2006). *Your guide to lowering your blood pressure with DASH.* NIH Publication No. 06-4082. Bethesda, MD: National Institutes of Health.

9. Smith, P. J., and others. (2010). Effects of the dietary approaches to stop hypertension diet, exercise, and caloric restriction on neurocognition in overweight adults with high blood pressure. *Hypertension, 55*(6), 1331–1338.

Blumenthal, J. A., and others. (2010). Effects of the dietary approaches to stop hypertension diet alone and in combination with exercise and caloric restriction on insulin sensitivity and lipids. *Hypertension, 55*(5), 1199–1205.

Azadbakht, L., Mirmiran, P., Esmaillzadeh, A., Azizi, T., & Azizi, F. (2005). Beneficial effects of a Dietary Approaches to Stop Hypertension eating plan on features of the metabolic syndrome. *Diabetes Care, 28*(12), 2823–2831.

10. Dietary Guidelines Advisory Committee. (2010). *Report of the Dietary Guidelines Advisory Committee on the dietary guidelines for Americans, 2010.* Retrieved from http://www.cnpp.usda.gov/DGAs2010-DGAC Report.htm

11. Institute of Medicine. (2006). *Addressing Foodborne Threats to Health: Policies, Practices, and Global Coordination Workshop Summary.* Washington D.C.: National Academy Press.

12. Byrd-Bredbenner, C., Maurer, J., Wheatley, V., Schaffner, D., Bruhn, C., & Blalock, L. (2007). Food safety self-reported behaviors and cognitions of young adults: Results of a national study. *Journal of Food Protection, 70*(8), 1917–1926.

Abbot, J. M., Byrd-Bredbenner, C., Schaffner, D., Bruhn, C. M., & Blalock, L. (2009). Comparison of food safety cognitions and self-reported food-handling behaviors with observed food safety behaviors of young adults. *European Journal of Clinical Nutrition, 63*(4), 572–579.

13. Abbot, J. M., Byrd-Bredbenner, C., Schaffner, D., Bruhn, C. M., & Blalock, L. (2009). Comparison of food safety cognitions and self-reported food-handling behaviors with observed food safety behaviors of young adults. *European Journal of Clinical Nutrition, 63*(4), 572–579.

14. FoodSafety.gov. (2010). *Seafood.* Retrieved from http://www.foodsafety.gov/keep/types/seafood

15. Dietary Guidelines Advisory Committee. (2010). *Report of the Dietary Guidelines Advisory Committee on the dietary guidelines for Americans, 2010.* Retrieved from http://www.cnpp.usda.gov/DGAs2010-DGAC Report.htm

16. Guan, T. Y., & Holley, R. A. (2003). Pathogen survival in swine manure environments and transmission of human enteric illness—A review. *Journal of Environmental Quality, 32,* 383–392.

17. Alternative Farming Systems Information Center, U.S. Department of Agriculture. (2008). *Should I purchase organic foods?*

Retrieved from http://www.nal.usda.gov/afsic/pubs/faq/BuyOrganicFoodsIntro.shtml

Benbrook, C. (2008). *Simplifying the Pesticide Risk Equation: The Organic Option.* Boulder, Col.: The Organic Center.

Dietary Guidelines Advisory Committee. (2010). *Report of the Dietary Guidelines Advisory Committee on the dietary guidelines for Americans, 2010.* Retrieved from http://www.cnpp.usda.gov/DGAs2010-DGAC Report.htm

Dangour, A. D., Lock, K., Hayter, A., Aikenhead, A., Allen, E., & Uauay, R. (2010). Nutrition-related health effects of organic foods: A systematic review. *American Journal of Clinical Nutrition, 92*(1), 203–210.

Alali, W. Q., Thakur, S., Berghaus, R. D., Martin, M. P., & Gebreyes, W. A. (2010). Prevalence and distribution of Salmonella in organic and conventional broiler poultry farms. *Foodborne Pathogens and Disease, 7*(11), 1363–1371.

18. Centers for Disease Control and Prevention. (2005). *Food irradiation.* Retrieved from http://www.cdc.gov/ncidod/dbmd/diseaseinfo/foodirradiation.htm

19. Sacks, F. M., and others. (2009). Comparison of weight-loss diets with different compositions of fat, protein, and carbohydrates. *New England Journal of Medicine, 360*(9), 859–873.

Foreyt, J. P., and others. (2009). Weight-reducing diets: Are there any differences? *Nutrition Reviews, 67*(Suppl1), S99–S101.

Gardner, C. D., and others. (2007). Comparison of the Atkins, Zone, Ornish, and LEARN diet for change in weight and related risk factors among overweight premenopausal women. *JAMA, 297*(9), 969–977.

Dansinger, M. L., Gleason, J. A., Griffith, J. L., Selker, H. P., & Schaefer, E. J. (2005). Comparison of the Atkins, Ornish, Weight Watchers, and Zone diets for weight loss and heart disease risk reduction. *JAMA, 293*(1), 43–53.

20. Alhassan, S., Kim, S., Bersamin, A., King, A. C., & Gardner, C. D. (2008). Dietary adherence and weight loss success among overweight women: Results from the A to Z weight loss study. *International Journal of Obesity, 32*(6), 985–991.

21. Randles, A., & Liguori, G. (2010). Does SES influence healthy eating promotions in restaurants? Abstract presented at the 2010 American Public Health Association annual meeting.

22. Artinian, N. T., and others. (2010). Interventions to promote physical activity and dietary lifestyle changes for cardiovascular risk factor reduction: A scientific statement from the American Heart Association. *Circulation, 122*, 406–441.

23. Burke, L. E., Sereika, S. M., Music, E., Warziski, M., Styn, M. A., & Stone, A. (2008). Using instrumented paper diaries to document self-monitoring patterns in weight loss. *Contemporary Clinical Trials, 29*(2), 182–193.

24. American Dietetic Association. (2009). Position of the American Dietetic Association: Weight management. *Journal of the American Dietetic Association, 109,* 330–346.

25. Wing, R. R., & Phelan, S. (2005). Long-term weight loss maintenance. *American Journal of Clinical Nutrition, 82*(1 Suppl), 222S–225S.

Catenacci, V. A., and others. (2008). Physical activity patterns in the National Weight Control Registry. *Obesity, 16*(1), 153–161.

26. Larson-Meyer, D. E., Redman, L., Heilbronn, L. K., Martin, C. K., & Ravussin, E. (2010). Caloric restriction with or without exercise: The fitness versus fatness debate. *Medicine and Science in Sports and Exercise, 42*(1), 152–159.

27. International Congress on Obesity. (2010). *News release: New research finds no evidence that popular slimming supplements facilitate weight loss.* Retrieved from http://www.ico2010.org/media.htm

28. Bent, S., Tiedt, T. N., Odden, M. C., and Shlipak, M. G. (2003). The relative safety of ephedra compared with other herbal products. *Annals of Internal Medicine, 138*(6), 468–471.

29. ConsumerReportsHealth.org. (2010). *Dangerous supplements: What you don't know about these 12 ingredients could hurt you.* Retrieved from http://www.consumerreports.org/health/natural-health/dietary-supplements/overview/index.htm

30. U.S. Food and Drug Administration. (2010). *"Dietary supplements" that contain undeclared prescription ingredients or other chemicals.* Retrieved from http://www.fda.gov/Drugs/ResourcesForYou/Consumers/BuyingUsingMedicineSafely/MedicationHealthFraud/ucm207647.htm

31. American Dietetic Association. (2009). Position of the American Dietetic Association: Weight management. *Journal of the American Dietetic Association, 109,* 330–346.

32. Ibid.

33. U.S. Food and Drug Administration. (2010, May). Weight-loss drugs and risk of liver failure. *Consumer Updates.* Retrieved from http://www.fda.gov/ForConsumers/ConsumerUpdates/ucm213401.htm

34. American College of Sports Medicine. (2009). Progression models in resistance training for healthy adults. *Medicine and Science in Sports and Exercise, 41*(3), 687–708.

35. Birmingham, C. L., Su, J., Hlynsky, J. A., Goldner, E. M., & Gao, M. (2005). The mortality rate from anorexia nervosa. *International Journal of Eating Disorders, 38*(2), 143–146.

36. National Institute of Mental Health. (2009). *Eating disorders.* Retrieved from http://www.nimh.nih.gov/health/publications/eating-disorders/complete-index.shtml

37. Borzekowski, D. L., Schenk, S., Wilson, J. L., & Peebles, R. (2010). e-Ana and e-Mia: A content analysis of pro-eating disorder Web sites. *American Journal of Public Health, 100*(8), 1526–1534.

CHAPTER 10

1. Dunser, M. W., & Hasibeder, W. R. (2009). Sympathetic overstimulation during critical illness: Adverse effects of adrenergic stress. *Journal of Intensive Care Medicine, 24*(5), 293–316.

2. Lee, H. J., Macbeth, A. H., Pagani, J. H., & Young, W. S. (2009). Oxytocin: The great facilitator of life. *Progressive Neurobiology, 88*(2), 127–151.

3. Player, M. S., King, D. E., Mainous, A. G., & Geesey, M. E. (2007). Psychosocial factors and progression from prehypertension to hypertension or coronary heart disease. *Annals of Family Medicine, 5*(5), 403–411.

Gouin, J. P., Kiecolt-Glaser, J. K., Malarkey, W. B., & Glaser, R. (2008). The influence of anger expression on wound healing. *Brain, Behavior, and Immunity, 22*(5), 699–708.

Stewart, J. C., Fitzgerald, G. J., & Kamarck, T. W. (2010). Hostility now, depression later? Longitudinal associations among emotional risk factors for coronary heart disease. *Annals of Behavioral Medicine, 39*(3), 258–266.

4. Williams, R., & Williams, V. (1994). *Anger kills.* New York, NY: Harper Paperbacks.

5. Niaura, R., Todaro, J. F., Stroud, L., Spiro III, A., Ward, K. D., & Weiss, S. (2002). Hostility, the metabolic syndrome, and incident coronary heart disease. *Health Psychology, 21*(6).

6. Gitau, R., Cameron, A., Fisk, N. M., & Glover, V. (1998). Fetal exposure to maternal cortisol. *Lancet, 352*(9129), 707–708.

7. Taylor, S. E. (2000). A new stress paradigm for women. *Monitor on Psychology, 31*(7).

Taylor, S. E., Klein, L. C., Lewis, B. P., Gruenewald, T. L., Gurung, R. A. R., & Updegraff, J. A. (2000). Biobehavioral responses to stress in females: Tend-and-befriend, not fight-or-flight. *Psychology Review, 107*(3), 411–429.

8. Lee, H. J., Macbeth, A. H., Pagani, J. H., & Young, W. S. (2009). Oxytocin: The great facilitator of life. *Progressive Neurobiology, 88*(2), 127–151.

9. Taylor, S. E., Klein, L. C., Lewis, B. P., Gruenewald, T. L., Gurung, R. A. R., & Updegraff, J. A. (2000). Biobehavioral responses to stress in females: Tend-and-befriend, not fight-or-flight. *Psychology Review, 107*(3), 411–429.

10. Lazarus, R. S., & Folkman, S. (1984). *Stress, appraisal, and coping.* New York, NY: Springer.

11. Heider, F. (1958). *The psychology of interpersonal relations.* New York, NY: Wiley.

Weiner, B. (1986). *An attributional theory of emotion and motivation.* New York, NY: Springer-Verlag.

12. Lazarus, R. S., & Folkman, S. (1984). *Stress, appraisal, and coping.* New York, NY: Springer.

13. Chandola, T., Brunner, E., & Marmot, M. (2006). Chronic stress at work and the metabolic syndrome: Prospective study. *British Medical Journal, 332*(7540), 521–525.

Bose, M., Olivan, B., & Laferre, B. (2009). Stress and obesity: The role of the hypothalamic-pituitary-adrenal axis in metabolic disease. *Current Opinion in Endocrinology, Diabetes, and Obesity, 16*(5), 340–346.

14. McEwen, B. S. (2000). Allostasis and allostatic load: Implications for neuropsychopharmacology. *Neuropsychopharmacology, 22*(2), 108–124.

15. Nyberg, A., Alfredsson, L., Theorell, T., Westerlund, H., Vahtera, J., & Kivimäki, M. (2009). Managerial leadership and ischaemic heart disease among employees: The Swedish WOLF study. *Occupational and Environmental Medicine, 66*(11), 51–55.

16. Mozumdar, A., Liguori G., Fountaine, C., Braun, S., & Muenchow, E. (2008). Working status, academic activity, leisure time activity, and BMI among first and second

year college students. [Abstract]. *Medicine & Science in Sports & Exercise, 40*(5), Supplement.

17. ACT. (2010). What works in student retention. *Research and policy issues.* Retrieved from http://www.act.org/research/policymakers/reports/retain.html

18. NASPA–Student Affairs Administrators in Higher Education. (2008). *Profile of the American college student, 2008.* Retrieved from http://www.naspa.org/divctr/research/profile/results.cfm

U.S. Department of Education, National Center for Education Statistics. (2009). *Digest of education statistics, 2008* (NCES 2009-020), Chapter 3.

19. Hansen, C. J., Stevens, L. C., & Coast, R. J. (2001). Exercise duration and mood state: How much is enough to feel better? *Health Psychology, 20,* 267–275

20. Hairston, K. G., and others. (2010). Sleep duration and five-year abdominal fat accumulation in a minority cohort: The IRAS family study. *Sleep, 33*(3), 289–295.

Donga, E., and others. (2010). A single night of partial sleep deprivation induces insulin resistance in multiple metabolic pathways in healthy subjects. *Journal of Clinical Endocrinology and Metabolism, 95*(6), 2963–2968.

21. Capuccio, F. P., D'Elia, L., Strazzullo, P., & Miller, M. A. (2010). Sleep duration and all-cause mortality: A systematic review and meta-analysis of prospective studies. *Sleep, 33*(5), 585–592.

22. MayoClinic.com. (2009). Causes. *Insomnia* (http://www.mayoclinic.com/health/insomnia/DS00187/DSECTION=causes).

23. Cohen, D. A., Wang, W., Wyat, J. K., Kronauer, R. E., Dijk, D.-J., Czeisler, C. A., & Klerman, E. B. (2010). Uncovering residual effects of chronic sleep loss on human performance. *Science Translational Medicine, 2*(14), 14ra3.

24. Benson, H., & Klipper, M. (1975). *The relaxation response.* New York, NY: HarperCollins.

25. Nidich, S. I., and others. (2009). A randomized controlled trial on the effects of the Transcendental Meditation program on blood pressure, psychological distress, and coping in young adults. *American Journal of Hypertension 22*(12), 1326–1331.

CHAPTER 11

1. American Heart Association. (2010). Heart disease and stroke statistics 2010 update: A report from the American Heart Association. *Circulation, 121,* e46–e215.

2. Humphries, S. E., Drenos, F., Ken-Dror, G., & Talmud, P. J. (2010). Coronary heart disease risk prediction in the era of genome-wide association studies: Current status and what the future holds. *Circulation, 121*(20), 2235–2248.

Dandona, S., Steward, A. F., & Roberts, R. (2010). Genomics in coronary artery disease: Past, present, and future. *Canadian Journal of Cardiology, 26*(Suppl A), 56A–59A.

3. American Heart Association. (2010). Heart disease and stroke statistics 2010 update: A report from the American Heart Association. *Circulation, 121,* e46–e215.

4. National Institute on Aging. (2005). *Aging hearts and arteries: A scientific quest.* NIH Publication No. 05-3738.

5. Pérez-López, F. R., Larrad-Mur, L., Kallen, A., Chedraui, P., & Taylor, H. S. (2010). Gender differences in cardiovascular disease: Hormonal and biochemical influences. *Reproductive Sciences, 17*(6), 511–531.

6. Berger, J. S., and others. (2009). Sex differences in mortality following acute coronary syndromes. *JAMA, 302*(8), 874–882.

7. American Heart Association. (2010). Heart disease and stroke statistics 2010 update: A report from the American Heart Association. *Circulation, 121,* e46–e215.

8. Kurian, A. K., & Cardarelli, K. M. (2007 Winter). Racial and ethnic differences in cardiovascular disease risk factors: A systematic review. *Ethnicity and Disease, 17*(1), 143–152.

9. Dietary Guidelines Advisory Committee. (2010). *Report of the Dietary Guidelines Advisory Committee on the Dietary Guidelines for Americans, 2010.* Retrieved from http://www.cnpp.usda.gov/DGAs2010-DGAC Report.htm

Stewart, D., Johnson, W., & Saunders, E. (2006). Hypertension in black Americans as a special population: Why so special? *Current Cardiology Reports, 8*(6), 405–410.

10. Wilson, P. W., D'Agostino, R. B., Sullivan, L., Parise, H., & Kannel, W. B. (2002). Overweight and obesity as determinants of cardiovascular risk: The Framingham Experience. *Archives of Internal Medicine, 162,* 1867–1872.

11. American Heart Association. (2010). Heart disease and stroke statistics 2010 update: A report from the American Heart Association. *Circulation, 121,* e46–e215.

12. U.S. Department of Health and Human Services. (2004). *The health consequences of smoking: A report of the Surgeon General.* Atlanta, GA: National Center for Chronic Disease Prevention and Health Promotion, Office on Smoking and Health.

13. Snow, W. M., Murray, R., Ekuma, O., Tyas, S. L., & Barnes, G. E. (2009). Alcohol use and cardiovascular health outcomes: a comparison across age and gender in the Winnipeg Health and Drinking Survey Cohort. *Age and Aging, 38*(2), 206–212.

14. Yap, S., Qin, C., & Woodman, O. L. (2010). Effects of resveratrol and flavonols on cardiovascular function: Physiological mechanisms. *Biofactors, 36*(5), 350–359.

15. Pletcher, M. J., and others. (2008). Prehypertension during young adulthood and coronary calcium later in life. *Annals of Internal Medicine, 149,* 91–99.

16. Pletcher, M. J., and others. (2010). Nonoptimal lipids commonly present in young adults and coronary calcium later in life: the CARDIA (Coronary Artery Risk Development in Young Adults) Study. *Annals of Internal Medicine, 153,* 137–146.

17. American Heart Association. (2010). Heart disease and stroke statistics 2010 update: A report from the American Heart Association. *Circulation, 121,* e46–e215.

18. Svensson, L., and others. (2010). Compression-only CPR or standard CPR in out-of-hospital cardiac arrest. *New England Journal of Medicine, 363*(5), 434–442.

19. American Cancer Society. (2010). *Cancer facts & figures 2010.* Atlanta, GA: ACS.

20. National Cancer Institute. (2010). *What is cancer?* Retrieved from http://www.cancer.gov/cancertopics/what-is-cancer, accessed August 20, 2010.

21. American Cancer Society. (2010). *Cancer facts & figures 2010.* Atlanta, GA: ACS.

22. Ibid.

23. Ibid.

24. U.S. Department of Health and Human Services. (2005). *National toxicology program 11th report on carcinogens.* Triangle Park, MD: National Toxicology Program.

25. American Cancer Society. (2010). *Cancer facts & figures 2010.* Atlanta, GA: ACS.

26. Singh, R., and others. (2009). Evaluation of the DNA damaging potential of cannabis cigarette smoke by the determination of acetaldehyde derived N2-ethyl-2'-deoxyguanosine adducts. *Chemical Research in Toxicology, 22*(6), 1181–1188.

Mehra, R., Moore, B. A., Crothers, K., Tetrault, J., & Fiellin, D. A. (2006). The association between marijuana smoking and lung cancer: A systematic review. *Archives of Internal Medicine, 166*(13), 1359–1367.

27. Hu, S., and others. (2009). Disparity in melanoma: A trend analysis of melanoma incidence and stage at diagnosis among whites, Hispanics, and blacks in Florida. *Archives of Dermatology, 145*(12), 1369–1374.

28. National Institute of Diabetes and Digestive and Kidney Diseases (NIDDK). (2008). National Diabetes Information Clearinghouse: National diabetes statistics. Retrieved from http://www.diabetes.niddk.nih.gov/dm/pubs/statistics/index.htm

29. Ibid.

30. National Institute of Diabetes and Digestive and Kidney Diseases (NIDDK). (2008). National Diabetes Information Clearinghouse: Diabetes overview. Retrieved from http://www.diabetes.niddk.nih.gov/dm/pubs/overview

31. Centers for Disease Control and Prevention. (2008). *National diabetes fact sheet: General information and national estimates on diabetes in the United States, 2007.* Atlanta, GA: CDC.

32. National Institute of Diabetes and Digestive and Kidney Diseases (NIDDK). (2007). *Type 2 Diabetes: What you need to know.* NIH Publication No. 07–6192.

CHAPTER 12

1. Winther, B., McCue, K., Ashe, K., Rubino, J. R., & Hendley, J. O. (2007). Environmental contamination with rhinovirus and transfer to fingers of healthy individuals by daily life activity. *Journal of Medical Virology, 79*(10), 1606–1610.

2. Wood, J. P., Choi, Y. W., Chappie, D. J., Rogers, J. V., & Kaye, J. Z. (2009). *Environmental persistence of a highly pathogenic avian influenza (H1N1) virus.* Research Triangle Park, NC: Environmental Protection Agency. Pub. No. EPA/600/R-09/054.

3. Smith-McCune, K. K., et al. (2010). Type-specific cervico-vaginal human papillomavirus infection increases risk of HIV acquisition independent of other sexually transmitted infections. *PLoS One, 5*(4), e10094.

de Jong, M. A., de Witte, L., Taylor, M. E., & Geijtenbeek, T. B. (2010). Herpes simplex virus type 2 enhances HIV-1 susceptibility by affecting Langerhans cell function. *Journal of Immunology, 185*(3), 1633–1641.

4. Sadeharju, K., Knip, M., Virtanen, S. M., et al. (2007). Maternal antibodies in breast milk protect the child from enterovirus infections. *Pediatrics, 119*(5), 941–946.

5. Centers for Disease Control and Prevention. (2010). Hepatitis C FAQs for health professionals (http://www.cdc.gov/hepatitis/HCV/HCVfaq.htm).

6. Aiello, A. E., Coulborn, R. M., Perez, V., & Larson, E. L. (2008). Effect of hand hygiene on infectious disease risk in the community setting: A meta-analysis. *American Journal of Public Health, 98*(8), 1372–1381.

White, C., Kolble, R., Carlson, R., et al. (2003). The effect of hand hygiene on illness rate among students in university resident halls. *American Journal of Infection Control, 31*(6), 364–370.

7. Surgeoner, B. V., Chapman, B. J., & Powell, D. A. (2009). University students' hand hygiene practice during a gastrointestinal outbreak in residence: What they say they do and what they actually do. *Journal of Environmental Health, 72*(2), 24–28.

Anderson, J. L., Warren, C. A., Perez, E., et al. (2008). Gender and ethnic differences in hand hygiene practices among college students. *American Journal of Infection Control, 36*(5), 361–368.

8. Fondell, E., Lagerros, Y. T., Sundberg, C. J., et al. (2010). Physical activity, stress, and self-reported upper respiratory tract infection. *Medicine and Science in Sports and Exercise,* June 23, epub ahead of print.

9. Pedersen, A., Zachariae, R., & Bovbjerg, D. H. (2010). Influence of psychological stress on upper respiratory infection—A meta-analysis of prospective studies. *Psychosomatic Medicine, 72*(8), 823–832.

10. Bennett, M. P., Zeller, J. M., Rosenberg, L., & McCann, J. (2003). The effect of mirthful laughter on stress and natural killer cell activity. *Alternative Therapies in Health and Medicine, 9*(2), 38–45.

11. Costelloe, C., Metcalfe, C., Lovering, A., Mant, D., & Hay, A. D. (2010). Effect of antibiotic prescribing in primary care on antimicrobial resistance in individual patients: Systematic review and meta-analysis. *British Medical Journal, 18*(340), c2096.

12. Centers for Disease Control and Prevention. (2010). How flu spreads (http://www.cdc.gov/flu/about/disease/spread.htm).

13. Centers for Disease Control and Prevention, National Center for Infectious Diseases. (2006). Epstein-Barr virus and infectious mononucleosis (http://www.cdc.gov/ncidod/diseases/ebv.htm).

14. Centers for Disease Control and Prevention. (2010). Fact sheet: Genital herpes (http://www.cdc.gov/std/herpes).

15. Giannini, C. M., Kim, H. K., Mortensen, J., Mortensen, J., Marsolo, K., & Huppert, J. (2010). Culture of non-genital sites increases the detection of gonorrhea in women. *Journal of Pediatric and Adolescent Gynecology, 23*(4), 246–252.

16. Cottrell, B. H. (2010). An updated review of evidence to discourage douching. *MCN: The American Journal of Maternal/Child Nursing, 35*(2), 102–107.

17. National Institute of Allergy and Infectious Diseases. (2009). *Pelvic inflammatory disease* (http://www.niaid.nih.gov/topics/pelvicinflammatorydisease).

18. Winer, R. L., Feng, Q., Hughes, J. P., O'Reilly, S., Kiviat, N. B., & Koutsky, L. A. (2008). Risk of female human papillomavirus acquisition associated with first male sex partner. *Journal of Infectious Diseases, 197*(2), 279–282.

19. Partridge, J. M., Hughes, J. P., Feng, Q., et al. (2007). Genital human papillomavirus infection in men: Incidence and risk factors in a cohort of university students. *Journal of Infectious Diseases, 196*(8), 1128–1136.

20. Winer, R. L., Hughes, J. P., Feng, Q., et al. (2006). Condom use and the risk of genital human papillomavirus infection in young women. *New England Journal of Medicine, 354*(25), 2645–2654.

21. Centers for Disease Control and Prevention. (2010). Diagnoses of HIV infection and AIDS in the United States and dependent areas. *HIV Surveillance Report, 200,* 20 (http://www.cdc.gov/hiv/topics/surveillance/resources/reports).

National Center for Health Statistics. (2010). Deaths: Leading causes for 2006. *National Vital Statistics Reports, 58*(14).

22. Joint United Nations Programme on HIV/AIDS (UNAIDS). (2010). *UNAIDS outlook report 2010.* Geneva: UNAIDS.

23. Trepka, M. J., & Kim, S. (2010). Prevalence of human immunodeficiency virus testing and high-risk human immunodeficiency virus behavior among 18 to 22 year-old students and nonstudents: Results of the National Survey of Family Growth. *Sexually Transmitted Diseases, 37*(10), 653–659.

24. Davis, K. R., & Weller, S. C. (1999). The effectiveness of condoms in reducing heterosexual transmission of HIV. *Family Planning Perspectives, 31*(6), 272–279.

Weller, S., & Davis, K. (2004). Condom effectiveness in reducing heterosexual HIV transmission (Cochrane Review). In *The Cochrane Library,* issue 2. Chichester, UK: Wiley.

25. Centers for Disease Control and Prevention. (2010). *Basic information about HIV and AIDS* (http://www.cdc.gov/hiv/topics/basic).

26. Ibid.

27. Centers for Disease Control and Prevention. (2006). Revised recommendation for HIV testing of adults, adolescents, and pregnant women in health-care settings. *MMWR Recommendations and Reports, 55*(RR14), 1–17.

28. Abdool, K. Q., Abdool, K. S. S., Frohlich, J. A., et al. (2010). Effectiveness and safety of tenofovir gel, an antiretroviral microbicide, for the prevention of HIV infection in women. *Science, 329*(5996), 1168–1174.

CHAPTER 13

1. Grant, J. E., Potenza, M. N., Weinstein, A., & Gorelick, D. A. (2010). Introduction to behavioral addictions. *American Journal of Drug and Alcohol Abuse, 36*(5), 233–241.

Potenza, M. N. (2006). Should addictive disorders include non-substance-related conditions? *Addiction, 101*(Suppl. 1), 142–151.

Holden, C. (2001). "Behavioral" addictions: Do they exist? *Science, 294*(5544), 980–982.

2. Grant, J. E. (2008) *Impulse control disorders: A clinician's guide to understanding and treating behavioral addictions.* New York, NY: Norton.

Chou, C., Condron, L., & Belland, J. C. (2005). A review of the research on Internet

Addiction. *Educational Psychology Review, 17*(4), 363–388.

3. National Institute on Drug Abuse. (2010). *Drugs, brains, and behavior: The science of addiction.* NIH Pub. No. 10-5605.

4. Substance Abuse and Mental Health Services Administration. (2010). *Results from the 2009 National Survey on Drug Use and Health.* Rockville, MD: Office of Applied Studies, Substance Abuse and Mental Health Services Administration.

5. American Psychiatric Association. (1994). *Diagnostic and statistical manual of mental disorders* (4th ed.). Washington, DC: APA.

6. National Institute on Drug Abuse. (2010). *Drugs, brains, and behavior: The science of addiction.* NIH Pub. No. 10-5605.

7. Frary, C. D., Johnson, R. K., & Wang, M. Q. (2005). Food sources and intakes of caffeine in the diets of persons in the United States. *Journal of the American Dietetic Association, 105*(1), 110–113.

8. Duchan, E., Patel, N. D., & Feucht, C. (2010). Energy drinks: A review of use and safety for athletes. *The Physician and Sportsmedicine, 38*(2), 171–179.

9. Salazar-Martinez, E., Willett, W. C., Ascherio, A., et al. (2004). Coffee consumption and risk for type 2 diabetes mellitus. *Annals of Internal Medicine, 140*(1), 1–8.

10. National Institute on Drug Abuse. (2010). *Research report series: Marijuana abuse.* NIH Pub. No. 10-3859.

11. Mittleman, M. A., Lewis, R. A., Maclure, M., Sherwood, J. B., & Muller, J. E. (2001). Triggering myocardial infarction by marijuana. *Circulation, 103*(23), 2805–2809.

12. Richer, I., & Bergeron, J. (2009). Driving under the influence of cannabis: Links with dangerous driving, psychological predictors, and accident involvement. *Accident Analysis and Prevention, 41*(2), 299–307.

13. Sewell, R. A., Poling, J., & Sofuoglu, M. (2009). The effect of cannabis compared with alcohol on driving. *American Journal of Addiction, 18*(3), 185–193.

14. Tetrault, J. M., Crothers, K., Moore, B. A., Mehra, R., Concato, J., & Fiellin, D. A. (2007). Effects of marijuana smoking on pulmonary function and respiratory complications: A systematic review. *Archives of Internal Medicine, 167*(3), 221–228.

15. Moore, T., Zammit, S., Lingford-Hughes, A., Barnes, T., Jones, P., Burke, M., & Lewis, G. (2007). Cannabis use and risk of psychotic or affective mental health outcomes: A systematic review. *Lancet, 370*(9584), 319–328.

16. Budney, A. J., Vandrey, R. G., Hughes, J. R., Thostenson, J. D., & Bursac, Z. (2008). Comparison of cannabis and tobacco withdrawal: Severity and contribution to relapse. *Journal of Substance Abuse and Treatment, 35*(4), 362–368.

17. National Institute on Drug Abuse. (2010). *Research report series: Marijuana abuse.* NIH Pub. No. 10-3859.

18. Centers for Disease Control and Prevention. (2010). Ecstasy overdoses at a New Year's Eve Rave—Los Angeles, California, 2010. *Morbidity and Mortality Weekly Report, 59*(22), 677–681.

19. Dumont, C. J., Wezenberg, E., Valkenberg, M. M., et al. (2008). Acute neuropsychological effects of MDMA and ethanol

co-administration in healthy volunteers. *Psychopharmacology, 197*(3), 465–474.

20. Warner, M., Chen, L. H., & Makuc, D. M. (2009). Increase in fatal poisonings involving opioid analgesics in the United States, 1999–2006. *NCHS Data Brief,* No. 22. Hyattsville, MD: CDC National Center for Health Statistics.

21. Centers for Disease Control and Prevention. (2005). *Behavioral Risk Factor Surveillance System, trends data, alcohol use: Binge drinking, 2005.* Atlanta, GA: CDC.

22. Office of Juvenile Justice and Delinquency Prevention. (2005). *Drinking in America: Myths, realities, and prevention policy.* Washington, DC: U.S. Department of Justice, Office of Justice Programs, OJJDP.

23. National Institute on Alcohol Abuse and Alcoholism. (2000). *Alcohol alert: Alcohol metabolism.* NIAAA Pub. No. 35; PH 271.

24. Department of Transportation, National Highway Traffic Safety Administration (NHTSA). (2009). *Traffic safety facts 2008: Alcohol-impaired driving.* Washington, DC: NHTSA. Available at http://wwwnrd.nhtsa .dot.gov/Pubs/811155.PDF

25. Swift, R., & Davidson, D. (1998). Alcohol hangover: Mechanisms and mediators. *Alcohol Health and Research World, 22*(1), 54–60.

26. McKinney, A., & Coyle, K. (2004). Next day effects of a normal night's drinking on memory and psychomotor performance. *Alcohol and Alcoholism, 39*(6), 509–513.

27. American Psychiatric Association. (1994). *Diagnostic and statistical manual of mental disorders* (4th ed.). Washington, DC: APA.

28. Centers for Disease Control and Prevention. (2007). Cigarette smoking among adults, United States, 2006. *Morbidity and Mortality Weekly Report, 56*(44), 1157–1161.

29. Centers for Disease Control and Prevention (2005). Tobacco use, access, and exposure to tobacco in media among middle and high school students—United States, 2004. *Morbidity and Mortality Weekly Report, 54*(12), 297–301.

30. U.S. Department of Health and Human Services. *The health consequences of smoking: A report of the Surgeon General.* Retrieved from http://www.surgeongeneral.gov/library/ smokingconsequences/

31. Akbartabartoori, M., Lean, M. E., & Hankey, C. R. (2005). Relationship between cigarette smoking, body size and body shape. *International Journal of Obesity, 29*(2), 236–242.

32. Barrett-Connor, E., & Khaw, K-T. (1989). Cigarette smoking and increased central adiposity. *Annals of Internal Medicine, 111*(10), 783–787.

33. Suminski, R. R., Wier, L. T., Poston, W., Arenare, B., Randles, A., & Jackson, A. S. (2009). The effect of habitual smoking on measured and predicted VO$_2$max. *Journal of Physical Activity and Health, 6*(5), 667–673.

34. Sépaniak, S., Forges, T., & Monnier-Barbarino, P. (2006). Cigarette smoking and fertility in women and men. *Gynecology, Obstetrics, and Fertility, 34*(10), 945–949.

Sepaniak, S., Forges, T., Fontaine, B., Gerard, H., Foliguet, B., Guillet-May, F., Zaccabri, A., & Monnier-Barbarino, P. (2004). Negative impact of cigarette smoking on male fertility: From spermatozoa to the offspring. *Journal of Gynecology, Obstetrics, and Biological Reproduction, 33*(5), 384–90.

35. National Cancer Institute. Smokefree.gov (n.d.). *Myths about smoking and pregnancy.* Retrieved from http://women.smokefree.gov/ topic-pregnancy-myths.aspx

36. Primack, B. A., Fertman, C. I., Rice, K. R., Adachi-Mejia, A. M., & Fine, M. J. (2010). Waterpipe and cigarette smoking among college athletes in the United States. *Journal of Adolescent Health, 46*(1), 45–51.

Eissenberg, T., Ward, K. D., Smith-Simone, S., & Maziak, W. (2008). Waterpipe tobacco smoking on a U.S. college campus: Prevalence and correlates. *Journal of Adolescent Health, 42*(5), 526–529.

37. Eissenberg, T., & Shihadeh, A. (2009). Waterpipe tobacco and cigarette smoking: Direct comparison of toxicant exposure. *American Journal of Preventive Medicine, 37*(6), 518–523.

38. National Cancer Institute. Health effects of exposure to environmental tobacco smoke. *Smoking and Tobacco Control Monographs,* 10. Retrieved from http://cancercontrol .cancer.gov/tcrb/monographs/10/index.html

39. Centers for Disease Control and Prevention. (2010). Vital signs: Nonsmokers' exposure to secondhand smoke—United States, 1999–2008. *Morbidity and Mortality Weekly Report, 59*(35), 1141–1146.

40. MedlinePlus.gov. (2009). Making the decision to quit tobacco. Retrieved from http:// www.nlm.nih.gov/medlineplus/ency/ article/002032.htm

Credits

.co.uk/Alamy; p. 241 (left): Comstock Images; p. 241(right): © Shutterstock; p. 243 (left): Justin Pumfrey/Getty Images; p. 243 (right) © David J. Green-people/Alamy; p. 244 (top): © Arthur Turner/Alamy; p. 244 (bottom left): Library of Congress, Prints & Photographs Division [LC-USZ62-78689]; p. 244 (bottom right): © Lars A. Niki; p. 245: © Stockbyte/Getty Images; p. 246: Scott Thuen; p. 248 (top to bottom): Scott Thuen; David Madison/Getty Images; Omron Healthcare; Courtesy Life Measurement, Inc.; GE Healthcare; p. 250: © Peter Banos/Alamy; p. 250 (video still): Brella Productions; p. 251: Brand X Pictures/PunchStock; © Photodisc/PunchStock; Burke/Triolo Productions/Getty Images; © Stockdisc/PunchStock; Blend Images/Getty Images; p. 252: Ingram Publishing/SuperStock; p. 253: © RF/Corbis; p. 255: Scott Thuen; p. 257: Scott Thuen

CHAPTER 8

p. 265: Plush Studios/Photodisc/Getty Images; p. 266 (video still): Brella Productionsp.267 top right): Jules Selmes/Dorling Kindersley/Getty Images; p. 267 (fig 8.1): ©iStockphoto.com/webphotographer; p. 268: © Stockdisc/PunchStock; p. 270: Photodisc Collection/Getty Images; p. 271 (top right): photosindia/Getty Images; p. 271 (middle): © PhotoAlto/PunchStock; p. 271 (bottom): Jules Frazier/Getty Images; p. 272: ©iStockphoto.com/Lauri Patterson; p. 273: © The McGraw-Hill Companies, Inc./Elite Images; p. 274: © Chris Kerrigan; p. 275 (clockwise): Judith Collins/Alamy; © Stockdisc/PunchStock; © Stockdisc/PunchStock; C Squared Studios/Getty Images p. 278: © Comstock/Jupiter Images; p. 279: Dorling Kindersley/Getty Images; p. 280 (left to right): © BananaStock/PunchStock; © Imagestate Media (John Foxx)/ Imagestate; Burke/Triolo Productions/Getty Images; ©iStockphoto.com/Jason Lugo; C Squared Studios/Getty Images; Burke/Triolo Productions/Getty Images; © Comstock/Jupiter Images; p. 282: C Squared Studios/Getty Images; p. 283: Burke/Triolo Productions/Getty Images; p. 285 (top): © The McGraw-Hill Companies, Inc./Jill Braaten, photographer; p. 285 (bottom): © Brand X Pictures/PunchStock; p. 287: © Getty Images; p. 288: © Image Club; p. 289: © J Marshall - Tribaleye Images/Alamy; p. 291: © Creatas/PunchStock; p. 292 (left): PRNewsFoto/Stonyfield Farm/AP Images; p. 292 (right): © David Young-Wolff/PhotoEdit; p. 294: © istockphoto.com/Magdalena Kucova; p. 295: The McGraw-Hill Companies, Inc./Christopher Kerrigan, photographer

CHAPTER 9

p. 305: Philip Koschel/Getty Images: p. 306: Rick Nease/MCT/Newscom; p. 309 (top to bottom):Richard Hutchings;© iStockphoto.com/Victor Burnside; ©iStockphoto.com/Onur Döngel; ©iStockphoto.com/Andrzej Burak; ©Ingram Publishing/Fotosearch; C Squared Studios/Getty Images; p. 310: Wave RF/photolibrary; p. 311: © Mark Richards/PhotoEdit; p. 312: Wang Leng/Asia Images/Getty Images; p. 313: Richard Hutchings/The McGraw-Hill Companies; p. 315: Davies and Starr/Getty Images; p. 316: picturegarden/Getty Images; p. 317: p. 319: © istockphoto.com/Diane Diederich; p. 320: © Brand X Pictures/PunchStock; p. 321 (left to right): © Royalty Free/Corbis; ©iStockphoto.com/Oleksii Akhrimenko; © istockphoto.com/Webking p. 322: © foodfolio/Alamy; p. 323: Corbis Super RF/Alamy; p. 326: Photodisc

Collection/Getty Images; p. 328: Gerard Fritz/Getty Images; p. 330: The McGraw-Hill Companies, Inc./Jacques Cornell photographer; p. 331: © Ingram Publishing/Fotosearch; p. 333: Brella Productions; p. 335: © The McGraw-Hill Companies, Inc./Jill Braaten, photographer

CHAPTER 10

p. 343:Andersen Ross/Getty Images; p. 344: C Squared Studios/Getty Images; p. 345: PM Images/Getty Images; p. 346: © Fuse/Getty Images; p. 348: JGI/Jamie Grill/Getty Images; p. 349: Sheer Photo, Inc./Getty Images; p. 350: Kablonk!/photolibrary; p. 353(top to bottom): © Ingram Publishing/AGE Fotostock; © BananaStock/PunchStock; Nathan Lau/Design Pics/Corbis; p. 355: © Sean Justice/Corbis; p. 356: Comstock Images/Jupiter Images; p. 358: Chapman Wiedelphoto/photolibrary; p. 359: Brella Productions; p. 363: Asia Images Group/Getty Images; p. 365: Somos RF/Getty Images; p. 366: George Doyle/Getty Images; p. 367 (top): Eye Candy Images/Getty Images; p. 367 (bottom): © Design Pics Inc./Alamy; p. 368: © Ashley Cooper/Corbis; p. 370: Steve Gorton, Matthew Ward/Getty Images; p. 372 (top): Maria Teijeiro/Getty Images; p. 372 (bottom): Rubberball/Getty Images; p. 373: © BananaStock/PunchStock

CHAPTER 11

p. 379: © Erika Larsen 2009/Redux Pictures; p. 382: The McGraw-Hill Companies, Inc./ /Photo by JW Ramsey; p. 383: © Ingram Publishing/Fotosearch; p. 384: Lael Henderson/Getty Images; p. 385: © iStockphoto.com/Roel Smart; p. 386: Brand X Pictures/PunchStock; p. 387: Thinkstock/Getty Images; p. 390: Andersen Ross/photolibrary; p. 392: © Photodisc/Getty Images; p. 393 (top): The McGraw-Hill Companies, Inc./Ken Karp photographer; p. 393 (bottom): The McGraw-Hill Companies, Inc./Rick Brady, photographer; p. 394: © Creatas/PunchStock; p. 395: Michael Hitoshi/Photodisc/Getty Images; p. 398: Radius Images/Alamy; p. 400: Comstock Images/Getty Images; p. 402: © The McGraw-Hill Companies, Inc./Elite Images; p. 405: Erik Isakson/Getty Images; p. 406: Seth Joel /Digital Vision; p. 407: Britt Erlanson /Getty Images; p. 410: © Banana Stock/photolibrary

CHAPTER 12

p. 415: Image Source/Getty Images; p. 416 (top to bottom): CDC/Cynthia Goldsmith; CDC/Janice Haney Carr; Centers for Disease Control; CDC/Dr. Stan Erlandsen; ©iStockphoto.com/© Karl Dolenc; p. 418 (left): © McGraw-Hill Companies/Ed-Imaging; p. 418 (right): © Stockdisc/PunchStock; p. 419: CDC/ James Gathany; p. 422 (top to bottom): © Stockbyte/PunchStock; ©iStockphoto.com/Christian Pound; ©iStockphoto.com/Ashok Rodrigues; p. 425: Stockbyte/PictureQuest; p. 426: Stockbyte/Getty Images; p. 428 (top): numb/Alamy; p. 428 (bottom): Rubberball/Getty Images; p. 430 (top): Stockbyte/Getty Images; p. 430 (bottom): George Doyle/Getty Images; p. 431: © Ingram Publishing/Fotosearch; p. 433: Gary Gardiner/Bloomberg via Getty Images; p. 435: The McGraw-Hill Companies, Inc./Christopher Kerrigan, photographer; p. 436: Footage supplied by Goodshoot/Punchstock; p. 438 (top): © Jeff Greenberg/agefotostock; p. 438 (bottom): The McGraw-Hill Companies, Inc./Christopher Kerrigan, photographer

CHAPTER 13

p. 441: Ian Spanier/Getty Images; p. 442: REUTERS/Toby Melville /Landov; p. 444: © Brand X Pictures/PunchStock; p. 446 (left to right): Stockbyte/Getty Images; Ryan McVay/ Getty Images; © PhotoAlto/PictureQuest; ©iStockphoto. com/Chris Bernard; Stockbyte/Getty Images; p. 448: © The McGraw-Hill Companies, Inc./Jill Braaten, photographer; p. 450 (left): McGraw-Hill Companies, Inc./Gary He, photographer; p. 450 (right): Drug Enforcement Agency; p. 451 (left to right): © iStockphoto.com/broken3; © iStockphoto. com/Bjorn Heller; © iStockphoto.com/plainview; ©iStock-photo.com/Serghei Platonov; p. 452: © iStockphoto.com/ Alexander Maksimenko; p. 453 (left): ©iStockphoto.com/ DNY59; p. 453 (right): Martin Diebel/Getty Images; p. 455 (top): © RF/Corbis; p. 455 (bottom): ©iStockphoto.com/ Murat Giray Kaya; p. 457: Tanya Constantine/Brand X Pictures/Jupiterimages; p. 458: © BananaStock/PictureQuest; p. 459: © Comstock Images/Alamy; p. 461: © i love images/ Alamy; p. 462: © simon de glanville/Alamy; p. 463: Brella Productions; p. 464: Amos Morgan/Getty Images; p. 465: UPPA /ZUMA Press/Newscom

Text and Figure Credits

TEXT AND FIGURE CREDITS

CHAPTER 1

Fig 1.5 UC Atlas of Global Inequality. Reprinted with permission.

CHAPTER 2

Fig 2.3 Adapted from PEP Kit: Physical Activity Precontemplation. Reprinted with permission from The Cooper Institute, Dallas, TX, www.cooperinst.org.

Fig 2.4 Adapted from PEP Kit: Physical Activity Precontemplation. Reprinted with permission from The Cooper Institute, Dallas, TX, www.cooperinst.org.

p. 41 Practical Prevention - What's My Stage? Adapted from Transtheoretical Model Constructs, Table 5.1 in Karen Glanz, Barbara K. Rimer, and K. Viswanath, eds., *Health Behavior and Health Education: Theory, Research, and Practice,* 4e San Francisco: Jossey-Bass. Used by permission of John Wiley & Sons, Inc.

p. 52 Fast Facts Adapted with permission from The Marist Institute for Public Opinion (2009). The Marist College Poll, *Turning the Page to 2010: New Year's Resolutions.*

CHAPTER 3

Lab 3.1 Physical Activity Readiness Questionnaire (PAR-Q) © 2002. Used with permission from the Canadian Society for Exercise Physiology. www.csep.ca/forms.asp.

Lab 3-3 p. 98 Centers for Disease Control, *Promoting Physical Activity: A Guide for Community Action* Campaign, IL: Human Kinetics.

CHAPTER 4

Fig 4-5 Reprinted with permission from Blair, S. N., and Wei, M. Sedentary Habits, Health, and Function in Older Women and Men. *American Journal of Health Promotion,* 2000:15(1): 1-8, figure 1, All-cause Mortality and Cardiorespiratory fitness in Women and Men 60 years of age.

Table 4-1 Adapted with permission from American College of Sports Medicine. (2009). *ACSM's Guidelines for Exercise Testing and Prescription,* 8e. Baltimore: Lippincott Williams & Wilkins, http://lww.com.

Lab 4.1 3-minute step test: McArdle, W.D, Katch, F.L., Pechar, G.S., Jacobson, L., & Ruck, S. (1972). Reliability and interrelationships between maximal oxygen intake, physical work capacity, and step-test scores in college women. *Medicine and Science in Sports and Exercise, 4*(4): 182-186. Used by permission of Wolters Kluwer Health.

Lab 4-2, p. 139 Adapted with permission from American College of Sports Medicine (2009). *ACSM's Guidelines for Exercise Testing and Prescription,* 8e. Baltimore: Lippincott Williams & Wilkins, http://lww.com.

CHAPTER 5

Lab 5.1, p. 184 Reprinted with permission from The Cooper Institute, Dallas, Texas from *Physical Fitness Assessments and Norms for Adults and Law Enforcement.* Available online at www.cooperinstitute.org.

Lab 5.1, p. 185 Reprinted with permission from The Cooper Institute, Dallas, Texas from *Physical Fitness Assessments and Norms for Adults and Law Enforcement.* Available online at www.cooperinstitute.org.

Lab 5.2, p. 187 *The Canadian Physical Activity, Fitness & Lifestyle Approach*: CSEP-Health & Fitness Program's Health-Related Appraisal and Counseling Strategy, 3e, © 2003. Used with permission from the Canadian Society for Exercise Physiology.

Lab 5.2, p. 188 *The Canadian Physical Activity, Fitness & Lifestyle Approach*: CSEP-Health & Fitness Program's Appraisal and Counseling Strategy, 3rd edition, © 2003. Adapted with permission from the Canadian Society for Exercise Physiology.

CHAPTER 6

Lab 6-1 Sit & Reach Test *The Canadian Physical Activity, Fitness & Lifestyle Approach*: CSEP-Health & Fitness Program's Appraisal and Counseling Strategy, 3rd edition, © 2003. Adapted with permission from the Canadian Society for Exercise Physiology.

Lab 6-1 Shoulder Flexibility Test Adapted from Nieman, D. (2003) Exercise Testing and Prescription: A Health-Related Approach (5e). NY: McGraw-Hill. © 2010 by The McGraw-Hill Companies, Inc. Reproduced by permission of The McGraw-Hill Companies.

CHAPTER 7

Fig 7-9 American College of Sports Medicine (2009). *ACSM's Resource Manual for Guidelines for Exercise Testing and Prescription,* 6e. Baltimore: Lippincott Williams & Wilkins, http://lww.com. Used with permission.

Lab 7.1, p. 258 Body Fat Estimate for Men: *The Physician and Sportsmedicine* is a registered trademark of JTE Multimedia,

LLC 1235 Westlakes Drive Suite 320, Berwyn PA, 19312 (610)889-3730. Used with permission.

Lab 7.1, p. 259 Body Fat Estimate for Women: *The Physician and Sportsmedicine* is a registered trademark of JTE Multimedia, LLC 1235 Westlakes Drive Suite 320, Berwyn PA, 19312 (610)889-3730. Used with permission.

Lab 7-1, p. 260 Percent Body Fat Standards for Men and Women: American College of Sports Medicine (2009). *ACSM's Resource Manual for Guidelines for Exercise Testing and Prescription,* 6e. Baltimore: Lippincott Williams & Wilkins, http://lww.com . Used with permission.

Lab 7-1, p. 261 Reprinted with permission from V.H. Heyward (2010). *Advanced fitness assessment and exercise and prescription,* 6e, p. 222, Table 8.8. Champaign, IL: Human Kinetics, p. 222. Adapted from G. A. Bray and D.S. Gray, 1988, Obesity: Part I—pathogenesis," *Western Journal of Medicine* 149: 429-441.

Lab 7-2 Waist-to-Hip Ratio and Health Risk: Reprinted with permission from V.H. Heyward (2010). *Advanced fitness assessment and exercise and prescription,* 6e, p. 222, Table 8.8. Champaign, IL: Human Kinetics, p. 222. Adapted from G. A. Bray and D.S. Gray, 1988, Obesity: Part I—pathogenesis," *Western Journal of Medicine* 149: 429-441.

CHAPTER 10

p. 362 Wellness Strategies: Ellis, A. (2004), Expanding the ABC's of rational-emotive therapy, In M.J. Mahoney & A. Freeman (eds.), *Cognition and psychotherapy,* pp. 313-323. NY: Plenum. Used with permission of Springer Publishing Company, via Copyright Clearance Center, Inc.

CHAPTER 11

Fig 11.4 American Heart Association (2010). Heart disease and stroke statistics 2010 update: A report from the AHA, *Circulation* 121(7): e46-e215, p. e121. Used with permission.

Fig 11.5 American Heart Association (2010). Heart disease and stroke statistics 2010 update: A report from the AHA, *Circulation* 121(7): e46-e215, p. e71 Feb. 2010. Used with permission.

Table 11. 9 American Cancer Society, *Cancer Facts and Figures* 2010. Atlanta: American Cancer Society, Inc. Used with permission.

Fig 11.11 Narayan, K.M.V., et al. 2007, "Effect of BMI on lifetime risk for diabetes in the U.S." *Diabetes Care* 30(6): 1562-66, June 2007. Copyright 2007 by the American Diabetes Association. Reproduced with permission of the American Diabetes Association via Copyright Clearance Center.

CHAPTER 13

Lab 13-1 Part 1 Saunders, J.B. et al., 1993, "Development of the Alcohol Use Disorders Identification Test (AUDIT): WHO Collaborative Project on Early Detection of Persons with Harmful Alcohol Consumption-II," *Addiction,* 88(6), 791-804. Published by John Wiley & Sons, www.interscience. wiley.com. Used with permission.

Index